COMMUNITY
ORAL HEALTH PRACTICE
for the DENTAL HYGIENIST

COMMUNITY ORAL HEALTH PRACTICE *for the* DENTAL HYGIENIST

Fifth Edition

CHRISTINE FRENCH BEATTY, RDH, BS, MS, PhD

Professor Emeritus
Dental Hygiene Program
Department of Communication Sciences and Oral Health
Texas Woman's University
Denton, Texas
United States

ELSEVIER

Elsevier
3251 Riverport Lane
St. Louis, Missouri 63043

COMMUNITY ORAL HEALTH PRACTICE FOR
THE DENTAL HYGIENIST, FIFTH EDITION

ISBN: 978-0-323-68341-8

Library of Congress Control Number : 2021930275

Content Strategist: Joslyn Dumas/Kelly Skelton
Director, Content Development: Ellen Wurm-Cutter
Senior Content Development Specialist: Kathleen Nahm
Publishing Services Manager: Deepthi Unni
Senior Project Manager: Manchu Mohan
Designer: Bridget Hoette

Printed in India

Last digit is the print number: 9 8 7 6 5 4 3

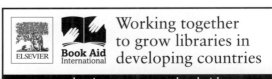

This textbook is dedicated to oral health professionals who have participated in community efforts to improve the oral health of all citizens. Oral health, as an integral component of the overall health and well-being of individuals, must be available to and attainable by all populations. Throughout my career working in the field of community oral health, I have observed how oral health professionals have demonstrated their dedication and commitment to this goal. They need to be commended and thanked and told to keep up their efforts. Many worthwhile programs and services have been provided, but there is still much to be accomplished.

Christine French Beatty, RDH, BS, MS, PhD
Professor Emeritus
Dental Hygiene Program
Department of Communication Sciences
    and Oral Health
Texas Woman's University, Denton
Texas
United States

Charlene B. Dickinson, RDH, BSDH, MS
Associate Clinical Professor
Program Director
Dental Hygiene Program
Department of Communication Sciences
    and Oral Health
Texas Woman's University, Denton
Texas
United States

Risa Handman-Nettles, BSDH, MDH, EdD
Associate Professor
Associate Department Chair and Program
    Director
Dental Hygiene Program
Health Professions Department
Georgia State University Perimeter College,
    Dunwoody
Georgia
United States

**Amanda M. Hinson-Enslin, BSDH, MPH,
PhD, CHES®**
Assistant Professor
Department of Population and Public
    Health Sciences
Boonshoft School of Medicine at Wright
    State University, Dayton
Ohio
United States

Beverly Ann Isman, RDH, MPH, ELS
Dental Public Health Consultant
Association of State and Territorial Dental
    Directors, Reno
Nevada
United States

**Faizan Kabani, PhD, MBA, MHA, RDH,
FAADH**
Assistant Professor
Caruth School of Dental Hygiene
Assistant Director for Diversity and Faculty
    Development
Office of Academic Affairs
Texas A&M College of Dentistry, Dallas
Texas
United States

Schelli Stedke, BSDH, MDH
Oral Health Consultant
Dental Hygiene Division
NSK Dental America Corporation, Hoffman
    Estates
Illinois
United States

Sharon C. Stull, BSDH, MS, BSDH, MS
Lecturer
Community Outreach Coordinator
Gene W. Hirschfeld School of Dental
    Hygiene
Old Dominion University, Norfolk
Community Adjunct Faculty
Eastern Virginia Medical School, Norfolk
Virginia
United States

Tiffany Baggs, CRDH, MSDH
Dental Hygiene Professor
Valencia College
Orlando, Florida

Kimberly G. Bastin, CRDH, RDH, CDA, EFDA
Assistant Professor and Program Director
Dental Hygiene
State College of Florida Manatee-Sarasota
Bradenton, Florida

Tammy S. Clossen, RDH, PHDHP, PhD
Assistant Professor
Dental Hygiene
Pennsylvania College of Technology
Williamsport, Pennsylvania

Lorinda L. Coan, MS, RDH
Associate Professor of Dental Hygiene
Dental Hygiene
University of Southern Indiana
College of Nursing and Health Professions
Evansville, Indiana

Darlene Jones, CDA, RDH, MPA
Clinical Lecturer
Dental Hygiene Program
University of Michigan
Ann Arbor, Michigan

Laurie A. Magill, RDH, ASDH
Professor
Dental Hygiene/Dental Assisting
Confederation College
Thunder Bay, Ontario

Kimberly A. J. Speicher, RDH, MS
Assistant Professor
Dental Hygiene
Pennsylvania College of Technology
Williamsport, Pennsylvania

"Why do I need to know anything about community oral health?"

Many dental hygiene students ask this question of their faculty at the beginning of the Community Oral Health course. The purpose of this textbook is to provide students with information about community oral health that is relevant to dental hygiene. It is my intention that, through reading the chapters and participating in the suggested activities, dental hygiene students can find the answer to this question. My aim is to help them develop an understanding of the importance of this integral component of their education to their future profession regardless of their career path or practice setting. Although this textbook is written specifically for dental hygiene students, it is also a valuable resource for all oral health professionals practicing their professional responsibility to improve the oral health of their community.

Community Oral Health, or Dental Public Health as it is called in some programs, is a required course for dental hygiene accreditation. In the *Accreditation Standards for Dental Hygiene Education Programs* effective as of January 2019, the Commission on Dental Accreditation (CODA) states that the curriculum in dental hygiene schools must include content in the following four general areas: general education, biomedical sciences, dental sciences, and dental hygiene science. CODA requires that these areas must be "integrated and of sufficient depth, scope, sequence of instruction, quality, and emphasis to ensure achievement of the curriculum's defined competencies." Furthermore, these CODA Standards state:

> Dental hygiene science content must include oral health education and preventive counseling, **health promotion**, patient management, clinical dental hygiene, provision of services for and management of patients with special needs, **community dental/oral health**, medical and dental emergencies, legal and ethical aspects of dental hygiene practice, infection and hazard control management, and the provision of oral health care services to patients with bloodborne infectious diseases.

The American Dental Education Association (ADEA) Council of Allied Dental Program Directors Administrative Board developed the *ADEA Compendium of Curriculum Guidelines Allied Dental Education Programs (Revised Edition), 2015–2016 (ADEA Curriculum Guidelines)* to assist dental hygiene and dental assisting schools in curriculum planning. The comprehensive competencies and learning objectives in that document serve as guidelines for individual programs in defining the abilities they want their graduates to possess and designing courses to achieve that goal.

At the end of each chapter in this textbook, competencies and learning objectives are listed that are from that document and are relevant to the chapter content. The complete list of community dental health competencies and learning objectives for dental hygiene programs from the *ADEA Curriculum*

Guidelines can be found in Appendix B. Using these resources, instructors and students can apply the information in *Community Oral Health Practice for the Dental Hygienist* to the goal of developing competencies in the profession of dental hygiene in relation to community oral health.

Chapter 1 defines community oral health for students through examples of public health problems and solutions. The core public health functions and essential public health services are defined, and the role of the government in community oral health is discussed. Chapter 2, on careers in public health, enables students to envision the future use of the information they are learning in this textbook and in the Community Oral Health course. It describes the various alternative dental hygiene career roles and options, and features profiles of dental hygienists who practice in alternative settings and in roles related to community oral health. Reviewing these featured career choices allows students to comprehend the relevance of the content in the forthcoming chapters.

Chapter 3, on assessment, and Chapter 4, on measuring oral health, emphasize the importance of these crucial steps in planning and evaluating community oral health programs and in oral health surveillance at the national and state levels. Dental hygienists involved in public health need to be knowledgeable about and proficient in using the tools of assessment and measurement of oral health, including common dental indexes. Chapter 5, on the burden of oral disease in the population, will help students become well informed about the current level of various oral diseases and conditions in the population to be able to prioritize the needs of different community groups. This chapter also describes the status of various issues that affect access to care, including workforce and financing of oral care. The *Healthy People 2030* framework, objectives, and leading health indicators are discussed in these three chapters to provide valuable context for assessment and the planning and development of community oral health programs.

Chapters 3, 4, and 5 are appropriately placed in the book as preparation for Chapter 6 on community oral health programs, which discusses the planning, implementation, and evaluation phases of program development as well as the funding of community oral health programs. Successful community oral health programs at the local, state, and national levels are featured in relation to various priority populations. Internet websites, resources, and updates on state oral health programs are incorporated. Also included is a description of the steps needed to set up a community program, which can assist students in developing community oral health projects for the Community Oral Health course, the American Dental Hygienists' Association (ADHA) student organization, or other service-learning activities. These steps will also be useful after graduation when working or volunteering in the community through ADHA or other means.

Chapter 7 covers the research process and statistics in a relevant, organized format, with application to community oral health. Criteria for reviewing oral health literature are included, as is a discussion of the use of research results for evidence-based decision-making in dental hygiene practice. Chapter 8 explains theories of health promotion and identifies strategies for developing and delivering oral health information to the public. Chapter 9 addresses the social responsibility of oral health providers and the role of government with respect to improving access to care for underserved populations and achieving health equity in the population. The importance of communication and leadership are discussed in relation to these social responsibilities.

In Chapter 10, cultural competence is discussed in relation to the cultural diversity of the nation and the importance of reducing oral health disparities. Also described are the development of cultural competence and models of ways to incorporate cultural competence into interactions with patients and in our community oral health promotion efforts. Chapter 11, on service-learning, defines the importance of the interface between the needs of the community and student learning. The benefits of service-learning, especially in relation to interprofessional collaboration, are discussed and ways are suggested to integrate service-learning into the student's community oral health experience.

Chapter 12 provides the student with practice in answering community oral health test questions similar to those on the National Board Dental Hygiene Examination (NBDHE). These community cases test the student's understanding of content in the textbook in relation to real-world community situations. The practice test also can assist the student in successfully answering this type of question on the NBDHE and potentially result in improved scores on the NBDHE in the area of community oral health. A discussion of the *Healthy People 2030* oral health objectives is threaded throughout the textbook as an important framework for community oral health practice.

Listings of knowledge-application activities can be found at the end of each chapter. These are suggestions for classroom activities and/or outside assignments that can bring the chapter content to life for greater overall understanding of community oral health. Instructors can assign the activities, or students can elect to pursue them on their own for enrichment.

Also, at the end of each chapter are sample community cases with test questions. The answers and rationales to these cases are on the Instructor section of the Evolve website. A second set of cases for each chapter is available on the Student section of the Evolve website (http://evolve.elsevier.com/Beatty/community/), which also contains practice quizzes for extra study. The cases are designed to assist students in their mastery of the material in each chapter and provide practice in answering case-type questions similar to those on the NBDHE. The answers/rationales to the questions in the second set of cases are also on the Student section of the Evolve website. In addition, a third set of cases with test questions and answers/rationales for each chapter are available on the Instructor section of the Evolve website, which can be used by instructors for testing or shared with the students for further practice/application.

Supplementary materials are located at the end of the textbook. Appendices A and D contain websites for various professional, nonprofit, community, health, and voluntary organizations; clearing houses and resource centers; foundations; policy and research centers; programs and initiatives; healthcare organizations; and government agencies that can serve as resources for oral health assessment and program planning. Appendix B lists the ADEA dental hygiene competencies and objectives for community dental health, and Appendices C and D include valuable information for forming community partnerships and performing community health assessments, respectively. Appendix E provides ideas for topics to address in community oral health assessments and programming, and Appendix F describes common dental indexes for use in assessment, program evaluation, and research. Because a vocabulary of terms is unique to community oral health practice, a Glossary is included for reference; key terms are bolded throughout the book and included in the Glossary. Studying the terms listed in the Glossary will facilitate the student's understanding of community oral health content.

I humbly submit this textbook to the profession with the goal of providing students with the information they need to begin their profession with a positive attitude toward community oral health and a willingness to contribute to the oral health of all persons in their community. The future of community oral health rests with the upcoming leaders who are currently studying and experiencing it as students. I hope the textbook can help to spark and/or cultivate a passion that will result in the same fulfillment from community oral health practice that I have experienced in my 57 years in the profession.

ACKNOWLEDGMENTS

Over the course of preparing this textbook for publication, many people have provided their support, guidance, and assistance. I want to acknowledge with sincere appreciation the following colleagues for their contributions and time, which went far beyond the scope of their chapters in providing assistance with moral support, project planning, research, content review. and manuscript preparation:

Charlene B. Dickinson, RDH, BSDH, MS, Associate Clinical Professor and Program Director, Dental Hygiene Program, Department of Communication Sciences and Oral Health, Texas Woman's University, Denton, Texas, United States

Amanda M. Hinson-Enslin, BSDH, MPH, PhD, CHES®, Assistant Professor, Department of Population and Public Health Sciences, Boonshoft School of Medicine at Wright State University, Dayton, Ohio, United States

The many students who have shared my enthusiasm for community oral health during my 44 years of teaching have inspired me, and I thank them for their commitment to the oral health of the public.

I especially appreciate family and friends who have supported this professional endeavor with their understanding, love, sacrifice, and prayers. I particularly want to recognize the following family members:

Husband Richard; our son Justin, his wife Connie, and our grandchildren Grace, Josiah, Piper, and Hudson; and our son Allen and his wife Ariane.

Christine French Beatty

CONTENTS

People's Health
An Introduction

Christine French Beatty

OBJECTIVES

1. Define public health terms and relate them to one another.
2. Compare the components of private practice and public health practice.
3. Identify public health problems and public health solutions and relate them to each other.
4. Define dental disease as a chronic public health problem with public health solutions.
5. Explain the role of government in public health practice.

6. Explain the role and importance of key national oral health initiatives.
7. Describe core functions of public health, the essential public health services, and the essential public health services to promote oral health; relate them to each other.
8. Describe the future potential and challenges of dental public health.

OPENING STATEMENTS: What Is Public Health?

- Influenza immunizations prevent epidemics, saving lives and money
- Research to develop a vaccine for coronavirus disease 2019 (COVID-19) is a top priority.
- Community water fluoridation is credited with substantial decreases in dental caries in the United States (U.S.) and Canada during the 20th century.
- Oral infection can contribute to life-threatening systemic diseases such as cardiovascular disease, stroke, and bacterial pneumonia.
- Public health officials in the U.S. and Canada promote tobacco cessation because of the associated serious health risks.
- Bioterrorism has put public health officials on alert for unusual diseases.
- Government agencies in the U.S. and Canada prevent work-related injuries by enforcing laws and providing education and training.
- The American Dental Hygienists' Association (ADHA) and the Canadian Dental Hygienists Association support alternative dental hygiene practice models to increase access to oral health care for underserved groups.
- US Public Health Service officers assisted with recovery after the 9/11 attack on the U.S.
- Legislation has increased dental coverage for children of low-income families in the U.S.

HEALTH, PUBLIC HEALTH, AND DENTAL PUBLIC HEALTH

The Opening Statements reveal the importance of people's **health** and help to show the wide range of activities involved. They also illustrate the meaning of key public-health-related terms (see Guiding Principles) and other concepts discussed in this chapter. Although various formal definitions exist for the terms presented here, these suffice within the scope of community oral health practice for the dental hygienist. In practice, the terms *population health*, *community health*, and *public health* are used interchangeably, as are the terms *community oral health*, *community dental health*, and *dental public health*.

Public Health/Private Practice

Oral health professional practice in the private dental office setting is integral to dental public health in the U.S. because it is where the majority of people are served.[11] Community oral health practice is unique in many ways, requiring the acquisition of specific knowledge and skills. Understanding the association between community oral health practice and private practice (Table 1.1) will help in grasping the concept of **community oral health**.

On the community level, oral health professionals focus on the community rather than the individual as the patient. Although individual patients are treated in community settings, the emphasis is on the community that the individual is part of. Community oral health practice extends the private-practice role of the dental hygienist to include the people of the community as a whole. The community setting (e.g., hospital, community clinic, school, or public health agency), rather than the private dental office, becomes the environment in which oral health care is provided.

The components of community oral health practice[12] parallel those of private practice. The patient's oral examination compares to the community survey as a means of assessment. Diagnosis and analysis are comparable in the process of identifying and prioritizing problems. Treatment planning and program planning for the community are similar; both include the many facets of preparation, such as determining various methods, strategies, and costs of choosing the best plan. Treatment compares to program implementation or program operation

GUIDING PRINCIPLES

Key Introductory Terms Related to People's Health

Health

- "A state of complete physical, mental, and social well-being and not merely the absence of disease."[1]

Public Health

- "Science of protecting and improving the health of people and their communities…by promoting healthy lifestyles, researching disease and injury prevention, and detecting, preventing, and responding to infectious diseases."[2]
- "Concerned with protecting the health of entire populations…as small as a local neighborhood, or as big as an entire country or region of the world."[2]
- "Promotes and protects the health of people and the communities where they live, learn, work and play."[3]
- Concerned with prevention, health education and marketing, recommending policies, administering services, conducting research, and limiting **health disparities** by promoting healthcare equity, quality, and accessibility.[2]

Community Health

- "Focuses on studying, protecting, and improving health within a community."[4]
- Includes a wide range of healthcare interventions, including health promotion, disease prevention, treatment, and management and administration of care.[4]

Population Health

- "Approach to health that aims to improve the health of an entire population."[5]
- Focuses on the implicit goal of improving health outcomes in the population, including the distribution of outcomes within the group.[6]
- Encompasses health status of a population and emphasizes the varied extent of factors that affect public health: environmental and individual factors that influence health, disparities, and inequities, **determinants of health**, and shared responsibility for accountability.[6]
- Requires **collaboration** of community partners to improve outcomes and an epidemiological approach to manage the health of the population, making measurement fundamental.[6]

Community Oral Health/Community Dental Health/Dental Public Health

- "The science and art of preventing and controlling dental diseases and promoting dental health through organized **community** efforts. It is the form of dental practice that serves the community as a patient rather than the individual. It is concerned with dental education of the public, with applied research, and with the administration of group dental care programs as well as the prevention and control of dental diseases on a community basis."[7]
- "That part of dentistry providing leadership and expertise in population-based dentistry, oral health surveillance, policy development, community-based disease prevention and health promotion, and the maintenance of the dental **safety net.**"[8] (See Chapter 2.)
- "Encompasses dental care and education, with an emphasis on the use of the dental hygiene sciences, delivered to a population."[9]

Community

- "All people within a geographical location or involved in a specific activity."[4]
- "A group of people who live in one area and have common interests."[9]

Target Population

- "A representation of a certain segment of the population."[9]

Public Health System

- "All public, private, and voluntary entities that contribute to the delivery of essential public health services within a jurisdiction,"[10] including state- and local-level public health agencies, healthcare providers, public safety agencies, human service and charity organizations, education and youth development organizations, recreation and arts-related organizations, economic and philanthropic organizations, and environmental agencies and organizations.

TABLE 1.1   Relationship of the Components in Private Practice and Public Health Practice

Private Practice	Public Health Practice
Patient	Community
Examination	Survey/assessment
Diagnosis	Analysis
Treatment planning	Program planning
Treatment	Program implementation/operation
Fee/payment	Program funding/financing/budget
Patient evaluation	Program evaluation/appraisal

---

as the plan is carried out. The fee or payment for dental services is equated with program funding; various methods of payment or financing are often explored in both cases. Evaluation of treatment is similar to program evaluation or appraisal and should occur during implementation and at the end of treatment or program operation.[13] This comparison can help clarify the concepts of assessment, analysis, program planning, implementation, evaluation, and financing in relation to community programs (see Chapters 3 and 6).

THE PUBLIC HEALTH PROBLEM AND THE PUBLIC HEALTH SOLUTION

Two further concepts of importance to comprehending public or people's health are the public health problem, also referred to as the public health issue, and the public health solution. The **public health problem**, as perceived by the public, usually brings to mind an infectious disease such as acquired immunodeficiency syndrome (AIDS) or influenza. The spectrum of problems, however, is vast and diverse. An issue is identified as a public health problem or issue based on how well it meets certain commonly suggested criteria[14,15] (see Guiding Principles).

GUIDING PRINCIPLES

Common Criteria Used to Identify Public Health Problems

- Burden of the disease or condition
- Prevalence of a risk factor for the disease or condition
- Ability of affecting the population as a whole
- Seriousness of the problem
- Economic or social impact
- Public health concern
- Political will to address the issue
- Availability of resources
- Requirement for group action to solve the problem
- Availability of current interventions
- Cultural appropriateness of the problem
- Degree to which it negatively affects **health equity**

Figure 1.1 depicts the steps in the public health approach used to identify problems. The characteristics of a public health problem are reflected in the steps of the process. Box 1.1 lists the 10 highest-ranking public health problems and concerns identified by the **Centers for Disease Control and Prevention** (CDC) in 2016, based on public health policies and practices in the 50 states and the District of Columbia.[16] These health issues also illustrate what constitutes a public health problem.

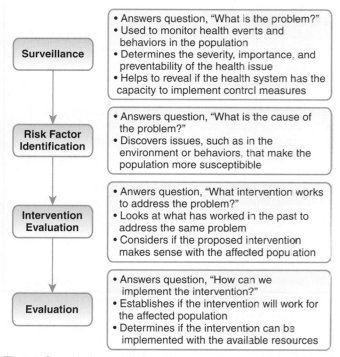

Fig 1.1 Steps in the public health approach to public health problems. (From Introduction to Epidemiology (Power Point Slide Presentation). Public Health 101 Series. Atlanta, GA: Centers for Disease Control and Prevention; 2018. Available at: <https://www.cdc.gov/publichealth101/epidemiology.html#anchor_resources>; [Accessed December 2, 2019].)

BOX 1.1 Ten Most Important Public Health Problems and Concerns Identified by the Centers for Disease Control and Prevention in 2016

- Alcohol-related harms
- Food safety
- Healthcare-associated infections
- Heart disease and stroke
- Human immunodeficiency virus
- Motor vehicle injury
- Nutrition, physical activity, and obesity
- Prescription-drug overdose
- Teen pregnancy
- Tobacco use

(From About the Prevention Status Reports. Atlanta, GA: Centers for Disease Control and Prevention; August 30, 2017. Available at: <https://www.cdc.gov/psr/overview.html>; [Accessed December 3, 2019].)

A **public health solution** is an answer to this problem designed to solve it.[13] Some familiar examples of solutions to public health problems are immunizations, water fluoridation, smoking ordinances, and early detection of disease. These public health solutions are concerned with health promotion and disease prevention. They are effective measures that address the problems of the community at large. The effectiveness of a public health solution depends on how well it possesses seven key characteristics (see Guiding Principles). Also, when proceeding with a public health solution, a community must unify to have collective impact through social and political support.[13]

GUIDING PRINCIPLES

Seven Characteristics of Public Health Solutions

- Safe; not hazardous to life or function
- Effective in reducing or preventing the targeted disease, condition, or practice
- Easily and efficiently implemented; minimum compliance required
- Potency maintained for a substantial period
- Attainable regardless of **socioeconomic status** (SES)
- Effective immediately upon application
- Affordable, cost-effective, and within the means of the community

Community water fluoridation (see Chapter 6) can be used to illustrate these characteristics of a public health solution. Fluoridation has been proven to be a safe, effective, and cost-effective solution to address the problem of dental caries in children and adults at the population level.[17] It is easily implemented by adding fluoride to the water supply, and the only compliance required is to drink the fluoridated water. Its potency is maintained as long as the fluoridated water is consumed, and it reaches all people regardless of SES. It is effective immediately upon initiation and costs far less than restorative treatment. Meeting all seven characteristics, it is considered by public health officials to be an effective solution to the public health problem of dental caries. [8]

SES is the social standing or position of a person or group in a community or society on a social-economic scale. It is measured by factors such as education, type of occupation, income, wealth, and place of residence. SES is important in public health because lower SES populations are generally at increased risk for dental disease, experience more oral health disparities, and have limited **access to oral health care** for a variety of associated reasons.[19]

Oral Disease as a Public Health Problem

Many oral diseases are significant universal, chronic problems that do not undergo remission and can result in expensive care or loss of teeth if left untreated. Dental caries is common and widespread for many Americans and Canadians, especially children from minority, racial, and ethnic groups, and low-SES individuals of all ages.[20,21] Older adults also have racial/ethnic and income disparities in relation to oral health-related quality of life.[22] Table 1.2 presents data for some of the oral diseases in selected groups of the population in the U.S. and Canada.

Dental disease has been described as a universal dental public health problem of the 21st century in the U.S. and Canada that is serious, can be alleviated, and can even be prevented with public health measures.[23] Thus, additional oral health education, promotion, prevention, and early treatment programs are needed.[19,24]

The public health solution of water fluoridation cited earlier has been applied to the problem of dental caries since 1945.[17] Organized community efforts have brought fluoridated drinking water to more than 210 million people in the U.S.[17] and to 13.9 million in Canada,[25] with significant reductions in dental caries in both countries.[17,25] Nevertheless, approximately 72 million Americans[17] and 22 million Canadians[25] do not have access to optimally fluoridated water. Thus, the oral health agendas of both nations aim to increase the percentage of the population that has access to optimally fluoridated water.[19,25]

Chapter 5 presents additional population data on dental caries and other significant oral diseases and conditions. Chapters 6, 8, and 11 describe health promotion programs that can be implemented as public health solutions to these problems within various sized communities, including additional information on water fluoridation in Chapter 6.

TABLE 1.2	Oral Disease Among American and Canadian Populations
American children ages 3-5 years (2013–2014 data)[a]	• 29.7% with caries experience in primary teeth • 14.1% with untreated caries in primary teeth
American children ages 6-9 years (2013–2014 data)[a]	• 51.7% with caries experience in primary or permanent teeth • 16.2% with untreated caries in primary or permanent teeth
American adolescents ages 13-15 years (2013–2014 data)[a]	• 49.9% with caries experience in permanent teeth • 17.9% with untreated caries in permanent teeth
American adults (2013–2014 data)[a]	• 31.3% aged 35-44 years with untreated caries • 72% aged 45-64 years missing a tooth from caries or periodontal disease • 37.4% aged 45-74 years with moderate to severe periodontitis
Older American adults	• 19.1% aged 65-74 years with untreated coronal caries (2013–2014 data)[a] • 37.9% aged ≥75 years with untreated root caries (1999–2004 data)[a] • 15.2% aged 65-74 years completely edentulous (2013–2014 data)[a] • Majority of aged ≥65 years taking medications, which is associated with xerostomia and dental caries (1990–2016 data)[b] • Older adults historically the primary group to experience oral and pharyngeal cancers[c]
Canadian children and adolescents (2007–2009 data)[d]	• 48% aged 6-11 years with caries experience in primary teeth; average decayed, missing, and filled teeth (DMFT) of 1.99 • 24% aged 6-11 years with caries experience in permanent teeth; average DMFT of 0.49 • 59% of aged 12-19 years with caries experience; average DMFT of 2.49
Canadian adults (2007–2009 data)[d]	• 96% with caries experience • 21% with moderate or severe periodontal problems • 6.4% aged 20-79 edentulous
Canadians ages 6-79 years (2007–2009 data)[e]	• 12% experienced dental pain within previous 12 months • Higher rates of dental pain experienced by adolescents and adults compared with other age groups

[a]Oral Health Objectives, 2020 Data for This Objective (OH-1, OH-2, OH-3, OH-4, OH-5). Healthy People 2020; November 27, 2019. Available at: <https://www.healthypeople.gov/2020/topics-objectives/topic/oral-health/objectives>; [Accessed December 2, 2019].
[b]Tan ECK, Lexomboon D, Sandborgh-Englund G, Haasum Y, Johnell K. Medications that cause dry mouth as an adverse effect in older people: A systematic review and metaanalysis. J Am Geriatr Soc 2018;66(1):76. <https://onlinelibrary.wiley.com/doi/full/10.1111/jgs.15151>; [Accessed December 2, 2019].
[c]Oral Cancer Facts. Newport Beach, CA: Oral Cancer Foundation; February 27, 2019. Available at: <https://oralcancerfoundation.org/facts/>; [Accessed December 2, 2019].
[d]Summary Report on the Findings of the Oral Health Component of the Canadian Health Measures Survey 2007–2009. Ottawa, Ontario, Canada: Health Canada; 2010. Available at: <http://www.caphd.ca/sites/default/files/CHMS-E-summ.pdf>; [Accessed December 2, 2019].
[e]Ravaghi V, Quiñonez C, Allison P. Oral pain and its covariates: Findings of a Canadian population-based study. J Can Dent Assoc 2018;79:d3. Available at: <http://www.jcda.ca/article/d3>; [Accessed December 2, 2019].

ROLE OF GOVERNMENT IN PUBLIC HEALTH

Government Agencies

As a dental hygienist you may choose a variety of ways to fulfill your ethical responsibility to contribute to the health of people in the community.[26,27] For example, you could participate in local community oral health promotion activities such as presenting an educational program at a school or conducting a cancer screening at a facility for older adults. The more formal public health programs, however, generally are supported by the government. Programs developed by government agencies focus on both prevention and the delivery of services.

In the U.S. the federal government's role in participating in oral health-related activities primarily falls under the jurisdiction of the **Department of Health and Human Services** (DHHS). The goals of the DHHS for the period 2018 to 2022 are the following:[28]

1. Reform, strengthen, and modernize the nation's healthcare system
2. Protect the health of Americans where they live, learn, work, and play
3. Strengthen the economic and social well-being of Americans across the lifespan
4. Foster sound, sustained advances in the sciences
5. Promote effective and efficient management and stewardship

The DHHS has 11 operating divisions, including eight agencies in the Public Health Service and three human services agencies (Figure 1.2).[29] Many of these federal agencies have programs that relate to oral health (Box 1.2). The primary involvement of the federal government in public health is to provide an infrastructure, research, **surveillance**, and funding for programs that are carried out at the state and local levels.

Other federal government agencies also have a role in oral health for specific populations. The related functions of the Department of Defense, the Veterans Health Administration, the Department of Agriculture, and the Indian Health Service are also described in Box 1.2.

At the state level, public health agencies have been charged with developing and coordinating oral health programs within their states. The **Association of State and Territorial Dental Directors** (ASTDD) has recommended best practices to assure that these programs have the infrastructure and capacity necessary to increase awareness of oral health issues, promote sound oral health policy development, and support initiatives to prevent and control oral diseases.[30]

At the local level, educational, preventive, and patient care oral health programs vary nationwide. These local programs are implemented through local government, nonprofit, faith-based, or other agencies or organizations. For example, local community health centers provide services for low-income families, and school-based programs provide oral health education and oral disease prevention services to children (see Chapters 5 and 6). State and local oral health programs collaborate with other entities such as the Medicaid-CHIP program, oral health coalitions, Head Start offices, maternal and child health offices, and professional dental and dental hygiene associations.[31]

Other countries also have government agencies that address oral health issues at various levels. For example, in Canada this is accomplished by Health Canada and the Public Health Agency of Canada, both part of the Health Portfolio under the direction of the Minister of Health.[32] The First Nations and Inuit Health Branch of Health Canada provides health promotion and dental health services to indigenous people groups.[32] The Canadian Institute of Health Information has valuable current data on

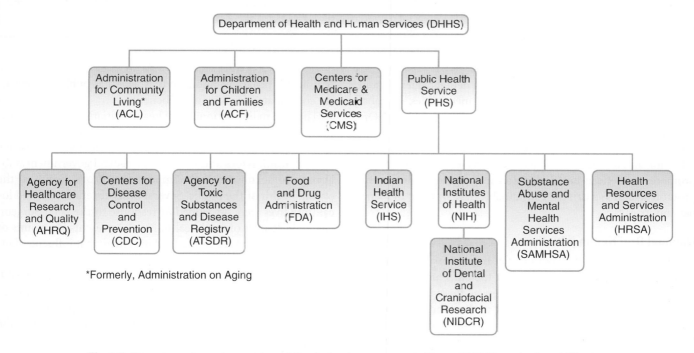

Fig 1.2 Departments and agencies of the federal government. (From HHS Organizational Chart. Washington DC: Department of Health & Human Services; September 23, 2020. Available at: <https://www.hhs.gov/about/agencies/orgchart/index.html>; [Accessed October 1, 2020].)

BOX 1.2   Federal Governmental Agencies of Interest in Community Oral Health

Administration for Children and Families (ACF; www.acf.hhs.gov/)

Manages the Head Start (HS) program that funds local HS programs that educationally prepare qualified preschool-age children for entry into school.

Agency for Healthcare Research and Quality (AHRQ; www.ahrq.gov/)

Supports research to improve the quality of health care, reduce its costs, address patient safety and medical errors, and increase access to care.

Centers for Disease Control and Prevention (CDC; www.cdc.gov/)

Works to protect people's health and safety by addressing a wide range of health threats, including oral diseases through the Division of Oral Health (DOH), focusing on disease prevention and wellness promotion, providing credible information to enhance health decisions, and encouraging strong community partnerships. CDC provides expertise, information, tools, and collaboration to assist agencies with community programming; administers funding for state and local health departments and community-based organizations for many varied public health programs, including oral health; provides surveillance data (e.g., water fluoridation and disease prevalence); provides leadership and direction in the prevention and control of diseases and other conditions; coordinates and implements national health policy on the state and local levels; responds to public health emergencies; and cooperates with other nations on health projects.

Centers for Medicare & Medicaid Services (CMS; www.cms.gov/)

Provides oversight for Medicare, the federal portion of Medicaid and the Children's Health Insurance Program (CHIP), and the Health Insurance Marketplace.

Department of Agriculture (USDA; www.usda.gov/wps/portal/usda/usdahome)

Administers the Women, Infants, and Children (WIC) program. Local WIC programs provide nutritional foods, education, screening, and referrals, including for dental care and education, for eligible women who are pregnant, are breastfeeding, or have young children under age 5 years.

Department of Defense (DoD; www.defense.gov/) and Veterans Administration (VA; http://www.va.gov/)

Provides direct care for specific armed services and veteran populations.

U.S. Food and Drug Administration (FDA; www.fda.gov/)

Enforces laws to ensure the safety and effectiveness of drugs, biological products, and medical devices (includes dental).

Health Resources and Services Administration (HRSA; www.hrsa.gov/)

The primary agency for improving access to health care for people who are uninsured, geographically isolated, or medically vulnerable through various means, including funding community and school-based health centers and programs that strengthen the healthcare workforce, build healthy communities, and help to achieve health equity.

Indian Health Service (IHS; www.ihs.gov/)

Provides direct comprehensive patient care and community health programming for Native American and Alaska Native populations, with opportunity for maximum tribal involvement in developing and managing the programs.

National Institutes of Health (NIH; www.nih.gov/)

Conducts and funds epidemiological, medical, and biomedical research; provides science transfer; trains researchers; and promotes acquisition and distribution of medical knowledge. Several institutes are relevant to oral health such as the National Institute of Dental and Craniofacial Research (NIDCR), National Cancer Institute (NCI), and National Institute on Aging (NIA).

Public Health Service (PHS or USPHS; www.usphs.gov/)

The principal operating division of DHHS responsible for protecting, promoting, and advancing the population's health and safety. The PHS provides activities to advance public health science; rapid, effective response to public health crises; and leadership and excellence in public health practices. Goals are executed by the Commissioned Core of Health Officers who, led by the Surgeon General, staff various federal agencies and clinics and respond to national emergencies.

---

the dental workforce in Canada, including dental hygienists and dental therapists, and on dental health inequalities.[33] Global oral health issues are addressed also by the World Health Organization,[1] working through regional offices worldwide to improve health outcomes in member countries. The regional office for the Americas, the Pan American Health Organization, promotes evidenced-based decision-making to improve and promote health as a driver of sustainable development in member countries.[1]

National Oral Health Initiatives

Whether an oral health program is at the national, state, or local level, the objectives should reflect the current national oral health initiatives. It is important to review these initiatives and their development to have a complete understanding of how to reflect the current national agenda in community programs. Even strategies and services implemented through the private sector should reflect current national initiatives. In this way all

oral health programs and activities, whether public or private, are coordinated for maximum benefit.

The first major national oral health initiative in the U.S. was the publication of the 2000 Surgeon General's Report, *Oral Health in America*.[23] This landmark report focused exclusively on oral health issues and was the first federal government publication to acknowledge the importance of oral health to the overall health of the public. Several other federal, state, and local initiatives were developed in response to the 2000 Surgeon General's Report on oral health. Box 1.3 presents key points of these and other important federal initiatives that influence dental public health in the U.S. today.

An updated 2020 Surgeon General's report on oral health was launched in November 2018 with an anticipated publication date of 2020.[34] This effort has the following purposes:

- Document progress in oral health since publication of the 2000 report
- Describe key issues that currently affect oral health

BOX 1.3   Significant Federal Oral Health Initiatives in the United States

Key Points of the Surgeon General's Report *Oral Health in America* (2000)[a]

- Oral health is essential to general health and well-being.
- General health factors (e.g., tobacco use, diabetes) affect oral health.
- Oral health can be achieved by all Americans.
- Profound and consequential oral health disparities exist.
- Dental public health programs are needed.

Principle Actions and Implementation Strategies Charged by *A National Call to Action to Promote Oral Health* (2003)[b]

- Take specific actions toward optimal oral health.
- Educate the public to change perceptions about oral health.
- Build the science and accelerate the transfer of the science.
- Increase collaborations (partnerships, coalitions).
- Increase workforce diversity, capacity, and flexibility.
- Overcome barriers by replicating effective programs.

Promoting and Enhancing the Oral Health of the Public: HHS Oral Health Initiative 2010[c]

- Developed as a coordinated effort of multiple DHHS agencies in response to the realization that many oral health challenges of the 1990s had not been addressed successfully.
- Key message: Oral health is integral to overall health.
- Purpose: To improve the nation's oral health by realigning existing resources and creating new activities to maximize outputs.

Goals:

- Emphasize oral health promotion and disease prevention.
- Increase access to care.
- Enhance the oral health workforce.
- Eliminate oral health disparities.

Strategies:

- Partnership of Office of Head Start and American Academy of Pediatric Dentistry to develop an infrastructure to recruit and support dentists to serve as dental homes for the underserved.
- Collaboration of NIDCR, CDC's DOH, and CDC's National Center for Health Statistics to enhance oral health surveillance.
- Endeavor of the CMS to increase access to dental care in state Medicaid programs by identifying and sharing best practices used successfully by some of these programs.
- Affiliation of DHHS and HRSA administrators to increase the visibility of existing DHHS oral health activities and improve awareness of oral health services available to the public.
- Collaboration of the National Research Council, the Institute of Medicine (IOM), the Board on Children, Youth and Families, and the Board on Health Care Services to develop a report on access of vulnerable and underserved groups to oral health care.
- Implementation and expansion of a multidisciplinary Early Childhood Caries Initiative by the IHS Division of Oral Health to promote prevention and early intervention of dental caries in young children by involving other agencies and community partners.
- Support and promotion by NIH of the building of a web-accessible national dental consortium research infrastructure network to facilitate the standardization of dental research.
- Launching of a new Cultural Competency E-Learning Oral Health Continuing Education Program by the Office of Minority Health to target oral health disparities.

- Incorporation of accurate oral health information into educational programs and highlighting of regional oral health activities by the Office on Women's Health to change the perception of oral health's impact on overall health.

Advancing Oral Health in America (2011)[d]

- Described the continuation of the problems of oral disease status and disparities.
- Reinforced the link of oral diseases to complications with medical diseases and conditions.

Recommendations:

- Establish high-level accountability.
- Emphasize disease prevention and oral health promotion.
- Improve oral health literacy and cultural competence.
- Reduce oral health disparities.
- Explore new models for payment and delivery of care.
- Enhance the role of nondental healthcare professionals.
- Expand oral health research and improve data collection.
- Promote collaboration among private and public stakeholders.
- Measure progress toward goals and objectives.
- Advance *Healthy People* goals and objectives.

Improving Access to Oral Health Care for Vulnerable and Underserved Populations (2011)[e]

- Highlighted the problem of oral health disparities.
- Suggested strategies to improve access to oral health care for those who need it the most.

Recommendations:

- Integrate oral health care into overall health care.
- Change laws and regulations such as **scope of practice**.
- Improve dental education in relation to treating diverse populations in various settings.
- Reduce financial and administrative barriers to care.
- Expand capacity of the oral healthcare system.

Outcomes of Integration of Oral Health and Primary Care Practice (2014)[f]

- Developed core clinical oral health competencies for use by primary care medical practitioners to increase oral healthcare access for safety net populations.
- Designed an infrastructure, payment policies, and evaluation strategies to implement the core clinical oral health competencies in primary care medical practices.

U.S. Department of Health and Human Services Oral Health Strategic Framework, 2014–2017 (2016)[g]

- Provides the context for leveraging current and planned oral health priorities and actions across HHS and partner agencies.
- Offers a guide to HHS, federal partners, and oral health stakeholders for working collaboratively to achieve greater impact in moving a national oral health agenda forward.
- Aligns key activities with five major goals and associated strategies in response to recommendations from IOM reports *Advancing Oral Health in America* and *Improving Access to Oral Health Care for Vulnerable and Underserved Populations*.
- Suggests strategies to fulfill each of the goals.

(Continued)

BOX 1.3   Significant Federal Oral Health Initiatives in the United States (*Cont.*)

Goals:

- Integrate oral health and primary health care.
- Prevent disease and promote oral health.
- Increase access to oral health care and eliminate disparities.
- Increase the dissemination of oral health information and improve health literacy.
- Advance oral health in public policy and research.

Reforming America's Healthcare System Through Choice and Competition (2018)[h]

Goals:

- Increase access to care, especially in underserved areas.
- Reduce cost of care.

Recommendations:

- Expand scope of practice and eliminate rigid collaborative practice and supervision requirements for dental hygienists and mid-level providers.
- Allow direct payment for services to dental hygienists and mid-level providers by private and public insurance carriers and through health reimbursement arrangements for dental benefits.
- Evaluate success of the dental therapy profession relative to increasing access to dental care and reducing costs while still ensuring safe, effective care.
- Consider ways to improve **license portability** to facilitate movement across state lines and provide interstate telehealth services.

[a] Oral Health in America: A Report of the Surgeon General. Rockville, MD: Department of Health and Human Services, National Institute of Dental and Craniofacial Research; 2000. Available at: <https://www.nidcr.nih.gov/research/data-statistics/surgeon-general>; [Accessed December 2, 2019].
[b] A National Call to Action to Promote Oral Health. Office of the Surgeon General, Publication No. 03-5303. Bethesda, MD: National Institute of Dental and Craniofacial Research; 2003. Available at: <https://www.ncbi.nlm.nih.gov/books/NBK47472/>; [Accessed December 2, 2019].
[c] Promoting and Enhancing the Oral Health of the Public: HHS Oral Health Initiative 2010. Washington, DC: Department of Health and Human Resources; 2010. Available at: <https://www.hrsa.gov/sites/default/files/oralhealth/hhsinitiative.pdf>; [Accessed December 2, 2019].
[d] Advancing Oral Health in America. Institute of Medicine of the National Academies, Committee on an Oral Health Initiative. Washington, DC: National Academies Press; 2011. Available at: <https://www.hrsa.gov/sites/default/files/publichealth/clinical/oralhealth/advancingoralhealth.pdf>; [Accessed December 2, 2019].
[e] Improving Access to Oral Health Care for Vulnerable and Underserved Populations. Institute of Medicine, National Research Council. Washington, DC: National Academies Press; 2011. Available at: <https://www.hrsa.gov/sites/default/files/publichttp://www.hrsa.gov/publichealth/clinical/oralhealth/advancingoralhealth.pdfhealth/clinical/oralhealth/improvingaccess.pdf.>; [Accessed December 2, 2019].
[f] Integration of Oral Health and Primary Care Practice. Rockville, MD: Health Resources and Services Administration; 2014. Available at: <https://www.hrsa.gov/sites/default/files/hrsa/oralhealth/integrationoforalhealth.pdf>; [Accessed December 2, 2019].
[g] U.S. Department of Health and Human Services Oral Health Coordinating Committee. U.S. Department of Health and Human Services Oral Health Strategic Framework, 2014–2017. Public Health Rep 2016;131(2):242-257. Available at: <https://www.ncbi.nlm.nih.gov/pmc/articles/PMC4765973/>; [Accessed December 2, 2019].
[h] Reforming America's Healthcare System Through Choice and Competition. Washington, DC: Department of Health and Human Services, Department of the Treasury, Department of Labor; December 2018. Available at: <https://www.hhs.gov/sites/default/files/Reforming-Americas-Healthcare-System-Through-Choice-and-Competition.pdf>; [Accessed December 2, 2019].

- Identify challenges and opportunities that have emerged since publication of the first report
- Convey a vision for the future
- Call upon the American public to take action

Some of the topics to be included in this report are oral health across the life span, integrating medical and dental care, how communities and the economy are affected by oral health, and the effects of the opioid epidemic.

Healthy People Initiative

As a major ongoing initiative of the DHHS, ***Healthy People*** provides science-based goals and measurable objectives for the U.S. designed to improve the health of the public.[19] Also included are targets and guidance for reaching the targets. These objectives and targets direct the agenda of government health programs based on a 10-year framework for health promotion and disease prevention. In addition, states and localities are invited to use the national framework and objectives for their own community health programming. These *Healthy People* objectives and targets are organized by various health topics, oral conditions being one of them.[19] A driving force of dental public health is achieving the *Healthy People* national oral health and related goals, following the principles and practices described throughout this textbook.

At the end of each decade the DHHS applies scientific insights and lessons learned from the past decade, along with new knowledge of current data, trends, and innovations, to create *Healthy People* reports with new objectives and targets for the next decade. In this way, "*Healthy People* has established benchmarks and monitored progress over time to encourage collaborations across communities and sectors, empower individuals toward making informed health decisions, and measure the impact of prevention activities."[19]

The first *Healthy People* goals were set in 1979 for the next decade. Work on the fifth version, *Healthy People 2030*, began in 2016, and it was launched in August 2020.[19] Current *Healthy People* objectives are discussed in detail in Chapter 4 and referred to in relation to other topics throughout this book.

Other countries develop oral health initiatives specific to their own population. Several initiatives listed in Box 1.4 will be of interest to readers in Canada. These national oral health initiatives in the U.S. and Canada have the common goals of increasing access to oral health care, improving oral health, eliminating oral health disparities, and expanding quality of life. **Stakeholders** must work together to achieve the vision, goals, and objectives of the national oral health initiatives of their own country, although the outcomes of some initiatives can be extrapolated to the oral health needs of other countries.

BOX 1.4 Significant Canadian Oral Health Initiatives

Canadian Oral Health Strategy (2005)[a]
- Reflects goals and objectives meant to improve Canadians' oral health.
- Lists actions to achieve the goals that can be promoted and undertaken by oral healthcare professionals or organizations, government agencies, and other entities.
- Has provided a foundation for Canada's dental public health efforts.

Summary Report on the Findings of the Oral Health Component of the Canadian Health Measures Survey 2007–2009[b]
- Provides the most recent oral health status data in Canada.

Improving Access to Oral Health Care for Vulnerable People Living in Canada (2014)[c]
- Describes inequalities in oral health status and oral care for this population. Recommends ways to address core problems and achieve equity in access to oral health care.

The State of Oral Health in Canada (2017)[d]
- Suggests ways the private oral healthcare sector can collaborate to address dental public health problems.

National Health Expenditure Trends, 1975 to 2018[e]
- Provides data on dental expenditures.

Canadian Community Health Survey[f]
- Has been conducted annually since 2000 as a collaborative effort of several Canadian health agencies.
- Contains an oral health component.

[a] Canadian Oral Health Strategy. Federal, Provincial, and Territorial Dental Directors; 2005. Available at: <http://www.caphd.ca/sites/default/files/Canadian%20Oral%20Health%20Strategy%20-%20Final.pdf>; [Accessed December 2, 2019].
[b] Summary Report on the Findings of the Oral Health Component of the Canadian Health Measures Survey 2007-2009. Ottawa, Ontario, Canada: Health Canada; 2010. Available at: <http://www.caphd.ca/sites/default/files/CHMS-E-summ.pdf>; [Accessed December 2, 2019].
[c] Improving Access to Oral Health Care for Vulnerable People Living in Canada. Ottawa, Ontario, Canada: Canadian Academy of Health Sciences; 2014. Available at: <https://www.cahs-acss.ca/wp-content/uploads/2014/09/Access_to_Oral_Care_FINAL_REPORT_EN.pdf>; [Accessed December 2, 2019].
[d] The State of Oral Health in Canada. Ottawa, Ontario, Canada: Canadian Dental Association; 2017. Available at: <https://www.cda-adc.ca/stateoforalhealth/_files/TheStateofOralHealthinCanada.pdf>; [Accessed December 2, 2019].
[e] National Health Expenditure Trends, 1975 to 2018. Ottawa, Ontario, Canada: Canadian Institute of Health Information; 2018. Available at: <https://www.cihi.ca/sites/default/files/document/nhex-trends-narrative-report-2018-en-web.pdf>; [Accessed December 2, 2019].
[f] Canadian Community Health Survey – Annual Component, 2018. Ottawa, Ontario, Canada: Statistics Canada; 2018. Available at: <http://www23.statcan.gc.ca/imdb/p2SV.pl?Function=getSurvey&SDDS=3226>; [Accessed December 2, 2019].

Core Functions and Essential Services of Public Health

Federal, state, and local programs have been charged with improving the health of the people through the **core functions of public health**, which are **assessment, policy development**, and **assurance**.[10] The purposes of the core public health functions

BOX 1.5 Core Functions of Public Health Agencies at All Levels of Government

Assessment
- Includes systematic collection, analysis, and sharing of information on the health of the community.
- Comprises epidemiological data on health status, community health needs, and health problems.
- Depends on essential intergovernmental and interagency teamwork to manage and share data.
- Reflects responsibility of each public health agency to ensure that assessment is achieved (cannot be delegated).

Policy Development
- Demonstrates responsibility of each public health agency to develop comprehensive public health policies.
- Encompasses the use of a scientific knowledge base in making public health decisions.
- Requires a strategic approach.
- Is based on the democratic political process.

Assurance
- Entails reassurance of each public health agency that services necessary to achieve agreed-upon goals are provided by one of the following means:
  - Encouraging actions by other private- or public-sector entities.
  - Requiring such action through regulation.
  - Providing services directly.
- Involves key agency policymakers and the general public in determining high-priority personal and community-wide health services that governments will guarantee.
- Provides subsidization or direct provision of high-priority personal health services by public health agencies for people unable to afford them.

From The Future of the Public's Health in the 21st Century. Washington, DC: Institute of Medicine. National Academies Press; 2003. Available at: <https://doi.org/10.17226/10548>; [Accessed December 2, 2019]. With permission.

are to protect and promote health, wellness, and the quality of life and to prevent disease, injury, disability, and death. They are described in detail in Box 1.5.

Ten **essential public health services** have been identified to represent the activities that all communities should undertake (Table 1.3). These services are considered vital to the achievement of healthy people in healthy communities and are an integral part of public health practice.[10] Figure 1.3 demonstrates the relationship of the essential public health services to the core public health functions, also providing further understanding of the core functions.[10] Basically, the essential services operationalize the core functions. Successful provision of these services requires collaboration among members of the public health system.[31]

Building on the framework of the core public health functions and the essential public health services, ASTDD developed comparable **essential public health services to promote oral health**[35] (see Table 1.3). The core public health functions, the essential public health services, and the essential public health services to promote oral health provide guidelines and direction for dental public health professionals working in national, state, and local oral health programs (see Chapters 4, 5, and 6). They are reflected in past and current public health initiatives and in the future plans for dental public health discussed in the next section.

TABLE 1.3   Comparison of the Essential Public Health Services to Promote Health and Oral Health in the United States, Organized around the Core Public Health Functions

10 Essential Public Health Services (CDC)	10 Essential Public Health Services to Promote Oral Health (ASTDD)
Assessment	**Assessment**
1. Assess and monitor population health status, factors that influence health, and community needs and assets	1. Assess oral health status and implement an oral health surveillance system
2. Investigate, diagnose, and address health problems and hazards affecting the population	2. Analyze determinants of oral health and respond to health hazards in the community
	3. Assess public perceptions about oral health issues and educate/empower them to achieve and maintain optimal oral health
Policy Development	**Policy Development**
3. Communicate effectively to inform and educate people about health, factors that influence it, and how to improve it	4. Mobilize community partners to leverage resources and advocate for/act on oral health issues
4. Strengthen, support, and mobilize communities and partnerships to improve health	5. Develop and implement policies and systematic plans that support state and community oral health efforts
5. Create, champion, and implement policies, plans, and laws that impact health	**Assurance**
6. Utilize legal and regulatory actions designed to improve and protect the public's health	6. Review, educate about, and enforce laws and regulations that promote oral health and ensure safe oral health practices
Assurance	7. Reduce barriers to care and assure utilization of personal and population-based oral health services
7. Assure an effective system that enables equitable access to the individual services and care needed to be healthy	8. Assure an adequate and competent public and private oral health workforce
8. Build and support a diverse and skilled public health workforce	9. Evaluate effectiveness, accessibility, and quality of personal and population-based oral health promotion activities and oral health services
9. Improve and innovate public health functions through ongoing evaluation, research, and continuous quality improvement	10. Conduct and review research for new insights and innovative solutions to oral health problems
10. Build and maintain a strong organizational infrastructure for public health	

From 10 Essential Public Health Services. Atlanta, GA: Centers for Disease Control and Prevention; 2020. Available at: <https://www.cdc.gov/publichealthgateway/publichealthservices/essentialhealthservices.html>; [Accessed October 1, 2020]; Essential Public Health Services to Promote Health and Oral Health in the United States. Reno, NV: Association of State & Territorial Dental Directors. Available at: <https://www.astdd.org/docs/essential-public-health-services-to-promote-health-and-oh.pdf>; [Accessed December 3, 2019].

FUTURE OF DENTAL PUBLIC HEALTH

What Needs to Be Done

Although dental disease has significantly improved over the last decades,[22,36] it persists as a public health problem.[37] Significant disparities in oral health also continue to occur.[37,38] Knowledge exists to alleviate the problem; however, constraints and a lack of resources have continued to prevent its application toward the goal of freeing communities from dental disease and achieving oral health equity.[37,39]

Despite the fact that dental utilization rates have increased for children,[40] significant numbers of all ages in the U.S. have not had a dental visit within the last year.[41,42] Insurance coverage,[43] Medicaid coverage,[44] and the number of Medicaid dental providers[45] have all increased; yet, significant numbers of the population do not have insurance coverage, and access to dental care continues to be a public health problem,[46,47] especially for older adults.[42] The Affordable Care Act (ACA) that passed in 2010, also known as Obamacare, increased dental coverage; however, 48% of children on Medicaid still did not receive any dental care in 2017.[37] In addition, early figures indicate that although 9.8 million adults gained dental benefits through

2017 as a result of the ACA,[44] adults who have dental coverage through Medicaid do not fully use the benefits.[48] Also, even with the ACA, gaps have remained for many low-income adults[49] and most older adults.[42]

The ongoing need to emphasize the importance of oral health continues. It is the responsibility of oral health professionals to advocate for oral health care, **access to care**, and cost-reduction measures to the policymakers of the nation (see Chapter 9).[26,50] The following strategies have been suggested to address the aforementioned dental public health problems and shape the future of oral health care in the U.S.:

- Increase the number of oral health professionals who can provide high-quality oral health care to low-income children.[51]
- Authorize dental therapists and other mid-level oral health-care workforce models to extend dental care to underserved populations.[46] (See Chapter 2.)
- Increase the utilization of evidence-based preventive services such as sealants and silver diamine fluoride.[37] (See Chapter 6.)
- Seek changes in regulations in states that still limit **direct access** of dental hygienists to the public to be able to

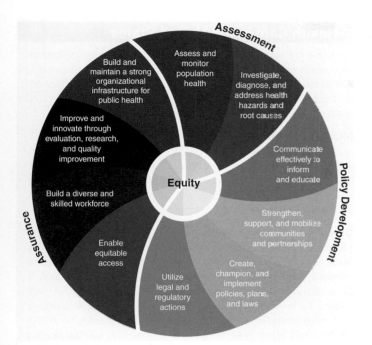

Fig 1.3 Core public health functions and essential public health services. (Adapted from The 10 Essential Public Health Services. Public Health Professionals Gateway. Atlanta, GA: Centers for Disease Control and Prevention; 2020. Available at: <https://phnci.org/uploads/resource-files/EPHS-Graphic-English.pdf>; [Accessed October 1, 2020].)

provide important services in community programs.[46] (See Chapter 2.)

- Transform scope-of-practice laws to allow all oral health-care providers to practice to the "top of their license."[46] (See Chapter 2.)
- Address reasons for poor utilization of dental care other than the cost barrier.[48]
- Ensure the effectiveness of interprofessional collaborative education for all oral healthcare providers to secure the success of interprofessional collaborative practice (ICP)[52,53] as a means of more effectively addressing the multifactorial nature of oral diseases.[54] (See Chapter 2.)
- Persevere in advocating for states to allow direct Medicaid reimbursement to dental hygienists to be able to accommodate more people who have Medicaid dental coverage.[46] In 2018, only 18 states provided for direct Medicaid reimbursement to dental hygienists.[55] (See Chapter 2.)
- To help control costs, decrease the number of expensive hospital emergency room visits for dental treatment that could be provided in dental offices.[42] Because use of emergency departments for dental care is associated with poor oral health, the solution should also be aimed at increasing utilization of routine dental care by those that currently depend on emergency departments for their dental care.[42]
- Improve oral health literacy in our society through health marketing.[56] (See Chapter 8.)
- Continue to stress the need for broad collaborations of committed oral health professionals, dental public health officials, and lawmakers to promote new initiatives that can improve the oral health of underserved populations and that all communities of interest can support.[10,19,31]

- Persist in seeking new ways to increase access to dental care for underserved groups, especially adults and older adults.[42,46,48]

Going in the Right Direction

Even though changes are needed to improve the oral health of the public, it appears that progress is being made in that direction. In 2020 and again in 2030, a *Healthy People* oral health objective was identified as one of the leading health indicators.[19] This indicates a more profound understanding by others of the importance of oral health compared to the past.[57]

Water fluoridation was identified by the CDC as one of the 10 most important public health accomplishments of the 20th century.[58] More recently the CDC listed the 10 great public health accomplishments of the first decade of the 21st century.[59] In addition to providing strong support for and promotion of water fluoridation, dentistry and dental hygiene have had a role in several of these latest public health successes, for example:

1. ADHA and the American Dental Association (ADA) have contributed to the significant decrease in tobacco use by adopting policy, establishing standards of practice, and providing resources related to tobacco cessation.[60,61]
2. The professions' attention to and training of office personnel for safe practices have helped to reduce work-related injuries.[9,62]
3. Oral health professionals have contributed to the reduction of cardiovascular disease by screening for high blood pressure and promoting the importance of oral health in relation to cardiovascular health.[60,63]

There has been a major effort in recent years by oral health organizations, policymakers, and advocacy groups to take action to address access to care for American citizens. Dental hygiene and dental organizations have participated diligently in these efforts, thus fulfilling an ethical and social responsibility to participate in activities that can result in effective and efficient community oral health practice becoming an important achievement in the 21st century.[2,50] Some of these latest actions are described in Box 1.6. Social responsibility in relation to community oral health is discussed further in Chapter 9.

Dental Public Health Specialty Training for Oral Health Professionals

Oral health professionals and public health officials share a vision of optimal oral health for citizens and universal access to comprehensive oral health care. Toward this aim, oral health professionals enter the field of public health by providing volunteer efforts or accepting employment within programs that include oral health promotion, community oral disease prevention, and provision of dental care to selected groups of people.

The DHHS has recommended public health training for all oral health professionals who direct state dental public health programs in the U.S.[19] Dentists can become recognized specialists in the field of dental public health through specialty certification with the American Board of Dental Public Health by meeting required competencies.[7]

In most states, dental hygienists have no required formal or specialty education to work in the community. However, the basic dental hygiene educational program includes essential community oral-health-practice goals, objectives, and competencies (see

BOX 1.6 Recent Actions to Improve Access to Oral Health Care in the United States

Dental Hygiene Education

In 2015 the ADHA developed a strategic plan to address dental hygiene curriculum changes needed to prepare future dental hygienists for the expanded roles required as a result of the current national oral health agenda, changes in the healthcare environment, shifting societal needs, the increasing understanding of the need to focus on the relevance of oral health to systemic health, and the growing emphasis on interprofessional collaborative practice.[a]

Interprofessional Collaborative Practice

In 2016 the Interprofessional Education Collaborative (IPEC), with ADEA as a charter member organization, reaffirmed the value and impact of the core competencies for **interprofessional collaborative practice** (ICP) that were developed by IPEC in 2011 and implemented nationwide in educational programs of six health professions, including dentistry and dental hygiene.[b] The 2016 update report described the headway made in **interprofessional education** (IPE), the inclusion in IPEC of additional health professions, and the vital collaborations that will forge the future of IPE and ICP. The report also presented the reorganized and broadened competencies and sub-competencies that were designed to "improve the patient experience of care, improve the health of populations, and reduce the per capita cost of health care."[b] (See Chapters 2 and 11 for more information on ICP.)

Direct Access for Dental Hygienists

ADHA has continued to advocate for direct access of the public to oral healthcare services provided by a dental hygienist to address the access-to-care problem (see Chapter 2). In 2018, 42 states allowed direct access in community-based settings.[c]

New Competencies for Dental Public Health Specialists

To reflect the changing landscape of dental public health practice, the American Board of Dental Public Health, in partnership with the American Association of Public Health Dentistry and others, developed new competencies for the 21st-century dental public health specialist that went into effect in 2018.[d]

Action for Dental Health Act

In December 2018 President Trump signed into law the Action for Dental Health Act. Supported by ADA, the bill was aimed at improving the status of oral health and access to dental care by[e]

- Improving oral health education and dental disease prevention
- Reducing the use of emergency rooms for dental care
- Helping patients establish dental homes
- Reducing barriers to receiving care, including language and cultural barriers
- Facilitating dental care to nursing home residents

Reforming America's Healthcare System Through Choice and Competition

In December 2018 the White House released a landmark report *Reforming America's Healthcare System Through Choice and Competition*.[f] The report was a response to President Trump's directing his administration to "facilitate the development and operation of a healthcare system that provides high-quality care at affordable prices for the American people by promoting choice and competition."[f] Recommendations have the potential to significantly impact oral health care and the practice of dental hygiene (see Box 1.3).

Mid-level Oral Health Practitioners

In 2018 the ADHA reaffirmed its support for utilizing mid-level oral health practitioners and advocated for a dental hygiene-based workforce model for them.[c] The White House report *Reforming America's Healthcare System Through Choice and Competition* called for utilizing dental hygienists, dental therapists, and other mid-level providers at the "top of their license."[f]

Dental Care for Older Adults

Dental and medical professionals have taken greater notice of the unmet oral health needs of seniors in the last few years.[g] Momentum has increased for the idea of dental benefits under Medicare. Discussions occurred at a Santa Fe Group salon in 2016 and continued at a symposium cosponsored by Oral Health America, the DentaQuest Foundation, and the American Dental Association in 2017, which resulted in a white paper published by Oral Health America in 2018, *An Oral Health Benefit in Medicare Part B: It's Time to Include Oral Health in Health Care*.[g] Greater attention has been given to promoting the idea, recruiting a broad base of stakeholders for it, and exploring innovative dental payment and delivery models to make the proposal a reality. In January 2019, legislation was introduced to cover routine dental services under Medicare Part B[h] (Figure 1.4).

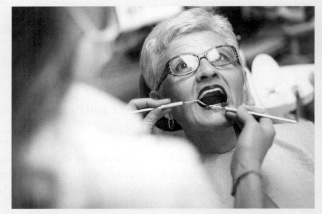

Fig 1.4 Efforts to increase access to dental care have targeted the older adult population by proposing to add dental benefits to Medicare. (@ iStock.com/danchooalex.)

[a] Transforming Dental Hygiene Education and the Profession for the 21st Century. Chicago, IL: American Dental Hygienists' Association; 2015. Available at: <https://www.adha.org/resources-docs/Transforming_Dental_Hygiene_Education.pdf>; [Accessed December 2, 2019].

[b] Core Competencies for Interprofessional Collaborative Practice: 2016 Update. Washington, DC: Interprofessional Education Collaborative; 2016. Available at: <https://www.unthsc.edu/interprofessional-education/wp-content/uploads/sites/33/Core-Competencies-for-Interprofessional-Collaborative-Practice.pdf>; [Accessed December 2, 2019].

[c] Facts about the Dental Hygiene Workforce in the United States. Chicago, IL: American Dental Hygienists' Association; November 2019. Available at: <http://www.adha.org/resources-docs/75118_Facts_About_the_Dental_Hygiene_Workforce.pdf>; [Accessed December 2, 2019].

[d] Altman D, Mascarenhas AK. New competencies for the 21st century dental public health specialist. J Public Health Dent 2016;76(S1):S18-S28. Available at: <https://onlinelibrary.wiley.com/doi/full/10.1111/jphd.12190>; [Accessed December 2, 2019].

[e] Garvin J. Action for Dental Health Act is now law. ADA News; December 11, 2018. Available at: <https://www.ada.org/en/publications/ada-news/2018-archive/november/action-for-dental-health-act-is-now-law>; [Accessed December 2, 2019].

[f] Reforming America's Healthcare System Through Choice and Competition (Press Release). Washington, DC: HHS Press Office; December 3, 2018. Available at: <https://www.hhs.gov/about/news/2018/12/03/reforming-americas-healthcare-system-through-choice-and-competition.html>; [Accessed December 2, 2019].

[g] Aravamudhan K, Burroughs M, Chaffin J, Chávez EM, Goldberg J, Jones J... Yarbrough C. An Oral Health Benefit in Medicare Part B: It's Time to Include Oral Health in Health Care. Oral Health America; 2018. Available at: <https://www.justiceinaging.org/wp-content/uploads/2018/07/Medicare-Dental-White-Paper.pdf>; [Accessed December 2, 2019].

[h] Senator Cardin Introduces Bill to Add Oral Health Coverage to Medicare. Washington, DC: Center for Medicare Advocacy; 2019. Available at: <https://medicareadvocacy.org/medicare-oral-health-cardin-bill/>; [Accessed December 15, 2020].

Appendix B) that were adopted by the American Dental Education Association (ADEA),[9] an organization that is a driving force of change within dentistry and dental hygiene. These goals, objectives, and competencies are reflected throughout the content of this book. In addition, the Commission on Dental Accreditation (CODA) has included a strong community oral health curriculum requirement for accreditation of dental hygiene programs.[12]

In some cases, dental hygienists with an interest in community oral health practice have pursued advanced degrees or certification in public health or community health. Others have sought a graduate degree in dental hygiene with a focus in community health. Competencies for the graduate dental hygiene degree were developed jointly by the ADHA and ADEA.[64] These proficiencies are based on the recognition that further education in public health prepares the dental hygienist to meet the challenges of community oral health practice. An advanced degree or certification is required for some public health positions as described later in this chapter.

ADHA has suggested advanced community-based education for dental hygienists who are filling the expanded roles of innovative workforce models.[65] Most states that have advanced certification for dental hygienists have established this requirement.[65] In 2015 the Commission on Dental Accreditation adopted accreditation standards for dental therapy programs that include requirements for community-based learning experiences to be able to serve in a community setting.[66] (See Chapter 3 for more information about the community-based education requirements for dental hygienists.)

SUMMARY

People's health is the health of the public living within a community, state, or nation. An understanding of people's health includes learning the basic terminology of the field and being able to identify public health problems and solutions. Comparison of private practice to community oral health practice demonstrates the similarities and prepares dental hygienists for the assessment, planning, implementation, and evaluation phases of community oral health programs, as does an understanding of core public health functions and essential public health services. The government's role in people's health is mentioned briefly as an introduction to the programs to be discussed in more detail in future chapters. National oral health initiatives lay the foundation to understand past progress and future needs to be able to address the problems. As healthcare providers, dental hygienists have a calling and an ethical duty to serve the communities in which they live. Oral health professionals who have chosen careers in public health contribute to the advancement of community oral health, but much more needs to be accomplished by all members of the dental professional community. Collaboration of all stakeholders is required to develop creative solutions to the significant problems of widespread oral diseases, unmet dental needs, oral health disparities, and limited access to oral health care for certain underserved groups. The community oral health educational preparation of oral health professionals puts them in a position to participate in this process.

APPLYING YOUR KNOWLEDGE

1. Evaluate a health issue in the news and discuss in class what the problem is and how it is being addressed. To evaluate the issue, use the criteria for identifying public health problems and the characteristics of public health solutions described in this chapter.
2. Choose a government public health program and further investigate its purpose and success in accomplishing this purpose.
3. Identify a local community oral health program and analyze how it reflects the vision, goals and objectives of the national oral health initiatives.
4. Read and report on one of the national oral health initiatives described in the chapter.
5. Search the Oral Health Atlas online, and report on dental disease as a worldwide public health problem; use maps and charts in this atlas for comparison.

LEARNING OBJECTIVES AND COMPETENCIES

This chapter addresses the following community oral health learning objectives and competencies for dental hygienists that are presented in the revised May 2015-2016 *ADEA Compendium of Curriculum Guidelines for Allied Dental Education Programs*:

Learning Objectives
- Define community dental health/dental public health.
- List the government departments and agencies related to oral health and dental hygiene.
- Compare the federal, state/provincial, and local presence of government in dental care delivery.
- List and define the international professional organizations involving dental public health.
- Describe current epidemiological trends of oral conditions and diseases.
- List and describe the publications reporting oral epidemiology and use appropriate information resources in community dental health.
- Describe various government-related opportunities for dental public health programs.

Competencies
- Promoting the values of good oral and general health and wellness to the public and organizations within and outside the professions.
- Advocating for consumer groups, businesses, and government agencies to support healthcare issues.
- Accepting responsibility for solving problems and making decisions based on accepted scientific principles.

COMMUNITY CASE

As the Oral Health Program Coordinator at the State Health Department, you are asked to conduct a statewide screening project to determine the oral health status of school-age children. After collecting the survey data, you will analyze it to identify and prioritize the problems reflected by the data. Then you will participate with other stakeholders to select and plan oral health programs for local implementation that will address the needs of children across the state.

1. Which core public health function is addressed through the initial phase of this project?
   a. Assurance
   b. Assessment
   c. Policy development
   d. Planning

2. All of the following essential public health services to promote oral health EXCEPT one would apply to this venture. Which is the EXCEPTION?
   a. Assess oral health status and implement an oral health surveillance system
   b. Develop and implement policies and systematic plans that support state and community oral health efforts
   c. Reduce barriers to care, and assure utilization of personal and population-based oral health services
   d. Promote and enforce laws and regulations that encourage oral health and ensure safe oral health practices

3. Which major DHHS agency would have the most possibilities for funding the programs you select to conduct?
   a. PHS (Public Health Service)
   b. ACF (Administration for Children and Families)
   c. CMS (Centers for Medicare & Medicaid Services)
   d. WIC (Women, Infants, and Children)

4. The last phase of the project as described in the scenario relates to which private-practice function?
   a. Diagnosis
   b. Evaluation
   c. Examination
   d. Treatment
   e. Treatment planning

5. If the programs you select are to be effective public health solutions, they will need to have all EXCEPT one of the following characteristics. Which is the EXCEPTION?
   a. Not hazardous to life or function
   b. Easily and efficiently implemented
   c. Attainable by those who can afford the dental care
   d. Effective immediately upon application

REFERENCES

1. Constitution of the World Health Organization: Principles. Geneva, Switzerland: World Health Organization; 2019. Available at: <https://www.who.int/>; [Accessed December 2, 2019].

2. What is Public Health? Atlanta, GA: CDC Foundation; 2019. Available at: <http://www.cdcfoundation.org/content/what-public-health>; [Accessed December 2, 2019].

3. What is Public Health? Washington, DC: American Public Health Association; 2019. Available at: <https://www.apha.org/what-is-public-health>; [Accessed December 2, 2019].

4. Polozkova V. Community Health: Definition & Care. Human Biology Study Guide, Chapter 17, Lesson 8. Available at: <https://study.com/academy/lesson/community-health-definition-care.html>; [Accessed December 2, 2019].

5. Introduction to Epidemiology, Public Health 101 Series. Atlanta, GA: Centers for Disease Control and Prevention; November 15, 2018. Available at: <https://www.cdc.gov/publichealth101/epidemiology.html#anchor_resources>; [Accessed December 2, 2019].

6. What is Population Health? Population Health Training in Place Program. Atlanta, GA: Centers for Disease Control and Prevention; July 23, 2019. Available at: <https://www.cdc.gov/pophealthtraining/whatis.html>; [Accessed December 2, 2019].

7. Altman D, Mascarenhas AK. New competencies for the 21st century dental public health specialist. J Public Health Dent 2016;76(S1):S18–28.

8. ASTDD Orientation Module: Dental Public Health 101. Reno, NV: Association of State & Territorial Dental Directors; March 23, 2016. Available at: <https://www.astdd.org/docs/dph-101-with-slide-notes-04-06-2016.pptx>; [Accessed December 2, 2019].

9. ADEA Compendium of Curricular Guidelines (Revised Edition) Allied Dental Education Programs May 2015-2016. Washington, DC: American Dental Education Association; 2015. Available at: <file:///C:/Users/Admin/AppData/Local/Temp/ADEA%20COMPENDIUM%202005%20GUIDELINES%20-%20Revised%20May%202016-5.pdf>; [Accessed December 2, 2019].

10. The Public Health System & the 10 Essential Public Health Services. Public Health Professional Gateway. Atlanta, GA: Centers for Disease Control and Prevention; June 26, 2018. Available at: <https://www.cdc.gov/publichealthgateway/publichealthservices/essentialhealthservices.html>; [Accessed December 2, 2019].

11. Supply of Dentists in the U.S.: 2001-2018. Chicago, IL: American Dental Association, Health Policy Institute; February 2019. Available at: <https://www.ada.org/en/science-research/health-policy-institute/data-center/supply-and-profile-of-dentists>; [Accessed December 2, 2019].

12. Accreditation Standards for Dental Hygiene Education Programs. Chicago, IL: Commission on Dental Accreditation; February 2018. Available at: <https://www.ada.org/~/media/CODA/Files/2019_dental_hygiene_standards.pdf?la=en>; [Accessed December 2, 2019].

13. Some Methods for Evaluating Comprehensive Community Initiatives. Chapter 38, Community Tool Box; 2019. Lawrence, KS: University of Kansas. Available at: <https://ctb.ku.edu/en>; [Accessed December 2, 2019].

14. Facilitating Public Health Problems: Facilitator Guide. Atlanta, GA: Centers for Disease Control and Prevention; 2013. Available at: <https://www.cdc.gov/globalhealth/healthprotection/fetp/training_modules/4/prioritize-problems_fg_final_09262013.pdf>; [Accessed December 2, 2019].

15. List of Public Health Issues Continues to Grow: No Consensus on Criteria for Framing an Issue as a Public Health Issue. The Epidemiology Monitor; 2018. Available at: <http://www.epimonitor.net/Public-Health-Issues-2018.htm>; [Accessed December 2, 2019].

16. About the Prevention Status Reports. Atlanta, GA: Centers for Disease Control and Prevention; August 30, 2017. Available at: <https://www.cdc.gov/psr/overview.html>; [Accessed December 3, 2019].

17. Hannan C, Espinoza L. Statement on the Evidence Supporting the Safety and Effectiveness of Community Water Fluoridation. Atlanta, GA: Centers for Disease Control and Prevention, Community Water Fluoridation; June 6, 2018. Available at: <https://www.cdc.gov/fluoridation/guidelines/cdc-statement-on-community-water-fluoridation.html>; [Accessed December 2, 2019].

18. U.S. Department of Health and Human Services Federal Panel on Community Water Fluoridation. U.S. Public Health Service recommendation for fluoride concentration in drinking water for the prevention of dental caries. Public Health Rep 2015, July1;130(July-Aug):318-331.

19. Healthy People 2020. Rockville, MD: Department of Health and Human Services, Office of Disease Prevention and Health Promotion; November 27, 2019. Available at: <https://www.healthypeople.gov/>; [Accessed December 2, 2019].

20. Dental Caries (Tooth Decay). Bethesda, MD: National Institute of Dental and Craniofacial Research; July 2018. Available at: < https://www.nidcr.nih.gov/research/data-statistics/dental-caries >; [Accessed December 2, 2019].

21. Ravaghi V, Quiñonez C, Allison P. Oral pain and its covariates: Findings of a Canadian population-based study. J Can Dent Assoc 2013;79:d3.

22. Oral Health for Older Americans. Atlanta, GA: Centers for Disease Control and Prevention, Oral Health; May 22, 2019. Available at: <https://www.cdc.gov/oralhealth/basics/adult-oral-health/adult_older.htm>; [Accessed December 2, 2019].

23. 2000 Surgeon General's Report on Oral Health in America. Bethesda, MD: National Institute of Dental and Craniofacial Research; January 2019. Available at: <https://www.nidcr.nih.gov/research/data-statistics/surgeon-general>; [Accessed December 2, 2019].

24. The State of Oral Health in Canada. Ottawa, Ontario, Canada: Canadian Dental Association; 2017. Available at: <https://www.cda-adc.ca/stateoforalhealth/_files/thestateoforalhealthincanada.pdf>; Accessed December 2, 2019.

25. The State of Community Water Fluoridation across Canada. Ottawa, Ontario, Canada: Government of Canada; 2017. Available at: <https://www.canada.ca/en/services/health/publications/healthy-living/community-water-fluoridation-across-canada-2017.html>; [Accessed December 2, 2019].

26. Code of Ethics for Dental Hygienists. In Bylaws & Code of Ethics, pp. 32-38. Chicago, IL: American Dental Hygienists' Association; June 2018. Available at: <https://www.adha.org/resources-docs/7611_Bylaws_and_Code_of_Ethics.pdf>; [Accessed December 2, 2019].

27. Dental Hygienists' Code of Ethics. Ottawa, Ontario, Canada: Canadian Dental Hygienists Association; June 2012. Available at: <https://www.cdha.ca/pdfs/Profession/Resources/Code_of_Ethics_EN_web.pdf>; Accessed December 2, 2019.

28. Strategic Plan FY 2018-2022. Washington, DC: Department of Health and Human Services; January 30, 2019. Available at: <http://www.hhs.gov/strategic-plan/priorities.html>; [Accessed December 2, 2019].

29. HHS Agencies & Offices. Washington, DC: Department of Health and Human Services, HHS Family of Agencies; May 24, 2016. Available at: <http://www.hhs.gov/about/agencies/hhs-agencies-and-offices/index.html>; [Accessed December 2, 2019].

30. Best Practice Approaches. Reno, NV: Association of State and Territorial Dental Directors. Available at: <https://www.astdd.org/best-practices/>; [Accessed December 2, 2019].

31. Collaboration. Reno, NV: Association of State & Territorial Dental Directors; 2014. Available at: <https://www.astdd.org/collaboration/>; [Accessed December 2, 2019].

32. Government of Canada: Health, Ottawa, Ontario, Canada; November 25, 2019. Available at: <https://www.canada.ca/en/services/health.html>; [Accessed December 2, 2019].

33. Canadian Institute for Health Information, Ottawa, Ontario, Canada. Available at: <https://www.cihi.ca/en>; [Accessed December 2, 2019].

34. National Institute of Dental and Craniofacial Research. Surgeon General commissions 2020 report on oral health. NIDCR News; March 2019. Available at: <https://www.nidcr.nih.gov/news-events/nidcr-news/surgeon-general-commissions-report-oral-health>; [Accessed December 2, 2019].

35. Essential Public Health Services to Promote Health and Oral Health in the United States. Reno, NV: Association of State & Territorial Dental Directors. Available at: <https://www.astdd.org/docs/essential-public-health-services-to-promote-health-and-oh.pdf>; [Accessed December 2, 2019].

36. Oral Health Objectives, 2020 Data for This Objective (OH-1, OH-2, OH-3, OH-4, OH-5). Healthy People 2020; November 27, 2019. Available at: <https://www.healthypeople.gov/2020/topics-objectives/topic/oral-health/objectives>; [Accessed December 2, 2019].

37. Koppelman J, Corr A. Children's Dental Health Month Is an Opportunity to Assess Progress: States and Advocates Work to Increase Access to Effective Care. Washington, DC: Pew Charitable Trusts; February 15, 2019. Available at: <https://www.pewtrusts.org/en/research-and-analysis/articles/2019/02/15/childrens-dental-health-month-is-an-opportunity-to-assess-progress>; [Accessed December 2, 2019].

38. Racial Disparities in Untreated Caries Narrowing for Children. Chicago, IL: American Dental Association, Health Policy Institute; June 2017. Available at: <http://www.ada.org/~/media/ADA/Science%20and%20Research/HPI/Files/HPIgraphic_0617_1.pdf?la=en>; [Accessed December 2, 2019].

39. Oral Health and Well-Being Among Medicaid Adults by Type of Medicaid Dental Benefit. Chicago, IL: American Dental Association, Health Policy Institute; 2018. Available at: <https://www.ada.org/~/media/ADA/Science%20and%20Research/HPI/Files/HPIgraphic_0518_1.pdf?la=en>; [Accessed December 2, 2019].

40. Dental Care Use Among Children: 2016. Chicago, IL: American Dental Association, Health Policy Institute; July 2018. Available at: <https://www.ada.org/~/media/ADA/Science%20and%20Research/HPI/Files/HPIGraphic_0718_1.pdf?la=en>; [Accessed December 2, 2019].

41. Dental Care Utilization in the U.S. Chicago, IL: American Dental Association, Health Policy Institute; 2015. Available at: <https://www.ada.org/~/media/ADA/Science%20and%20Research/HPI/Files/HPIgraphic_1117_2.pdf?la=en>; [Accessed December 2, 2019].

42. Freed M, Neuman T, Jacobson G. Drilling Down on Dental Coverage and Costs for Medicare Beneficiaries. San Francisco, CA: Kaiser Family Foundation; March 13, 2019. Available at: <https://www.kff.org/medicare/issue-brief/drilling-down-on-dental-coverage-and-costs-for-medicare-beneficiaries/>; [Accessed December 2, 2019].

43. Dental Benefits Coverage in the U.S. Chicago, IL: American Dental Association, Health Policy Institute; 2015. Available at: <https://www.ada.org/~/media/ADA/Science%20and%20Research/HPI/Files/HPIgraphic_1117_3.pdf?la=en>; [Accessed December 2, 2019].

44. Medicaid Expansion and Dental Benefits Coverage. Chicago, IL: American Dental Association, Health Policy Institute; November 2018. Available at: <https://www.ada.org/~/media/ADA/Science%20and%20Research/HPI/Files/HPIgraphic_1218_3.pdf?la=en>; [Accessed December 2, 2019].

45. Dentist Participation in Medicaid or CHIP. Chicago, IL: American Dental Association, Health Policy Institute; 2016. Available at: <https://www.ada.org/~/media/ADA/Science%20and%20Research/HPI/Files/HPIGraphic_0318_1.pdf?la=en>; [Accessed December 2, 2019].

46. Reforming America's Healthcare System Through Choice and Competition. Washington, DC: U.S. Department of Health and Human Services, U.S. Department of the Treasury, U.S. Department of Labor; December 3, 2018. Available at: <https://www.hhs.gov/sites/default/files/Reforming-Americas-Healthcare-System-Through-Choice-and-Competition.pdf>; [Accessed December 2, 2019].

47. Is Medicaid Expansion Easing Cost Barriers to Dental Care for Low-Income Adults? Chicago, IL: American Dental Association, Health Policy Institute; 2016. Available at: <https://www.ada.org/~/media/ADA/Science%20and%20Research/HPI/Files/HPIgraphic_1016_1.pdf?la=en>; [Accessed December 2, 2019].

48. Manchir M. Study: Results of Medicaid expansion on adult dental services mixed. ADA News; April 17, 2017. Available at: <https://www.ada.org/en/publications/ada-news/2017-archive/april/study-results-of-medicaid-expansion-on-adult-dental-services-mixed>; [Accessed December 2, 2019].

49. Nasseh K, Vujicic M, O'Dell A. Affordable Care Act Expands Dental Benefits for Children but Does Not Address Critical Access to Dental Care Issues. Chicago, IL: American Dental Association, Health Policy Institute; April 2013. Available at: <https://pdfs.semanticscholar.org/2869/63a5839bf9bbddf4d1c3b79f2f9a8d876ace.pdf?_ga=2.220728795.210825787.1575307944-891776938.1574182065>; [Accessed December 2, 2019].

50. Principles of Ethics & Code of Professional Conduct. Chicago, IL: American Dental Association; November 2018. Available at: <https://www.ada.org/~/media/ADA/Member%20Center/Ethics/Code_Of_Ethics_Book_With_Advisory_Opinions_Revised_to_November_2018.pdf?la=en>; [Accessed December 2, 2019].

51. Health Resources and Services Administration, National Center for Health Workforce Analysis. National and State-Level Projections of Dentists and Dental Hygienists in the U.S., 2012-25. Rockville, MD: Department of Health and Human Services; 2015. Available at: <https://bhw.hrsa.gov/sites/default/files/bhw/nchwa/projections/nationalstatelevelprojectionsdentists.pdf>; [Accessed December 2, 2019].

52. Core Competencies for Interprofessional Collaborative Practice: 2016 Update. Washington, DC: Interprofessional Education Collaborative; 2016. Available at: <https://www.unthsc.edu/interprofessional-education/wp-content/uploads/sites/33/Core-Competencies-for-Interprofessional-Collaborative-Practice.pdf>; [Accessed December 2, 2019].

53. Transforming Dental Hygiene Education and the Profession for the 21st Century. Chicago, IL: American Dental Hygienists' Association; 2015. Available at: <https://www.adha.org/resources-docs/Transforming_Dental_Hygiene_Education.pdf>; [Accessed December 2, 2019].

54. Andrews EA. The future of interprofessional education and practice for dentists and dental education. J Dental Educ 2017;81(8):eS186. <https://doi.org/10.21815/JDE.017.026>; [Accessed December 2, 2019].

55. 2017-2018 Annual Report. Chicago, IL: American Dental Hygienists' Association; 2018. Available at: <http://www.adha.org/resources-docs/2018_ADHA_Annual_Report.pdf>; [Accessed December 2, 2019].

56. What is Health Literacy? Atlanta, GA: Centers for Disease Control and Prevention; October 23, 2019. Available at: <https://www.cdc.gov/healthliteracy/learn/index.html>; [Accessed December 2, 2019].

57. George MC. Public policy and legislation for oral health: A convergence of opportunities. J Dent Hyg 2013;87(Suppl 1):50. Retrieved from: <https://jdh.adha.org/content/87/suppl_1/50>; [Accessed December 2, 2019].

58. Centers for Disease Control and Prevention. Ten great public health achievements – United States, 1900-1999. MMWR April 2, 1999;48(12):241. Retrieved from: <https://www.cdc.gov/mmwr/preview/mmwrhtml/00056796.htm>; [Accessed December 2, 2019].

59. Centers for Disease Control and Prevention. Ten great public health achievements, United States, 2001-2010. MMWR, May 20, 2011;60(19):619-623. Available at: <http://www.cdc.gov/mmwr/preview/mmwrhtml/mm6019a5.htm>; [Accessed December 2, 2019].

60. Standards for Dental Hygiene Practice. Chicago, IL: American Dental Hygienists' Association; 2016. Available at: <https://www.adha.org/sites/default/files/2016-Revised-Standards-for-Clinical-Dental-Hygiene-Practice_0.pdf>; [Accessed December 2, 2019].

61. Policies and Recommendations on Tobacco Use. Chicago, IL: American Dental Association; 2016. Available at: <https://www.ada.org/en/advocacy/advocacy-issues/tobacco-use>; [Accessed December 2, 2019].

62. Employer Obligations after Exposure Incidents OSHA: Introduction: A Guide to Employer Obligations. Chicago, IL: American Dental Association; 2019. Available at: <http://www.ada.org/en/science-research/osha-standard-of-occupational-exposure-to-bloodbor>; [Accessed December 2, 2019].

63. Jeong C. Dental professional update: Blood pressure guidelines changed. Dentistry IQ. December 19, 2017. Retrieved from: <https://www.dentistryiq.com/dental-hygiene/clinical-hygiene/article/16366105/dental-professional-update-blood-pressure-guidelines-changed>; [Accessed December 2, 2019].

64. ADEA Core Competencies for Graduate Dental Hygiene Education. Washington, DC: American Dental Education Association; 2011. Available at: <https://www.adea.org/uploadedFiles/ADEA/Content_Conversion_Final/about_adea/governance/ADEA_Core_Competencies_for_Graduate_Dental_Hygiene_Education.pdf>; [Accessed December 2, 2019].

65. Expanding Access to Care through Mid-Level Oral Health Practitioners. Chicago, IL: American Dental Hygienists' Association; March 2018. Available at: <https://www.adha.org/sites/default/files/Expanding_Access_to_Care_through_Mid-Level_Oral_Health_Practitioners_March_2018.pdf>; [Accessed December 2, 2019].

66. Accreditation Standards for Dental Therapy Education Programs. Chicago, IL: Commission on Dental Accreditation; 2015. Available at: <http://www.ada.org/~/media/CODA/Files/dt.pdf>; [Accessed December 2, 2019].

ADDITIONAL RESOURCES

Association of State & Territorial Dental Directors
www.astdd.org
Canadian Association of Public Health Dentistry
http://www.caphd.ca/
Department of Health and Human Services
www.hhs.gov
Office of the Surgeon General
https://www.hhs.gov/surgeongeneral/index.html

Careers in Public Health for the Dental Hygienist

Christine French Beatty and Charlene B. Dickinson

OBJECTIVES

1. List and explain public health career options for dental hygienists.
2. Discuss public health careers as a means of addressing the problem of access to oral health care.
3. Compare and contrast various alternative oral health careers in alternative practice settings.
4. Discuss stages of prevention and regulatory changes, including scope of practice, direct access, levels of supervision, direct reimbursement, and license portability, in relation to alternative practice settings and access to care.

5. Identify and describe various careers to do with innovative alternative workforce models and define scope of practice, supervision, and educational requirements for each.
6. Discuss and provide examples of interprofessional collaborative practice (ICP) in public health practice.
7. Discuss the disconnect between oral health care and overall health care in relation to the future of ICP.
8. Identify and describe public health careers in relation to specific dental hygiene career paths and roles categorized by the American Dental Hygienists' Association (ADHA).

OPENING STATEMENT: Dental Public Health Career Possibilities

- Public health hygienist at a local health department
- Statewide coordinator for a school-based fluoride varnish program
- Dental hygienist at a Veterans Affairs hospital
- Dental hygienist working with a state migrant farm worker program
- Dental hygienist at a state correctional facility
- State dental director in a state health department
- Coordinator of oral health programs with a university community outreach department
- Dental health educator with a school system
- Manager of a dental sealant team operated by a nonprofit organization
- Administrator of a U.S. Department of Health and Human Services (DHHS) federal health program
- Dental hygienist contracting for services in a nursing home
- Consultant to a Head Start program
- Dental hygienist U.S. Public Health Service (USPHS) officer with an Indian Health Service (IHS) clinic
- Dental clinic director in a community-based health center
- Dental hygiene therapist with a rural dental public health mobile clinic
- Coordinator of a regional oral health coalition operated by a metropolitan children's hospital
- Chief officer of a nonprofit dental organization
- Coordinator of a community-based program operated by a for-profit corporation
- Grant manager in an oral health department of a federal health agency.
- Entrepreneurial owner of a program to deliver dental care to an underserved population

COMMUNITY ORAL HEALTH PRACTICE AS A CAREER

Dr. Alfred C. Fones initiated the development of the dental hygiene profession and established its original public health focus. When he started the first dental hygiene school in 1913, Dr. Fones placed students in the public schools (Figure 2.1) and trained them to work in the community (Figure 2.2), where they provided education and preventive services in their role as an advocate for dental public health.[1] Dr. Fones had a vision for what we now refer to as the oral-systemic link when he spoke of a connection between oral health and systemic health and the dental hygienist's role in addressing systemic conditions of the schoolchildren by implementing preventive oral health programs.[1]

Public health careers for dental hygienists now run the gamut from high-level administrative posts to providing dental hygiene care for various populations in a local community, and are located in a variety of settings[2] (see Opening Statement). Dental hygienists in public health positions can have an entry-level degree or an advanced degree, depending on the responsibilities of the position and the requirements of the organization or agency.[3] Many dental hygienists with advanced degrees working in public health began with the minimum level of education. They chose to continue their education as their interests developed, their challenges expanded, and their desire

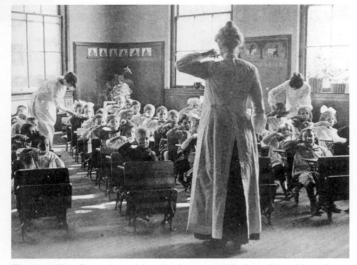

Fig 2.1 The first dental hygienists provided oral health education in public schools. Pictured here are dental hygiene students teaching brushing to children who were seated at their desks in the classroom. The dental hygiene student at the front of the classroom demonstrated while other students circulated to provide hands-on assistance as the children practiced the correct brushing technique. (Courtesy University of Bridgeport, Fones School of Dental Hygiene.)

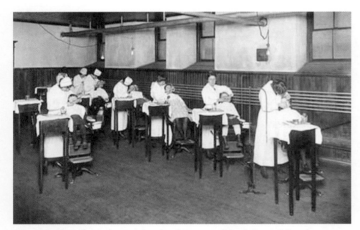

Fig 2.2 The first dental hygienists provided dental hygiene services in community settings. (Copyright University of Rochester Libraries. All Rights Reserved.)

grew to do more for the oral health of their community. A career in community oral health practice offers a variety of rewarding experiences that tend to feed the desire to make a difference in the oral health of all people and provide job satisfaction for dental hygienists.[4]

This career chapter has been placed in the beginning of the textbook to allow students to connect with the role they might play in performing the functions discussed in later chapters. Public health has the potential to take the dental hygienist into the realm of program development, implementation, and evaluation; present a chance to work with various populations, other professionals, agencies, financing mechanisms, and rules and regulations; provide a variety of activities that reflect diverse

roles; and offer career opportunities to advance to higher level administrative and management positions.[2,3,4]

FUTURE TRENDS FOR DENTAL HYGIENISTS IN PUBLIC HEALTH

Potential of the Dental Hygienist to Address the Access to Oral Health Care Problem

Chapter 1 introduced the issues of ongoing high rates of oral diseases in the population, inadequate access to oral health care, profound disparities among specific population groups in oral health status and access to oral health care, and the problem of dental disease as a chronic problem among low-income populations. Also presented were ways that federal agencies, state governments, and oral health professional organizations are addressing these gaps in access to oral health care through legislation, policy development, and refocusing of programs.

Some of the actions resulting from these processes relate to dental hygiene careers, thus laying a foundation for this chapter (see Guiding Principles). Several of these achievements are concerned with expanding and creating new roles for the dental hygienist in the oral health workforce. Future initiatives such as those described in Chapter 1 and associated follow-up strategies and action plans are expected to increase the demand for dental hygienists working in community oral health practice.[5]

GUIDING PRINCIPLES
Summary of Actions Resulting From Recent Government and Professional Oral Health Initiatives

- Allocating additional funds for dental programs and services
- Expanding treatment for special populations
- Creating volunteers and donated dental services
- Providing service programs
- Providing additional dental benefits through existing public insurance programs
- Extending educational loans and loan forgiveness for oral health professionals
- Creating tax credits for providers
- Forming career ladders for dental providers
- Increasing flexible licensure requirements
- Increasing the scope of practice for dental hygienists
- Decreasing supervision of dental hygienists in community settings
- Allowing Medicaid and insurance reimbursement of dental hygienists
- Expanding coverage for provider services
- Developing innovative oral health workforce models, including dental hygiene-based mid-level providers (e.g., dental therapists)
- Increasing interprofessional collaborative practice (ICP)

The ADHA has been an advocate for issues related to dental public health (Box 2.1),[6,7] including issues that involve increased utilization of dental hygienists in public health practice to address the unmet needs of underserved, vulnerable populations. These groups include low-income children, pregnant women, older adults, and persons who are developmentally, physically, mentally, or medically compromised. Dental hygienists have demonstrated their ability to reach these disenfranchised groups.[8] Research has demonstrated that fully utilizing dental hygienists by expanding their professional practice environment, reducing supervision requirements, and increasing their insurance reimbursement potential improves access to oral health services, utilization of oral health services, and oral health outcomes.[8]

A recent federal policy change that reflects sustained advocacy input from ADHA over many years is the reclassification of dental hygienists in the Standard Occupational Classification (SOC) system.[7] The SOC system is part of the U.S. federal statistical system that is coordinated by the White House Office of Management and Budget. It is used by federal agencies to classify workers into occupational categories for the purpose of collecting, calculating, or disseminating data. Users of SOC occupational data include government program managers, labor relations practitioners, and employers wishing to set salary scales. All workers are classified into one of 867 detailed occupations according to their occupational definition.[9] Detailed occupations in the SOC with similar job duties, and in some cases skills, education, and/or training, are grouped together.

As of 2018, dental hygienists are newly classified as *Healthcare Diagnosing or Treating Practitioners,* in the same grouping

as dentists, in contrast to the 2010 SOC, in which dental hygienists were classified as *Health Technologists and Technicians.* This important elevation of the dental hygiene profession at the federal level can significantly impact the full utilization of dental hygienists in solving public health problems of oral health and access to oral health care. It is an important acknowledgment of the role of dental hygiene in addressing access to care.

Dental hygienists are expected to have increased opportunities to improve the nation's oral health through expanded roles in a greater number and variety of community-based oral health settings such as hospitals, long-term care facilities, clinics, public health agencies, state oral health programs, and interprofessional practice settings.[5] Advances in **teledentistry** will also make it easier for dental hygienists to provide care in off-site clinics and community centers[10] (see Chapter 5). To realize this potential, a 2018 federal government report, *Reforming America's Healthcare System Through Choice and Competition,* called for by President Trump and developed by the DHHS, Department of the Treasury, and Department of Labor, recommended the following major changes:[11]

1. Expanding dental hygienists' scope of practice.
2. Eliminating rigid collaborative practice and supervision requirements for dental hygienists.
3. Allowing direct reimbursement for services, to dental hygienists by third-party payers.
4. Increasing **license portability** for oral health professionals.

Alternative Practice Settings

Public health settings are frequently described as **alternative practice** settings.[8] Delivering oral health services in a traditional private practice setting does not address the need for services for those without access to oral health care. Alternative settings can increase access to care by bringing oral health care to underserved, vulnerable populations. Examples of alternative practice settings include a community-based clinic, a migrant health center, a mobile van, a school-based oral health program, a hospital, a long-term care facility, a nursing home, and individual homes of homebound individuals (Figures 2.3 and 2.4). Dental hygienists can provide preventive services in these settings, reaching large numbers of people who might not otherwise receive care.

Different stages or levels of prevention are reflected in the various services provided by oral health practitioners[12] (Table 2.1). Services at the **primary prevention** stage are more effective, less costly, and involve less technology than **secondary prevention** and **tertiary prevention** services. Often, primary prevention strategies do not require a dentist,[13] thus allowing the dental hygienist to work directly (unsupervised) with underserved populations to provide these services. Primary preventive services and screening, which is classified as secondary prevention, are typically provided by dental hygienists in public health programs in alternative settings.

Regulatory Changes Related to Dental Hygiene Practice

Government agencies and government-authorized regulatory boards are responsible for licensing and regulating healthcare professionals based on state statutes that define minimum education

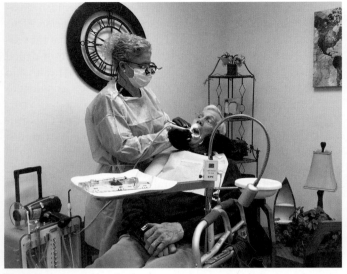

Fig 2.3 A dental hygienist can transport portable dental equipment to homebound patients' homes to provide treatment. (Courtesy Charlene Dickinson and Amy Teague.)

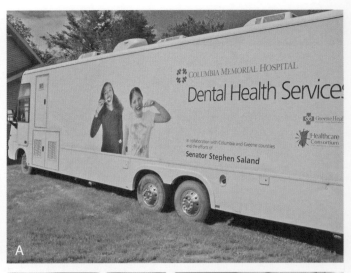

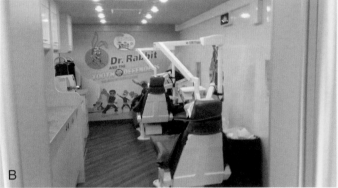

and training requirements, and scope of practice, supervision, and other regulations for these healthcare professions. The purpose of these regulations is to minimize the risk of consumer harm; the regulations are justified for healthcare professionals when consumers are at risk if treated by unqualified individuals.[11]

Inadequate access to oral health care caused by dental professional shortages and maldistribution and by geographic and financial barriers prevents people from attaining improved oral health status and quality of life.[5] Because of the need for services in alternative practice settings that do not already have oral health programs, dental hygienists are initiating programs in these situations. They are also filling community positions beyond those connected with existing public health facilities where there is a dentist available to provide supervision.

To facilitate these efforts to increase access for underserved populations, public health professional organizations and government agencies have advocated regulatory changes that will allow dental hygienists and dental therapists to provide public health preventive programs for these populations in these settings.[11,14] The ADHA has also advocated regulatory changes nationwide that will maximize the effectiveness of dental hygienists in alternative practice settings to bring oral health care

Fig 2.4 A, A mobile dental van operated by GreeneHealth in partnership with Columbia Memorial Hospital provides primary preventive services as well as dental examinations and x-rays, restorations, and simple extractions to children in dentally underserved rural school districts in Columbia and Greene Counties in New York. (Courtesy Columbia Memorial Health.) **B,** The inside treatment area of a mobile dental van for screening. Dental vans used for comprehensive dental treatment are outfitted with a full dental unit, x-ray machine, and other necessary equipment. (Courtesy Colgate Oral Pharmaceuticals.)

to underserved populations that do not have access.[6,15] These regulatory changes relate to supervision and direct access, direct reimbursement, and scope of practice (Box 2.2).

TABLE 2.1	**Stages of Prevention**		
Stage	**Description**		**Examples**
Primary	Prevents the disease before it occurs; includes health education, disease prevention, and health protection		Dental prophylaxis, sealants, fluoride varnish application, water fluoridation, oral health education
Secondary	Eliminates or reduces diseases in the early stages; includes screening to detect and treat changes before onset of symptoms to control disease progression; requires more technology and is more costly than primary prevention		Restorations of all types, including crowns; nonsurgical periodontal therapy; extractions; radiation or chemotherapy; dental and oral cancer screening; silver diamine fluoride application to arrest caries
Tertiary	Seeks to reduce the impact of a disease on the patient's function, longevity, and quality of life after treatment at the acute stage; most costly stage and requires highly trained professionals		Dentures, implants, bridge work, prostheses, reconstructive surgery, periodontal surgery

---

BOX 2.2   Regulatory Changes That Can Maximize Dental Hygienists' Effectiveness in Public Health Practice Settings

Direct Access

The dental hygienist's right to initiate treatment based on their assessment of a patient's needs without the specific authorization of a dentist, to treat the patient without the presence of the dentist, and to maintain a provider-patient relationship.

Direct Reimbursement

The dental hygienist's right to file and be reimbursed for services directly from third-party payers such as Medicaid and private dental insurers.

Scope of Practice

The procedures that a dental hygienist or another oral health professional is permitted to practice according to the state statute.

Supervision and Direct Access

Direct supervision, indirect supervision, general supervision, and **unsupervised practice** are described in Table 2.2. The ADHA has advocated reduced supervision levels for dental hygienists to improve access to oral health care for underserved, vulnerable populations. This has been based on their 2014 and 2015 policies that in combination communicate the stance that dental hygienists who have graduated from accredited dental hygiene programs can be fully used in all public and private practice settings to deliver preventive and therapeutic oral health care safely and effectively without supervision.[15]

Required dental supervision levels for dental hygienists have decreased nationwide over time, with more states adopting fewer supervision regulations in recent years.[13] In addition, the number of states with **direct access** (Box 2.2) has increased.[16] In 2018, 82.4% of states allowed the public to have direct access to the oral healthcare services of a dental hygienist, which is 27.5% more than in 2008.[16] Practice regulations for direct access vary by state. Various states have different forms of direct access, some in only certain public health settings, some for only certain services, and some for only a specified period of time before the patient must be seen by a dentist.[17]

TABLE 2.2   Levels of Supervision

Supervision Level	Description
Direct	The dentist must be present, examines the patient to authorize the work to be performed, and inspects it after to ensure quality.
Indirect	The dentist must be present, generally authorizes the work to be performed, examines the patient, either before or after work is performed, and is available for consultation during treatment.
General	The dentist must authorize the work to be completed before services but does not need to be present during treatment; the patient must be one of record.
Direct access	The dental hygienist can provide services as they determine appropriate without specific authorization or supervision, also referred to as unsupervised practice.

Specific examples of supervision regulations for dental hygienists can help clarify the variety of direct access arrangements and the impact of direct access. In New Mexico, dental hygienists are allowed to practice in any setting without the oversight of a dentist, through a **collaborative practice** agreement with a dentist.[17] In Washington, dental hygienists may be employed, retained, or contracted to practice unsupervised in hospitals, nursing homes, home health agencies, group homes, state institutions, and public health facilities, provided the hygienist refers to the dentist for treatment and meets a requirement of clinical experience. Also, in senior centers in Washington, dental hygienists may provide limited dental hygiene services under the *off-site supervision* of a dentist.[17] In Maine, an *independent practice dental hygienist* may practice with no dentist oversight, but a written practice agreement with a dentist is required to expose dental radiographs.[17]

The Health Resources and Services Administration (HRSA) defines a **dental health professional shortage area** (dental HPSA) for the purpose of funding for public health programs.[18] One of the criteria used for this designation is the population-to-provider ratio. Because of the shortage of dentists in these areas, dental HPSAs are particularly in need of regulatory changes that allow dental hygienists and dental therapists to have direct access. Thus, the call to relax supervision regulations to help alleviate the access-to-care problem is coming also from public health professional organizations and government agencies.[11]

Direct Reimbursement

Some dental hygienists initially volunteer to provide services in alternative settings. However, more and more have found creative ways to be reimbursed for working in these settings. Writing grants, seeking school board funds, collecting Medicaid payments through an accepted provider, or contracting with a facility in states that allow it are a few of the innovative reimbursement plans currently being used.

With less restrictive dental hygiene supervision and an increased number of dental hygienists seeking public health careers, changes are being made in restrictive regulations that prevent dental hygienists from receiving **direct reimbursement** for dental hygiene services (see Box 2.2), as recommended by federal agencies.[11] The ADHA also has advocated these changes and has provided dental hygienists with resources to pursue direct insurance reimbursement in their states.[7,19,20] Currently, 18 states allow dental hygienists to receive direct reimbursement.[21]

Scope of Practice

Within the medical and dental fields, various models of workforce delivery have been developed to provide the public with access to quality health care. **Scope of practice** regulations (see Box 2.2) in professions with overlapping skill sets often impose unnecessary restrictions, and do not address legitimate consumer concerns.[1] These restrictions are familiar to health professions that are regulated by another profession and provide complementary and overlapping services. Healthcare workforce examples include advanced practice registered nurses and physician assistants. Dental hygienists and dental therapists are examples in dentistry. Federal government initiatives have recommended reducing scope-of-practice restrictions to allow these health professionals to practice to the full extent of their abilities to improve the capacity of the overall healthcare system.[11]

In dentistry, overly restrictive scope of practice of dental hygienists and other nondentist oral healthcare providers can increase the cost of care and limit patients' access to care.[5] Initial reports describe the same cost-reduction benefits from increasing their scope of practice as seen in medicine, while maintaining the high quality of dental care that is provided by dentists in this nation.[11] In addition, there is a lack of consistency in the scope of practice of dental hygienists and dental therapists across states,[5] which limits mobility and challenges teledentistry practices. To improve access, federal government agencies have recommended addressing the problem of scope-of-practice inconsistency across states.[11]

The ADHA advocates the expansion of dental hygienists' scope of practice.[7] They also provide scope-of-practice resources to help dental hygienists advocate scope-of-practice changes in their states. This information can be viewed on the ADHA website at https://www.adha.org/scope-of-practice.

Data for regulatory changes achieved by states change continually as more states succeed in these efforts. Current information on supervision and direct access, direct reimbursement, and scope of practice by state can be viewed on the ADHA website at https://www.adha.org/advocacy.

Impact of Dental Hygiene Practice Regulations on Population Oral Health Outcomes

A dental hygiene professional practice index (DHPPI) was developed in 2001, rescored in 2014, and revised in 2016, with financial support from HRSA.[22] The DHPPI comprises numerous legal-parameter variables that represent improved opportunity for dental hygienists, both individually and as a profession, to provide preventive oral health services in public health settings. The variables are organized according to four categories: regulation, supervision, tasks, and reimbursement.

An optimal total DHPPI score is 100, and a higher composite score reflects a more permissive scope of practice and less restrictive regulations for dental hygienists in public health settings in a state.[22] Thus, the DHPPI provides a comparative and quantitative tool that can be used to assess the impact of dental hygiene scope of practice and practice regulations on oral health outcomes in the population. Research with the DHPPI in both 2001 and 2014 revealed that more autonomous dental hygiene practice in a state was positively and significantly associated with utilization of services and oral health outcomes in the population[22] (Figure 2.5). DHPPI scores for all states can be viewed in the DHPPI project report listed in the Additional Resources at the end of this chapter.

The 2016 revision of the DHPPI also includes variables that describe the current practice of dental hygiene in public health settings and capture the new roles available to them in some states.[22] It accommodates emerging workforce models and newly permitted reversible and irreversible functions for dental hygienists that were not included in the first version of the DHPPI. It is anticipated that these additional variables in the DHPPI should enable more accurate future assessment of the impact of dental

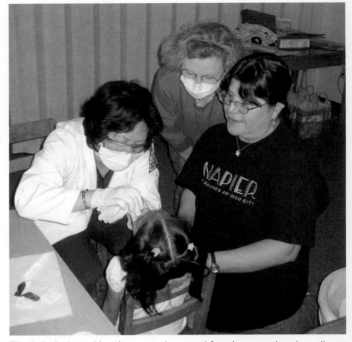

Fig 2.5 A dental hygiene student and faculty member in a direct access state provide dental screening, education, fluoride varnish treatment, and dental referral for a preschool age child in a school-based oral health program, with the assistance of the child's teacher. (Courtesy Connie Beatty.)

hygiene scope of practice and practice regulations on oral health outcomes in the population.[22]

Innovative Workforce Models

Various dental workforce delivery models have been developed to serve the populations that cannot easily access dental services as the result of problems of geographic location, poor financial resources, no dental insurance, a lack of understanding about disease prevention measures, a shortage of dentists to meet the needs of the population, and low dentist participation in Medicaid programs. Most of the new workforce models in dentistry are various forms of a dental therapist, similar to the physician assistant as part of the healthcare team.[23]

Dental Therapist

More than 50 countries worldwide have developed **dental therapist** programs to meet the dental needs of their people.[24] The dental therapist is meant to be an extension of the dental team and expand its capacity to provide oral healthcare services to underserved populations.[23] Services provided by the dental therapist vary by country. In 1921, a dental therapist program was first introduced in New Zealand, called the *dental nurse* at that time. Dental therapists in New Zealand are required to complete a bachelor's degree in an approved oral health major and a dental therapy training program that results in certification.[25]

Dental Therapy in the U.S. The *dental health aide therapist* (DHAT) was the first dental therapist model in the U.S., approved in 2004 by the Alaska Native Tribal Health Consortium.[26] Authorized by the native tribal government rather than the state government, DHATs can provide dental care only for the Alaska native population on tribal lands.

DHATs provide community-based oral health preventive care and education, examinations and x-rays, cleanings, basic restorations, nonsurgical extractions, and referral for care beyond their scope of practice.[26] The post-high school DHAT training is equivalent to a 3-year program, consisting of didactic and preclinical phases and a clinical preceptor phase under direct supervision of clinical instructor dentists. According to Dr. Mary E. Williard, Director of the Alaska Dental Therapy Educational Program, the DHAT curriculum includes a strong emphasis in participatory community-based programs (personal communication, December 9, 2019). Graduation from the training program results in certification, and the DHAT must apply for recertification every 2 years. In Alaska, the DHAT certification is through the Alaska Community Health Aide Program certification board.[26]

DHATs provide services to people in the most isolated rural regions of Alaska, in which little-to-no care was previously provided, under remote general supervision via teledentistry (Figure 2.6). To improve access to care in these rural communities, candidates with strong ties to rural areas of Alaska are selected for the DHAT program. Nearly 80% of DHATs return to their home regions to practice, and the program has an 81% retention rate.[26]

Over the 15 years of existence of the program, DHATs have increased access to preventive and restorative oral health care for over 40,000 citizens of Alaska's remote, rural communities. The DHAT program has proven to be economically viable and sustainable. A 2-year intensive evaluation by the Research

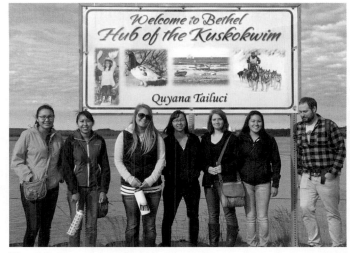

Fig 2.6 Dental health aide therapist students in a remote area of Alaska, where they experience community oral health in action as they receive their clinical preceptor training in the Alaska Dental Therapy Educational Program. (Courtesy Alaska Native Tribal Health Consortium.)

Triangle Institute in 2010 demonstrated that Alaska's DHATs provided safe, competent, and appropriate dental care.[27]

Recently, other states have approved the use of DHATs on tribal lands (Table 2.3). In some states, the DHATs are trained

TABLE 2.3   Dental Therapy Workforce Models in the United States Approved Since the Alaska Dental Health Aide Therapist

State/Name/Date Signed into Law	Education/Licensure	Practice Settings	Supervision	Scope of Practice
Minnesota: Dental Therapist (DT); Advanced Dental Therapist (ADT), 2009	May be dually licensed as Registered Dental Hygienist (RDH) and DT but not required DT—bachelor's degree and DT license ADT—master's degree in ADT and 2,000 hours practice as DT for ADT certification	Primarily settings that serve low-income, uninsured, and underserved patients, or are located in designated public health or private sector dental health professional shortage areas (HPSAs)	DT—general for primary preventive and noninvasive services; indirect for invasive services ADT—Presence of a dentist not required for DT services; general for others, including with teledentistry Collaborative management agreement with dentist required for ADT	DT—primary preventive and restorative scope and extraction of primary teeth ADT—all the services of a DT and the following procedures, pursuant to a written collaborative management agreement with a dentist: oral assessment, treatment planning and routine, nonsurgical extractions of certain diseased teeth, and more
Maine: Dental Hygiene Therapist (DHT), 2014; amended 2019	Dual licensure as RDH and DHT required CODA approved DT education required	Schools, healthcare facilities, clinical facilities, and various public health programs that serve underserved patients	Direct supervision by licensed dentist Written practice agreement required	Primary preventive and restorative scope
Vermont: DT, 2016	Dual licensure as RDH and DT Graduation required from Commission on Dental Accreditation (CODA)-accredited DT program	Practice setting contracted into a collaborative agreement	General supervision	Primary preventive and restorative scope
Washington: DHAT, 2017	Same as Alaska	Limited to tribal lands	Same as Alaska	Same as Alaska

(Continued)

TABLE 2.3   Dental Therapy Workforce Models in the United States Approved Since the Alaska Dental Health Aide Therapist (*Cont.*)

State/Name/Date Signed into Law	Education/Licensure	Practice Settings	Supervision	Scope of Practice
Arizona: DT, 2018	Dual licensure as RDH and DT required	Tribal settings, **federally qualified health centers** (FQHCs) and lookalike facilities, community health centers, and private dental practices that contract with FQHCs	Direct; can be reduced as specified in a collaborative practice agreement after 1,000 hours of practice experience	Primary preventive and restorative scope; nonsurgical extraction of permanent teeth only under direct supervision
Michigan: DT, 2018	Licensure as DT required Graduation from CODA-accredited DT school	Community health centers and private dental practices	General under a written practice agreement with a dentist after practicing 500 clinical hours under direct supervision	Primary preventive and restorative scope
New Mexico: DT, 2019	Dual licensure as RDH and DT required	Traditional office settings, schools, nursing homes, community health centers, rural care clinics, and in tribal communities	General under a dental therapy practice agreement with a dentist	Primary preventive and restorative scope Full scope requires completing DT postgraduate clinical experience approved by the Board
Idaho: DT, 2019	Graduation from CODA-accredited DT school	Limited to tribal lands	To be determined by negotiated rulemaking by the dental board	Primary preventive and restorative scope and other minor procedures
Montana: DHAT, 2019	Same as Alaska DHAT	Limited to tribal lands	Same as Alaska DHAT	Same as Alaska DHAT with exclusion of extractions and invasive procedures
Nevada: DT, 2019	Dual licensure as RDH and DT required; must obtain a Public Health Endorsement	Rural health clinics, FQHCs, tribal health clinics, school-based health clinics, mobile dental units and any other clinics that primarily serve Medicaid patients or other low-income, uninsured individuals	Determined by required written practice agreement following completion of 500, 1,000, or 1,500 hours of clinical practice, depending on experience, under direct supervision	Primary preventive and restorative scope
Connecticut: DT, 2019	Licensure as RDH required with additional required certification as DT	Public health settings	Under collaborative agreement after 1,000 clinical hours under direct supervision and 6 hours of DT continuing education	Preventive and restorative scope

(From Expanding Access to Care Through Dental Therapy. American Dental Hygienists' Association; July 2019. Available at: <https://www.adha.org/resources-docs/Expanding_Access_to_Dental_Therapy.pdf>; [Accessed December 21, 2019]; Brickle CM, Self KD. Dental therapists as new oral health practitioners: increasing access for underserved populations. J Dent Educ 2017;81(9)eS65-eS72. Available at: <https://doi.org/10.21815/JDE.017.036>; [Accessed December 21, 2019]; Dental Therapy in Minnesota: Issue Brief. Minnesota Department of Health, Minnesota Board of Dentistry; 2018. Available at: <https://www.health.state.mn.us/data/workforce/oral/docs/2018dtb.pdf>; [Accessed December 21, 2019]; ADEA State Update: Washington State Signs into Law Dental Health Aide Therapy Bill. American Dental Education Association; 2017. Available at: <https://www.adea.org/Blog.aspx?id=36283&blogid=20132>; [Accessed December 21, 2019]; New Arizona law limits dental therapists to tribal settings, underserved areas. ADA News; May 30, 2018. Available at: <https://www.ada.org/en/publications/ada-news/2018-archive/may/new-arizona-law-limits-dental-therapists-to-tribal-settings-underserved-areas>; [Accessed December 21, 2019]; New Mexico's Passage of Dental Therapy Law Builds National Momentum for Changing Provision of Dental Care Amid Oral Health Crisis. Community Catalyst; March 29, 2019. Available at: <https://www.communitycatalyst.org/news/press-releases/new-mexicos-passage-of-dental-therapy-law-builds-national-momentum-for-changing-provision-of-dental-care-amid-oral-health-crisis>; [Accessed December 21, 2019]; Update: Public Act 463–Dental Therapists Licensed in Michigan. Oral Health in Michigan; 2018. Available at: <http://www.midentalaccess.org/>; [Accessed December 21, 2019]; Michigan Board of Dentistry Board of Dentistry Rules Committee Work Group Meeting. State of Michigan Department of Licensing and Regulatory Affairs; June 13, 2019. Available at: <https://www.michigan.gov/documents/lara/6-13-19_Dentistry_Rules_Work_Group_minutes_with_attachments_661509_7.pdf>; [Accessed December 21, 2019]; Senate bill No. 1062. Legislature of the State of Idaho; 2019. Available at: <https://legislature.idaho.gov/wp-content/uploads/sessioninfo/2019/legislation/S1062.pdf> [Accessed December 21, 2019]; House Bill No. 599. 2019 Montana Legislature; 2019. Available at: <https://leg.mt.gov/bills/2019/billhtml/HB0599.htm>; [Accessed December 21, 2019]; Messerly M. Mid-level dental providers to only practice in underserved areas under amended legislation. Nevada Independent; May 28, 2019. Available at: <https://thenevadaindependent.com/article/mid-level-dental-providers-to-only-practice-in-underserved-areas-under-amended-legislation>; [Accessed December 21, 2019]; Andrews E. 2019 Connecticut legislative session – what happened and what didn't happen. Connecticut Health Policy Project; June 6, 2019. Available at: <https://cthealthpolicy.org/index.php/2019/06/06/2019-connecticut-legislative-session-what-happened-and-what-didnt-happen/>; [Accessed December 21, 2019].)

in a program that is under tribal government authority. In other states, graduation from a program accredited by the Commission on Dental Accreditation (CODA) is required.

Two initiatives encouraged the growth and expansion of dental therapy to multiple states. In 2009, Minnesota approved dental therapy practice statewide (not limited to tribal lands),[28] and in 2015, CODA implemented accreditation standards for dental therapy education programs.[29] As of 2019, 11 states had authorized the practice of dental therapy in the U.S. since 2009, and 6 more states had pending legislation to authorize the practice of dental therapy[28] (see Table 2.3). In some of these states, dental therapists practice statewide, and in some, their practice is limited to tribal lands (see Table 2.3). Current dental therapists are educated, trained, and prepared to work under general supervision and collaborative practice agreements that allow for the expansion of the dental practice far outside the office.[24]

As of 2019, no dental therapy educational programs are listed as accredited by CODA.[29] However, program sessions at major dental conferences in 2018 and 2019 were designed to encourage the expansion of dental therapy and assist with CODA accreditation of current and future dental therapy programs.[30,31] It can be anticipated that programs will soon seek and acquire CODA accreditation status, and that this process will lead to consistency in educational requirements for dental therapists in the U.S.[32]

The need for the dental therapy workforce model, the expansion of the dental hygienists' scope of practice, and the relaxation of practice regulations for dental hygienists and dental therapists are highlighted by the fact that "nearly 58 million people live in areas designated by the federal government as dental shortage areas."[33] Looking at this critical need on a state level, the New Mexico Dental Therapy Coalition reported that in New Mexico "nearly 900,000 live in areas without enough dentists, with the burden falling heaviest on rural, tribal, and low-income communities."[34] In response to this crisis, New Mexico authorized the practice of dental therapy in 2019.[33] Other states that have authorized or are seeking to authorize dental therapy have a similar access-to-care crisis.

The outcomes of implementing the dental therapy workforce model statewide in terms of improving access to care have been evaluated in Minnesota (Box 2.3). These results support the federal government agency recommendations to expand dental therapy programs.[11]

Dental Hygiene-Based Dental Therapy Workforce Model.
The ADHA supports the development and implementation of new dental therapy workforce models and has policy specifically supporting oral healthcare workforce models that culminate in graduation from an accredited institution, professional licensure, and direct access to patient care.[28] At the same time, for the following reasons, the ADHA advocates a **dental hygiene-based dental therapist** workforce model rather than nonhygiene-based:[28]

1. The dental hygiene workforce is available and ready, with over 185,000 licensed dental hygienists in the U.S. as of 2019.
2. The educational infrastructure is developed, with over 300 entry-level dental hygiene programs in 2019.
3. The public will benefit from providers that have a broad range of skill sets, including preventive and restorative.

BOX 2.3 Evaluation Results for Dental Therapy in Minnesota

Facts of Interest:

- As of April 2018, there were 86 licensed dental therapists (DTs), working in 54 different community settings.
  - 34 (39%) were dually licensed in both dental hygiene and dental therapy.
  - 48 (55%) had achieved certification as Advanced Dental Therapists (ADTs).
- The primary practice setting for 49% of DTs in 2017 was a dental clinic; 47% worked in community-based nonprofit organizations, community health centers, FQHCs, hospitals, schools, and mobile clinics. The remaining 4% reported working in academic settings.
- DTs also provided services in community and rural settings at more than 370 mobile dental sites throughout the state in schools, Head Start programs, community centers, Veterans Affairs facilities, and nursing homes.
- DTs were geographically distributed in proportion to the state's population:
  - 55% of the state's population lived in the seven-county Greater Twin Cities metropolitan area, where 59% of working DTs were employed.
  - 45% of Minnesotans lived outside this metropolitan area, where 41% of working DTs were employed.
- In 2017, 93% of licensed DTs reported being employed as compared with 74% in 2014, indicating greater integration of DTs.
- 98% of DTs indicated career satisfaction in the previous 12 months, and 96% were satisfied with their careers overall; 84% planned to practice for 10 years or more.

Access to Care:

- General supervision of ADTs made it economically viable for dental clinics to provide routine dental care in schools, rural communities, Head Start programs, nursing homes, and other community settings.
- A 2014 evaluation by the Minnesota Department of Health and the Minnesota Board of Dentistry determined that DTs improved access for underserved patients, resulting in reduced wait times and travel distances.
- The Minnesota Department of Health catalogued 35 reports, peer-reviewed journal articles and studies documenting the growth and impact of DTs on oral health access in the state.
- The Wilder Foundation's case studies noted that the addition of a DT at one study clinic decreased wait time from 3 or 4 weeks to 1 week, and increased the volume of patients with public insurance at two rural dental clinics.
- The Pew Foundation's 2017 case studies with Apple Tree Dental concluded that an ADT at a veteran's home increased the number of diagnostic and restorative services provided at the home.

(From Dental Therapy in Minnesota (Issue Brief). Department of Health; 2018. Available at: <https://www.health.state.mn.us/data/workforce/oral/docs/2018dtb.pdf>; [Accessed December 21, 2018].)

The goal of these policies is to improve and enhance the oral healthcare delivery system by providing complete direct access, thus opening the door for direct care to underserved, vulnerable populations by dental hygienists and dental therapists in school systems, nursing homes, and other community programs.[24] In 2019 dental therapists were dental-hygiene based in 6 of the 11 states that had authorized dental therapy to date and in 3 of the 5 states that authorized it that year. Dental therapy was also proposed as dental-hygiene based in the six states that had pending authorization at that time.[28]

Community Dental Health Coordinator

To support the existing dental workforce in reaching out to underserved communities, the American Dental Association (ADA) developed the **community dental health coordinator** (CDHC) workforce model in 2006 and piloted it in 2009.[35] CDHCs work under the supervision of the dentist and within the confines of state statutes to promote oral health for communities and to assist patients in navigating through the healthcare system to establish a dental home. They function in private practices, FQHCs, hospital emergency rooms, senior centers, Head Start and Early Head Start centers, schools, Lamaze and other classes for pregnant women, and anywhere that patients need education and care coordination.[36] Depending on the setting, CDHCs provide a variety of services to increase health knowledge and self-sufficiency, including outreach, community education, informal counseling, advocacy, and limited primary preventive procedures such as fluoride treatments and sealants.[35] To reduce cultural, language, and other barriers that might reduce their effectiveness, CDHCs are typically recruited from the same types of communities in which they would serve, often the actual communities in which they grew up.[35]

Experts in education developed the CDHC curriculum in public health and dentistry to meet core competencies. Although CDHC training programs are designed for online delivery, the CDHC student is also required to complete an internship in a community clinic or FQHC that consists of a series of in-person sessions for student skill development and evaluation.[36]

In 2012, the ADA conducted an evaluation of both the individual CDHC's value and the degree to which they are helping increase access to dental care in their communities. Results exceeded expectations, and interest in the CDHC grew.[36] According to the ADA, as of 2019, CDHCs were working in underserved communities in 40 states, and more than 150 students were in training.[35] CDHC training programs were available in all 50 states,[35] and the ADA and state dental societies were working with state governments, the higher education community, and the charitable and private sectors to create new CDHC programs.[36]

INTERPROFESSIONAL COLLABORATIVE PRACTICE

One of the characteristics of public health practice is the use of **interprofessional collaborative practice** (ICP). The World Health Organization declared in 2010 that "interprofessional healthcare teams understand how to optimize the skills of their members, share case management, and provide better health services to patients and the community" and asserted that "the resulting strengthened health system leads to improved health outcomes."[37] This method of practicing health care can enable the integration of oral health into overall health at the level of healthcare delivery. **Collaboration** and communication among dental, medical, social services, and other health professionals can enable the sharing of data, resources, health education materials, and general community information relevant to all health needs, including oral health.[37]

As alternative workforce models in dental hygiene emerge, the need for ICP is becoming imperative. This interprofessional team approach is considered to be comprehensive and cost-effective, and has the potential to improve healthcare outcomes of individuals served in a community health center.[38] Community health centers in urban and rural areas, school-based health centers, clinics in local public health departments, hospital-based clinics, and other comprehensive community healthcare settings lend themselves to the ICP approach.[38] Examples of this approach are presented in the Guiding Principles.

GUIDING PRINCIPLES

Examples of Interprofessional Collaborative Practice

- A dental hygienist with an IHS community health center dental clinic collaborates with the medical staff to develop a tobacco cessation program that connects oral health and overall health effects of using tobacco.
- In a community-based health clinic, a dental hygienist and a member of the medical staff collaborate to develop and implement referrals and health educational materials that associate oral health and diabetes for use with patients in a diabetes prevention program.
- A dental hygienist partners with mental health professionals in a community clinic to address the oral healthcare effects of various psychological problems treated in the clinic, including substance abuse.
- A dental hygienist and public health nutritionist in a local health department work together to develop a nutritional education program that links dietary choices to oral health issues and obesity for use with at-risk patients.
- In a school-based oral health program, a dental hygienist and school nurse team up to establish oral health programs for the schoolchildren that will also improve their overall health and educational outcomes.
- A public health hygienist works with other staff in a local health department to develop programs and educational materials for individuals served in the well-baby clinic and the Women, Infants, and Children (WIC) program.
- A dental hygienist working in a corporate medical facility provides oral health education to medical professionals and patients, delivers preventive oral health services, and serves as an advocate to help families navigate the oral healthcare system.

In ICP settings, effective interaction of dental hygienists with other health professionals can increase the awareness and importance of the relationship between oral health and overall health. This can result in collaboration to identify risk, make preventive recommendations, and implement treatments that integrate oral and general health. In addition, oral health and primary care practitioners can design and deliver integrated health messages that address the health issues relevant to the **priority population** in a way that reflects the oral-systemic link.

Interprofessional resources have been developed to assist with ICP. One example is *Bright Futures Guidelines*, a national health promotion initiative launched by the HRSA Maternal and Child Health Bureau and spearheaded in its third edition by the American Academy of Pediatrics. This online program provides comprehensive health information and resources, including oral health guidelines from pregnancy to adolescence and a periodicity schedule, that can be used by public health teams to achieve optimal health for these priority populations.[39] Another example is the *National Interprofessional Initiative on Oral Health* (NIIOH), which is a foundation-funded consortium of funders, health professionals, and national organizations focused on integrating oral health into primary care education and practice.[40] NIIOH provides easily accessible online, downloadable oral health education materials and resources to health professionals for use in this endeavor.

One of the resources available on the NIIOH website is *Smiles for Life*, a free online curriculum of 11 independent modules that extend across the lifespan, address core areas of oral health relevant to medical practitioners, and include assessment of user competencies.[41] The modules can be completed online for continuing education credit by health professionals or downloaded for use by healthcare education programs. Produced by the Society of Teachers of Family Medicine, *Smiles for Life* was designed to help integrate oral health into primary care. The *Smiles for Life* curriculum is endorsed and commended by multiple health and oral health professional organizations in the U.S. and Canada, including the ADHA, ADA, American Academy of Pediatric Dentistry, Association of State and Territorial Dental Directors, and American Association of Public Health Dentistry.

Another resource is the Oral Health Toolkit from the American Academy of Pediatrics.[42] This resource provides healthcare professionals with necessary information to treat patients and to inform policymakers about children's oral health issues. The online toolkit helps to provide conversation tactics to healthcare providers and oral health resources to prenatal patients and families with infants so these populations can get the oral health answers they need.

Disconnect of Oral Health Care and Overall Health Care

Even though there is increasing recognition of the relationship between oral health and overall health, oral health is still perceived as less critical.[37] In addition, although the movement to integrate oral health and overall health has progressed, there continues to be a disconnect between the two.[37] This is apparent in differences in education, policies, and reimbursement mechanisms.[43] The insurance system, financing structure, and coverage of treatment are not equally matched.[44] This problem has been presented as an ethical issue in the American Medical Association *Journal of Ethics*. According to Simon, the movement toward ICP is an acknowledgment that "continued separation of these two fields disproportionately burdens vulnerable populations of patients"[45] and that "low-income people, people of color, people with disabilities, rural-dwellers, and formerly incarcerated people are all more likely to suffer from dental disease and pain and to report difficulty gaining access to (oral health) care."[45]

The continued development of infrastructure and payment policies within the healthcare system that will enhance ICP and address access-to-care issues has been recommended.[11] For example, the dental home and medical home concepts have resulted in earlier and more effective health care. However, they have not adequately connected oral health care and overall health care.[46] Thus, the *U.S. Department of Health and Human Services Oral Health Strategic Framework, 2014-2017* called for the support of initiatives that recognize the value and integration of oral health into healthcare homes that provide patient-centered medical health care.[46] One such change has been the reimbursement of primary healthcare providers for early oral examinations and application of fluoride varnish in infants and toddlers and the support by the American Academy of Pediatrics in this process through the *Bright Futures Guidelines*.[39]

Future of Interprofessional Collaborative Practice in Oral Health Care

Comprehensive application of ICP to the delivery of oral health care is being promoted to address the disconnect of oral health care and overall health care.[47] As health care continues to evolve, it is critical that all healthcare professional students receive education and clinical experiences interacting with other healthcare team members in treating and educating a diverse population. This process is referred to as **interprofessional education** (IPE).

The Interprofessional Educational Collaborative (IPEC) is a consortium of national associations of schools of health professions formed to promote and encourage constituent efforts that would advance substantive ICP learning experiences.[47] The goal is to help prepare future health professionals for enhanced team-based care of patients and improved population health outcomes. The collaborative represents multiple health professions, including dentistry and dental hygiene through membership of the American Dental Education Association (ADEA). In 2016, IPEC released core competencies for ICP to guide curriculum development across health professions schools.[47]

Another collaborative related to IPE is the Health Professions Accreditors Collaborative (HPAC).[48] This is an organization of accrediting bodies for healthcare professions with a broad representation of 23 healthcare professions. The member organizations have been independently creating accreditation policies, processes, and/or standards for IPE. Dentistry and dental hygiene are represented in HPAC by CODA. In 2019, the HPAC released a report, *Guidance on Developing Quality Interprofessional Education for the Health Professions*,[48] to support individuals charged with implementing IPE. The report states, "In order to provide quality and cost-effective care, health professionals must be better prepared to lead and collaborate in interprofessional teams."[48]

The oral health professions have taken steps to embrace IPE. In August 2016, CODA implemented a requirement in the *Accreditation Standards for Dental Hygiene Education Programs* that focuses on IPE.[28] In a survey to determine the effects of this new standard on IPE in dental hygiene curricula, dental hygiene program directors indicated that it has been the driving force for increasing participation in IPE activities and rated IPE as less challenging than in the past[49] (Figure 2.7). A requirement for IPE is reflected also in CODA accreditation standards for both predoctoral dental education and dental therapy education.[28]

The future of IPE looks promising. It is anticipated that the growth of ICP will bring about changes in the practice delivery systems for oral healthcare practitioners and result in

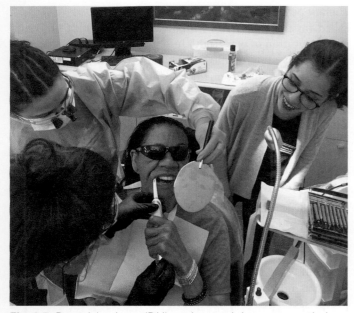

Fig 2.7 Dental hygiene (DH) and speech-language pathology (SLP) students collaborate in an interprofessional education program at a stroke center. Pictured are DH students providing oral hygiene instructions to a post-stroke patient with an SLP student engaging to understand the patients' needs. In this program DH students learn speech-language assessment of post-stroke patients to facilitate communication for oral health promotion. SLP students learn the importance of oral health, oral care, and daily oral hygiene for post-stroke patients who are at higher risk for oral complications as a result of the stroke. (Courtesy Charlene Dickinson.)

improved oral health care.[37] In addition, the offering of IPE by dental and dental hygiene schools will allow dentistry and dental hygiene to highlight their roles as healthcare providers, potentially increasing opportunities for dental hygienists to have a role in medical settings such as hospitals and medical clinics.[50] These changes will require, and result in, a greater incorporation of public health principles, practices, and priorities into the practice of dentistry and dental hygiene in the private and nonprofit sectors.[50]

CAREERS IN PUBLIC HEALTH

The ADHA has described various career paths for dental hygienists, some of which are public health careers and some of which are not.[2] Regardless of the path, it has been suggested that public health is embedded because all dental hygiene careers relate to improving the oral health of the public.[51] This relationship of public health to the various career paths and roles is illustrated in Figure 2.8 and described in Table 2.4 with further examples provided in the Opening Statements. The dental hygienist who has a concern for improving and protecting the oral health of the public can make a difference regardless of the dental hygiene career path selected.

In this section, various dental hygiene career paths are described as they apply to public health. Most public health positions require a combination of skills defined in these multiple roles. Dental hygienists who hold positions in alternative

practice settings are also highlighted to illustrate the variety of career possibilities and inspire the reader.

Public Health

Dental hygienists who pursue a clearly defined career path in public health will be associated with one of a variety of settings that are geared to the underserved populations that are unable to access dental care through private dental offices. These various settings make up what is commonly referred to in public health circles as the **safety net**, a group of unrelated entities that deliver care to vulnerable populations that have no or limited insurance.[52] The dental safety net includes community health centers, school-based health centers, state and local health departments, nonprofits and civic organizations that operate oral health programs, private facilities that offer pro bono services, dental and dental hygiene school clinics, and hospital emergency rooms that will not turn away Medicaid beneficiaries and patients who are in pain and cannot afford care. Millions of citizens receive dental services through the dental safety net.[52]

Because the dental safety net is a patchwork of institutions, clinics, and oral healthcare providers supported by a variety of sometimes dissimilar financing options, it is not uniform from one community to another and is not always financially secure. It is affected by the general political environment, the number of uninsured people, and the types of oral healthcare institutions in the area.[53] Dental hygienists working in public health settings are part of this dental safety net.

Public health opportunities include a variety of roles and settings. Some examples are clinicians, administrators, and researchers in local, state, or federal public health departments

Professional Roles of the Dental Hygienist

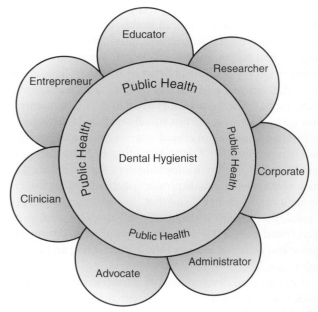

Fig 2.8 Public health is embedded in all dental hygienist career paths. (Modified from American Dental Hygienists' Association. Professional Roles of the Dental Hygienist. Available at: <https://www.adha.org/resources-docs/714112_DHiCW_Roles_Dental_Hygienist.pdf>; [Accessed December 5, 2019].)

TABLE 2.4   Relationship of Public Health to Various Dental Hygiene Career Paths

Career Path	Description Related to Dental Public Health	Examples of Public Health–Related Activities
Clinician	Provides clinical care in a variety of settings, in line with public health priorities, objectives, recommendations, and best practices.	• Provides clinical services in a community health center dental clinic in a dental health professional shortage area (HPSA). • Treats Medicaid patients in a hospital-based clinic.
Educator	Dental hygiene (DH) educator: Educates DH students and practicing hygienists about dental public health topics. Oral health educator: Educates about and promotes oral health to patients and various target groups to improve the oral health of the public.	• DH educator: Writes a grant as a professor in a DH program to create a COH program for DH student participation. • Oral health educator: Conducts community oral health (COH) education programs on topics that are relevant to specific priority populations.
Corporate	Supports the oral health industry through the promotion and sale of products and services and the education of oral health professionals regarding those products and services with the end goal of improving the health of the public.	• Presents educational programs on preventive and therapeutic products to DH students and practitioners to enhance their use in COH programs. • Contributes financially to COH programs; underwrites or donates supplies to specific COH projects.
Advocate	Sees problems related to achieving optimal oral health and attempts to develop a solution; supports, recommends, and/or campaigns for a specific cause or policy to improve the oral health of the public.	• Participates in a local school board campaign to control the availability of cariogenic snacks and drinks in school vending machines. • Lobbies for a change in state nursing home licensure requirements to improve the oral health services they are required to provide to residents.
Researcher	Conducts research related to health and disease within a population, preventive procedures, dental utilization, public health infrastructure, assessment of population needs, program evaluation, workforce models, public health outcomes, and other central public health topics.	• Conducts a comprehensive oral health community needs assessment to be able to plan relevant programs. • Collects data on program outcomes to evaluate the success of a school-based sealant program.
Administrator	Creates and directs dental public health programs.	• Directs the oral health unit of a state health department. • Coordinates preventive programs for state or local health departments, faith-based or other nonprofit organizations, or for-profit corporations.
Entrepreneur	Uses imagination and creativity to initiate or finance commercial enterprises that will provide oral health services or programming for underserved populations.	• Establishes a business to take dental hygiene care to an underserved population. • Starts a nonprofit to build a new safety net dental clinic in the community.

or agencies; rural and inner-city community clinics; IHS clinics and programs; Head Start programs; and school sealant and fluoride programs. Dental hygienists can serve in some of these roles by joining the Public Health Service or National Health Service Corps.

Positions in public health can involve varied levels of responsibility. Thus, different educational requirements, skills, and experience are necessary, depending on the position. Many public health positions require a bachelor's degree. In more advanced, nonclinical positions, a master's or doctoral degree in community health, public health, or healthcare administration will be necessary, depending on the responsibilities. This will be discussed in subsequent career paths of this section.

To seek employment in a public health setting, a dental hygienist can research available positions with federal agencies, state and local health departments, nonprofit organizations, hospitals, and corporations. Much of this search can be accomplished on the web. In addition, **networking** with other oral health professionals in public health positions can be beneficial. Common sources of available public health positions with government agencies are USAJOBS at www.usajobs.gov for federal postings and Government Jobs at www.governmentjobs.com for government jobs at all levels. Positions in federally funded

community health centers are posted at the local and state levels where the centers are located. Table 2.5 presents some of the primary federal agencies and programs that are significant employers of dental hygienists.

Clinician

In the familiar role of **clinician**, the public health dental hygienist provides evidence-based clinical services to priority populations, including assessment of oral health conditions; delivery of preventive, periodontal, and restorative care within the regulated scope of practice for the state; and evaluation of treatment outcomes (see Table 2.4). The characteristics, values, and prevalent oral diseases of lower socioeconomic status (SES) groups that seek care in public health clinics can influence the utilization of dental services offered in these clinics.

The clinician role in public health can require a variety of skills depending on the specific expectations of the position and the population served. For example, specialized clinical skills may be required to work with a medically compromised population with various complex diseases and to manage other special populations such as patients with physical and mental disabilities. Additional skills needed include the ability to assess the patient's perceived dental needs and to recognize the social

TABLE 2.5 Selected Public Health Career Opportunities for Dental Hygienists in Federal Agencies and Programs

Agency	Dental Hygiene Professional Role	Description
U.S. Public Health Service (USPHS) www.usphs.gov/	• Various roles depending on the position • Begin as clinician and oral health educator; can advance to other roles	• A Commissioned Corps of officers—one of the seven uniformed services for the federal government (not an armed service) • Excellent benefits, including retirement similar to the military • Federal school-loan-repayment programs available if working in an underserved area • Work as clinician and educator in clinics located on Indian reservations, in federal prisons, and in immigrant detention facilities • Can advance to administrator and advocate positions with various federal agencies, including HRSA • Work as researcher with various federal agencies, including Centers for Disease Control and Prevention (CDC) and HRSA • Can be deployed to areas in need of emergency response (e.g., 9/11, Liberia's 2014 Ebola outbreak, and various hurricanes) • Internships available for dental hygiene students (COSTEP)
Health Resources and Services Administration (HRSA) www.hrsa.gov	• Administrator • Researcher	• Work in various positions related to improving access to oral health services for the country • Can serve as a civil service hire or USPHS officer (see earlier in this table)
National Health Service Corps (NHSC) nhsc.hrsa.gov/	• Clinician • Oral health educator	• Serve primarily low-income and underserved populations • Work in community clinics, clinics at federal prisons, Indian reservations, and immigrant detention facilities that have been classified as dental HPSAs • Established by HRSA as a federal school-loan-repayment program • Healthcare equivalent of the Peace Corps
Indian Health Service (IHS) www.ihs.gov/	• Clinician • Oral health educator • Administrator of a community-based program	• Work in clinical facilities with the Native American and Alaska Native populations, in urban or rural settings • Can serve as a tribal hire, military transfer, civil service hire, or USPHS officer (see earlier in this table) • Benefits vary according to type of hire • Federal school-loan-repayment programs available
Department of Justice (DOJ) www.justice.gov/	• Clinician • Oral health educator • Administrator	• Work in clinical facilities at federal prisons • Can serve as civil service hire, USPHS officer (see earlier in this table), NHSC clinician (see earlier in this table), or military transfer • Benefits vary according to type of hire • Federal school-loan-repayment programs available
Department of Veterans Affairs (VA) www.va.gov/	• Clinician • Oral health educator • Administrator • Researcher	• Full-time, part-time, and on-call work • Work in VA hospitals and with various veteran's programs, including homeless programs for veterans • May be assigned to supervise other dental hygienists • Federal school-loan-repayment programs may be available
Department of Defense (DOD) www.defense.gov/	• Clinician • Oral health educator • Administrator • Researcher	• Work as employee of DOD, not a member of the military • Provide primarily clinical and oral health education on military bases and other DOD facilities • May be assigned to supervise other dental hygienists • Can function at both domestic and overseas locations
Community, Homeless, and Migrant Health Programs/ Centers	• Clinician • Oral health educator • Advocate for population served • Administrator	• Work in federally qualified community health centers funded by HRSA and/or the USPHS • May be assigned to supervise other dental hygienists • Can advance to administrative role • Can be part of the NHSC (see earlier in this table)

and economic barriers to successful oral health outcomes (see Chapter 3). Also, some populations served in public health clinics have language barriers and present the need for cultural competency skills (see Chapter 10).

A public health clinician may treat many types of patients and perform various activities during a given week, providing care to infants, children, adults, and older adults. For example, a dental hygienist may place varnish on infants' teeth during a nutrition clinic one day. On another day they may provide periodontal treatment to pregnant women coming to the health department for prenatal care visits. Another day the hygienist may go to a local elementary school to participate in a survey as part of an ongoing assessment of the prevalence of dental disease in the state, and follow up with the required **referral** component of the screening. Another part of the clinician's job may be to visit a long-term care facility on a monthly basis to provide clinical care to bedridden residents.

Clinicians in public health learn to be flexible with their dental environment. Clinical facilities may be similar to a dental office or may be in stationary school dental trailers or mobile dental vans that can be moved to multiple locations within a geographic area. Also, a clinical facility may consist of portable dental equipment moved from one school, facility, or home to another.

Clinical dental hygiene positions are available in many community settings, for example, health department clinics, community health centers and clinics, hospitals, university dental clinics, schools, nursing homes, residential facilities for older adults, and prison facilities. Because these facilities also provide medical care, interprofessional practice is characteristic of the clinician role in public health. Some locations offer the additional challenges of complex medical histories and patients with physical or mental disabilities.

Federal and state agencies have established clinical dental hygiene positions (e.g., the IHS, the National Health Service Corps, Community and Migrant Health Programs, the USPHS, military bases, Bureau of Prisons, and state oral health programs). In addition, local clinical care programs may be supported by nonprofit volunteer or faith-based organizations. Many of these positions involve ICP by the nature of the setting. As the economy fluctuates, the number of public health dental programs and clinics will vary. In nonprofit and publicly funded programs, clinicians must be accountable with the most cost-effective means of providing quality dental services to the most people.

Educational requirements for a public health clinical position may vary from an associate's degree with 1 year of experience to a bachelor's degree with several years of experience, depending on the requirements of the agency and the position. Additional certification may be required, according to the workforce models authorized in the state. If the public health position involves a combination of clinical treatment and program coordination or management, coursework in business and public health may be required. Positions that require some administrative or management skills (see later section) may require a master's degree. Depending on the position, experience as a clinician with specific populations and in various aspects of public health and ICP experience may be required also.

Educator

Dental Hygiene Faculty

A dental hygienist with a focus in community oral health in a faculty role may concentrate their career on teaching community oral health/dental public health courses and supervising dental hygiene students in community projects, rotations, and practicums (see Table 2.4). This educator can help students understand how public health is integrated into all aspects of dental hygiene practice, become aware of the segment of society that does not have access to oral health care, and become knowledgeable of disparities in dental disease and dental utilization and how to help solve these problems. Incorporating community involvement and service learning (see Chapter 11) into the dental hygiene student's experience will promote civic engagement, reinforce humanitarian ideals, build skills in cultural competence, and influence the student's interest after graduation in treating low-income patients in clinical practice, volunteering with community oral health projects, or pursuing a full-time career in dental public health.

Educational requirements for dental hygiene faculty are a bachelor's or master's degree, depending on the college and on the teaching responsibilities and clinical dental hygiene experience. Dental hygiene educators need knowledge of curriculum development, program development, and program evaluation. They also need effective human relations and communication skills. Advanced education and professional practice experience in public or community health and volunteer experience in the community are important also for an educator who is responsible for teaching community courses and coordinating community learning experiences.

Oral Health Educator

A second educator role in community oral health is the delivery of oral health education to the public (see Table 2.4). This is important to accomplish with individual patients as a clinician and with groups in the community. Oral health education is used to inform patients and clients about scientifically based methods for preventing oral diseases, promoting total wellness by reinforcing the relationship of oral health to overall health, encouraging clients to become responsible for personal oral health, and empowering clients' adoption of behaviors and practices to improve health.

The **oral health educator** in public health collaborates with other health professionals on the public health team. They share information about a common population, explore the relationship of oral health and other health problems of the population, plan ways to include oral health education in programs planned to intervene in other chronic medical conditions, and collaborate in the community health program planning process of assessment, planning, implementation, and evaluation (see Chapters 3 and 6) to deliver health education programs.

Oral health education programs can address a wide variety of oral health topics and can be directed to diverse target groups. Examples of oral health education programs include a smokeless tobacco intervention program related to prevention of oral cancer, promotion of dental sealants for schoolchildren, education about prevention of early childhood caries for daycare providers, denture-care classes for nursing home staff, and promotion of the use of mouth guards for athletes and coaches in a school district.

Oral health education programs can be associated effectively with health promotion events and campaigns sponsored by

---

BOX 2.4   Examples of Health Campaigns With Which to Associate Oral Health Education

- Great American Smokeout sponsored annually by the American Cancer Society on the third Thursday of November
- American Heart Month in February each year, identified by the American Heart Association
- March for Babies sponsored by the March of Dimes throughout the year in different locations
- National Children's Dental Health Month sponsored annually by the American Dental Association (ADA) in February
- Oral Cancer Awareness Month promoted annually by the Oral Cancer Foundation in April
- National Dental Hygiene Month sponsored annually by the American Dental Hygienists' Association (ADHA) in October
- Give Kids a Smile sponsored annually by the ADA during February

---

health and oral health organizations and professional associations (see Box 2.4). Oral health educators can collaborate with local dental hygiene societies, dental hygiene educational programs, and others on plans for these special events.

Oral health education is crucial to maximize the efficiency of the dental hygienist in a public health setting. By educating staff, teachers, and others who work directly with individuals, dental hygienists can have a greater impact. The professionals can pass on or apply the information to the individuals they work with. This concept is referred to as *train the trainer*.

Educational requirements for oral health educator positions vary from an associate's degree to a graduate degree, depending on the hiring agency or organization and the specific job responsibilities and requirements. Certification in health education or as a Certified Health Education Specialist (CHES) can be valuable also. The oral health educator in the community needs organizational skills, current scientific knowledge, excellent written and oral communication skills, creativity, and flexibility to meet the challenges of community health improvement (see Chapter 8). Also helpful is experience with patients who have special healthcare needs and experience with a diverse patient population and their parents, guardians, and caregivers.

Corporate Educator

A third educator role is as a corporate educator (see Table 2.4). In this role the dental hygienist is employed by industry to educate oral health professionals on the science and appropriate use of their oral health products. Many larger companies also have corporate educators who focus on academic relations, making presentations to students and faculty. Corporate educators can be a resource for oral health educators and dental hygiene faculty who are teaching community courses or coordinating students' community experiences.

Educational requirements for corporate educators vary. Usually a bachelor's or master's degree is required, depending on the job responsibilities. Professional experience and other requirements will also vary according to the specific job requirements and may parallel those of a dental hygiene educator or an administrator.

Advocate

The dental hygienist has a professional responsibility to take a leadership role in advocating oral health and access to care for the underserved (see Chapter 9). The role of advocate will most likely be part of one of the other dental hygiene professional roles or career paths (see Table 2.4). **Advocacy** can take several forms, depending on the needs of the community.

Dental hygienists will become aware of individuals or groups in the local community that have oral health disparities and lack access to oral health care. For example, older adults in long-term care facilities and senior living communities and individuals with developmental, physical, and intellectual disabilities served by community agencies may have difficulty accessing dental care for a variety of reasons, including problems with mobility and transportation, financial barriers, and limited oral health literacy (Figure 2.9). The dental hygienist can be an advocate for these individuals by representing them in seeking community resources and in developing special programs to meet their needs. Also, by bringing such consumer issues to the attention of local media or powerful citizens, the dental hygienist is able to influence changes that might lead to resolution of the access problems, ultimately improving their oral health.

Another form of advocacy is to provide technical assistance to nondental community groups interested in oral health issues. Some states and regions have active oral health coalitions that have consumers ready to work on access-to-care issues. These coalitions welcome the participation of a dental hygienist. Also, nonprofit organizations can benefit from the expertise of a dental hygienist on their boards, especially if the organization is small and has limited staff to implement oral health programs. Some examples of ways for a dental hygienist to contribute to a

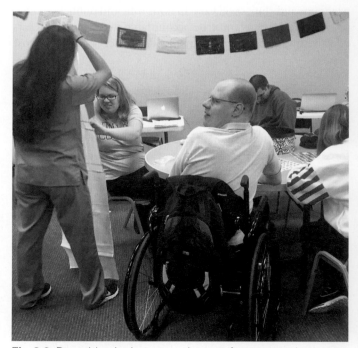

Fig 2.9 Dental hygienists can advocate for community groups with special needs, which can take several forms, depending on the needs of the community. (Courtesy Charlene Dickinson.)

coalition or to other community organizations are to establish and plan oral health programs for the population served by the organization; seek funding for oral health programs, including grant writing; recruit volunteers for oral health initiatives; and provide guidance on the appropriateness of oral health educational materials. Although these activities involve other professional roles described in this section, they are accomplished in the role of advocating for the population being served by the coalition or organization.

Consumer advocacy can also encompass protection of the public. A dental hygienist who serves on a state dental board is certifying individuals for licensure to practice dental hygiene, reviewing any problems or complaints regarding individual dental hygienists or their practices, and enforcing the laws regulating the practice of dental hygiene. Serving on a regional examining board involves evaluation of new practitioners' skills to endorse them for licensure to practice dental hygiene. Serving on committees to develop the National Board Dental Hygiene Examination relates to the certification of new practitioners as well. Dental hygiene faculty who serve as consultants to CODA evaluate dental hygiene programs to assure the potential qualifications of their graduates. All these are examples of activities that protect the public by assuring the competence of practicing dental hygienists who are serving the public.

Membership in the ADHA, its state constituents, and local component societies guarantees a platform to be an advocate for dental hygiene. A request for expert testimony on oral health issues might come from state legislative bodies, state and local boards of health, city councils, and other government entities. In this advocacy role the dental hygienist is advocating for the health of the public through legislation and public policy changes.

On the other hand, an advocate dental hygienist could be proactive as a change agent, for example, by being involved in a local fluoridation campaign (see Chapter 6). Another way that dental hygienists are proactive is by lobbying at the state level for the relaxation of dental hygiene supervision laws, changes in regulations regarding direct reimbursement of dental hygienists, expansion of the dental hygienists' scope of practice, implementation of a new dental workforce model in the state, or portability of licensure (Figure 2.10). Successful attempts in other states can serve as models for such changes, and the ADHA can provide resources to assist with the process (see Additional Resources at the end of this chapter). Most of the state-level changes related to these issues described earlier in this chapter have resulted from dental hygiene's advocacy efforts.

The required educational level to function effectively as an advocate depends on the nature of the advocacy role. To be an advocate for the public we serve, a specific educational degree beyond dental hygiene may not be required, but a bachelor's or master's degree in health, community health, public health, healthcare management, healthcare policy, social services or the equivalent could be helpful. A master's or law degree would be preferred for a lobbyist or legislative representative and helpful for a dental hygienist wishing to run for office as a legislator.

Change can be a slow process so advocacy can require patience and tenacity. An effective advocate is current in

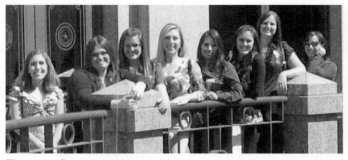

Fig 2.10 Dental hygiene students attend the state dental hygiene association lobby day at the state capitol to experience political advocacy first-hand. (Courtesy Christine French Beatty.)

scientific knowledge and public health issues, familiar with legislative and other government processes, confident, a good communicator, able to influence change, and eager for all citizens to have optimal oral health. Advocacy requires experience working with special needs populations; facilitating connections between individuals and oral health services; and strong computer competency, including knowledge of electronic medical records, computerized appointment/billing programs, and Microsoft Office programs. Ability to speak a foreign language can be helpful as well. Dental hygienists who become advocates may have several years of experience in the profession and the ability to visualize the "big picture" of dental hygiene in relation to the complexities of dental public health.

Researcher

As a **researcher** a dental hygienist uses scientific methods and knowledge to identify and pursue a specific area of interest (see Chapter 7). Dental hygienists in a research career path work in various settings such as state health departments, colleges and universities, dental schools, hospitals, other government agencies, nonprofit organizations, health professional associations, and private industry.

Some examples of the dental hygienist in research are presented in Table 2.4 and Box 2.5. As evident from these examples, the role of researcher is frequently part of another professional role. In many positions the dental hygienist may work part-time as a researcher, with the remainder of the job description being one of the other professional roles discussed in this section.

The epidemiology of dental diseases is one possible research area of interest. In this role, the public health dental hygienist might coordinate statewide or local needs assessments. Knowledge of research methods and assessment tools, including dental indices, is required to survey the prevalence of oral diseases; biostatistics skills are important for analyzing data; and critical thinking is necessary for interpretation and application of research results. In addition, because much epidemiological research is conducted in the field, it is important to possess interpersonal skills to be able to work with representatives and administrators of various community and government organizations, such as school districts and other government agencies.

BOX 2.5 Examples of the Dental Hygienist in a Researcher Role

- At a dental school, participating in a periodontal research project to study the effectiveness of a new antimicrobial product.
- With a microbiology department of a university, conducting research on the microbial etiology of periodontal disease.
- As part of the expectations of a dental hygiene faculty position, involved in the conduct of a variety of research projects, the written or oral presentation of research results, or the writing of textbooks.
- As an employee of a Veterans Affairs hospital, studying therapeutic procedures for patients with head and neck cancer.
- On staff with a dental clinic associated with a children's hospital, studying pediatric patient management techniques.
- Employed by HRSA, involved in research related to the adequacy and effectiveness of the dental workforce nationwide.
- As part of a research team of a dental product company, participating in research to scientifically determine the effectiveness of new methods and products.

BOX 2.6 Examples of Administrator Positions in Public Health

- Coordinator of a state or regional oral health coalition.
- Director of a children's hospital dental clinic.
- Executive director of a nonprofit dental organization.
- Coordinator of a local, regional, or statewide school-based sealant or fluoride varnish program associated with a health department, school district, or Head Start program.
- Manager of a community-based dental clinic.
- Coordinator of an oral health program in a state prison system.
- President and owner of a mobile nursing home practice.
- Assistant administrator of a DHHS operating division.
- Administrator of an oral health program with a federal agency such as the CDC or the Office of the Assistant Secretary of Health.
- Public health-emphasis staff position with a dental hygiene or dental public health professional organization or a state dental board.

The role of researcher is involved in the required accountability for public funds used by public health programs at all levels. Oral health data must be continually gathered to evaluate and demonstrate the effectiveness of public health programs in improving oral health and reducing barriers to oral health care. Epidemiological research is crucial in maintaining existing oral health programs or initiating new ones.

Educational requirements for researcher positions include a bachelor's degree with several years of relevant experience and a research-based master's or doctoral degree, depending on the type of research position and the job responsibilities. Also crucial are critical thinking skills and knowledge of research design and methodology, biostatistics, data analysis, standard statistical software packages and other computer skills, and project cost estimation. The researcher role involves the sharing of research results with other oral health professionals and the public, which requires strong writing and oral presentation skills (see Chapter 8). Depending on the type of research, it may also be important to have knowledge of assessment tools and dental indices, medical terminology, and medical procedures. Certification by the Research Administrators Certification Council has value for the researcher who is developing and administering projects; it will increase credibility and improve employment and advancement opportunities. A researcher involved in epidemiological research will benefit from certification through the Association for Professionals in Infection Control and Epidemiology (https://apic.org/).

Administrator

The expanded coordination of community-wide oral health programs creates the need for an administrator role (see Table 2.4). In this role, the dental hygienist initiates, develops, organizes, and/or manages a dental public health program at the local, state, or federal level. If the oral health program is implemented for a large population or within a large geographic area, supervision of other professional and technical staff may be required.

Dental hygienists fill **administrator** positions at various levels. The type of oral health program managed depends on the needs of the population. Some examples of public health administrator positions held by dental hygienists are presented in Table 2.4 and Box 2.6.

Most of these positions are in government or nonprofit settings. Some are in for-profit healthcare settings such as hospitals or nursing homes. In addition, some corporations also focus on community oral health programs and employ dental hygienists to coordinate these programs. For example, Colgate Oral Pharmaceuticals, a for-profit company leading the oral care market with both over-the-counter and therapeutic professional products, has a presence in the community by supporting and coordinating community oral health programs. Through their Bright Smiles, Bright Futures® program, Colgate provides free dental screening and oral health education globally. In the U.S., a fleet of mobile dental vans travel to underserved rural and urban communities, reaching over 1000 towns and more than 10 million children each year (Figure 2.11). Their award-winning oral health education curriculum is available in 30 languages and in 80 countries. In the U.S., it has reached nearly 90% of kindergarten students each year, 3.5 million children in all 50 states, and over 750,000 preschool children through a partnership with Head Start.[54] Dental hygienists are employed by Colgate to coordinate these community programs.

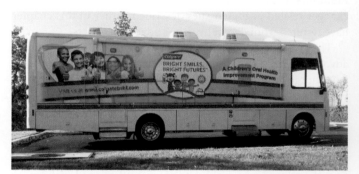

Fig 2.11 The Colgate Bright Smiles, Bright Futures® dental van is used to provide free dental screening and oral health education to children globally. (Courtesy Colgate Oral Pharmaceuticals.)

An administrator will often have additional professional roles. This individual may be required to provide some consulting, become an advocate for changing public policy, or be involved with social marketing for a new oral health initiative. Administrators frequently are called on to collaborate with leaders of other programs.

Educational requirements of this administrative role are a bachelor's or master's degree in dental hygiene or a related field. Especially helpful would be a master's degree in public health, community health, public administration, or healthcare administration. Higher level administrator positions may require a doctoral degree in one of these disciplines.

Required skills to function effectively as an administrator vary according to whether it is a state or local position and the magnitude of the program. Necessary skills can include leadership, personnel management, program development and implementation, project management, program evaluation, oral and written communication, collaboration, grant writing, and organizational skills. It can be important also to have current knowledge of dental and dental hygiene sciences; dental public health issues, practices, and operations; and business management such as budget development, supply ordering and inventories, and record keeping. Experience in local, city, and county public assistance dental programs; state Medicaid programs; dental policy development; and provider relations can be of value too. Several years of experience are generally needed to perform successfully as an administrator.

Entrepreneur

The **entrepreneur** applies imagination and creativity to initiate or finance a new enterprise (see Table 2.4). Many entrepreneurial ventures that dental hygienists might pursue will relate to

> ### BOX 2.7 Examples of Entrepreneurial Positions
>
> - Consulting with communities or professional organizations that are establishing community oral health programs.
> - Founding a business to provide oral care to a vulnerable, underserved population, such as homeless individuals or residents of nursing homes.
> - Establishing a collaborative dental hygiene practice to provide school-based preventive oral health care.
> - Authoring a community oral health textbook.
> - Public speaking on dental public health topics.
> - Writing a community oral health column for a dental hygiene periodical.

dental public health. Some also will cross over to other career paths, such as administrator or researcher. Some examples of public health entrepreneurial positions are presented in Table 2.4 and Box 2.7.

Educational requirements depend on the entrepreneurial undertaking. For example, becoming a public speaker or author related to community oral health topics would necessitate an advanced degree to gain knowledge and establish credibility. On the other hand, establishing a nonprofit dental organization could be accomplished with the minimum dental hygiene education as long as the dental hygienist has the experience and contacts needed to accomplish the task. Some ventures could necessitate a business degree, for example, operating a business or nonprofit. Establishing a collaborative dental hygiene practice may necessitate specific requirements as set by individual state statutes.

Required characteristics for the dental hygienist entrepreneur include ingenuity, inspiration, and resourcefulness. Experience in the profession and networking are also important to successfully initiate a new venture.

DENTAL HYGIENIST MINI-PROFILE

Public Health/Clinician/Advocate

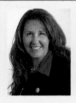

Name
Christy Jo Fogarty, RDH, ADT, BSDH, MSOHP

Position and Place of Employment
Licensed dental hygienist (RDH) and advanced dental therapist (ADT), Children's Dental Services, Minneapolis, Minnesota

Description of Organization
Children's Dental Services (CDS; http://childrensdentalservices.org/) is a not-for-profit organization providing dental services to children that, in 2019, celebrated its 100-year anniversary. CDS serves children through community-based clinics that focus on a diverse population of children under the age of 21 years. The main clinic is in the inner city of Minneapolis, and CDS also serves several schools with onsite school-based clinics and mobile outreach programs in Minneapolis and St. Paul. In addition, CDS has outreach mobile clinics in rural areas throughout the state. ADTs and RDHs travel from the main clinic to these rural sites to treat children using mobile equipment, providing services that include examination, radiographs, prophylaxis, sealants, and fluoride.

Responsibilities of Position
As ADT: Perform examinations, all types of restorations, stainless steel crowns on permanent and primary teeth, extract on of primary teeth and permanent teeth with class III or IV mobility
As RDH: Perform prophylaxis and nonsurgical periodontal therapy (not allowed with only ADT license), radiographs, sealants, and fluoride

Required Qualifications and Experience
Bachelor's degree with both RDH and ADT licenses; Oral Hygiene Practitioner master's degree

Personal Comment
I began my career as a dental hygienist employed in private practice in Minneapolis. About 20% of our clients were on public assistance, so I spent much of my time working with that population. I also worked closely with, and provided care to, teens at a drug treatment facility. Then I spent 7 years as an independent contractor in the Minneapolis/St. Paul area. When I got the opportunity to expand my dental knowledge and scope of practice to serve those who could not gain access to care, I knew I had found my lifelong calling. I started in the first ADT class even before the legislation passed to allow the practice of dental

(Continued)

DENTAL HYGIENIST MINI-PROFILE (*Cont.*)
Public Health/Clinician/Advocate

therapy, taking a leap of faith in relation to the amazing success of dental therapy in Minnesota.

Being the first ADT in this organization, I faced various challenges and had to overcome numerous trials. Many dentists held latent feelings of mistrust created by the ADA and the Minnesota Dental Association. Thus, I had to prove my knowledge and skills to several dentists that I worked with. In the meantime, CDS was faced with the logistics of how to incorporate the ADT position into the office. Also, we had to educate everyone on both my scope of practice and my supervision level. Even setting up billing was challenging; many insurers were not sure in what category of provider the ADT should be entered because mid-level providers were new to dentistry.

As I transitioned from dental hygiene into more of the dental therapy scope of practice, I worked more closely with the dentists, and they came to realize the strong restorative skills that I had. Today, I practice in a very fluid and seamless way with the dentists and other dental therapists in my office. The staff is well versed in the ADT scope of practice and the level of supervision needed. I collaborate on treatment continually with my supervising dentist, but rarely at the same site. We communicate regularly, and I can use her knowledge and skills remotely whenever necessary. I am treated as a valuable member of the team, and most of the dentists can no longer imagine working without a dental therapist.

In addition, I have functioned in the role of advocate for legislative proposals related to dental hygienists as mid-level providers in other states. I have talked with dozens of legislators across the nation about how dental therapy is effectively and efficiently benefiting the citizens of Minnesota in terms of increased access to dental care and improved oral health. In May of 2014, Maine became the second state to codify a mid-level dental practitioner, and several other states have followed since.

Advice to Future Dental Hygienists
Spend time honing your clinical skills and practicing in public health. It is hard work and will challenge you on many levels, but it also has huge payoffs. If you would like to provide more for your patients as a clinician, consider continuing your training by becoming an ADT as well. Not many jobs allow one to get paid in both money and hugs... mine does!

DENTAL HYGIENIST MINI-PROFILE
Entrepreneur/Administrator/Public Health

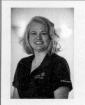

Name
Terri Chandler, RDH, EFDA, CDA

Position and Place of Employment
Founder/CEO/Executive Director, Future Smiles, Las Vegas, Nevada

Description of Organization
Established in 2009, Future Smiles (https://www.futuresmiles.net/) is a nonprofit organization that has the mission to provide the essential resources and infrastructure to increase access to oral health care for underserved populations. It also serves to generate public health opportunities for dental hygienists. Through school-based care, Future Smiles applies a systems approach to remove common barriers of cost, transportation, lost income resulting from time off work, and lost school time for learning. The ultimate goal is to change the way children and their families think and act regarding their personal oral health and at the same time to instill positive oral health behaviors that can last a lifetime.

Future Smiles delivers school-based services in the Clark County School District with three types of operational delivery modes: (1) a dental hygiene model, (2) a dentist model, and (3) a school-based sealant team. The school-based dental hygiene settings are referred to as Education and Prevention of Oral Disease (EPOD) programs. An EPOD is a hybrid of a traditional dental sealant program that includes additional dental hygiene services. Typically, an EPOD operates in a school-based health center but is sometimes set up in a classroom, nurse's office, lunch room, modular building, or other available space.

The Clark County School District provides the space at no cost for one EPOD, which operates year-round. Our new Nevada Women's Philanthropy (NWP) Dental Wellness Center is home to a dentist and a community dental health coordinator (CDHC) and is where comprehensive dental restorative treatment is provided and Medicaid enrollment and care navigation are coordinated. Dental hygiene "carry-in-and-carry-out" portable dental units are used in the school-based sealant team EPOD. Weighing 50 pounds or less, these mobile units fold into suitcase containers and are on wheels for easy transport from school to school throughout the school year.

Using a positive consent form signed by a parent or guardian, Future Smiles offers dental hygiene services to all at-risk students enrolled in the school. These services include screening, oral health education, prophylaxis, sealants, fluoride varnish, digital x-rays (at limited locations), and case management through a referral system for restorative dentistry. Children are referred to our NWP Dental Wellness Center, community-based clinics, the local dental schools, and area dentists through a network of dentists who are Medicaid providers or have offered pro bono dental care to the students who have untreated dental caries. Further impact is achieved through oral health education presentations, "brush at lunch" presentations, health fairs, and program services provided at various community health clinics.

Responsibilities of Position
My role is primarily administrative, which involves financial planning, public relations, program development, grant writing, public health advocacy, oral health consulting, and public speaking. In addition, I provide leadership for a staff of 16 oral health professionals and our Associate Director to set the tone and establish a culture of collaborative teamwork in this community oral health program.

Required Qualifications and Experience
Personal qualities that made it possible to create this nonprofit were my passion, determination, enthusiasm, careful planning, strong sense of possibility, and profound belief that we can make a difference. Eight years with the Nevada State Health Division's Oral Health Program as the statewide sealant coordinator and the oral health coalition coordinator provided in-depth knowledge of oral health issues in Nevada and innovative solutions to foster long-term change.

Personal Comment
While practicing clinically, I came to a crossroad in my life, at which point I clearly saw a way to impact the oral health of disadvantaged youth through my personal life experience. One might ask why I left private practice in a great dental office that offered financial security and respect to form a nonprofit to

DENTAL HYGIENIST MINI-PROFILE (*Cont.*)

Entrepreneur/Administrator/Public Health

address dental wellness for the underserved. It's simple: to make a difference in the lives of others! I was at a point in my life when the reward and challenge of developing a dental hygiene-based program was possible for me, and I took the opportunity and ran with it.

In mid-2009, I left private practice employment and devoted my time and energy to developing Future Smiles. My goal was to increase access to dental hygiene services for at-risk children and their families with a school-based program. Today, my focus is as the executive director of Future Smiles, a Nevada, 501(c)(3) nonprofit organization.

As an oral health professional for over 35 years, I had never been in business for myself. Thus, forming this nonprofit organization required a lot of learning for example, about insurance, financial planning, state/local licenses, and the Internal Revenue Service (IRS) application process for a nonprofit. After 10 years, many of these new business elements are now part of our standard operating procedures, and we have learned to embrace annual audits, renewal dates, and financial reviews.

As a public health entity, Future Smiles was under the scrutiny of the dental community. They had many questions concerning what Future Smiles was offering the public and how that "fit into" the business culture of private dental practices. Fortunately, Future Smiles had a solid business plan that allowed our school-based services to operate under the Nevada State Board of Dental Examiners Public Health Dental Hygiene Endorsement. The dental hygienists and dentists who work with Future Smiles are contracted as providers with Medicaid and private dental insurance companies.

I believe it is important for all dental hygienists to be acknowledged as registered professionals with the National Plan & Provider Enumeration System (NPPES) at https://nppes.cms.hhs.gov. A dental hygienist is registered as a dental health professional through NPPES and receives a National Provider Identification number (NPI). The NPI is attached to all dental hygiene licenses and can be used as an identifier for Medicaid and private insurance contracting.

The best part of my work with Future Smiles is going into a school to serve the students. It is also gratifying to hear stories from our dental professionals about their positive and rewarding experiences serving the children and making a difference within the profession.

Advice to Future Dental Hygienists

As dental hygienists, we often think that what we do only involves clinical treatment. However, with a nonprofit like Future Smiles, we become a collective group with many talents and the ability to make a long-term impact on the oral health of the population we serve. The work of the nonprofit is exponential, touching many lives and continuing beyond its individual founders. The real joy of working with a nonprofit is the hope and compassion that result, providing the inspiration that serves as the true essence of a nonprofit.

DENTAL HYGIENIST MINI-PROFILE

Public Health/Entrepreneur/Administrator

Name
Tammy L. Allen, RDH

Position and Place of Employment
Co-owner, LifeCycle Dental, Fort Worth, Texas

Description of Organization
LifeCycle Dental (https://www.lifecycledental.com/) is a privately owned, mobile provider of dental and dental hygiene services to older adult residents of long-term care facilities, a population that continues to be underserved. The mission of LifeCycle Dental is, "We believe that everyone deserves excellence in dental service throughout all phases of life. We are committed to caring for oral health, self-esteem, and dignity in geriatric dental care" (www.lifecycledental.com). Based on a genuine belief that prevention is the key to maintaining oral health, the organization was established in 2002 to implement a preventive dental model for this population. LifeCycle Dental began by transporting mobile clinics to three long-term care facilities. We have expanded to over 55 facilities in the North Texas area in 17 years.

Responsibilities of Position
We deliver clinical dental hygiene and dental services to the residents of long-term care facilities. As co-owner, I serve as administrator. Our office staff does the billing and insurance, and I navigate cases that involve complicated medical histories.

Required Qualifications and Experience
Personal qualities that were essential to establish this business were having a passion for the provision of oral health care for older adults, being willing to sacrifice the time necessary to learn what was needed to launch the business, and exhibiting determination and focus. Extensive knowledge and experience in providing oral care for older adults were necessary. Also, knowledge of regulations related to caring for this population and advocacy skills were vital. Some of this was acquired through the experience of developing the business and is an ongoing endeavor.

Personal Comment
Oral health remains a tremendous concern for residents of long-term care facilities and their families. Although most mobile dental companies work on the basis of emergency pain referrals, I believe that optimum dental care should focus on prevention, not alleviation of pain. My love for older people has guided my professional journey to care for this population. During part of this journey, I was a member of the Texas State Board of Dental Examiners. It was then that I became aware of Texas's critical need for a preventive oral health model for long-term care facilities. I was instrumental in changing Texas law to allow dental hygienists to provide care in long-term care facilities.

Along the way, I have faced many challenges, mostly with time commitments. It takes a great deal of time to set up and operate an organization to serve this segment of the population. Therefore, for a time, I eliminated all extracurricular activities to focus my energy on learning how to care for and deliver care to residents of long-term care facilities.

Currently, no regulations exist in this state that require nursing homes to provide dental examinations, professional dental hygiene services, or dental care for their long-term care residents. In addition, daily oral care is still viewed as relatively unimportant in long-term care facilities. Oral hygiene is usually last on the priority list of regular care, even below hair appointments and nail polishing.

There continues to be a dearth of oral health knowledge among most long-term care facility staff, especially concerning the significance of oral care in relation to the overall health, comfort, and quality of life of long-term care residents. Our team of dentists and dental hygienists are challenged by this daily. After

(Continued)

DENTAL HYGIENIST MINI-PROFILE (*Cont.*)
Public Health/Entrepreneur/Administrator

18 years of providing care in long-term care facilities, we believe that oral health professionals must take the responsibility of daily oral care. Ultimately, an oral health professional employed as part of the long-term care facility team would solve the issue of poor dental care in the facility. Until laws are changed to require this level of care, we are forced to rely on the inadequate resources available.

The current role of the certified nurse aide does not allow enough time for daily oral care. Thus, we believe the duty of regular oral care should be delegated to the hydration aid. The Food and Hydration Aid is central to the interdisciplinary team and is responsible for accurately identifying nutrition and hydration problems and assessing the need to increase food and fluid intake. It seems natural to add the responsibility for daily oral care, with the goal of providing care that is individualized for each resident. Also, daily oral care can be completed during shower and bath times. In our experience, these two changes in procedure have been effective solutions to the problem of inadequate daily oral care in nursing homes.

Daily oral care is a simple task but viewed as complicated. We have found that keeping things simple will most likely result in success. Nurse aides report that daily oral care is avoided because it takes too much time to find the toothbrush and supplies in the residents' room. We recommend a prepasted disposable brush that can be handed to the resident in their bed, in the bathroom, or wherever it is convenient. This brushing regimen saves significant time, allowing the aid to implement the care into the daily care plan easily. Finally, an oral health professional must monitor the regular care program every 3 months and suggest any changes that are indicated for each resident and in the overall program. Fortunately, facilities are mandated to have a dentist as a vendor, and most residents have a benefit that allows dental cleaning two times a year.

As a licensed dental hygienist, I continue to think outside the box to find solutions within the given restraints. Whereas brushing, flossing, and using a mouth rinse are optimal practices twice a day, it has not become a priority for the long-term care industry. Until dental care is viewed as a priority among other life-threatening diagnoses, we will continue to look outside the box.

Advice to Future Dental Hygienists
Learn about and, as needed, get involved in changing the laws and regulations related to oral health care in your state before pursuing an entrepreneurial endeavor to provide oral health care to a specific population. For example, until regulations are changed, I believe dental hygienists are called to be advocates consistently for oral care for geriatric residents in long-term care facilities.

DENTAL HYGIENIST MINI-PROFILE
Public Health/Administrator/Educator/Clinician

Name
Joyce Bartle Flieger, BSDH, MPH, RDH, EFDH

Position and Place of Employment
- Oral Health Professional, First Smiles Program, University of Arizona College of Agriculture and Life Sciences Cooperative Extension, Tucson, Arizona
- First Smiles Matter, Pima County Health Department (Arizona), Oral Health Division, Consultant (to educate dentists, dental hygienists, pediatricians, obstetricians, nurse practitioners, and medical assistants about oral screening, applying fluoride varnish on children aged 0–5 years, and referring pregnant women to dentists to improve birth outcomes), funded by a grant from First Things First in Arizona (https://www.firstthingsfirst.org/).

Description of Organizations
As an outreach arm of The University of Arizona and the College of Agriculture and Life Sciences, the office of the Arizona Cooperative Extension is a statewide not-for-profit nonformal education network that provides a link between the university and the citizens of Arizona, "bringing research-based information into communities to help people improve their lives" (https://extension.arizona.edu). Their vision is to be "a vital national leader in creating and applying knowledge to help people build thriving, sustainable lives, communities, and economies." Their mission is "to engage with people through applied research and education to improve lives, families, communities, environment, and economies in Arizona and beyond." The First Smiles program operated by the Cooperative Extension serves the oral health needs of at-risk children and their families in a rural Arizona county on the Mexican border. This county has medical and dental healthcare professional shortages; in some parts of the county, a 1- to 3-hour drive is required to access a dental or medical provider. This grant-funded program provides oral health education to parents and their children and delivers preventive services to infants, children, and pregnant women.

The Pima County Health Department is dedicated to help the residents of Pima County achieve and maintain on optimal level of wellness. The Health Department and its partners are committed to embracing and promoting diversity throughout our programs. They encourage an active network of public health and safety professionals and community-based organizations. They are the community voice of public health based on their knowledge, experience, skills, and accessibility.

Responsibilities of Positions
I provide oral health assessments, preventive services such as fluoride varnish, and dental referrals as needed for children aged 0 to 5 years and pregnant women. In addition, oral health education is provided for these groups and their families and childcare providers.

Required Qualifications and Experience
Licensure as a dental hygienist and Affiliated Practice Dental Hygienist (APDH) certification were required for this position. In addition, working with this population requires experience managing young children who have never had any type of dental service or assessment. Also, to competently refer children, knowledge is required of oral pathology/abnormalities in young children and infants; how these abnormalities can affect breast feeding, speech, and success later in life; when and to which health professionals to refer for a workup of these conditions; and the health professionals available for referral in the rural community. The oral health professional must be able to do it all in a rural community where funds and other resources are limited. This position requires skills in clinical procedures, data gathering, data recording, and data storage. In addition, traits such as confidentiality, creativity, and especially trustworthiness are required.

Personal Comment
The journey to my current position has taken many different turns. Upon graduation with honors in 1973 from the University of Southern California Dental

DENTAL HYGIENIST MINI-PROFILE (*Cont.*)
Public Health/Administrator/Educator/Clinician

Hygiene program, I took a position in public health with the Los Angeles County Health Department and worked on a community water fluoridation campaign for the city of Los Angeles. As a dental hygienist, I practiced in community health centers and parochial schools, providing dental hygiene services to children and pregnant women, and in an American Indian health center. My experiences as a public health dental hygienist prompted me to pursue a Master of Public Health degree from the University of Michigan.

After graduate school, I also pursued an academic career as a professor, clinic coordinator, dental hygiene program director, and department chair. Throughout my years as a dental hygiene educator, I continued to satisfy my love for clinical dental hygiene with part-time clinical practice. I also supported my local dental hygiene associations and encouraged students to participate in community service activities.

When I moved to Arizona, I became certified as an Expanded Function Dental Hygienist (EFDH) in California to qualify for local anesthesia. More recently, I served the State of Arizona as the Office Chief with the Arizona Department of Health Services, Office of Oral Health. This position allowed me to participate in many new state-level initiatives, including being part of the new landscape for the APDH in Arizona. I personally earned the APDH certification so I could organize dental sealant programs in the schools for state and county health departments without dentist supervision. Also, I worked on state projects to provide dental services for rural communities and other underserved populations and to procure grant funding to pilot teledentistry in Arizona.

Currently, I administer the First Smiles program, for which I helped with the groundwork at the state level. This qualified me to apply for the county-level position when the funding became available. Thus, I have experienced the "boots-on-the-ground" work of this state initiative, learning what works and what does not work. As a result, I have concluded that it is important to get out of the office after developing and implementing a new program to experience its strengths and weaknesses.

The barriers I have encountered in the First Smiles program were more entrenched in the community than I had imagined. False doctrines were abundant, such as "children do not need to see a dentist until age 2 or 3," "fluoride is not healthy," and "tooth decay in primary teeth is fine because those teeth come out anyway." The First Smiles project started with a strong educational program based on the established needs of this rural community, which helped dispel these myths. I developed age-appropriate messages about oral health for the children, and I learned quickly that these messages were successful as well to educate the adults that were present during the children's education.

A tight-knit rural community can be a difficult place to affect change in behaviors. Every interaction matters! Developing trust among community members is important to the success of any program. Providing a model professional oral health program that truly benefits the community is important to establish trust.

Advice to Future Dental Hygienists
Learn as much as you can about the scientific evidence that will support your program and what will make it an effective program. Knowing how to collect data and how to apply that data in a grant report is invaluable when it comes to successfully acquiring funding to continue a program. Know how to advocate change and make evidenced-based decisions.

DENTAL HYGIENIST MINI-PROFILE
Corporate Educator

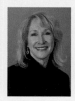

Name
Annette Wolfe, RDH, BS

Position and Place of Employment
Academic Manager, Southwest Region, Colgate Oral Pharmaceuticals, New York, New York (retired November 13, 2020)

Description of Organization
Colgate-Palmolive is a leading global consumer products company, tightly focused on oral care, personal care, home care, and pet nutrition with business in over 200 countries and territories around the world. As part of Colgate-Palmolive, Colgate Oral Pharmaceuticals is a leader in the oral care market with both over-the-counter and therapeutic professional dental products. Colgate is committed to doing business with integrity and respect for all people and for the world. Their three fundamental values—Caring, Global Teamwork, and Continuous Improvement—are part of everything they do. They demonstrate their Caring value by supporting community programs around the world including their flagship program, Colgate Bright Smiles, Bright Futures® (https://www.colgate.com/en-us/bright-smiles-bright-futures).

Colgate Bright Smiles, Bright Futures® is among the most far-reaching, successful children's oral health initiatives in the world. With long-standing partnerships with governments, schools, and communities, Colgate Bright Smiles, Bright Futures® has reached more than 500 million children and their families in 80 countries with free dental screenings and oral health education.

Responsibilities of Position
I presented scientific technology and product lectures and seminars at dental colleges and dental hygiene programs; delivered continuing education programs to practicing oral health professionals; assisted in developing various presentations; and participated as a vendor and educational representative at continuing education events, dental and dental hygiene conventions, and other professional meetings. I also assisted in training field representatives. In relation to community oral health, I participated with my team in Bright Smiles, Bright Futures® initiatives (see earlier), as well as partnering with dental hygiene education programs and dental hygiene professional associations to help implement community-based programs that served underserved population groups.

Required Qualifications and Experience
Necessary qualifications included being a Registered Dental Hygienist with a minimum of 2 to 5 years of experience in an academic setting or visiting academic institutions. A master's degree or equivalent experience was required. Strong interpersonal, organizational, and communication skills were also a must.

Personal Comment
In 1978, I received my Associate of Science degree and was licensed as a dental hygienist in Florida, where I practiced for 8 years. Later, I completed a Bachelor of Science degree in dental hygiene through the degree completion program at Texas Woman's University, minoring in business. Before graduating I responded

(*Continued*)

DENTAL HYGIENIST MINI-PROFILE (*Cont.*)
Corporate Educator

to a newspaper advertisement that read, "Wanted: Dental Hygienist to sell dental equipment" and was hired by EMS/Electro Medical Systems, manufacturer of the Piezon ultrasonic scaler.

During my time with EMS, I gained experience in many areas including training, program development, marketing, internal auditing, and sales. It was during this time that I got my first opportunity to be a presenter and learned to overcome my fear of public speaking, which was one of my biggest career challenges. The networking opportunities here paved the way for my further professional development.

After my stint at EMS, Dentsply presented an opportunity to be a clinical educator. I developed and managed an 11-state territory and continued to develop my presentation skills. After that I spent 2 years as Professional Services Specialist and trainer for D4D Technologies, a manufacturer of chairside CAD/CAM systems. This was another great learning experience and networking opportunity. Finally, in 2009 I was hired by Colgate Oral Pharmaceuticals as an Academic Manager.

My clinical experience was invaluable in my corporate positions. It made training students and dental personnel more efficient and practical. As a result of my experience, I understood patient care, motivation, and the possible challenges involved in both. In addition, it provided me with credibility in the field.

Advice to Future Dental Hygienists

Get as much clinical experience as possible, as that is the foundation of a dental hygiene career in other roles. Make sure to maintain your membership in ADHA and network, network, network! To seek a corporate position within the dental industry, whether in sales, as an educational representative, or another aspect, attend meetings, talk to dental company representatives, introduce yourself to speakers at continuing education programs, have a business card to pass out, develop computer skills, and get trained in public speaking. Pursuing a career in education can simultaneously enhance your dental hygiene knowledge and speaking skills. Finally, never say "never," don't try to predict what life will bring your way, and work hard to follow your dream.

DENTAL HYGIENIST MINI-PROFILE
Public Health/Administrator

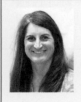

Name
Stacy P. Redden, RDH, MS

Position and Place of Employment
Practice Administrator, Dental and Orthodontic Clinics, Children's Health Specialty Center, Children's Medical Center, Dallas, Texas

Description of Organization

Children's Health^{SM}, formerly known as Children's Medical Center Dallas, has the mission "to make life better for children" (www.childrens.com). The organization encompasses a full range of pediatric health, wellness, and acute care services for children from birth to age 18, built around academic medical centers, specialty care, primary care, home health, a pediatric research institute, and community outreach services, among other forms of healthcare delivery. Children's Health^{SM} is the seventh-largest pediatric healthcare provider in the country and the only academically affiliated pediatric hospital in the area.

The hospital is home to numerous outpatient affiliated clinics that represent interdisciplinary collaboration in treating patients; the dental clinic and orthodontics clinic are two of them. The dental and orthodontics clinics address the entire range of needs, from routine and preventive oral health care to treatment for complex dental problems, and from conventional orthodontics for the purpose of straightening teeth to specialized strategies for a variety of particular needs and situations such as cleft palate.

Responsibilities of Position

As the Practice Administrator, I manage the day-to-day operations of the dental and orthodontics clinics of the hospital, including supervision of 23 staff members and management of almost 300 patients each week. I am the "go to" person for my Division Director and other dental school faculty who supervise the pediatric dentistry residents who actually provide the dental treatment for our patients. I serve as the intermediary and communicator of information from our leadership team to my staff. Finally, I function in an interdisciplinary collaborative capacity with administrators of other clinics to work on initiatives aimed at assuring that excellent service is provided by our staff to our patients.

Required Qualifications and Experience

Master's degree and management experience are needed. Children's Health^{SM} preferred a Master of Business Administration or Master of Health Administration degree for the Practice Administrator position. However, because my predecessors held the same degrees as mine (Bachelor of Science and Master of Science in Dental Hygiene [MSDH]), my credentials were accepted.

Personal Comment

I practiced dental hygiene in private dental offices for several years before I returned to school to get my MSDH. I decided to return because, even though I loved my patients and where I worked, I felt stagnant. At the time, I had several patients diagnosed with cancer, discovered that I had a passion for working with that patient population, and equally enjoyed researching ways to make them more comfortable. This draw in addition to an interest in clinical teaching after I visited with the Dental Hygiene Department at Baylor College of Dentistry prompted me to pursue graduate education.

While in my graduate program I did an internship at Children's Health^{SM} under the supervision of the Dental Clinic Practice Administrator at that time. This experience resulted in my falling in love with the hospital and the Practice Manager position. Because of my interest, I did my master's thesis on the provision of daily oral care by nurses in hospitals. After my internship I continued to volunteer through graduate school and beyond until I was employed in 2012.

The program was developed already when I came to Children's Health^{SM} so my focus has been to continue to expand our services, market our clinics to parents of children who require our specialized care, and identify new community partners who can assist us with this. Our biggest challenge is in relation to working with dental insurance. Many of our patients are covered by Medicaid, with its cumbersome reimbursement mechanisms and continual changes in benefits and other provisions. Another challenge is being diligent about careful interviewing and medical consults before treatment to assure that we have complete medical information for our children, some of whom are exceptionally medically compromised. Our chief concern is to keep our patients happy and healthy while they are in our care.

DENTAL HYGIENIST MINI-PROFILE (*Cont.*)
Public Health/Administrator

Advice to Future Dental Hygienists

Regardless of the professional role that appeals to you, I recommend working in clinical practice first to hone your skills and gain experience working with patients outside of the school environment. Take as many continuing education courses as possible relative to subjects or patient populations of interest so you can solidify the areas that appeal to you for your professional career long term. Then find someone working in the area or role that you are drawn to, visit with them about their career, and ask if you can do an internship or volunteer to shadow them to experience what they do on a day-to-day basis. I also recommend pursuing graduate education. Even though I did a MSDH, I believe a Master of Health Administration or Master of Business Administration would be more beneficial for the dental hygienist interested in pursuing a management role in a hospital setting.

DENTAL HYGIENIST MINI-PROFILE
Public Health/Clinician/Administrator

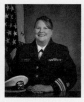

Name

Cynthia Chennault, RDH, BSDH, MPH, Lieutenant Commander, USPHS Commissioned Corps

Position and Place of Employment

Senior Public Health Analyst, Health Resources and Services Administration (HRSA), Rockville, Maryland

Description of Organization

Overseen by the Surgeon General, the USPHS Commissioned Corps is a diverse team of more than 6500 highly qualified public health professionals. The USPHS is one of the seven U.S. uniformed services, and our officers hold ranks equivalent to, and wear uniforms similar to, the U.S. Navy or Coast Guard, with special PHS Commissioned Corps insignia on the uniform. Driven by a passion to serve the underserved, USPHS officers fill essential public health leadership and clinical service roles with federal government agencies. Stationed in various federal agencies worldwide, they protect, promote, and advance the health and safety of the nation. When called upon, they selflessly serve as first responders to public health crises and national emergencies such as natural and man-made disasters, disease outbreaks, and terrorist events—both stateside and overseas. Some recent examples are the earthquake in Haiti (2010), the Ebola response in West Africa (2014), and the COVID-19 pandemic (2020).

Dental hygienists serve as commissioned officers in the USPHS. As such, they have the opportunity to be employed in the following varied federal agencies: Indian Health Service (IHS) and tribal facilities, Bureau of Prisons, U.S. Food and Drug Administration, Centers for Disease Control and Prevention, Health Resources and Services Administration (HRSA), National Institutes of Health, Centers for Medicare and Medicaid, and Office of the Assistant Secretary for Health. USPHS Commissioned Corps officers qualify for retirement on a par with military service retirement.

Currently, I am employed by HRSA (see Chapter 1). HRSA manages its programs through five bureaus and eleven offices; I work in the Bureau of Health Workforce (BHW), which is responsible for administering programs designed to strengthen the health workforce and connect skilled professionals to rural, urban, and tribal underserved communities nationwide. I work specifically in the Oral Health Branch of the Division of Medicine and Dentistry of the BHW. My branch manages the bureau's primary training and workforce programs for oral health professions. The purposes of these programs are to (1) increase the supply, education, and training of a qualified health workforce to improve access and distribution of oral healthcare services and (2) support states in developing and implementing innovative programs to address the dental workforce needs of designated dental HPSAs (see earlier in this chapter and Chapter 5).

Previously, I was employed by the IHS, which provides a comprehensive health service delivery system for approximately 2.6 million American Indians and Alaska Natives (AI/AN) who belong to 574 federally recognized tribes in 37 states. Care is provided directly and through community-based clinics on the reservations, which are staffed by a combination of USPHS Commissioned Corps officers, federal Civil Service employees, and direct tribal hires. A dental hygienist can follow any of these three routes to work for the IHS, all of which provide excellent employment benefits.

Responsibilities of Position

My roles and responsibilities as a Senior Public Health Analyst for HRSA include monitoring and assisting federal awardees in dental and dental hygiene training and workforce grant programs. I regularly interact with dental training institutions and monitor their progress on goals and statutory compliance, and provide technical assistance as needed. I also collaborate on projects with other internal and external stakeholder organizations and collect qualitative and quantitative information for use in future program decisions.

Prior to my move to HRSA, I had two positions with the IHS. In the first I provided clinical dental hygiene services to an appreciative, medically underserved patient population. Of special significance, I established a mobile school-based sealant and fluoride varnish program, through which over 500 AI/AN children received preventive services. During the school year, I provided care in the clinic on the reservation 1 to 2 days a week and preventive care in the schools the rest of the week.

The second position was serving a population of 2000 patients as a clinical dental hygienist and oral health promotion/disease prevention coordinator at an IHS dental clinic. Responsibilities included all aspects of direct patient dental hygiene care, assessing community oral health needs, and establishing community oral health programs, including planning, implementing, and evaluating the programs. Additional collateral duties included developing local safety training programs associated with fire safety, hazardous waste, occupational safety, blood borne pathogens, and infection control, and working on interagency collaborative health projects.

Required Qualifications and Experience

Becoming part of the USPHS Commissioned Corps Health Service requires U.S. citizenship, being less than 44 years of age (may be adjusted upward for current or prior active duty), and meeting current medical and security conditions. Also required is a qualified bachelor's degree from an accredited college or university. Dental hygienists must have graduated from a CODA-accredited dental hygiene program and have a current, unrestricted, and valid dental hygiene license to practice in one of the 50 states, Washington, D.C., the Commonwealth of Puerto Rico, the U.S. Virgin Islands, or Guam.

Qualifications for a HRSA Public Health Analyst position include completion of all requirements for an associate, bachelors, master's, doctorate, vocational, or technical degree from an accredited institution with a cumulative GPA of 3.5 or higher and demonstration of specialized experience in five public health, healthcare administration, and written and oral communication competencies. When seeking employment by IHS, prior clinical experience and a background in community oral health program planning can be beneficial but is not required.

(Continued)

DENTAL HYGIENIST MINI-PROFILE (*Cont.*)
Public Health/Clinician/Administrator

Some federal agencies have intern programs for students interested in public health. The Junior and Senior Commissioned Officer Student Training and Externship Programs with the USPHS can lead to early careers in the Commissioned Corps. The HRSA Public Health Student Intern Program provides an opportunity for professional growth and development in public health practice by serving as an ambassador for HRSA's mission in one's professional discipline, work setting, education, or community.

Personal Comment

I wanted my dental hygiene career to be professionally fulfilling and rewarding, and I was drawn to public health as my desired path to accomplish this goal. I enjoy contributing to the improvement, protection, and advancement of the oral health of our nation. I chose the USPHS for my career because it provides many different options that use our education and talents. USPHS dental hygiene officers have a unique opportunity to expand their skills beyond the boundaries of the dental clinic and can have a significant impact on improving health outcomes in the population, particularly for individuals from low-income, underserved, uninsured, underrepresented minority, health disparity, and rural population groups.

The majority of IHS locations are rural and remote, offering exciting opportunities for those who seek the "great outdoors" lifestyle. One of the joys of working with IHS was learning about the culture of the populations I served. My first assignment was at the Fort Belknap Indian Reservation in Montana, home to two tribes, Gros Ventre (People of the White Clay) and Assiniboine (Nakoda). The people of this rural community had a deep respect for the land and their culture and heritage. Their main industry is cattle ranching and agriculture. My second assignment was with the Catawba Tribe in South Carolina who also has a long history and a rich culture. Their greatest legacy is their traditional pottery that is made following strict standards. It is made from their local clay, which comes from the Catawba River and is hand rubbed with smooth river rock. Some of these river rocks are passed down to future potters through the generations. The pottery is hand formed, all natural from start to finish, never glazed or painted, and pit fired using oak wood. The Catawba Native American pottery is on display in the White House, in museums throughout the state of South Carolina, and in the Smithsonian Museum.

Advice to Future Dental Hygienists

A career with the USPHS is extremely rewarding and provides amazing benefits such as professional development, advanced education and degrees, student loan repayment, health care, and retirement. Also, you can work with multiple federal agencies in a variety of positions with diverse job descriptions. You can select an agency, community, and position that matches your personal and professional needs and preferences. It is also possible to move from one agency to another to vary your professional experiences. Be patient and persistent as you pursue a career with the USPHS and the agencies that employ USPHS officers. The application process can be cumbersome, lengthy, and slow, but it is well worth the wait and the effort.

Disclaimer

The views expressed in the article are solely the opinions of the author and do not necessarily reflect the official policies of the Department of Health and Human Services (HHS) or the Health Resources and Service Administration (HRSA), nor does mention of the names of HHS or HRSA imply endorsement by the United States government.

DENTAL HYGIENIST MINI-PROFILE
Public Health/Researcher/Educator/Advocate/Entrepreneur

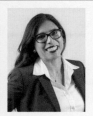

Name
Josefine Ortiz Wolfe, BSDH, MPH, PhD, RDH, CHES

Position and Place of Employment
- Assistant Professor, A.T. Still University, College of Graduate Health Studies, Kirkland, Missouri
- Consultant, Oral Health Program, Texas Health Institute, Austin, Texas
- Owner, Informed Dental Solutions PLLC, Austin, Texas

Description of Organizations
A.T. Still University College of Graduate Health Studies provides online education to prepare healthcare professionals with comprehensive health management and administrative degrees for a variety of settings.

Texas Health Institute (THI; https://www.texashealthinstitute.org/) is a nonprofit, nonpartisan public health institute. As a member of the National Network of Public Health Institutes, THI is connected with more than 8,000 subject-matter experts and organizational partners across the nation.

Informed Dental Solutions is my own business which provides me a platform for public speaking and dental consulting to provide current evidence-based education and support to oral health professionals and the general public.

Responsibilities of Positions
At A.T. Still University I teach dental public health courses in a graduate public health program that has an oral health emphasis. A variety of students are enrolled in my classes, some of whom do not have an oral health background, providing an opportunity for IPE. Some are dental students pursuing a Certificate in Public Health or a Master's in Public Health (MPH) degree. Many are practicing dental hygienists or foreign-trained dentists pursuing a MPH.

As a consultant with the Oral Health Program at THI, I am involved in oral health research, advocacy, and community engagement. What makes this work exciting is working alongside THI's partners to identify knowledge gaps and disseminate emerging evidence. In some cases, the partners are focused on oral health, and THI's research fortifies their efforts. In other cases, the partner's focus is not oral health, and THI's research informs their efforts by making the connection between oral health and overall health. The work of a researcher is the most valuable when we can translate the research into action. My background as a clinical dental hygienist gives me an understanding of patients' and providers' needs and limitations, allowing me to interpret the research into easy-to-understand, clear reports and research briefs for dental providers and oral health advocates to share with their diverse communities.

THI's research linking social determinants of health and oral health positions oral health as a critical social justice issue and demonstrates that oral health is a core component of health equity. This work allows me to work alongside nonoral partners to equip them with evidence-based research to strengthen their work and amplify their impact while concurrently advocating for oral health. The current research emphasis of the Oral Health Program at the Institute is to conduct research related to the economic impact and disparities associated with patients who seek oral care through hospital settings. Related issues are rural versus urban distribution of this care, the economic value related to lost workdays resulting from this care, and the financial burden to the healthcare system.

DENTAL HYGIENIST MINI-PROFILE *(Cont.)*

Public Health/Researcher/Educator/Advocate/Entrepreneur

Among other things, these results will provide data to advocate dental benefits for adults with disabilities and older adults.

Utilizing my platform through Informed Dental Solutions PLLC, I provide education via presentations at local, state, and national oral health conferences. I also provide consulting services to dental practices seeking support to implement current evidence-based prevention recommendations. This role also affords me the opportunity to serve as a brand ambassador and keynote speaker to bring the message of the importance of oral health to a variety of groups.

Required Qualifications and Experience

I earned a Bachelor of Science in Dental Hygiene from the University of Texas Health Science Center at San Antonio. My researcher and educator roles require an advanced degree. I hold a Master of Science in Public Health (MSPH) and a PhD in Community Health Education and Health Promotion from Walden University, and I am a CHES. My clinical experience and background in dental public health helped me understand the systems that affect access to care in our communities and allows me to offer pragmatic guidance and instruction to students. Working in private dental offices increased my understanding of the varying levels of application of evidence into dental practice.

Leadership involvement is an essential part of a career in dental public health and higher education. I serve as Chair of the Oral Health Section of the American Public Health Association. This section promotes the importance of oral health, increased access to oral health services, and advancing an interprofessional approach to oral health care. It also actively develops and promotes national policies to improve the public's oral health and overall health.

Personal Comment

My passion for community oral health was sparked by working with the Head Start program while in dental hygiene school. Upon graduation I immediately enrolled in my master's program while I also served in the National Health Service Corps (NHSC) for 2 years. I was assigned to a clinical community dental health setting within a major city health department where I worked with primarily Spanish-speaking pregnant women and children. After that I developed and coordinated a school-based sealant program for a city health department, which, over 5 years, grew to be one of the largest programs of its kind in the nation.

While completing my dissertation for my PhD, I worked as a clinical dental hygienist, temping in private dental offices. It was then that I came to appreciate the different levels of practice and gained an understanding of the challenges associated with implementing evidence-based research into a clinical setting. Because of this realization, I made it a goal to communicate data and research results to practitioners and partners in a way that it can be clearly understood, implemented, and shared with others.

My dental public health career has brought me satisfaction, knowing my work improves the lives of vulnerable, underserved, and marginalized communities. It has also afforded me many opportunities, including serving as a thought leader and in many other leadership roles and passing on opportunities to my children, both of whom I consider my greatest successes, to also follow their dreams.

Advice to Future Dental Hygienists

My work is rewarding and fulfilling, but it did not come without its challenges. I was a nontraditional student; I took my first college course in my late 20s. I was the first in my family to attend college, and navigating the education system was a challenge. I am not a native English speaker, and as a graduate student, I struggled with writing. Through most of my education, I was a full-time student and also worked full-time because I was the only parent of two young children. I believe each of us has a unique timeline and a distinctive path. Through my journey, I have learned that the things in life that are the most valuable will require the most effort. My advice to future dental hygienists is not to be discouraged by the inevitable failures or changes in your path. Forge on and stay focused on your goal. Surround yourself with professionals who are passionate about their work and mentors who will challenge you to be the best version of yourself.

DENTAL HYGIENIST MINI-PROFILE

Public Health/Clinician/Advocate/Entrepreneur/Educator

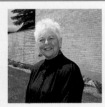

Name
Lynda McKeown, RDH, HBA, MA

Position and Place of Employment
- Independent practice dental hygienist and Owner, Oral Care, Thunder Bay, Ontario, Canada
- Oral Health Demonstrator (faculty position), Confederation College, Thunder Bay, Ontario, Canada

Description of Organizations

Oral Care is my dental hygiene independent practice (http://www.oralcare.ca/index.htm), through which I provide care in long-term care (LTC) facilities.

Confederation College has a 3-year advanced dental hygiene diploma program. It is fully accredited by CODA.

Responsibilities of Positions

As an entrepreneurial independent practice fee-for-service provider in LTC homes, I deliver hands-on palliative dental hygiene care on site to residents of LTC homes. The care consists of performing assessments, updating oral/dental care plans, and removing debris from the oral cavity using oral physiotherapy tools twice monthly to daily, depending on the needs of the individual. Frail LTC residents are no longer able to perform this task themselves. I have provided care in LTC homes for over 20 years.

As a faculty member at Confederation College, I supervise dental hygiene students participating in an externship in LTC homes. I facilitate their transfer of knowledge and skills to a community setting as they provide oral health care to residents in the LTC home rather than in a clinical setting. The students assess residents' needs and compare the results to the intake assessment data collected by nondental LTC facility staff. Oral care plans are modified as needed and shared with the staff. Through experiential learning, students also acquire the skills they need to care for this priority population that has complex medical and oral health needs.

This experience helps students realize the need for dental hygienists in nursing homes. They see and experience the deficiencies in oral assessments performed by, and daily oral hygiene care plans developed by performed by, non-dental staff. They grasp that achieving improved oral health for this population involves overcoming complex political, legislative, organizational, institutional, and financial barriers. Finally, they gain an appreciation for the reality that working with this population requires advocating their special needs. They learn that the provisions for oral/dental care required by the Long-Term Care Homes Act of 2007 in Ontario do not require the utilization of oral health professionals. The required assessment of oral/dental status, twice-daily oral hygiene, and oral care to maintain the integrity of oral tissues are assigned to a nondental personal support worker with little or no knowledge of the mouth nor experience providing oral care.

DENTAL HYGIENIST MINI-PROFILE (*Cont.*)
Public Health/Clinician/Advocate/Entrepreneur/Educator

Required Qualifications and Experience

Minimum clinical experience of 5 years and advanced education are required and necessary for faculty to effectively guide students in developing clinical skills, gaining knowledge, and integrating theory into practice. For independent practice in LTC, homes in Ontario, registration as a dental hygienist and authorization to self-initiate are required by the regulatory board, the College of Dental Hygienists of Ontario (CDHO). My learning experiences with indigenous and special needs populations, such as patients with dementia, including Alzheimer's disease, my development of the skills needed to work in LTC, and my broad dental hygiene career experience with all ages in private practice, public health, LTC, breath odor treatment, research, education, leadership in professional organizations, and advocacy have proven valuable in both teaching and my specialized entrepreneurial practice.

Personal Comment

I began my career as an independent contractor clinical dental hygienist providing periodontal treatment and oral health education. The dentist had a vision for this unique contractual arrangement to engage me as the first dental hygienist in our community. When he died, the group's vision changed and I decided to pursue a master's degree and refocus my dental hygiene career. At that time, Canada was seeking self-regulation for dental hygiene. I gained skills and confidence to be an effective advocate through my master's program, and I used the dental hygiene self-regulation struggle as the subject for my master's thesis. I also served as Chair of the Transitional Council and first President of the CDHO.

After that, I pursued many different professional roles, including serving as President of the Canadian Dental Hygienists Association, working in public health, managing and delivering treatment in a program that provided individualized treatment to patients with severe halitosis, teaching an applied sociology course to dental hygiene students, and participating in a fluoride varnish efficacy study led by University of Toronto dental faculty to address the alarming increase in early childhood caries, which resulted in the introduction of fluoride varnish into public health programs and to indigenous communities. I served as the CDHO representative to the Quality Palliative Care in Long

Term Care Alliance, which established a framework for providing palliative care and developed resources that are available free of charge on the project website (www.palliativealliance.ca). I also collaborated with a registered nurse serving as the Long-Term Care Best Practices Coordinator for the Thunder Bay District on a quality improvement initiative to advance oral care in a local LTC facility. Conference presentations, articles, and textbook chapters resulted, which have helped to strengthen understanding of best practices for LTC residents.

Throughout my dental hygiene career, I have advocated the dental hygienist's nontraditional role, finding it important to help the public and dentistry understand the value of dental hygienists functioning in alternative practice settings. By returning to Dr. Fones's vision for dental hygienists working in community settings, the profession can greatly impact access to care for marginalized and vulnerable populations.

Advice to Future Dental Hygienists

In terms of working in a community setting, my advice is to earn an advanced degree. Advanced education provides a broad understanding of communities, thus better preparing dental hygienists to promote changes in the profession to be able to meet the needs of vulnerable groups in the population. As dental hygienists we have a responsibility to be active in dental hygiene organizations, partially to advocate change. Advocating for underserved priority populations frequently requires working with government representatives and being politically engaged to influence legislative changes.

To provide oral health services for frail older adults, it is important that you enjoy working with this population. Spending time in a nursing home will expose you to their unique situation and needs. Knowledge is needed in the needs and management of frail individuals, including end-of-life medical issues; palliative care; stabilization of teeth; pharmacology in the LTC home; and strategies for effective communication, safety, and confidence to deliver patient-centered oral care to individuals with dementia. ICP experience is valuable, and connecting with a colleague who has experience working with this population will be helpful.

SUMMARY

Various career options exist for dental hygienists in the public health arena. Public health career options offer many challenges and opportunities for the dental hygienist to become actively involved in providing optimal oral health for the community. The trend of less restrictive dental hygiene regulations to facilitate the dental hygienist's desire to provide preventive treatment to underserved populations is explored, in relation to scope of practice, direct access, supervision, and reimbursement.

Workforce models are defined, which may provide an advanced career path that students can pursue to address the problems of access to oral health for underserved populations. Public health career options and public health positions for dental hygienists are available in a variety of settings. The dental hygienist may choose to develop and apply public health skills in a career path as a clinician, educator, advocate, researcher, or administrator in a public health, corporate, or entrepreneurial position. The skills and education necessary to fulfill these roles are delineated in the chapter, and dental hygienists in these various roles and positions are highlighted.

APPLYING YOUR KNOWLEDGE

1. Check with your state health department to determine if public health dental hygiene positions are available in your community. Obtain a job description, and evaluate the skills needed for this position using the dental hygiene roles and positions described in the chapter.

2. Research all available dental resources in your community for older adults who are unable to afford or travel to private dental offices. Consider whom you would contact to find out the location of these dental services. Write a job description for a position to treat older adult residents unable to have access to care in private offices.

3. Research dental supervision laws in several states including your own, and compare and contrast your state's supervision regulations to other states to determine a need for change in your state. Which populations might benefit from a change? How might you be involved in initiating a change? Report your findings in class.

4. Participate in a community rotation/service project that is considered an alternative practice setting. Report your experience and reflections about it to your class.

5. Read the law in your or another state concerning a dental hygiene-based oral health mid-level provider, and interview someone who is one. Determine how they are addressing the oral health needs of the underserved. Consider if this career option would appeal to you. Report this to your class.

6. Research current and proposed dental therapist workforce models in the U.S. Add to the information in Table 2.3 in relation to the stage of development, education and training, regulation and licensure, practice settings, supervision, and preventive, periodontal, restorative, and additional scope of practice for each model. Report this to your class.

LEARNING OBJECTIVES AND COMPETENCIES

This chapter addresses the following community oral health learning objectives and competencies for dental hygienists that are presented in the revised May 2015-2016 *ADEA Compendium of Curriculum Guidelines for Allied Dental Education Programs:*

Learning Objectives

- Explain the history of dental hygiene in relation to dental public health.
- Describe dental labor force use of and access to dental care.
- Describe the rules and regulation of the dental hygiene scope of practice.
- Advocate the use of a dental hygienist without restrictive barriers in scope of practice.
- Describe the responsibilities of dental hygienists in the U.S.
- Explain the role of dental providers, with emphasis on the dental hygienist, in activities related to the practice of public health.

- Identify target populations to whom dental hygienists may provide services.
- Describe dental public health careers.
- Describe various government-related opportunities for dental public health programs.
- Define dental hygiene positions in the areas of public health and government.

Competencies

- Providing dental hygiene services in a variety of settings, including offices, hospitals, clinics, extended care facilities, community programs, and schools.
- Providing health education and preventive counseling to a variety of population groups.
- Advocating for consumer groups, businesses and government agencies to support healthcare issues.

COMMUNITY CASE

In your position as the oral health program coordinator for the Division of Dental Health, State Health Department, you are assigned the task of developing an educational campaign to promote oral health as critical to overall health. You are also in charge of setting up a dental sealant program in a part of the state that is classified as a dental HPSA. You will be responsible for selecting schools to participate in the dental sealant program and for organizing the project, including planning all meetings, ordering supplies, supervising personnel, and arranging the schedule.

1. According to the laws of this state, a dentist must screen the children to approve the teeth for dental sealants before a dental hygienist places the sealants; the dentist does not have to be present at the time that the dental sealants are placed. Based on this information, which of the following is correct?
   a. This is an example of direct supervision.
   b. This describes a direct access state.
   c. This describes general supervision.
   d. Assessment is within the scope of practice for dental hygienists in this state.

2. You decide to set up a committee to help develop the "healthy mouth, healthy body" campaign and invite a public health nurse, a nutritionist, a mental health specialist, and a chronic disease health educator to join. This step is an example of which of the following?

   a. Advocating for policy changes
   b. Interprofessional collaborative practice
   c. Working under remote supervision
   d. Secondary prevention strategies

3. What professional career path is represented by your responsibility for the school-based sealant program?
   a. Clinician
   b. Researcher
   c. Administrator
   d. Educator

4. All of the following factors EXCEPT one relates to the determination of the location for the sealant program. Which is the EXCEPTION?
   a. The ratio of dental providers to population
   b. The number of people who do not have access to dental care
   c. The number of elementary, middle, and high schools
   d. The number of dental therapists

5. The educational campaign would be categorized as a primary prevention measure. The sealant program would be a secondary method of prevention.
   a. Both statements are true.
   b. Both statements are false.
   c. The first statement is true, the second is false.
   d. The first statement is false, the second is true.

REFERENCES

1. Nathe CN. Dental public health & research. 4th ed. New York, NY: Pearson; 2017.

2. Career Paths. American Dental Hygienists' Association. Available at: <https://www.adha.org/professional-roles>; [Accessed December 20, 2019].

3. Thinking Outside the Box: The Path to a New Career. American Dental Hygienists' Association; August 2016. Available at: <http://www.adha.org/resources-docs/72615_The_Path_to_a_New_Career.pdf>; [Accessed December 20, 2019].

4. Hartley M. Career satisfaction survey: Besides relationships with patients, what's important to dental hygienists? Dentistry IQ; April 4, 2017. Available at: <https://www.dentistryiq.com/dental-hygiene/salaries/article/16366312/career-satisfaction-survey-besides-relationships-with-patients-whats-important-to-dental-hygienists>; [Accessed December 20, 2019].

5. Fried JL, Maxey HL, Battani K, Gurenlian JR, Byrd TO, Brunick A. Preparing the future dental hygiene workforce: Knowledge, skills, and reform. J Dent Educ 2017;81(9):eS45–52. Available at: <http://www.jdentaled.org/content/81/9/eS45.long>; [Accessed December 20, 2019].

6. Public Health. American Dental Hygienists' Association. Available at: <https://www.adha.org/public-health>; [Accessed December 20, 2019].

7. Advocacy. American Dental Hygienists' Association. Available at: <https://www.adha.org/advocacy>; [Accessed December 21, 2019].

8. Facts about the Dental Hygiene Workforce in the United States. American Dental Hygienists' Association; May 2019. Available at: <http://www.adha.org/resources-docs/75118_Facts_About_the_Dental_Hygiene_Workforce.pdf>; [Accessed December 20, 2019].

9. Standard Occupational Classification. Bureau of Labor Statistics. Available at: <https://www.bls.gov/soc/>; [Accessed December 201, 2019].

10. Facts about Teledentistry. American TeleDentistry Association; 2019. Available at: <https://www.americanteledentistry.org/facts-about-teledentistry/>; [Accessed December 20, 2019].

11. Reforming America's Healthcare System Through Choice and Competition. Washington, DC: Department of Health and Human Services, Department of the Treasury, Department of Labor; December 2018. Available at: <https://www.hhs.gov/sites/default/files/Reforming-Americas-Healthcare-System-Through-Choice-and-Competition.pdf>; [Accessed December 20, 2019].

12. Faller RV. Caries process and prevention strategies: Prevention (CE Course No. 375). Dentalcare.com; September 15, 2017. Available at <https://www.dentalcare.com/en-us/professional-education/ce-courses/ce375>; [Accessed December 20, 2019].

13. Dental Hygiene Practice Act Overview: Permitted Functions and Supervision Levels by State. American Dental Hygienists' Association; July 2019. Available at: <https://www.adha.org/resources-docs/7511_Permitted_Services_Supervision_Levels_by_State.pdf>; [Accessed December 20, 2019].

14. AAPHD Policy Statements. American Association of Public Health Dentistry. Available at: <https://www.aaphd.org/policy-statements>; [Accessed December 20, 2019].

15. ADHA Policy Manual. American Dental Hygienists' Association; June 2018. Available at: <https://www.adha.org/resources-docs/7614_Policy_Manual.pdf>; [Accessed December 20, 2019].

16. Direct Access. American Dental Hygienists' Association. Available at: <https://www.adha.org/direct-access>; [Accessed December 20, 2019].

17. Direct Access States. American Dental Hygienists' Association; June 2019. Available at: <https://www.adha.org/resources-docs/7513_Direct_Access_to_Care_from_DH.pdf>; [Accessed December 20, 2019].

18. Bureau of Health Workforce. Bethesda, MD: Health Resources and Services Administration; June 2019. Available at: <https://www.hrsa.gov/about/organization/bureaus/bhw/index.html>; [Accessed December 2, 2019].

19. Dental Hygiene: Reimbursement Pathways. American Dental Hygienists' Association; November 2013. Available at: <https://www.adha.org/resources-docs/7529_Report_Reimbursement_Pathways.pdf>; [Accessed December 20, 2019].

20. Getting Started: How a Dental Hygienist May Achieve Direct Reimbursement. American Dental Hygienists' Association; November 2014. Available at: <https://www.adha.org/resources-docs/7528_Reimbursement_At_A_Glance.pdf>; [Accessed December 20, 2019].

21. Direct Medicaid Reimbursement 2018, 18 States. American Dental Hygienists' Association; November 2019. Available at: <https://www.adha.org/resources-docs/7526_Medicaid_Map.pdf>; [Accessed December 20, 2019].

22. Langelier M, Baker B, Continelli T. Development of a New Dental Hygiene Professional Practice Index by State, 2016. Rensselaer, NY: Oral Health Workforce Research Center, Center for Health Workforce Studies, School of Public Health, SUNY Albany; November 2016. Available at: <https://www.chwsny.org/wp-content/uploads/2016/12/OHWRC_Dental_Hygiene_Scope_of_Practice_2016.pdf>; [Accessed December 20, 2019].

23. Bianchi T, Borgida S, Brunton C, Monopoli M, Yee A. Dentistry's Newest Profession: Expanding Access, Creating Equity, Improving Health. Washington, DC: Grant Makers in Health; 2018. Available at: <http://www.gih.org/Publications/ViewsDetail.cfm?ItemNumber=9605>; [Accessed December 20, 2019].

24. Minjarez J, Nuzzo S. Dental Therapists: Sinking Our Teeth into Innovative Workforce Reform. Tallahassee, FL: The James Madison Institute; 2018. Available at: <https://www.jamesmadison.org/wp-content/uploads/2019/01/PolicyBrief_DentalTherapy_2019_v01.pdf/>; [Accessed December 20, 2019].

25. Scopes of Practice for Dental Therapists. Dental Council of New Zealand; 2018. Available at: <http://www.dcnz.org.nz/i-practise-in-new-zealand/dental-therapists/scopes-of-practice-for-dental-therapists/>; [Accessed December 20, 2019].

26. Alaska Dental Therapy Educational Program. Alaska Native Tribal Health Consortium; 2019. Available at <https://anthc.org/alaska-dental-therapy-education-programs/>; [Accessed December 20, 2019].

27. Wetterhall S, Bader JD, Burrus BB, Lee JY, Shugars DA. Evaluation of the Dental Health Aide Therapist Workforce Model in Alaska. Research Triangle Institute International; December 20, 2019. Available at: <http://anthc.org/wp-content/uploads/2016/02/DHAT_2010EvaluationDHATWorkforce.pdf>; [Accessed December 20, 2019].

28. Expanding Access to Care through Dental Therapy. American Dental Hygienists' Association; July 2019. Available at: <https://www.adha.org/resources-docs/Expanding_Access_to_Dental_Therapy.pdf>; [Accessed December 20, 2019].

29. Commission on Dental Accreditation; 2019. Available at: <https://www.ada.org/en/coda/current-accreditation-standards>; [Accessed December 20, 2019].

30. 2018 ADEA Annual Session Program. American Dental Education Association; 2018. Available at: <https://www.eventscribe.

com/2018/ADEA/assets/ADEA_AS2018_Program_FINAL.pdf>; [Accessed December 20, 2019].

31. 2019 National Oral Health Conference Program. American Association of Public Health Dentistry and Association of State and Territorial Dental Directors; 2019. Available at: <http://www.nationaloralhealthconference.com/pdfs/2019-NOHC-program-book.pdf>; [Accessed December 20, 2019].

32. Brickle CM, Self KD. Dental therapists as new oral health practitioners: increasing access for underserved populations. J Dent Educ 2017;81(9):e65–72. Available at: <https://doi.org/10.21815/JDE.017.036>; [Accessed December 20, 2019].

33. New Mexico's Passage of Dental Therapy Law Builds National Momentum for Changing Provision of Dental Care Amid Oral Health Crisis. Boston, MA: Community Catalyst; March 29, 2019. Available at: <https://www.communitycatalyst.org/news/press-releases/new-mexicos-passage-of-dental-therapy-law-builds-national-momentum-for-changing-provision-of-dental-care-amid-oral-health-crisis>; [Accessed December 20, 2019].

34. Bonner BL. Will House Bill 308 help solve rural NM's dental health crisis? Riudoso News; February 12, 2019. Available at: <https://www.ruidosonews.com/story/news/local/community/2019/02/12/dental-therapy-legislation-clears-first-hurdle-new-mexico-passes-house-health-and-human-services-com/2849408002/>; [Accessed December 20, 2019].

35. Solutions: About CDHCs. American Dental Association; 2019. Available at: <http://www.ada.org/en/public-programs/action-for-dental-health/community-dental-health-coordinators>; [Accessed December 20, 2019].

36. Community Dental Health Coordinator: The Value of Dental Case Management. American Dental Association; 2018. Available at: <http://media.news.health.ufl.edu/misc/cod-oralhealth/docs/conferences/2018OHF/Community%20Dental%20Health%20Coordinator.pdf>; [Accessed December 20, 2019].

37. Cole JR, Dodge WW, Findley JS, et al. Interprofessional collaborative practice: How could dentistry participate? J Dent Educ 2018;82(5):442–5. Available at: <http://www.jdentaled.org/content/jde/82/5/441.full.pdf>; [Accessed December 21, 2019].

38. Maxey HL, Farrell C, Gwozdek A. Exploring current and future roles of non-dental professionals: Implications for dental hygiene education. J Dent Educ 2017;81(9):e53–8. Available at: <http://www.jdentaled.org/content/81/9/e53.long>; [Accessed December 21, 2019].

39. Bright Futures Guidelines. American Academy of Pediatrics; 2019. Available at: <https://brightfutures.aap.org/Pages/default.aspx>; [Accessed December 21, 2019].

40. Oral Health Integration in Whole Person Care. National Interprofessional Initiative on Oral Health; 2017. Available at <https://www.niioh.org/>; [Accessed December 21, 2019].

41. Smiles for Life: A National Oral Health Curriculum, 3rd ed. Leawood, KS: Society of Teachers of Family Medicine; June 2010. Available at: <https://www.smilesforlifeoralhealth.org/buildcontent.aspx?pagekey=101552&lastpagekey=62948&userkey=15096135&sessionkey=5307429&tut=555&customerkey=84&custsitegroupkey=0>; [Accessed December 21, 2019].

42. Oral Health Toolkit. American Academy of Pediatrics; 2019. Available at: <https://www.aap.org/en-us/about-the-aap/aap-press-room/campaigns/tiny-teeth/Pages/default.aspx>; [Accessed December 21, 2019].

43. National Advisory Committee on Rural Health and Human Services. Improving Oral Health Care Services in Rural America. Washington, DC: Department of Health and Human Services; December 2018. Available at: <https://www.hrsa.gov/sites/default/files/hrsa/advisory-committees/rural/publications/2018-Oral-Health-Policy-Brief.pdf>; [Accessed December 21, 2019].

44. Halas Y, Doonan M. Integrating Oral and General Health: The Role of Accountable Care Organizations (Issue Brief). Massachusetts Health Policy Forum; 2016. Available at: <https://www.hcfama.org/sites/default/files/yara_-_white_paper_final.pdf>; [Accessed December 21, 2019].

45. Simon L. Overcoming historical separation between oral and general health care: Interprofessional collaboration for promoting health equity. AMA J Ethics 2016;18(9):941–9. Available at <https://journalofethics.ama-assn.org/article/overcoming-historical-separation-between-oral-and-general-health-care-interprofessional/2016-09>; [Accessed December 21, 2019].

46. U.S. Department of Health and Human Services, Oral Health Coordinating Committee. U.S. Department of Health and Human Services Oral Health Strategic Framework, 2014-2017. Public Health Rep 2016;131:242-257. Available at: <https://www.ncbi.nlm.nih.gov/pmc/articles/PMC4765973/pdf/phr131000242.pdf>; [Accessed December 21, 2019].

47. Core competencies for interprofessional collaborative practice. Washington, DC: Interprofessional Education Collaborative; 2016. Available at: <https://hsc.unm.edu/ipe/resources/ipec-2016-core-competencies.pdf>; [Accessed December 21, 2019].

48. Guidance on Developing Quality Interprofessional Education for the Health Professions. Chicago, IL: Health Professions Accreditors Collaborative; 2019. Available at: <https://healthprofessionsaccreditors.org/wp-content/uploads/2019/02/HPACGuidance02-01-19.pdf>; [Accessed December 21, 2019].

49. Furgeson D, Inglehart MR. Interprofessional education in U.S. dental hygiene programs: Program director responses before and after introduction of CODA Standard 2-15. J Dent Educ 2019;83(1):5–15. Available at: <http://www.jdentaled.org/content/83/1/5>; [Accessed December 21, 2019].

50. Hamil LM. Looking back to move ahead: Interprofessional education in dental education. J Dent Educ 2017;81(8):e74–80. Available at: <http://www.jdentaled.org/content/jde/81/8/e74.full.pdf>; [Accessed December 21, 2019].

51. Nathe C. Public health remains a part of dental hygiene career paths. RDH May 1, 2013;33:5e. Available at: <http://www.rdhmag.com/articles/print/volume-33/issue-5/columns/public-health-remains-a-part-of-dental-hygiene-career-paths.html>; [Accessed December 21, 2019].

52. Contreras OA, Stewart D, Vlachovic RW. Examining America's Dental Safety Net. American Dental Education Association, Office of Policy, Research, and Diversity; March 2018. Available at: <https://www.adea.org/policy/white-papers/Dental-Safety-Net.aspx>; [Accessed December 21, 2019].

53. Safety Net Dental Clinic Manual. Georgetown University, National Maternal and Child Oral Health Resource Center. Available at: <https://www.dentalclinicmanual.com/index.php>; [Accessed December 21, 2019].

54. Bright Smiles, Bright Futures®. Colgate-Palmolive; 2019. Available at: <http://www.colgate.com/app/BrightSmilesBrightFutures/US/EN/Our-Commitment.cvsp>; [Accessed December 21, 2019].

ADDITIONAL RESOURCES

A Qualitative Case Study of the Legislative Process of the Hygienist-therapist Bill in a Large Midwestern State, Dollins, Bray, & Fadbury-Amyot (dental therapy legislation)
https://jdh.adha.org/content/87/5/275

Bills into Law 2017; American Dental Hygienists' Association (dental therapy legislation)
https://www.adha.org/resources-docs/75110_Bills_Signed_Into_Law.pdf
Dental Hygiene Professional Practice Index project report
https://www.chwsny.org/wp-content/uploads/2016/12/OHWRC_Dental_Hygiene_Scope_of_Practice_2016.pdf
Groundbreaking Legislation, J. Rethman (dental therapy legislation)
https://dimensionsofdentalhygiene.com/article/groundbreaking-legislation/
Information on innovative workforce models and practice issues
https://www.adha.org/practice-issues

Resources to advocate change related to dental hygiene practice issues and innovative workforce models
www.adha.org/resources
The History of Introducing a New Provider in Minnesota: A Chronicle of Legislative Efforts 2008-2009, American Dental Hygienists' Association (dental therapy legislation)
http://www.adha.org/resources-docs/75113_Minnesota_Story.pdf
The Origins of Minnesota's Mid-level Dental Practitioner: Alignment of Problem, Political and Policy Streams, Gwozdek, Tetrick, & Shaefer (dental therapy legislation)
https://jdh.adha.org/content/88/5/292

Assessment for Community Oral Health Program Planning

Amanda M. Hinson-Enslin and Christine French Beatty

OBJECTIVES

1. Discuss the mission of public health and how various organizations have worked together to enhance the recognition and validity of public health professions.
2. Explain the importance of assessment as a core public health function.
3. Describe public health professionals' roles in assessment.
4. Apply basic epidemiology concepts to assessment.
5. Describe the conceptual models that illustrate the determinants of health.

6. Identify the determinants of health for individuals and communities, especially recognizing the importance of social determinants; apply to public health practice.
7. Apply the community oral health improvement process.
8. Describe the main steps followed and key activities undertaken in a community oral health assessment.
9. Compare and contrast the different types of data and methods of data collection used in community oral health assessments.

OPENING STATEMENT: Community Snapshot

- Population of 87,214 with 25,431 households
- Sex: 57.2% male; 42.8% female
- Race/ethnicity: 58% Hispanic; 19% white; 15% African American; 5% Asian; 3% other
- Median resident age: 28.3 years
- Geography: 62% rural and 38% urban; 789 square miles of land
- Industry: tobacco farming area; majority of population are migrant farm workers
- Median household income level: $39,000; range of $18,000 to $82,000
- Education level of people age 25 and older: 10% completed college; 19% completed some college; 45% completed only high school; 26% did not complete high school
- Language: 48% Spanish speaking
- Environment:
  - No community water fluoridation
  - Access to oral health care: limited because of lack of dental workforce; area identified by the U.S. Department of Health and Human Services Health Resources and Services Administration (HRSA) as a **dental health professional shortage area** (see Chapters 2 and 5)
  - Income: 45% below the **federal poverty level** and qualify for Medicaid
  - No dental sealant programs in the schools; fluoride varnish program present in all public schools
  - One community-based health clinic with a dental component
  - Limited public transportation to community-based health clinic
- Oral health attributes:
  - No dental visit for 45% of elementary schoolchildren within the last year and 33% within the last 5 years
  - Untreated dental caries in 42% of 3- to 9-year-old children
  - At least one sealant present on a permanent molar in 7% of 6- to 9-year-old children and 9% of 13- to 15-year-old adolescents
- Resource availability:
  - Grant funding available for school-based sealant program
  - Mobile dental equipment available at community-based clinic
  - Oral health workforce available one Thursday and one Friday a month to place sealants and treat dental caries
  - Three local business leaders willing to assist with funding and facilities

PUBLIC HEALTH PRACTICE

Professional work in community health is dynamic because the environment changes continually. Community health is affected by social, demographic, political, economic, and technological changes. Public health practitioners perform a broad array of duties focused on entire populations, with the overarching goal that people are healthy and live in healthy communities.[1,2] The mission of public health focuses on preventing disease and providing an environment in which people can live and function healthily (see Chapter 1). Public health services incorporate the roles of a myriad of public health professionals in various sectors and from diverse disciplines that form the public health workforce in the U.S. (see Chapters 2 and 5).[1,2] The focus of this chapter is assessment in relation to epidemiology and public health practice. It is supported by the definitions and explanation of terminology specific to assessment and epidemiology in the Glossary.

Professional Preparation of the Public Health Workforce

Public health professionals have expertise in diverse public health practices.[1,2] Several organizations and agencies have met the charge to increase the workforce and visibility of public health; however, there is still a need to build a comprehensive public health workforce across several health disciplines.[3] As a result, collaborative efforts have been undertaken to enhance the recognition of the public health professions by measuring and improving the competency and consistency of public health workers nationwide. Several credentialing examinations serve the purpose of improving and boosting the recognition of the

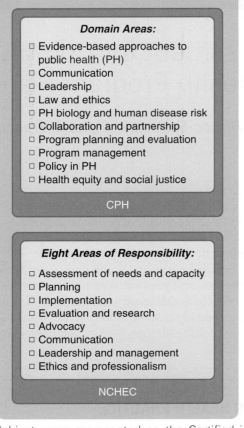

Domain Areas:

□ Evidence-based approaches to
  public health (PH)
□ Communication
□ Leadership
□ Law and ethics
□ PH biology and human disease risk
□ Collaboration and partnership
□ Program planning and evaluation
□ Program management
□ Policy in PH
□ Health equity and social justice

CPH

Eight Areas of Responsibility:

□ Assessment of needs and capacity
□ Planning
□ Implementation
□ Evaluation and research
□ Advocacy
□ Communication
□ Leadership and management
□ Ethics and professionalism

NCHEC

Fig 3.1 Subject areas represented on the Certified in Public Health (CPH) and National Commission for Health Education Credentialing, Inc (NCHEC) examinations. (From CPH Content Outline. Washington, DC: National Board of Public Health Examiners; 2019. Available at: <https://www.nbphe.org/cph-content-outline/>; [Accessed April 2020]; HESPA II 2020: Eight Areas of Responsibility. Whitehall, PA: National Commission for Health Education Credentialing, Inc.; 2020. Available at: <https://www.nchec.org/responsibilities-and-competencies>; [Accessed February 2020].)

public health professions by ensuring that graduates of undergraduate and graduate public health programs and schools have mastered the knowledge and skills relevant to contemporary public health practice.

First, the Certified in Public Health (CPH) examination, established and administered by the National Board of Public Health Examiners, ensures competency of graduates from public health schools and programs accredited by the Council on Education for Public Health (CEPH).[4] This national examination covers ten domains or knowledge areas relevant to contemporary public health and is offered in CEPH-accredited schools and programs[4] (Figure 3.1).

Second, the National Commission for Health Education Credentialing, Inc. (NCHEC) provides a Certified Health Education Specialist (CHES) certification and an advanced credentialing, the Master Certified Health Education Specialist (MCHES).[5] Health educators strive to promote healthy behaviors and empower individuals, groups, and communities to adopt healthy behaviors and maintain those healthy behaviors

throughout life.[5] The tasks necessary to fulfill mastery of the CHES and MCHES national examinations are organized within eight areas of responsibility[5] (see Figure 3.1).

In addition, the Council on Linkages Between Academia and Public Health Practice developed a set of core competencies for public health professionals to help strengthen public health workforce development.[6] These competencies guide academic institutions and training providers to develop curricula and course content and to evaluate public health education and training programs. The competencies are divided into eight domains:[6]

• Analytical/assessment skills
• Policy development/program planning skills
• Communication skills
• Cultural competency skills
• Community dimensions of practice skills
• Public health sciences skills
• Financial planning and management skills
• Leadership and systems thinking skills

The core competencies were crafted to transcend the boundaries of specific disciplines, to help unify the public health professions and to assure that necessary skills are built for the provision of these services. Academic institutions and health departments nationwide, the Centers for Disease Control and Prevention (CDC), the Centers for Public Health Preparedness (CPHP), and the HRSA-funded Public Health Training Centers have used the core competencies to extend capacity and to ensure that public health professionals have expertise in key public health services.[6]

Public Health Preparation of the Oral Health Workforce

The American Dental Association[7] and other definitions of dental public health (see Guiding Principles in Chapter 1) reflect the domains, areas of responsibilities, and competencies of public health practice as they relate to oral health. The American Dental Education Association (ADEA) and the Commission on Dental Accreditation (CODA) have developed competencies and accreditation standards, respectively, that emphasize dental public health in the education of the oral health workforce. According to the ADEA *Competencies for the New General Dentist,* dentists should be able to "provide prevention, intervention, and educational strategies" and "recognize and appreciate the need to contribute to the improvement of oral health beyond those served in a traditional practice setting."[8] Compared with previous standards, current CODA accreditation standards for the dental curriculum more strongly emphasize community in terms of advocacy.[9] The new CODA dental therapy education accreditation standards include requirements to prepare dental therapists to practice in community-based programs.[10] CODA also has established accreditation standards for the specialty program in dental public health.[11]

The CODA accreditation standards and ADEA curriculum guidelines for dental hygiene have greater emphasis on community oral health than those for prespecialty dental education programs and dental therapy education programs. According to CODA standards, dental hygiene graduates must be able to assess the needs of a community, plan and implement an oral health program, and evaluate its effectiveness.[12] The ADEA dental hygiene curriculum guidelines include objectives and competencies specifically related to community oral health[13] (see Appendix B), some of which are highlighted in each chapter of this textbook. These overlap the public health domains, areas of responsibility, and competencies described in the previous section. The accreditation standards and curriculum guidelines reflect high community oral health practice expectations for the dental hygiene profession. In addition, the ADEA competencies for graduate-level dental hygiene education have an even stronger emphasis on community oral health in terms of advocacy, public health policy, program development and administration, health promotion, facilitation of collaborative partnerships, and other related content areas.[14]

Collaboration in Public Health Practice

Successful provision of public health services requires collaboration among public, nonprofit, and private partners within a given community, across various levels of government, and across disciplines.[15,16] To accomplish this, partnerships must have broad-based representation of constituency and **stakeholder** groups, including private, voluntary, nonprofit, and public agencies or organizations involved in overall health, mental health, substance abuse, environmental health protection, oral health, and public health.[15,16]

A **coalition** is a type of collaboration; it is an alliance of multiple groups, organizations, and individuals whose combined actions are aimed at accomplishing a specific, common goal.[15] Coalitions exist to bring broader attention and action to a goal that affects many stakeholders and may disband when the goal is achieved.[16,17] There is power in the combined efforts of the members of the coalition to provide the capacity to mobilize resources to approach community oral health problems and to identify and implement solutions. Figure 3.2 provides

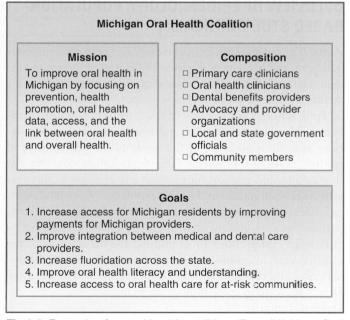

Fig 3.2 Example of an oral health coalition. (From Michigan Oral Health Coalition; 2018. Available at: <http://www.mohc.org/>; [Accessed February 2020].)

an example of a statewide oral health coalition. Appendix C provides a framework that can guide the process of creating a community oral health coalition, and a *Coalition Building Toolkit* is available in the Additional Resources at the end of this chapter. Examples of organizations, agencies, and other groups that can be engaged in coalitions and collaborative partnerships to improve the oral health of communities are presented in Appendix A and Appendix C. Partnerships will be discussed in more detail later in this chapter.

ASSESSMENT: A CORE PUBLIC HEALTH FUNCTION

Three core public health functions, assessment, policy development, and assurance, shape the basic practice of public health at the federal, state, and local levels[18] (see Box 1.5 in Chapter 1). Health agencies and departments must perform these functions to protect and promote health, wellness, and quality of life and to prevent disease, injury, disability, and death. This chapter emphasizes the core public health function of assessment.

Public health agencies promote, facilitate, and—when necessary and appropriate—perform community health assessments, as well as **monitor** changes in key measures to evaluate program performance. **Assessment** is defined as the regular and systematic collection, assemblage, and analysis of data resulting in communication regarding the health of the community.[15,16] Assessment, also referred to as needs assessment, includes statistics on health **status** and **trends**, community health needs, epidemiologic and other studies of health problems, **determinants of health**, and related factors.[15,16] The continual assessment of needs, which is considered surveillance, is discussed in Chapter 4. Chapter 5 explains the outcomes of surveillance, presenting the status and trends of oral health and related factors for the U.S. population. This provides useful data for a community health assessment.

Roles of Public Health Professionals in Assessment

The effective use of information in the 21st century is crucial to ensure that healthy children and adults are living in healthy communities. Technologies available to public health professionals influence their capacity and ability to generate and access a vast amount of information. In addition, evidence-based decision-making is shaping the development of public health policies, programs, and practices. Therefore, it is essential for public health practitioners to have skills in collecting, analyzing, disseminating, and effectively using data and information.[16] In addition, public health professionals must be able to perform certain functions (Figure 3.3).

Dental hygienists in public health are expected to play a leadership role in community oral health assessments.[19] As agencies and organizations take on greater responsibility in conducting periodic assessments, public health dental hygienists will be involved in evaluating assets, needs, problems, and resources of the **populations** they serve in the community. Dental public health professionals working at the national, state, and local levels will be responsible for community oral health assessment.[12] The essential public health services for oral health (see

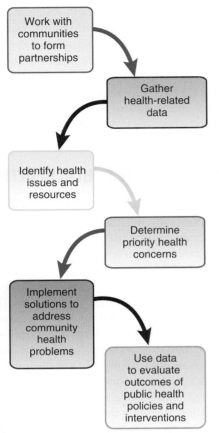

Fig 3.3 Public health workers need the knowledge, skills, and attitudes to perform these functions. (From Guidelines for State and Territorial Oral Health Programs Part II. Reno, NV: Association of State and Territorial Dental Directors; 2018 Jan. Available at: <https://www.astdd.org/docs/astdd-guidelines-section-II-matrix-for-state-roles-examples-and-resources-1-2018-revisions.pdf>; [Accessed April 2020].)

Chapters 1, 4, and 6) can be applied to assessment and evaluation (see Guiding Principles).

GUIDING PRINCIPLES

Essential Public Health Services for Oral Health Related to Assessment and Evaluation

- Assess oral health status and needs of the community.
- Assess public perceptions about oral health issues.
- Analyze determinants of identified oral health needs, including resources.
- Assess the fluoridation status of water systems and other sources of fluoride.
- Implement an oral health surveillance system to identify, investigate, and monitor oral health issues, problems, and risk factors.
- Evaluate the effectiveness, accessibility, and quality of population-based and personal oral health services.
- Conduct and support research projects to gain new insights and applications of innovative solutions to oral health problems.

Dental hygienists working within the public, private, or nonprofit sectors must have the skills to assess community oral health problems and to evaluate outcomes of population-based and personal oral health services. Dental hygienists working in

BOX 3.1   Examples of Roles of Public Health Dental Hygienists in Assessment

- A public health dental hygienist serves on a committee with the state oral health coalition. The committee collaborates with the state oral health program to develop a comprehensive document describing the burden of oral disease in the state. The report includes sections on the prevalence of disease and unmet needs, oral health disparities, and the societal impact of oral disease.
- An oral health program director evaluates the State Oral Health Plan by assessing the attainment of goals and objectives related to oral health promotion, disease prevention and control, and risk factors.
- An oral health policy analyst determines the number and geographic distribution of dentists statewide who participate in Medicaid and the state Children's Health Insurance Program (CHIP) to provide oral health care to children.
- An oral health program administrator with a city health department assesses the oral health assets, needs, and resources of a metropolitan area.
- An oral health educator assesses the knowledge, attitudes, and opinions of a community about water fluoridation to develop an oral health promotion campaign.
- A public health dental hygienist from a county health department assesses the occurrence of dental sealants in third-grade children in schools within the county.
- An oral health program manager evaluates the quality and outcomes of clinical preventive services in a school-based oral health program.
- An oral health services provider monitors oral health indicators in the neighborhood surrounding a community health center.
- A dental hygienist appointed to a state oral health advisory committee evaluates the performance measures in a work plan to implement state-level programs for water fluoridation and school-based dental sealants.

community settings generally participate in a variety of assessment and evaluation activities. Examples of some of these roles and potential activities are presented in Box 3.1.

OVERVIEW OF EPIDEMIOLOGY: POPULATION-BASED STUDY OF HEALTH

Public health dental hygienists involved in assessment and evaluation should become well versed in the basic concepts of epidemiology, which is a core science of community health. This section provides a broad overview of epidemiology.

Epidemiology is the study of the distribution and determinants of health-related states and events in specified populations and the application of this study to the prevention and control of health problems.[20] Epidemiologists consider the interactions and relationships among the multiple factors that influence health status and health problems.[16,20] Methods used in epidemiology and research are combined to focus on comparisons among groups or defined populations. Epidemiologists make comparisons by examining the occurrences of the health events, locations, times, and variations to assess the distribution and determinants of health events.[16,20] The principal factors analyzed in epidemiology are as follows:

- Distribution
- Population dynamics
- Occurrences
- Affected populations

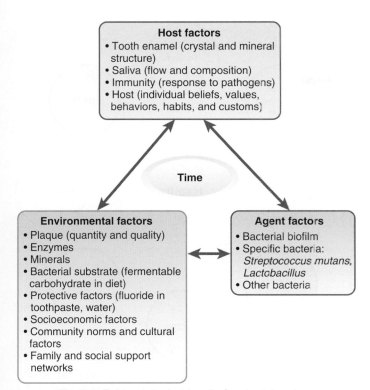

Host factors
- Tooth enamel (crystal and mineral structure)
- Saliva (flow and composition)
- Immunity (response to pathogens)
- Host (individual beliefs, values, behaviors, habits, and customs)

Time

Environmental factors
- Plaque (quantity and quality)
- Enzymes
- Minerals
- Bacterial substrate (fermentable carbohydrate in diet)
- Protective factors (fluoride in toothpaste, water)
- Socioeconomic factors
- Community norms and cultural factors
- Family and social support networks

Agent factors
- Bacterial biofilm
- Specific bacteria: *Streptococcus mutans, Lactobacillus*
- Other bacteria

Fig 3.4 Epidemiologic triangle for dental caries.

- Place characteristics
- Time
- Determinants

Common terms that describe the **occurrence** of disease in the population are **endemic, epidemic**, and **pandemic**. For example, most oral diseases such as dental caries and periodontitis are endemic in the U.S. population. The ideal is the **eradication** of a disease, which requires a firm understanding of the causative agents and factors.

Epidemiologic Triangle

Epidemiology is based on a **multifactorial approach**, with consideration given to the interacting relationships among host factors, agent factors, and environmental factors.[16,20] Disease or health status depends on multiple factors such as exposure to a specific agent, the strength of the agent, susceptibility of the host, and environmental conditions.[16,20] Health represents a general balance among these factors. Health problems occur when the balance is threatened by changes in the host, agent, or environment over time. Prevention is concerned with maintaining or initiating a balance of these factors over time.

The **epidemiologic triangle** depicts disease as the outcome of these multiple factors.[21] As an example, Figure 3.4 portrays the epidemiologic triangle in relation to dental caries, depicting the multifactorial nature of the disease influenced by host, agent, and environmental factors over time.[22]

Host Factors

The host is the individual potentially affected by the disease in question. **Host factors** (see Figure 3.4) relate primarily to susceptibility and resistance through biologic immunity, knowledge and cognition, behavior modification, screening, and

personal power. Age, gender, **socioeconomic status** (SES), race, ethnicity, culture, genetic endowment, behavior, physiologic condition, nutritional state, previous exposure, and other factors influence susceptibility and resistance.[16,20]

Agent Factors

Agent factors (see Figure 3.4) are the biologic or mechanical means of causing disease, illness, injury, or disability, such as microbial, parasitic, viral, or bacterial pathogens or vectors; physical or mechanical irritants; chemicals; drugs; trauma; and radiation. Biology, marketing, engineering, regulations, and legislation can influence agent factors.[16,20]

Environmental Factors

Environmental factors (see Figure 3.4) include physical, sociocultural, sociopolitical, and economic components. The media, beliefs, occupation, food sources, geography, climate, housing, social roles, technology, and other factors can influence environmental conditions.[16,20]

Time

In the center of the triangle is **time** (see Figure 3.4). This can represent the length of time it takes for damage or symptoms to occur, before death or recovery occurs, or from infection to the threshold of an epidemic for a population.[21] In this respect, time varies for different diseases, conditions, and individuals.[20]

Uses of Epidemiology

Epidemiology can be used to provide different types of data and information.[20] Epidemiologists in public health agencies are responsible for surveillance, investigation, analysis, and evaluation.[20] The various uses of epidemiology are presented in Box 3.2.

Changing Perspectives of Health

Major transformations have taken place during the last century in the concepts of health and the understanding of the **etiology** of diseases, disabilities, and injuries. These expanded visions

---

BOX 3.2 Uses of Epidemiology

- Describe patterns among groups.
- Describe normal biologic processes.
- Elucidate mechanisms of disease transmission.
- Describe the trends of **acute** and **chronic** diseases.
- Test hypotheses for prevention and control of diseases, injuries, disabilities, and deaths through population studies.
- Evaluate services (e.g., community preventive services, population-based health promotion services, and clinical health services).
- Study nondisease health and social problems (e.g., occurrences of intentional and unintentional injuries).
- Measure distributions of health status, diseases, injuries, disabilities, births, and deaths in populations.
- Identify determinants (e.g., protective and risk factors, social factors, policies) for death or acquiring diseases, injuries, and disabilities.
- Evaluate interventions and strategies to prevent and control diseases, disabilities, injuries, and deaths.
- Predict trends of diseases, disabilities, injuries, and deaths.
- Identify health assets, gaps, needs, problems, resources, solutions, and partnerships within the context of a community assessment.

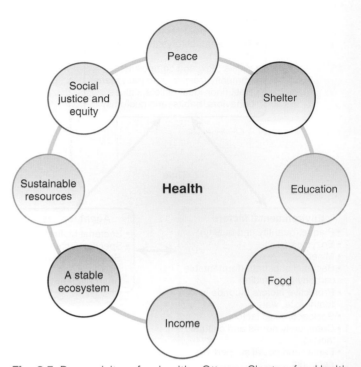

Fig 3.5 Prerequisites for health, Ottawa Charter for Health Promotion. (From Health Promotion: The Ottawa Charter for Health Promotion. Geneva: World Health Organization; 2019. Available at: <http://www.who.int/healthpromotion/conferences/previous/ottawa/en/>; [Accessed September 2019].)

continue to contribute to changes in clinical health care and public health practice. Box 3.3 outlines broad trends influencing the conceptions of health and health practice in the 21st century.

Many factors have been identified as influences on the health of individuals and populations.[16,20,23] Several are generally recognized as broader **risk factors** in relation to health (e.g., employment, educational levels, environmental state, income, economic factors, shelter, food, social justice and equity, relationships with family and friends, social supports, peace and safety, culture, and race relations). Other factors (e.g., language, learning, meaningful work, recreation, self-esteem, personal control) are considered contributors to well-being. Some factors are circumstantial, whereas others are genetic. [16,20]

As a result, there has been an expansion of the concepts of health and disease prevention from an individual focus toward a human **ecologic approach**.[24] First, health has become more than just the absence of disability and disease. The 1948 **World Health Organization** (WHO) definition of health, "a state of complete physical, social and mental well-being, and not merely the absence of disease or infirmity,"[25] is considered a standard today.[16] Second, the fundamental conditions and resources for health that were first described in 1986 by the WHO in the Ottawa Charter for Health Promotion[26] (Figure 3.5) are still considered the foundational components of maintaining and improving health.[16,26] These concepts are reflected in the multifactorial approach to health.[27]

Health promotion was discussed in the Ottawa Charter as the process of enabling people to increase control over and to improve their health.[26] To reach a state of complete physical, mental, and social well-being, an individual or group must be able to identify and realize aspirations, satisfy needs, and change or cope with the environment. Health was therefore seen as a resource for everyday life rather than the objective of living. Health was viewed as a positive concept emphasizing social and personal resources and physical capacities.[26] These principles of health promotion are still accepted today.[16]

As a result, health promotion has moved past a focus on only individual behavior toward encompassing a wide range of social and environmental interventions.[16,28] Currently, health promotion theory uses a complex, holistic, interactive approach, with a systems orientation focused on healthy people living in healthy communities. Health promotion approaches embrace the principles of population health, social ecology, epidemiology, and community participation. Thus it is no longer just the responsibility of the health sector,[27] and it goes beyond healthy lifestyles to well-being.[28,29]

DETERMINANTS OF HEALTH

Many models describing the multiple factors that influence the extensive dimensions of health in individuals and populations were developed in the second half of the 20th century as multicausal perspectives of health and disease began to take precedence over monocausal models.[16,20] The concept of a "web of causation" emerged as multifactorial perspectives grew. The far-reaching range of multiple factors that contribute to the health status of individuals and populations has come to be referred to as determinants of health.[23]

The recognition of a broader view of health has resulted in placing greater importance on these determinants of health.[23,28,30,31] They are described as having a comprehensive influence on collective and personal well-being with a profound impact on the health of individuals, families, communities, nations, and the world. In other words, whether people are healthy or not is determined largely by circumstances and environment, and the context of people's lives influences their health. Also, individuals are unlikely to be able to directly control many of the determinants of health.

BOX 3.4 Determinants of Health

Policymaking:

Definition: Local, state, and federal level laws and regulations that affect individual and population health.

Examples:

- A city ordinance that prohibits smoking in public and government buildings to prevent second-hand smoke inhalation.
- State law requirement that seat belts be worn in cars to protect people in the event of a car accident.
- Community water fluoridation to prevent dental caries.

Social:

Definition: Also known as social and physical determinants; the social factors and physical conditions in the environment in which people are born, live, learn, play, work, and age; they impact a wide range of health, functioning, and quality of life outcomes.

Examples:

- Social determinants: Socioeconomic conditions, such as concentrated **poverty**, transportation options to reach healthcare and oral healthcare clinics, quality of schools.
- Physical determinants: Housing, parks, sidewalks, biking lanes, ramps and sidewalk cuts to accommodate individuals with physical disabilities trying to access oral healthcare services.

Health Services:

Definition: Access to health services and the quality of health services

Examples:

- Availability of the oral health workforce in rural areas.
- Access to healthcare providers who speak the same language as the patient.
- Insurance and dental insurance coverage.

Individual Behavior:

Definition: Actions of individuals that influence their personal health.

Examples:

- Quitting smoking, resulting in reduction of risk for cancer and other conditions, including periodontal disease.
- Changing one's diet to improve overall health and reduce the risk of developing dental caries.
- Practicing adequate oral hygiene, which depends on, among other things, access to suitable and sufficient oral hygiene tools and supplies.

Biology and Genetics:

Definition: Basic biological and organic make-up of the human body; also, the inherited predispositions to specific diseases and conditions.

Examples:

- Age
- Sex
- Inherited conditions (e.g., congenitally missing teeth, tooth morphology)
- Family history of a condition (e.g., cancer, heart disease, or diabetes; familial transmission of bacteria associated with dental caries)
- Birth defects (e.g., physical and mental disabilities, cleft lip, cleft palate)

(From Determinants of Health, Healthy People 2020. Rockville, MD: Office of Disease Prevention and Health Promotion; 2019. Available at: <http://www.healthypeople.gov/2020/about/foundation-health-measures/Determinants-of-Health>; [Accessed September 2019].)

Box 3.4 presents one way to organize the categories of the determinants of health, including definitions and examples of each category. The specific categories interact and influence each other continuously, do so differently during different stages of human development, and vary in importance in different situations.[28] To improve health in the future, plans, policies, and programs should be directed toward these health determinants.[16,31]

Social Determinants of Health

One of the categories of the determinants of health is social determinants. A greater emphasis has developed on the **social determinants of health.**[28,30–33] These social determinants are shaped by the distribution of money, power, and resources at global, national, state, and local levels, which are themselves influenced by policy choices.[28,30,32,33] Social determinants affect a wide range of health risks and outcomes and are primarily responsible for **health inequities**[28,30,33]—the unfair, unjust, unnecessary, and avoidable differences in health status seen among various populations.[34] Social determinants have become the targets for refocused strategies for population health in the U.S.[28,30,32] and have a much greater focus in *Healthy People 2030* than in previous editions of *Healthy People*[28,30] (see Guiding Principles).

GUIDING PRINCIPLES

Key Areas to Address to Impact Social Determinants of Health

1. Economic stability
   - Poverty
   - Employment
   - Food security
   - Housing stability
2. Education
   - High school graduation
   - Enrollment in higher education
   - Educational attainment in general
   - Language and literacy
   - Early childhood education and development
3. Social and community context
   - Social cohesion
   - Civic participation
   - Discrimination
   - Conditions within the workplace
   - Incarceration
4. Health and health care
   - Access to health care
   - Access to primary care
   - Health insurance coverage
   - Health literacy
5. Neighborhood and built environment
   - Availability of healthy foods
   - Access to transportation
   - Quality of housing
   - Neighborhood crime and violence
   - Quality of the water or air

(From Social Determinants of Health: Frequently Asked Questions: How are the Healthy People domains defined? Atlanta, GA: Centers for Disease Control and Prevention; 2019 Sep. Available at: <https://www.cdc.gov/socialdeterminants/faqs/index.htm>; [Accessed April 2020].)

Determinants of Health in Relation to Oral Health

The same principles of health determinants that relate to various other health conditions also apply to oral health.[35] The determinants of health described in Box 3.4 are illustrated in Figure 3.6 with oral health examples of the determinants for greater understanding. The community snapshot in the Opening Statement also depicts determinants of health and their impact on oral health inequities in a population.

The Association of State and Territorial Dental Directors has highlighted numerous recent efforts that include strategies that apply determinants of health to oral health.[36] These include initiatives that focus on cultural competence, emphasize health literacy, and establish frameworks to assess and create partnerships to improve social determinants related to oral health. Toolboxes are included also for use in reframing oral health in light of health determinants. In addition, the American Academy of Pediatric Dentistry has recently adopted a policy that supports professional education, professional practices, research, and policies that address the effects of determinants of health on oral health,[37] and in 2019, CODA proposed incorporating the determinants of health into the accreditation standards for advanced dental education programs in pediatric dentistry.[38]

Transformations in relation to the meaning of health, importance of quality of life, multiple causation, and the oral-systemic link necessitate a collaborative approach to solving oral health problems within communities. By adopting a holistic approach to improving oral health, emphasizing interprofessional collaborative practice, and working with partner agencies and organizations, dental public health professionals can achieve the aim of improving both the oral health and overall health of populations by addressing **health disparities**.

THE COMMUNITY HEALTH PROGRAM PLANNING PROCESS

The **program planning process** is a model commonly used in public health practice, providing a basic flowchart of steps to (1) **assess** a community to identify the primary health issues, (2) **plan** a measurable process and outcome objectives to measure progress in addressing the health issues, (3) select and plan effective health **interventions** to help achieve the objectives, (4) **implement** the selected health interventions, and (5) **evaluate** the selected interventions based on objectives and use the evaluation results to improve the oral health program.[15] Also referred to as the *community health improvement process*, the community health program planning process can serve as the framework to develop an oral health plan, design a dental public health intervention, and measure oral health outcomes to quantify the performance of a program at a population level.

The program planning process is continuous, and each step can be further subdivided into detailed steps for a long-term health improvement process in the community.[15] Figure 3.7 illustrates the community health program planning process with these detailed steps outlined. This process can be applied to any size program, whether on a large scale at the state or community level, or on a smaller scale with a priority group, such as a school, residential facility for older adults, Head Start program, or community-based health center.

Following a process for community health program planning is critical; however, it is also essential to understand the need for flexibility in public health practice. Because of the dynamics in community health, new circumstances can arise, making it necessary to adjust a plan. Sometimes activities initially outlined in a plan may not be followed sequentially, necessitating modifications in the work plan. Even so, all the steps of the program planning process should be included in a plan to guide the process and assure effective community oral health programs.[15,16]

Following such a program planning process for community oral health programs allows a methodical approach of assessing different factors; considering various options for actions, policies, programs, and initiatives in the planning phase; implementing well-thought-out ideas; and evaluating outcomes to track progress and determine long-range actions. Thus, this process can support a coordinated community effort of assessment, planning, implementation, and evaluation. When these efforts are established over time into the community fabric, long-term oral health benefits are likely to be achieved by the community.

The Division of Oral Health of the CDC has developed a page called Oral Health Programs on their website.[39] The materials on this resource page focus on standards and priorities of the CDC for surveillance, monitoring, and evaluation. Their purpose is to assist dental public health programs in the

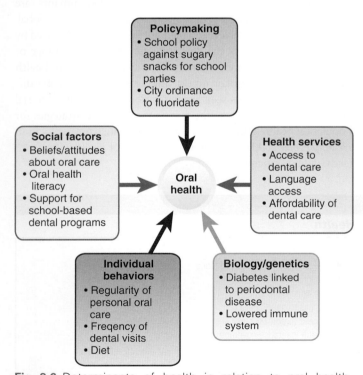

Fig 3.6 Determinants of health in relation to oral health. (Modified from Determinants of Health, Healthy People 2020. Rockville, MD: Office of Disease Prevention and Health Promotion; 2019. Available at: <http://www.healthypeople.gov/2020/about/foundation-health-measures/Determinants-of-Health>; [Accessed September 2019].)

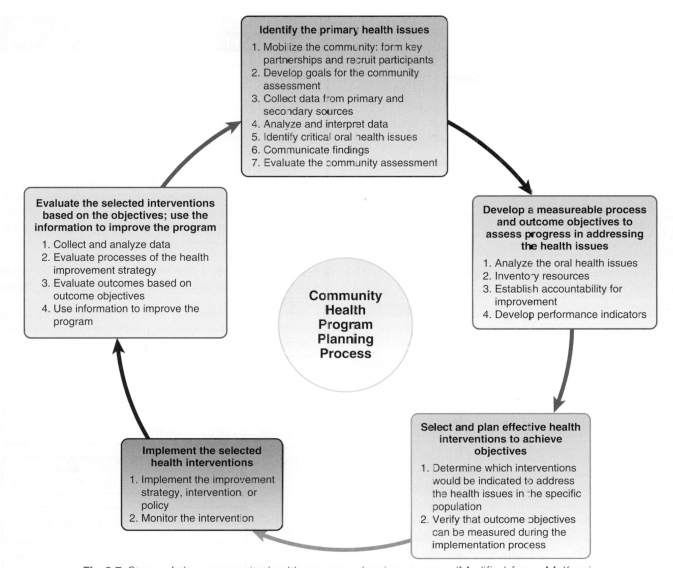

Fig 3.7 Steps of the community health program planning process. (Modified from: McKenzie JF, Neiger BL, Thackeray R. Planning, Implementing & Evaluating: Health Promotion Programs: A Primer, 7th ed. Glenview, IL: Pearson Education, Inc; 2017; Community Tool Box. Lawrence, KS: Work Group for Community Health and Development, University of Kansas; 2019 Available at: <https://ctb.ku.edu/en>; [Accessed September 2019].)

planning, designing, implementation, and evaluation of programs, using practical and increasingly comprehensive evaluation of oral health promotion and disease prevention efforts. "How-to" guides are provided for planning and implementing assessment activities using logic models for guidance.

Assessment of Oral Health in Communities

The planning of a community oral health program follows the same process that is used to plan any other community health program.[40] The first step of the community health program planning process is to identify the primary health issues by conducting a community assessment.[15,16] A **community oral health assessment** should be developed on the basis of the specific aims of the assessment and the available resources, special circumstances, and expertise in the community. The essential components that are reviewed in this section should be included in all

community oral health assessments, regardless of the size of the community or the purpose of the assessment. The upcoming content provides an overview of assessment as a key component within a comprehensive process that communities can adopt to improve oral health.

A community oral health assessment is a multifaceted process that is community-oriented and community-directed. An oral health assessment considers assets, gaps, needs, problems, resources, solutions, and partnerships within the context of the community. Its purposes are to identify factors that affect the oral health of a population and to determine the availability of resources and interventions that can be used to impact these factors to improve oral health.[15,16] Communities are better served and improved outcomes are more sustainable when assets-oriented assessment methods are used, in contrast to deficiency-based approaches that focus only on needs and

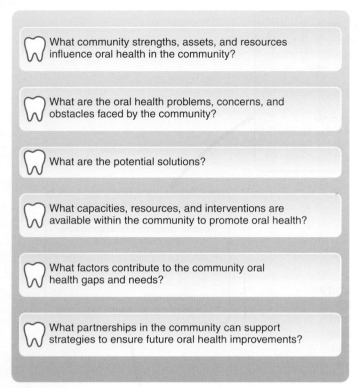

Fig 3.8 Questions to answer during a broad-based community oral health assessment.

problems. For example, *assets-oriented* assessment focuses on what assets the community has available, such as funding, workforce, materials, and facilities. However, a *deficiency-based* approach concentrates solely on the problems without taking into account the big picture of what strengths and assets the community has available to solve the problem. By engaging and fostering the community in a community-building process, one can gain insight about the specific factors in the community that influence health. Through a participatory framework for action and capacity development, a better understanding of opportunities for health enhancements can emerge over time.[15,16]

To know and understand the community's needs and resources, certain questions need to be answered during a community assessment (Figure 3.8). Answers to these questions will provide a better understanding of the oral health needs of the community and how to approach the program planning process.[15,16] These answers can assist in the final determination of critical oral health issues and priorities.

No single formula exists for conducting a community oral health assessment. Examples of community health assessment models are provided in Box 3.5. All these models share common characteristics, which are presented in Figure 3.9 as a basic guide of specific phases that are required in the assessment process. This basic guide can be applied to assess the oral health status of an entire community or a specific segment of the population within the community. Discussion of the community assessment process in this chapter will focus on this basic model. Only a summary of the highlights of the process will be presented in this chapter. A comprehensive discussion of different models

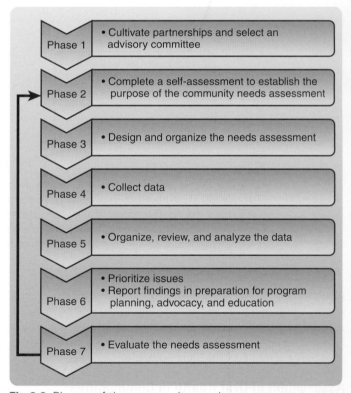

Fig 3.9 Phases of the community needs assessment process.

can be referred to if needed (see Box 3.5 and References and Additional Resources at the end of this chapter).

Phase 1: Cultivate Partnerships and Select an Advisory Committee

The first phase of the community needs assessment is to cultivate partnerships and select an advisory committee[15,16] (see Figure 3.9). Looking to the public, private, and nonprofit sectors will offer opportunities for potential champions of the assessment mission and process. A **community partnership** is an arrangement between or among agencies, organizations, businesses, and people that collaborate and combine resources to work toward a unified, common goal. Mobilization of community partnerships and coalitions (see earlier in chapter) to identify and solve oral health problems has been identified as a key public health activity and a prominent strategy for all phases of community health improvement, including assessment.[15,16] Community partners can broaden the scope, approaches, and perspectives during the process of an assessment, providing community input, data sources, resources, expertise, sponsorship, and political support that can assist with the common goal.[15,16]

Engaging community partners in the assessment process is also critical to the process of building support for community oral health improvement plans and initiatives that will arise from the assessment outcomes.[15,16] Examples of this kind of support are financial support for communication of the findings and promotion of the strategies identified by the assessment. Thus, involvement and support of partnering agencies and organizations throughout the assessment process can have a positive influence on the attainment of mutual missions and goals upon completion of the assessment.[15,16]

Community action and community-building efforts can engage and empower a community, which can have positive outcomes when sustained over time.[14,16] **Empowerment**, as it pertains to community health, is enabling the community to take control and make decisions as a whole about the achievement of health in their own community. This provides the appropriate tools and knowledge to the community members to enable them to make decisions for the community where they had previously been unable to. One of the principles of public health practice is that **interdisciplinary collaboration** (across disciplines) and broad community involvement are crucial to the empowerment of communities in relation to health improvement.[15,16] It is important to consider ways to identify and recruit partners that will result in an inclusive and empowering process.

In the course of finding support in the community, it is strongly recommended that an advisory committee be developed to plan and conduct the needs assessment.[15,16] Through the forming of partnerships and gaining support from the community members, organizations, and agencies, individuals can be identified who can serve on and lead an advisory committee to guide the needs assessment process. Successful and effective needs assessment and program planning are determined by the organizations and partnerships that are represented on the advisory committee. People and organizations should be selected that share the desire to accomplish the same goals.[15,16]

Broad-based community partnerships should be engaged and participants enlisted that reflect the cultural, racial, ethnic, gender, economic, and linguistic diversities of the community.[15,16] It is essential to involve diverse community partners, including a cross-section of the community, such as technical staff, program managers, and leaders from business, media, religious,

civic, philanthropic, community, and political realms.[15,16] They should represent diverse perspectives and be active in various disciplines to increase the opportunities to develop innovative approaches for the needs assessment.[15,16] In addition, they should represent the demographics of the community and consist of participants, community leaders, agency and organization leaders, service providers, and policymakers.[15,16]

The community partners involved in an assessment may vary according to the overall focus of the assessment process. Appendix A consists of a list of various community and professional organizations, and Appendix C provides a list of potential constituents and stakeholders, both of which should be considered when selecting community partners for specific initiatives of common interest. The coalition framework in Appendix C also can serve as a guide to selecting members for a community oral health assessment advisory committee.

Mechanisms for community mobilization, active involvement, input, and dialog must be incorporated throughout the assessment process.[15,16] Procedures should be in place to ensure opportunities to communicate with, get feedback from, and sustain support of the community throughout the process, and to evaluate the assessment process and results.[15,16]

Resource materials in the *Community Tool Box* can be helpful by offering additional innovative ideas about building effective collaborative partnerships.[15] Many of these resources discuss indepth ways to initiate and sustain collaborative relationships. Specific factors and conditions that are conducive to effective collaborative partnerships should be supported and nurtured for measurable and lasting results.[15,16]

Describing the community. The advisory committee must develop a clear description of the community at the onset of the assessment process.[15,16] Communities are a collection of people, places, and systems that define how people and places interact on an ongoing basis.[15,16] It is necessary to clearly identify the targeted community in an overview or *community snapshot*. This snapshot describes the community traits and profiles the health of the community by reporting on a spectrum of health indicators. Data collected for a snapshot briefly describe the features of the community but do not provide detailed statistics.[15,16] (see Guiding Principles and the Opening Statement for an example).

GUIDING PRINCIPLES

Factors to Consider in Understanding and Describing a Community

- People (socioeconomics, demographics, health status, risk profiles, cultural and ethnic characteristics)
- Location (geographic boundaries)
- Connectors (shared values, interests, motivating factors)
- Power relationships (communication patterns, social and political networks, formal and informal lines of authority and influence, stakeholder relationships, resource flows)

More comprehensive, detailed community data should be compiled during the data collection phase of the community assessment. This will be discussed in a later step in the process.

Phase 2: Complete a Self-Assessment to Establish the Purpose of the Community Needs Assessment

The second phase of the community needs assessment is to complete a self-assessment [15,16] (see Figure 3.9). Self-assessment is accomplished to identify the goals; this will define the purpose of the needs assessment through consensus of the advisory committee.[15,16] Before beginning the assessment process, the community partners must understand why the community is conducting an assessment, what the community hopes to achieve from it, and what will be gained through the assessment process.[16] There are many possible reasons to conduct a community oral health assessment, and a community may have more than one purpose. A few of the many potential purposes for conducting a community oral health assessment are listed in Figure 3.10.

This self-reflective step will thus guide the necessary scope and size of the assessment and influence other decisions relative to planning the needs assessment.[15,16] In addition, when necessary, this self-assessment phase can include internal evaluation of the organization and its role; external evaluation of the missions and roles of other organizations in the community that can affect the oral health assessment process or the future oral health improvement plan; and consideration of the organizational capacity, power structures, strategic plans, commitment, and resources available.[15,16]

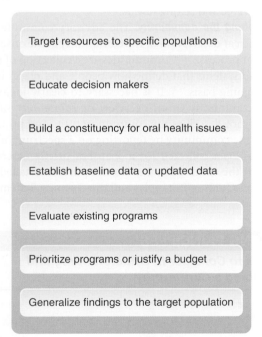

Fig 3.10 Potential purposes for conducting a community oral health assessment. (Modified from: McKenzie JF, Neiger BL, Thackeray R. Planning, Implementing & Evaluating: Health Promotion Programs: A Primer, 7th ed. Glenview, IL: Pearson Education, Inc; 2017; and Community Tool Box. Lawrence, KS: Work Group for Community Health and Development, University of Kansas; 2019. Available at: <https://ctb.ku.edu/en>;[Accessed September 2019].)

Phase 3: Design and Organize the Needs Assessment

The third phase of the community needs assessment is designing and organizing the needs assessment[15,16] (see Figure 3.9). Different types, sources, and levels of information are needed for a comprehensive health assessment.[15,16] It is vital to collect and evaluate data related to the current status of assets, gaps, needs, problems, resources, solutions, and partnerships in the community. Examples of information needed for a community assessment are included in Appendix D. In addition, Appendix E provides a comprehensive list of oral conditions and factors influencing oral health that can be included in a community assessment. Based on the goals and resources identified in the self-assessment, the advisory committee can resolve what information needs to be collected for the assessment and how it should be gathered. During the planning step a priority-based structure is developed to identify realistic means of obtaining the required data. This involves developing data collection methods.[15,16]

A standard element of an assessment is the compilation and synthesis of existing data from secondary sources.[16] These secondary sources will likely provide much of the needed information, but generally some gaps exist in the available data. Thus, after existing information is assessed, a decision can be made about the collection of new information from primary sources. These activities that are undertaken to achieve the goals of the assessment must be refined continually as information is collected and in light of available resources.[16]

Identifying sources of existing data. Multiple resources of information are widely available to the general public. The data sources used in an oral health assessment should be diverse to ensure a broad portrayal of the factors influencing oral health in the community.[15,16] Examples of sources are as follows:

- Government agencies and private and nonprofit organizations compile data and produce excellent reports on oral health status and trends and on the various determinants of overall health and oral health.
- Sources of local information include local reports, literature reviews, magazines, newspapers, newsletters, maps, and marketing data.
- Previous assessments that have been conducted in the community can provide valuable information, insights, and a historical perspective.

Table 3.1 outlines examples of various sources of information for community oral health assessments. In addition, Appendix A provides a list of specific community and professional resources, and government resources for health data are listed in Appendix D. Other resources are included in the References and Additional Resources at the end of this chapter and Chapters 4 and 5.

Types of data. Regardless of whether the data to be collected are *secondary data* (previously collected data) or *primary data* (data collected directly from the source such as through interviews and surveys), different types of information are necessary to ensure that a complete assessment accurately describes the factors influencing oral health in the community.[15,16] Which specific forms to collect will depend on the purposes of the assessment and the desired outcomes. For example, the assessment might be

TABLE 3.1   Sources of Information for a Community Oral Health Assessment

Potential Source	Examples
Federal, state, and local government agencies (see Appendix D)	• Health department, human services department, and social services department; department of aging; department of disabilities and special needs; highway safety department; police departments (documents, reports, surveys, statistics) • Population surveys • National, state, and local health surveys • Surveillance system reports and records • Population-based registries • Health agency records and reports of participants enrolled in programs • Agency records and reports of health professionals; health professional shortage areas; community health centers • State or local child protection agency records • Environmental agency records and reports
Private and public (community) health, healthcare (clinical or personal healthcare), social, and human service programs	Hospitals; health plans (health insurance claims data); healthcare systems (health charts and dental records, pathology reports); professional associations; trade groups; community advisory committees; community collaborative groups and coalitions (community surveys); health and social service groups; professional and community organizations, societies, and associations (documents, reports, surveys, statistics)
Philanthropic, nonprofit, and charitable organizations	Religious organizations and groups; voluntary agencies; civic organizations; service and voluntary groups; community organizations; advocacy groups (documents, reports, surveys, statistics, local information, referral service inventories)
Schools and colleges	School districts; school boards; school campuses; colleges; universities (student statistics, school health reports, school entry records)
Businesses, employers, and business organizations	Major employers or chambers of commerce; marketing data and survey data (e.g., Nielsen Claritas); economic statistics and financial records; corporate annual reports (e.g., sales of drugs, foods, tobacco)
Media	Media sources (newspapers, magazines, newsletters, radio, television, Internet, social media)

designed to evaluate determinants of health in the community, assess the needs and assets, and/or quantify disparities and inequities among population groups, all of which would require different types of data and measurement methods.[15,16] The following two main classes of data can be used to describe a community and to characterize dimensions of health within the community[15,16]:

1. **Quantitative data** refer to information that is objective and measurable. The data can be expressed as a quantity or amount, numerically representing the size of a problem. Examples are demographic information, vital statistics such as numbers of births or deaths, **incidence** or **prevalence rates** of disease, number of schools in a county, and employment statistics.
2. **Qualitative data** refer to information that cannot be numerically measured or analyzed; rather, the quality or nature of factors influencing a health problem is reflected. Qualitative data add meaning to the quantitative data and help answer questions of why problems exist in communities. Examples of these data are information gathered from personal interviews, participant observations, focus groups, descriptions of traditions, and the history of a community.

See Chapter 7 for more detail on quantitative and qualitative data.

Phase 4: Collect Data

The fourth phase of the community needs assessment is collecting data[15,16] (see Figure 3.9). **Data collection** is a gathering of information that the community can use to make decisions and set priorities. This is the actual implementation of the community oral health assessment, which consists of collecting the data that were identified as important in the assessment planning phase.[15,16] During secondary data collection, it is important to methodically conduct a broad search of available information and to organize an inventory of this information. Information from secondary sources should be carefully compiled to establish a system to record, process, and organize the data.

Determining the necessity of primary data collection. After the existing data from secondary sources are assessed, a decision can be made about the necessity to collect new data from primary sources.[15,16] Collecting original data is important when gaps in information needs still exist. This key decision should be made based on the following:

1. An analysis of the findings from the secondary data sources
2. A reevaluation and possible refinement of the assessment goals
3. Available resources to support primary data collection

The members of the advisory committee determine and prioritize information needs and evaluate alternative methods of data collection.[15,16]

Planning and collecting primary data. When it is necessary to collect primary data, the advisory committee must develop a plan that outlines objectives, activities, roles, responsibilities, a budget, and a timetable for this activity.[15,16] Examples of tasks that should be considered for conducting primary data collection are listed in Appendix D. Decisions about what primary data are required and what data collection methods and instruments will be used are crucial to the primary data collection plan. These decisions will depend on the aims of the community oral health assessment and the resources available.[15,16]

It is essential to study the many alternative ways by which primary data can be collected, considering both the advantages and limitations of the data collection options in light of the goals of the community assessment.[15,16] Based on this analysis, the committee can strategically determine the final primary data collection plan according to identified priorities and resources. After this is accomplished the group will need to develop data collection instruments, such as surveys and questionnaires, along with detailed instructions for their implementation.[15,16] One option might be to integrate specific measures into ongoing surveys and assessments.

Appendix D includes a description of assorted nonclinical data collection methods that can be used to collect primary data. Sometimes a clinical oral health survey will be required to collect primary data for oral health diseases and conditions that exist in the community. Appendix F and Chapter 4 are resources for various measurements and dental indexes that can be used for an oral health survey.

Phase 5: Organize, Review, and Analyze the Data

The fifth phase of the community needs assessment is to organize, review, and analyze the data[15,16] (see Figure 3.9). Analysis and interpretation of data often require special knowledge and experience; this is where the background and experience of the advisory committee members, community partners, and other professionals in the community are invaluable. Enlisting their expertise and assistance in analyzing and validating impressions and interpretations of the assessment data is vital.

To analyze and interpret both primary and secondary data, numerous actions are necessary. After the data have been organized by topic for ease and clarity, the initial action is to synthesize the information and summarize the findings.[15,16] A critique of each data source is required to assess its trustworthiness.[16] Limitations of the data and data sources must be checked for potential errors or bias. It is important to consider the sampling technique of research reports that are reviewed, such as type of sample, sample size, participation of population segments, and generalization of findings to population groups[16,40,41] (see Chapter 7).

Because of the potential for human error, it is essential to review the methods and processes used to ensure that protocols were followed in collecting, recording, compiling, analyzing, and interpreting data.[40,41] This will enable reduction of any possible bias and errors in the results and/or interpretation of those results. Information should be reviewed carefully to consider the possibility of errors in coding and groupings of data, erroneous instructions, typographical errors, or misinterpretation.[40,41,42] When the data have been determined to be reasonably free of errors, they should be compared with other data. Trends can be analyzed by comparing current or new data with data from previous years. These comparisons may show changes in the community over time, which can be very useful for program planning purposes. Figure 3.11 provides some suggestions of data sources with which the community assessment data can be compared. Data used for comparison should be as alike as possible to allow for valid comparison.[42]

At this point, it can be determined whether opportunities exist to analyze the secondary data further. Additional analysis of existing data sets may generate new information to provide more insight. In addition, there may be value in adding or

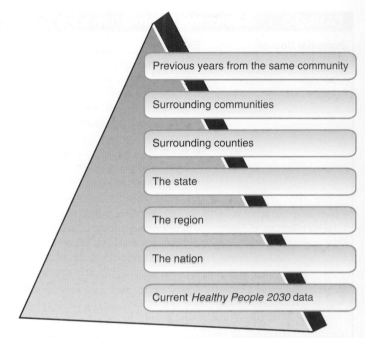

Fig 3.11 Assessment data can be compared with other data from various sources.

integrating the collection of new types of data into ongoing data collection efforts.[15,16]

The next action in the analysis process is to determine the meaning and significance of the data analysis.[15,16,41,42] The term *significance* means that the resulting information truly reflects that a problem exists in a community. Studying the data for significance involves identifying any possible misleading findings before conclusions can be drawn from the findings. An abundance of data that combines different types of data allows for a more accurate and meaningful determination of the significance of the findings.[41] See Chapter 7 for more detail on determining the significance of the data.

Feedback on the meaning of the findings can be provided by evaluating the implications of the data within the context and expectations of the community.[15,16] The findings from quantitative and qualitative data can provide direction for future actions that build on community assets. With potential strategies indicated, this action can help move the assessment step toward the planning step of a community oral health improvement process. At the same time, additional questions may arise that can direct the process toward the need for more information and supplementary assessment activities.[15,16]

Phase 6: Prioritize Issues and Report Findings in Preparation for Program Planning, Advocacy, and Education

The sixth phase of the community needs assessment is to prioritize issues and report findings in preparation for program planning, advocacy, and education.[15,16] As reflected in Figure 3.9, this step consists of two actions: (1) prioritize the issues and (2) report the findings. Completing these two actions leads to the development of programs that advocate for a change or that educate individuals and groups.[15,16]

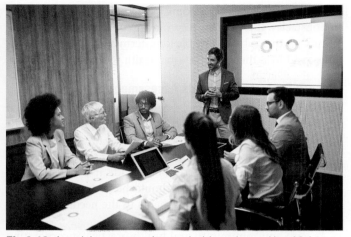

Fig 3.12 An advisory committee prioritizes the oral health issues of a community based on the assessment data. (© iStock.com/nd3000)

Prioritizing the issues. The issues that impact the oral health of the community are identified through the interpretation of the data in the previous phase (Phase 5). In Phase 6 these issues are prioritized to determine which must be addressed first.[15,16] *Prioritization* is a decision-making process that involves an impartial and balanced approach to deciding the order of importance of the issues.[15,16] Prioritization of issues is influenced in part by the availability of resources, including funding and workforce.[15,16] The advisory committee should be actively involved through a deliberative process in all aspects of identifying and prioritizing the critical issues that will be addressed later in the program planning process[15,16] (Figure 3.12). Key steps to follow in determining and prioritizing community oral health issues are outlined in Box 3.6.

Prioritizing oral health issues within a community can accomplish the following:

- Help oral health programs decide where to target resources based on sound evidence
- Assist underfunded and overworked agencies deal with the "crisis of the day" created by the public, media, or legislation
- Assure the rational distribution of resources
- Raise awareness of what the public wants or sees as important
- Increase the public's understanding of the critical oral health issues

Reporting the findings of the community oral health assessment. After the oral health issues have been prioritized, the results of the assessment should be presented to an intended target audience.[15,16] This audience could consist of personnel of health departments or community-based clinics, oral health and other health professionals, legislators, community leaders, members of the media or the public, or other groups that have an interest in the outcomes. The results can be used in program planning, advocacy efforts for policy changes and legislation, community education about oral health issues, and developing funding proposals to support future initiatives, all for the purpose of improving the oral health status of the community.[15,16]

The information presented to the intended target audience should address the issues that the audience considers important and pertinent.[15,16] The communication of a community oral health assessment to the community allows for further input by the community concerning how the results will be used and the critical oral health issues that will be addressed with program planning.

It is essential to establish a plan to communicate and disseminate the findings of the community oral health assessment.[15,16] These findings should be publicized and distributed widely to various community members, using diverse communication channels, such as public forums, news conferences, publications, electronic media, and social media. See Chapter 8 for contemporary strategies to communicate oral health findings and promote community oral health. The assessment outcomes should be communicated in a straightforward manner. To this end, it is important to prepare an executive summary that succinctly highlights key findings.[15,16]

The advisory committee should present the findings from the data collected and analyzed and share information about the overall assessment quest in a report similar to a research report[15,16] (see Chapter 7). Components of a report can include a statement of the purpose, materials and methods used to conduct the assessment, results, a discussion of the significance of the findings, conclusions, and a summary or abstract.[15,16] The report should include the outcomes of the inventory of community assets and resources to note their availability and limitations.[15,16] It is helpful to illustrate the findings through charts, graphs, tables, and maps (see Chapter 7 for ways to present data). In addition, partners can provide the audience with a frame of reference to show how the community data compare or contrast with similar local, state, or national data.[15,16] It is also vital to explain the limitations of the data.[15,16]

A detailed description of the community should be included in the report. The data gathered can expand on the initial community overview or snapshot and provide a comprehensive, detailed **community profile**.[16] Community profiles can be used to help stakeholders and funders visualize the community that was assessed and are essential when applying for grants. Examples of information in a community profile are presented in Box 3.7.

Preparing for program planning, education, and advocacy. The intended purpose of a community oral health assessment is to use the data to make plans for initiatives that can result in improving the oral health of the community. In the process of interpreting the findings of the assessment and communicating these to the community, the advisory committee can begin to engage the community in considering solutions to the problems and issues identified through the assessment.[15,16] In this way, Phase 6 leads naturally to the development of an oral health improvement plan.

At this point, the identified assets, gaps, needs, problems, resources, solutions, and partnerships in the community should be considered, and the advisory committee should communicate the community's assets and resources to create a shared vision of change.[15,16] Greater creativity is encouraged when community partners are engaged in building capacity to address problems and obstacles. It also helps to promote consensus among community partners about possible long-term and short-term solutions to address the identified oral health problems.[15,16]

Phase 7: Evaluate the Needs Assessment

After Phases 1 through 6 have been completed, there is a need to review and evaluate the needs assessment in Phase 7[15,16] (see Figure 3.9). The evaluation process provides the advisory committee the opportunity to determine whether the original goals of the needs assessment were met, decide if problems arose in the assessment process that should be addressed in future assessments, and make improvements to the needs assessment process for the future.

As with any community oral health practice, incorporating **formative evaluation** throughout the assessment process is also important. Throughout the assessment, the advisory committee should continually step back to systematically evaluate the process. Allowing time for this formative evaluation along the way can provide opportunity to implement changes that will improve the assessment results.[15,16]

A critique of the assessment at the end of the process, which is a form of **summative evaluation**, provides a record of lessons learned for future health assessments in the community.[15,16] Upon completion of the evaluation, the community needs assessment process loops back to Phase 2[15,16] (see arrow in Figure 3.9). The feedback loop provides the opportunity to use what is learned during the evaluation to improve the assessment,[15,16] thus creating a continual assessment process, similar to a surveillance system (see Chapter 4). This renders assessment and program planning dynamic, which contributes to a more effective and sustained oral health improvement process.[15,16]

Multiple ways exist to collect information that can be used to assess the health, determinants of health, and other related issues in a population, community, or priority group within the community. Numerous resources are available that describe methods and offer guidance for community health assessments. Use of these resources can assist in developing a methodical approach to a community oral health assessment. (See Box 3.5 and the References and Additional Resources at the end of this chapter for some of these resources.)

Next Steps: Developing and Implementing an Improvement Plan

With the published report of the assessment disseminated and the priorities identified, it is time to move to the next phase of the community oral health improvement process. At this stage oral health improvement strategies can be developed to address the prioritized oral health issues outlined in the oral health assessment. Concrete goals, objectives, policies, and programs can be planned and implemented (see Chapter 6) based on the findings, evidence, best practices, and priorities from the oral health assessment.[15,16] A community oral health assessment is virtually useless unless the information is used to develop and implement evidence-based oral health programs

---

BOX 3.7 Examples of Information for a Community Profile

Physical and Spatial Characteristics
Geographic boundaries and size, population size and density, community type, physical condition of neighborhoods, community assets, community layout, transportation, environmental conditions, water supply, water quality, community infrastructure, education resources and facilities, public commons and informal gathering places, number of places of worship, religious denominations, and signs of development or decay in the community.

Community Inventory
History of the community, community traditions, dominant values, beliefs, social norms, attitudes, political system, political and government structure, prominent political figures, formal and informal community leadership, community support systems through networks, support and community members, gatekeepers, communication channels, community organizations and associations, and capacities and inventories of community members and groups.

Sociodemographic Characteristics
Community Demographic Data: Population distribution by age, gender and gender ratios, race, ethnicity, social class, economic status, education levels, occupations, marital status, employment status, value of housing, household living conditions, religions, nationality, cultural characteristics, migration, immigration trends, and trends of change in size and composition.
Social Demographic Data: Social attributes, social structures, community stability, social cohesiveness, civic engagement, functioning of social networks, families and households, family values, individual beliefs, attitudes, opinions, social norms, cultural forces, religious beliefs, vulnerable population groups, quality of life, and enrollment in government and public assistance programs such as Medicaid, CHIP, Women, Infants, and Children (WIC) program, Head Start, and childcare support.

Vital Events
Birth rates, fertility rates, life expectancy, **mortality** rates, **morbidity** rates, cause-specific related morbidity and mortality rates, marriages, and divorces.

to address the needs identified. The Additional Resources at the end of this chapter and Chapters 4, 5, and 6 can provide guidance in the development of an oral health improvement plan.

SUMMARY

Epidemiology involves a multifactorial approach to analyzing the interacting relationships among host factors, agent factors, and environmental factors that contribute to health in populations. Attention to these multiple factors and determinants of health is essential in the oral health improvement process at global, national, state, and local levels.

Assessment is a core public health function, and dental hygienists involved in public health practice must be proficient in the various aspects of community oral health assessment. This chapter has reviewed the key elements necessary when a community undertakes an assessment. Community health assessment efforts are applied to evaluate assets, gaps, problems, resources, solutions, and partnerships in the community. This allows a community to assess the determinants of health, evaluate needs, quantify disparities and inequities among population groups, and measure preventable disease, injury, disability, and death. Data collection methods and instruments are varied, and their application depends on the overall aims of the assessment and resources available within and from outside the community. A systematic approach is crucial to this process to accomplish a comprehensive community oral health assessment.

Assessment is an integral component of the community oral health improvement process. Information gained from a community assessment can be used to plan, implement, and evaluate oral health improvement strategies and programs.

APPLYING YOUR KNOWLEDGE

1. Select three of the following groups and situations to illustrate the determinants of oral health, and present your results in class:
   a. Dental injuries among schoolchildren in a neighborhood
   b. Dental caries among adolescents in a city without fluoridated drinking water
   c. Oral cancer among older adults in a county
   d. Adults without access to annual dental visits in a rural county
   e. Periodontal disease among disabled young adults in a region of a state
   f. Early childhood caries among preschool children in a state
   g. Edentulism among adults in a region of the country and comparisons between multiple states
   h. Dental caries among children across nations on a global level

2. In a small group, discuss one of the following situations, and report to your class (see Appendices C and D for ideas):
   a. The social worker from the County Agency on Aging calls you to discuss the dental problems of older adults attending local nutrition sites near your community health center. The state health department has recently distributed the State Oral Health Improvement Plan, which notes a high rate of oral cancer among older men and a low rate of dental attendance for older edentulous adults. How would you maximize these "windows of opportunity" to initiate a community oral health assessment? Who would you contact? What steps would you take? Do you think these efforts could advance the development and implementation of a community oral health improvement plan?
   b. At a local childcare conference, a prominent speaker describes the high rate of early childhood caries among preschool children attending Head Start programs in the city. Also, during the conference, the new Director

   for the WIC Supplemental Food Program from the local health department highlights the need to improve the nutrition, health, and dental education for families enrolled in WIC. After the conference, the Community Coalition for Healthy Children (CCHC) asks you to join as a representative of the local component of the American Dental Hygienists' Association. How would you maximize this opportunity to focus on oral health and young children? Who would you contact? What steps would you take to initiate a community oral health assessment? How might the CCHC evaluate the assets, gaps, needs, problems, resources, solutions, and partnerships within the context of your community? How might this assessment promote the development and implementation of a community oral health improvement plan?

3. Perform a windshield survey (see Appendix D) of a neighborhood other than your own to assess oral health status and problems of the people and environment and the dental care resources in the community. Observe the oral status as far as you can tell from interacting with individuals in the community. Assess the number of dental care facilities, both private and public, and determine whether they are easily accessible. Is public transportation available and easily used to reach dental care facilities? What is the SES of the area? Record the details of your observation. Prepare a summary to report your observations, findings, and conclusions about the needs and resources of the community. Gather with other classmates and compare what you discovered.

4. Select three *Healthy People 2030* Oral Conditions objectives. For each one, what measures would you use to retrieve primary data for your local area population? How would you assess it in the coming year in the following situations: a) in an urban inner-city community for one objective, b) in a suburban community for another objective, and c) in a rural county for the final objective? Share your results with your class.

LEARNING OBJECTIVES AND COMPETENCIES

This chapter addresses the following community oral health learning objectives and competencies for dental hygienists that are presented in the revised May 2015-2016 *ADEA Compendium of Curriculum Guidelines for Allied Dental Education Programs*:

Learning Objectives

- Define the range of personal, social, economic and environmental factors that influence health status (i.e., determinants of health).
- Describe the responsibilities of dental hygienists in the U.S.
- Define oral health in relation to health education and promotion.
- Describe health education and promotion principles.
- Describe the various program planning paradigms.
- Perform a needs assessment of the target population.

- Compare qualitative and quantitative evaluation.
- Define oral epidemiology and related terms.
- Identify the role of host, agent and environment in the disease process.
- Describe oral epidemiology and its relationship to dental hygiene.
- Use appropriate information resources in community dental health.
- Describe the current epidemiologic issues of disease.

Competencies

- Assessing, planning, implementing and evaluating community-based oral health programs.
- Recognizing and using written and electronic sources of information.

COMMUNITY CASE

You are a dental hygienist serving on a health team at a community-based healthcare facility. The executive director has called a meeting about the need to plan a community health assessment in the surrounding neighborhood served by the community health center. This community health assessment is an essential component of the center's application to receive continued grant funding. Your role as a member of the planning committee is to provide input on the components of the community health assessment.

1. What is the first step the committee should take for the community health assessment?
   a. Collect data from existing resources.
   b. Identify critical health issues and select health priorities.
   c. Mobilize the community by forming key partnerships and recruiting participants to collaborate in the community health assessment.
   d. Plan and collect primary health data in the community.
2. During the data collection phase of the community health assessment, all of the following are government resources for health data that the committee could use EXCEPT one. Which is the EXCEPTION?
   a. Population surveys from the U.S. Census Bureau
   b. State health surveys
   c. Health and dental records from a private hospital
   d. CDC Cancer Registry

3. What is the name used for the comprehensive description of the community that includes comprehensive, detailed community data?
   a. Community asset map
   b. Community profile
   c. Primary data collection
   d. Community snapshot
4. Which of the following data collection methods would be the most costly and time-consuming?
   a. Windshield tour
   b. Mailed survey
   c. Person-to-person interview
   d. Telephone interview
5. The primary and secondary data included in this community assessment can be either qualitative or quantitative. The qualitative community assessment data are expressed as a quantity or amount.
   a. The first statement is true, and the second statement is false.
   b. The second statement is true, and the first statement is false.
   c. Both statements are true.
   d. Both statements are false.

REFERENCES

1. What is Public Health? Atlanta, GA: CDC Foundation; 2019. Available at: <http://www.cdcfoundation.org/content/what-public-health>; [Accessed September 2019].
2. What is Public Health? Washington, DC: American Public Health Association; 2018. Available at: <https://www.apha.org/what-is-public-health>; [Accessed September 2019].
3. Sellers K, Leider JP, Gould E, et al. The State of the US Governmental Public Health Workforce, 2014-2017. Am J Public Health 2019 May;109(5):674–80. Available at: <https://ajph.aphapublications.org/doi/10.2105/AJPH.2019.305011>; [Accessed October 2019].
4. CPH: Certified Public Health. Washington, DC: National Board of Public Health Examiners; 2019. Available at: <https://www.nbphe.org>; [Accessed August 2019].
5. National Commission for Health Education Credentialing. Whitehall, PA: National Commission for Health Education Credentialing, Inc. Available at: <http://www.nchec.org>; [Accessed August 2019].
6. Core Competencies for Public Health Professionals. Washington, DC: Council on Linkages Between Academia and Public Health

Practice; 2014 Jun 26. Available at: <http://www.phf.org/resourcestools/Documents/Core_Competencies_for_Public_Health_Professionals_2014June.pdf>; [Accessed September 2019].

7. Specialty Definitions: Dental Public Health. Chicago, IL: National Commission on Recognition of Dental Specialties and Certifying Boards; 2018 May. Available at: <https://www.ada.org/en/ncrdscb/dental-specialties/specialty-definitions>; [Accessed September 2019].

8. Competencies for the New General Dentist. Washington, DC: American Dental Education Association; 2008. Available at: <http://www.adea.org/about_adea/governance/Pages/Competencies-for-the-New-General-Dentist.aspx>; [Accessed September 2019].

9. Accreditation Standards for Dental Education Programs. Chicago, IL: Commission on Dental Accreditation; 2019. Available at: <https://www.ada.org/~/media/CODA/Files/pde.pdf?la=en>; [Accessed September 2019].

10. Accreditation Standards for Dental Therapy Education Programs. Chicago, IL: Commission on Dental Accreditation; 2015 Feb 6. Available at: <https://www.ada.org/~/media/CODA/Files/dental_therapy_standards.pdf?la=en>; [Accessed January 2020].

11. Accreditation Standards for Advanced Dental Education Programs in Dental Public Health. Chicago, IL: Commission on Dental Accreditation; 2018. Available at: <https://www.ada.org/~/media/CODA/Files/dph.pdf?la=en>; [Accessed September 2019].

12. Accreditation Standards for Dental Hygiene Education Programs. Chicago, IL: Commission on Dental Accreditation; 2018. Available at: <https://www.ada.org/~/media/CODA/Files/2019_dental_hygiene_standards.pdf?la=en>; [Accessed September 2019].

13. Dental Hygiene Curriculum Guidelines. In ADEA Compendium of Curriculum Guidelines for Allied Dental Education Programs (Revised Edition). Washington, DC: American Dental Education Association; 2015-2016 May. Available at: <https://www.adea.org/about_adea/governance/ACAPDToolkit/Allied_Dental_Education_Resources(Older_Version).html>; [Accessed September 2019].

14. Core Competencies for Graduate Dental Hygiene Education. Washington, DC: American Dental Education Association/American Dental Hygienists' Association; 2011. Available at: <http://www.adea.org/uploadedFiles/ADEA/Content_Conversion_Final/about_adea/governance/ADEA_Core_Competencies_for_Graduate_Dental_Hygiene_Education.pdf>; [Accessed August 2019].

15. Community Tool Box. Lawrence, KS: Work Group for Community Health and Development, University of Kansas; 2019. Available at: <https://ctb.ku.edu/en>; [Accessed September 2019].

16. McKenzie JF, Neiger BL, Thackeray R. Planning, Implementing & Evaluating: Health Promotion Programs: A Primer. 7th ed. Glenview, IL: Pearson Education, Inc; 2017.

17. Michigan Oral Health Coalition. Lansing, MI; 2018. Available at: <http://www.mohc.org/>; [Accessed September 2019].

18. Resources Organized by Essential Services. Atlanta, GA: Centers for Disease Control and Prevention; 2019 Mar 7. Available at: <https://www.cdc.gov/nceh/ehs/10-essential-services/resources.html>; [Accessed April 2020].

19. Career Paths. American Dental Hygienists' Association; 2017. Available at: <https://www.adha.org/professional-roles>; [Accessed September 2019].

20. Friis RH. Epidemiology 101 (Essential Public Health). 2nd ed. Burlington, MA: Jones and Bartlett Learning; 2018.

21. Understanding the Epidemiologic Triangle through Infectious Disease Working the Epidemiologic Triangle. Atlanta, GA: Centers for Disease Control and Prevention; 2018 Aug 28. Available at: <https://www.cdc.gov/healthyschools/bam/teachers/epi-triangle.html>; [Accessed September 2019].

22. Featherstone JDB, Rechmann P, Zellmer IH. Dental caries management by risk assessment. In: Bowen DM, Pieren JA, editors. Darby and Walsh Dental Hygiene Theory and Practice. 5th ed. Maryland Heights, MO: Elsevier; 2019. p. 265–84.

23. Determinants of Health. Geneva: World Health Organization; 2017 Feb 3. Available at: <https://www.who.int/news-room/q-a-detail/determinants-of-health>; [Accessed October 2020].

24. Williams L. Empowerment and the ecological determinants of health: three critical capacities for practitioners. Health Promot Int 2017;32(4):711–22. Available at: <https://doi.org/10.1093/heapro/daw011>; [Accessed April 2020].

25. Constitution. Geneva: World Health Organization; 2019. Available at: <https://www.who.int/about/who-we-are/constitution>; [Accessed September 2019].

26. The Ottawa Charter for Health Promotion. First International Conference on Health Promotion, Ottawa: November 21, 1986. Geneva: World Health Organization; 2019. Available at: <http://www.who.int/healthpromotion/conferences/previous/ottawa/en/>; [Accessed September 2019].

27. Public Health Law: A Tool to Address Emerging Health Concerns (video). Atlanta, GA: Centers for Disease Control and Prevention: Public Health Grand Rounds; 2016 Dec 16. Available at: <https://www.cdc.gov/grand-rounds/pp/2016/20161213-health-law.html>; [Accessed September 2019].

28. Report #7: Assessment and Recommendations for Proposed Objectives for Healthy People 2030. Secretary's Advisory Committee on National Health Promotion and Disease Prevention Objectives for 2030; 2019. Available at: <https://www.healthypeople.gov/sites/default/files/Report%207_Reviewing%20Assessing%20Set%20of%20HP2030%20Objectives_Formatted%20EO_508_05.21.pdf>; [Accessed April 2020].

29. What is Health Promotion? World Health Organization; 2019. Available at: <https://www.who.int/features/qa/health-promotion/en/>; [Accessed September, 2019].

30. Report #2: Recommendations for Developing Objectives, Setting Priorities, Identifying Data Needs, and Involving Stakeholders for Healthy People 2030. Secretary's Advisory Committee on National Health Promotion and Disease Prevention Objectives for 2030; 2017. Available at: <https://www.healthypeople.gov/sites/default/files/Advisory_Committee_Objectives_for_HP2030_Report.pdf>; [Accessed April 2020].

31. Healthy People 2030 Framework: What is the Healthy People 2030 Framework? Rockville, MD: Office of Disease Prevention and Health Promotion; 2020. Available at: <https://www.healthypeople.gov/2020/About-Healthy-People/Development-Healthy-People-2030/Framework>; [Accessed March 2020].

32. Social Determinants of Health. Atlanta, GA: Centers for Disease Control and Prevention; 2018 Jan 29. Available at: <https://www.cdc.gov/socialdeterminants/index.htm>; [Accessed September 2019].

33. Social Determinants of Health. Geneva: World Health Organization; 2019. Available at: <https://www.who.int/social_determinants/en/>; [Accessed September 2019].

34. National Academies of Sciences, Engineering, and Medicine. Communities in Action: Pathways to Health Equity. Washington, DC: The National Academies Press; 2017. Available at: <https://doi.org/10.17226/24624>; [Accessed September 2019].

35. Oral Health and the Social Determinants of Health (Policy Statement). Geneva, Switzerland: FDI World Dental Federation; 2013 Aug. Available at: <https://www.fdiworld-dental.org/resources/policy-statements-and-resolutions/oral-health-and-the-social-determinants-of-health>; [Accessed April 2030].

36. Oral Health Equity and Social Determinants of Oral Health. Reno, NV: Association of State and Territorial Dental Directors; n.d. Available at: <https://www.astdd.org/oral-health-equity-and-social-determinants-of-oral-health/>; [Accessed September 2019].

37. American Academy of Pediatric Dentistry (AAPD). Policy on Social Determinants of Children's Oral Health and Health Disparities; 2017. AAPD Reference Manual: Oral Health Policies; 2018-19;40(6):23-26. Available at: <https://www.aapd.org/glo-balassets/media/policies_guidelines/p_socialdeterminants.pdf>; [Accessed September 2019].

38. Proposed Revisions to Pediatric Dentistry Standards. Commission on Dental Accreditation; Summer 2019. Available at: <https://www.ada.org/en/~/media/CODA/Files/2019%20ADA%20Annual%20Meeting/Appendix_05_proposed_PED>; [Accessed September 2019].

39. Oral Health Programs. Atlanta, GA: Centers for Disease Control and Prevention, Division of Oral Health; 2019 Dec 19. Available at: <https://www.cdc.gov/oralhealth/funded_programs/index.htm>; [Accessed April 2020].

40. Nathe CN. Dental Public Health & Research. 4th ed. New York, NY: Pearson; 2017.

41. Beatty CF, Dickinson C. Oral epidemiology. In: Nathe CN, editor. Dental Public Health & Research,. 4th ed. New York, NY: Pearson; 2017. p. 233–62.

42. Beatty CF, Beatty CE. Biostatistics. In: Nathe CN, editor. Dental Public Health & Research,. 4th ed. New York, NY: Pearson; 2017. p. 201–32.

ADDITIONAL RESOURCES

American Association for Community Dental Programs (AACDP): A Model Framework for Community Oral Health Programs Based upon the Ten Essential Public Health Services: A guide for Developing and Enhancing Community Oral Health Programs.
www.aacdp.com/index.html

American Public Health Association
www.apha.org

Association for Community Health Improvement
https://www.healthycommunities.org/

Association of State and Territorial Dental Directors: Proven and Promising Best Practices for State and Community Oral Health Programs
https://www.astdd.org/best-practices/

Coalition Building Toolkit, Wisconsin Oral Health Coalition
https://www.chawisconsin.org/initiatives/oral-health/wisconsin-oral-health-coalition

HRSA Data Warehouse
http://datawarehouse.hrsa.gov/

Healthy Cities/Healthy Communities, Community Tool Box, University of Kansas Center for Community Health and Development
https://ctb.ku.edu/en/table-of-contents/overview/models-for-community-health-and-development/healthy-cities-healthy-communities/main

Healthy People 2030
https://health.gov/healthypeople

Mobilizing for Action through Planning and Partnerships (MAPP), National Association of County and City Health Officials
https://www.naccho.org/programs/public-health-infrastructure/performance-improvement/community-health-assessment/mapp

National Association of County and City Health Officials
www.naccho.org

Plans for State Oral Health Programs & Activities, CDC
https://www.cdc.gov/oralhealth/funded_programs/infrastructure/plan.htm

4

Measuring Oral Health Status and Progress

Charlene B. Dickinson and Christine French Beatty

OBJECTIVES

1. Discuss the national *Healthy People* initiative and its significance in relation to surveillance.
2. Apply the national oral health indicators, the leading health indicator related to oral health, and the national *Healthy People 2030* Oral Conditions objectives to oral health surveillance.
3. Describe the use of surveillance in relation to oral health.
4. Compare and contrast the procedures and methods used in oral health surveys.
5. Discuss measures used to assess oral diseases, oral conditions, and related factors in populations for the purpose of assessment, surveillance, and research.
6. Identify and use sources of oral health surveillance data for program planning purposes.
7. Discuss future considerations for oral health surveillance.

OPENING STATEMENT: Oral Health Indicators of the National Oral Health Surveillance System

Oral Health Indicator	Assessment Measure(s)
Adult Indicators	
Dental Visit	• Adults aged >18 years who have visited a dentist or dental clinic in the past year
	• Dental visit among adults aged ≥18 years
	• Dental visit among adults aged ≥18 years with diagnosed diabetes
Teeth Cleaning	• Adults aged >18 years who have had their teeth cleaned in the past year
	• Teeth cleaning among women before pregnancy
	• Teeth cleaning among women during pregnancy
Tooth Loss	• No tooth loss among adults aged 18–34 years
Cancer of the Oral Cavity and Pharynx	• Incidence and mortality **rates** of oral and pharyngeal cancer (OPC)
	• Incidence and mortality rates of invasive OPC
	• (Both are measured for adults and older adults)
Older Adult Indicators	
Tooth Loss	• Adults aged >65 years who have lost all of their natural teeth because of tooth decay or gum disease (complete tooth loss)
	• Adults aged 65+ who have lost six or more teeth because of tooth decay or gum disease
Dental Visit	• Dental treatment need among adults >65 years in long-term or skilled nursing facilities
	• Dental treatment need among adults >65 years attending congregate meal sites
Untreated Tooth Decay	• Untreated dental caries among adults >65 years in long-term or skilled nursing facilities
	• Untreated dental caries among adults >65 years attending congregate meal sites
Child Indicators	
Preventive Dental Services	• Preventive dental visit among children aged 1–17 years
	• Preventive dental service for children aged 1-20 years enrolled in Medicaid
	• Any dental service for children aged 1–20 years enrolled in Medicaid
Caries Experience	• Dental caries experience among children aged 3–5 years attending Head Start
	• Dental caries experience among children attending kindergarten
	• Dental caries experience among third-grade children
Untreated Tooth Decay	• Untreated dental caries among children aged 3–5 years attending Head Start
	• Untreated dental caries among children attending kindergarten
	• Untreated dental caries among third-grade children
Urgent Dental Needs	• Urgent dental treatment need among children aged 3–5 years attending Head Start
	• Urgent dental treatment need among children attending kindergarten
	• Urgent dental treatment need among third-grade children
Dental Sealants	• Children and adolescents aged 3–19 years with dental sealants on one of more primary or permanent molar teeth
	• Third-grade students with dental sealants on at least one permanent molar tooth
	• Dental sealant use among children aged 6–9 years and 10–14 years enrolled in Medicaid

Oral Health Indicator	Assessment Measure(s)
Fluoride and Fluoridation Indicators	• Population served by community water fluoridation • School-Based Health Centers that provide topical fluoride
Infrastructure and Capacity Indicators	• Population receiving oral health services at Federally Qualified Health Centers • School-Based Health Centers that provide dental sealants • School-Based Health Centers that provide dental care • States with an oral health surveillance system

(From National Oral Health Surveillance System. Atlanta, GA: Centers for Disease Control and Prevention; 2015. Available at: <https://www.cdc.gov/oralhealthdata/overview/nohss.htmlhttp://www.cdc.gov/nohss/index.htm>; [Accessed December, 2019]; Best Practice Approaches for State and Community Oral Health Programs. Reno, NV: Association of State and Territorial Dental Directors; 2017. Available at: <https://www.astdd.org/docs/BPASurveillanceSystem.pdf>; [Accessed May, 2020]; Healthy People 2030. Rockville, MD: Office of Disease Prevention and Health Promotion. Available at: <https://health.gov/healthypeople/objectives-and-data/browse-objectives/>; [Accessed September 2020].)

HEALTH ASSESSMENT: ESSENTIAL IN MONITORING COMMUNITY HEALTH

The previous chapter focused on assessment for community profiling and program planning to improve the health of the community. The emphasis of this chapter is assessment for the purpose of population surveillance. Both chapters highlight the protection, promotion, and improvement of the health of communities but emphasize different relevant processes.

Public health **surveillance** is the *ongoing systematic collection, analysis,* and *interpretation* of health-related data essential to planning, implementing, and evaluating public health practice. Closely integrated is the timely *dissemination* of these data to those responsible for planning, implementing, and evaluating public health practices and programs designed to prevent and control diseases and conditions.[1] All four processes (data collection, analysis, interpretation, and dissemination) are critical to the fulfillment of the following functions of surveillance:[2]

1. Provide actionable health information to public health staff, government leaders, and the public to guide public health policy and programs.
2. Serve as an early warning system for impending public health emergencies.
3. Document the impact of an intervention.
4. Track progress toward specific goals.
5. Monitor and clarify the epidemiology of health problems.
6. Inform public health policy, the setting of priorities, and the identification of strategies.

Health and oral health disparities exist across the United States (U.S.) population, affecting all ethnicities and age groups.[3] Oral health diseases and problems and resulting dental treatment can place an economic burden on society by compromising the ability to perform well at home, school, or on the job, resulting in lost time from productive work.[4,5]

Multiple determinants influence oral health in populations[4] (see Chapter 3). In addition, various factors affect access of population groups to community preventive services and clinical dental services.[4] Community preventive services such as community water fluoridation can prevent oral diseases at a community level and improve population oral health. Clinical preventive dental services such as restorative treatment can prevent oral problems among individuals with access to dental clinics or offices. Also, oral health practices and healthy behaviors by individuals can affect oral health outcomes. When conducting population surveillance, it is important to evaluate disparities as well as these and other key determinants that influence oral health **status** and **trends**.[6]

The U.S. faces a crisis with the burden of chronic diseases, including oral diseases and conditions.[5] Agencies and organizations such as the National Institute of Health (NIH), the **Centers for Disease Control and Prevention** (CDC), the National Institute of Dental and Craniofacial Research (NIDCR), and the **Association of State and Territorial Dental Directors** (ASTDD) are committed to improving the oral health of the nation by expanding and improving community-wide oral health surveillance.[4]

HEALTHY PEOPLE

Health promotion and disease prevention are important concepts in the U.S.[7] Therefore, the nation has developed plans for the prevention of diseases and the promotion of health embodied in the initiative known as *Healthy People*.[8] This program is grounded in the notion that establishing objectives and providing benchmarks to track and monitor progress over time can motivate, guide, and focus action.[8]

Healthy People has been the nation's blueprint for disease prevention and health promotion since the Surgeon General issued the first landmark report of the *Healthy People* initiative in 1979.[8] Referred to as *Healthy People 1990*, it included comprehensive, measurable national 10-year health objectives to be achieved by 1990.[8] In subsequent decades, *Healthy People 2000, 2010, 2020,* and *2030* were developed by the Department of Health and Human Services (DHHS), setting similar objectives to be achieved by the end of each decade.[8]

Each decade's objectives shaped the health agenda, established priorities, and provided targets aimed at improving the health of Americans for that period.[8] *Healthy People* priorities are those aspects of health that are the most critical to overall health and well-being and can be improved using available knowledge.[9] Progress reviews have been conducted for past decades of *Healthy People* to provide senior DHHS officials, *Healthy People* stakeholders, and the public with information and data on the current status of objectives and changes in health status of the population.[9,10] The results of the progress reviews also inform each new decade's goals and objectives.[9]

Development of *Healthy People 2030*

In May 2017, a committee was formed by the DHHS to develop *Healthy People 2030*.[9] This fifth edition of the program targets new challenges to improve the nation's health, building on the information learned from the previous 4 decades of benchmarks. In addition, the national Oral Conditions objectives outlined for *Healthy People 2030* provide an important framework for the development of oral health assessments at the state and local levels for the purpose of surveillance during this decade.[8]

Healthy People 2030 is the outcome of a multiyear, extensive collaborative process that relied on input from a diverse collection of individuals and organizations, both within and outside the federal government, with a common interest in improving the nation's health.[11] The Federal Interagency Workgroup on *Healthy People 2030* (FIW) oversaw and managed its development using input from the Secretary of Health and Human Services' Advisory Committee on National Health Promotion and Disease Prevention Objectives for 2030 and other *Healthy People* stakeholders.[11] Representatives from agencies within the DHHS served on the FIW, and federal agencies outside DHHS also served in support of the *Healthy People 2030* framework. Additional involvement in its development came from a private-public alliance of nonprofit, voluntary, and professional organizations; businesses; communities; and individuals, in addition to national, state, and local agencies, including a broad range of state, territorial, and tribal public health and health agencies.[11]

Healthy People 2030 Framework

The *Healthy People 2030* framework consists of a vision statement, a mission statement, foundational principles, and overarching goals that provide structure and guidance for achieving the *Healthy People 2030* objectives (Box 4.1). The framework also includes a plan of action to improve the health and well-being of people in the U.S.[12] The purposes of the framework are to provide context and rationale for the initiative's approach, communicate the principles that underlie decisions about *Healthy People 2030*, and situate the initiative within the five-decade history of *Healthy People*.[12]

The framework design embraces the determinants of health as an approach to health improvement and promotes the integration of policies that advance health.[8] It is influenced by a perspective of risk factors as a guide to improving health and builds on past versions of *Healthy People*.[8] Although the framework is general in nature, it emphasizes important areas in which action must be taken if the U.S. is to achieve better health by the year 2030. The final section of the framework is the plan of action which builds on all other sections (see Guiding Principles).

BOX 4.1 *Healthy People 2030* Framework

Vision

A society in which all people can achieve their full potential for health and well-being across the lifespan.

Mission

To promote, strengthen, and evaluate the nation's efforts to improve the health and well-being of all people.

Foundational Principles

Foundational principles explain the thinking that guides decisions about Healthy People 2030.

- Health and well-being of all people and communities are essential to a thriving, equitable society.
- Promoting health and well-being and preventing disease are linked efforts that encompass physical, mental, and social health dimensions.
- Investing to achieve the full potential for health and well-being for all provides valuable benefits to society.
- Achieving health and well-being requires eliminating **health disparities**, achieving **health equity**, and attaining **health literacy**.
- Healthy physical, social, and economic environments strengthen the potential to achieve health and well-being.
- Promoting and achieving the nation's health and well-being is a shared responsibility that is distributed across the national, state, tribal, and community levels, including the public, private, and not-for-profit sectors.
- Working to attain the full potential for health and well-being of the population is a component of decision-making and policy formulation across all sectors.

Overarching Goals

- Attain healthy, thriving lives and well-being, free of preventable disease, disability, injury, and premature death.
- Eliminate health disparities, achieve health equity, and attain health literacy to improve the health and well-being of all.
- Create social, physical, and economic environments that promote attaining full potential for health and well-being for all.
- Promote healthy development, healthy behaviors, and well-being across all life stages.
- Engage leadership, key constituents, and the public across multiple sectors to take action and design policies that improve the health and well-being of all.

(From Healthy People 2030. Rockville, MD: Office of Disease Prevention and Health Promotion. Available at: <https://health.gov/healthypeople/objectives-and-data/browse-objectives/>; [Accessed September 2020].)

GUIDING PRINCIPLES

Healthy People 2030 Plan of Action

- Set national goals and measurable objectives to guide evidence-based policies, programs and other actions to improve health and well-being.
- Provide data that is accurate, timely, accessible, and can drive targeted actions to address regions and populations with poor health or are at high risk for poor health in the future.
- Foster impact through public and private efforts to improve health and well-being for people of all ages and the communities in which they live.
- Provide tools for the public, programs, policy makers and others to evaluate progress toward improving health and well-being.
- Share and support the implementation of evidence-based programs and policies that are replicable, scalable and sustainable.
- Report biennially on progress throughout the decade from 2020 to 2030.
- Stimulate research and innovation toward meeting *Healthy People 2030* goals and highlight critical research, data, and evaluation needs.
- Facilitate development and availability of affordable means of health promotion, disease prevention, and treatment.

(From Healthy People 2030. Rockville, MD: Office of Disease Prevention and Health Promotion. Available at: <https://health.gov/healthypeople/objectives-and-data/browse-objectives/>; [Accessed September 2020].)

An interactive graphic model planned for the *Healthy People 2030* framework will enable users to explore it in more detail. Actionable data, strategic resources, and evidence-based interventions will intertwine through each concept of the graphic model to enable achievement of the overarching goals.[13] The purposes of the framework graphic are to capture main components of the *Healthy People 2030* framework in an action model, allow users to drill down for more detailed information in the action model, and build a shared understanding of fundamental public health concepts for a range of users.[13]

Promoting Health Equity by Eliminating Health Inequities and Disparities

The elimination of health disparities and promotion of health equity are embedded in the *Healthy People 2030* framework and objectives.[12] Achieving these lofty goals will require actions to address all important determinants of health that can be influenced by institutional policies and practices.[12] The concept of promoting health equity and eliminating health disparities requires removing obstacles to health and health care such as poverty, discrimination, and their consequences. These obstacles include the powerlessness that is produced by lack of access to good jobs with fair pay, insufficient opportunity for a quality education, inability to secure quality housing, and other compromised determinants of health (see Chapter 3). Social policies related to income, education, and housing are also powerful influences on health because they affect factors such as the types of foods that can be purchased and the quality of housing and neighborhoods in which individuals can live (Figure 4.1).[9]

The concepts of health equity and health disparities are inseparable in their practical application. However, policies and practices aimed at promoting health equity do not immediately eliminate health disparities. The general public usually understands health disparities to mean any differences in health. However, as defined by the Secretary's Advisory Committee for *Healthy People 2030*, the term health disparity refers to a particular type of health difference between individuals or groups that is unfair because it is caused by social or economic disadvantage.[9]

Health equity is a desirable goal and standard that entails special efforts to improve the health of those who have experienced social or economic disadvantage. Health equity is oriented toward achieving the highest level of health possible for all groups. The *Healthy People 2030* framework emphasizes health equity and addresses historical and current structural and systematic discrimination that influences health instead of only disease outcomes attributed to individual behaviors. Approximately 30% of the objectives clearly address health equity.[9] The following primary categories were used to classify the objectives as health equity objectives:[9]

1. Strategies to remove obstacles to health.
2. Initiatives to address structural and systematic prejudice and discrimination.
3. Policies and practices that promote health equity, including preventive care.
4. Conditions and opportunities that would allow children and youth to attain their highest level of health and well-being throughout their lifespan.
5. Healthy physical, social, and economic environments.

Oral health inequities and disparities occur in defined populations categorized by race/ethnicity, socioeconomic status, gender, disability status, sexual orientation, and geographic location.[11] For example, low socioeconomic status (SES) groups, uninsured individuals, rural and isolated populations, older adults, children, and pregnant women are identified as vulnerable and underserved. Low-oral-health-literacy individuals also experience oral health inequities and disparities.[11]

National Health Objectives

The overarching goals of *Healthy People* each decade provide general direction for developing health objectives that can be used to track progress of population health within the decade.[8] The national *Healthy People* objectives over the years have called for action to promote healthy behaviors and healthy and safe communities; improve systems for personal health and public health; address determinants of health; and prevent diseases, injuries, disabilities, and disorders.[8,9]

Healthy People 2030 has 355 core measurable objectives as well as developmental and research objectives.[12] This is significantly fewer objectives than in *Healthy People 2020*.[9] The objectives are organized by 62 topic areas that are further ordered into categories (see Box 4.2).[12] Each topic area has objectives that represent various types of health-related conditions;[12] in Box 4.2 these are indicated by their acronyms beside each topic area in parentheses, and the acronyms are explained following the topics in the box.

The *Healthy People 2030* objectives were established by a diverse group of individuals and organizations, reviewed by

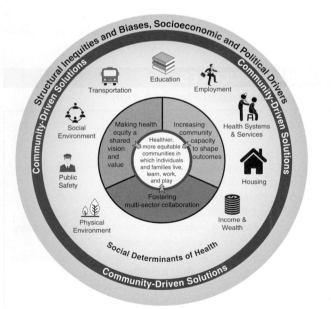

Fig 4.1 Conceptual model of community solutions to promote health equity. (From The Root Causes of Health Inequity. In: Communities in Action: Pathways to Health Equity. Washington, DC: The National Academies of Sciences, Engineering, and Medicine; 2017. Available at: <https://www.nap.edu/read/24624/chapter/5>; [Accessed May 2020].)

BOX 4.2   Topics by Which *Healthy People 2030* Objectives Are Organized

Health Conditions
- Addiction (SU)
- Arthritis (A)
- Blood Disorders (BDBS)
- Cancer (C & OH)
- Chronic Kidney Disease (CKD)
- Chronic Pain (A, CP, D & SU)
- Dementias (DIA)
- Diabetes (CKD, D, MPS, OA & V)
- Foodborne Illness (FS)
- Healthcare-Associated Infections (HAI)
- Heart Disease and Stroke (CKD, HDS & PREP)
- Infectious Disease (HAI, HOSCD & IID)
- Mental Health and Mental Disorders (AH, C, DH, EMC, IVP, LGBT, MHMD, MICH & MPS)
- **Oral Conditions (AHS, NWS & OH)**
- Osteoporosis (O)
- Overweight and Obesity (D, MICH & NWS)
- Pregnancy and Childbirth (FP, HIV, IID, MICH, STI & TU)
- Respiratory Disease (C & RD)
- Sensory or Communication Disorders (HOSCD, OSH & V)
- Sexually Transmitted Infections (HIV, IID & STI)

Health Behaviors
- Child and Adolescent Development (AH, ECBP, EH, EMC, HOSCD, IVP, MICH, PA, SDOH & SH)
- Drug and Alcohol Use (IID, IVP, LGBT, MHMD, MICH, MPS & SU)
- Emergency Preparedness (BDBS, GH, HC/HIT & PREP)
- Family Planning (FP, HIV & STI)
- Health Communication (AH, C, D & HC/HIT)
- Injury Prevention (IVP, MHMD, MICH & OA)
- Nutrition and Healthy Eating (AH, C, D, ECBP, HDS, MICH & NPS)
- Physical Activity (A, C, ECBP, HDS, NWS, OA & PA)
- Preventive Care (AH, AHS, C, D, ECBP, HDS, MHMD, HOSCD, MICH, O, OH, STI & V)
- Safe Food Handling (FS)
- Sleep (AH, EMC, MICH & SH)
- Tobacco Use (C, ECBP, MICH & TU)
- Vaccination (IID)
- Violence Prevention (AH, IVP & OSH)

Populations
- Adolescents (AH, C, CKD, DH, ECBP, EH, EMC, FP, HIV, HOSCD, IID, IVP, LGBT, MHMD, MICH, NWS, OH, PA, RD, SDOH, SH, STI, SU, TU & V)
- Children (AH, DH, ECBP, EH, EMC, FS, HOSCD, IID, IVP, LGBT, MHMD, MICH, NWS, OH, PA, PREP, RD, SDOH, TU & V)
- Infants (FS, HIV, HOSCD, IID, IVP, MICH & STI)
- LGBT (HIV & STI)
- Men (C, FP & STI)
- Older Adults (DIA, FS, IVP, O, OA, OH, RD & V)
- Parents or Caregivers (DH, CP, DIA, EMC, HC/HIT, PA, PREP & SDOH)
- People with Disabilities (A, AH, DH, HOSCD, MICH, OA & V)
- Women (C, FP, FS, IID, MICH, NWS, O, STI & TU)
- Workforce (AHS, ECBP, EH, OSH, PHI, TU & V)

Settings and Systems
- Community (AH, C, ECBP, FS, HDS, NWS, PA, PHI, PREP & V)
- Environmental Health (EH)
- Global Health (EH & GH)
- Health Care (A, AH, AHS, BDBS, C, CKD, D, DH, DIA, EMC, FS, HC/HIT, HDS, HIV, MHMD, HOSCD, IID, MICH, MPS, NWS, OH, SH, STI, SU, TU & V)
- Health Insurance (AHS, DH & TU)

- Health IT (AHS, HC/HIT & PHI)
- Health Policy (EH, OH & TU)
- Hospital and Emergency Services (AHS, CKD, DIA, HAI, HC/HIT, HDS, IVP, MICH, MPS, OA, RD & SU)
- Housing and Homes (DH, EH, MHMD, SDOH & TU)
- Public Health Infrastructure (DH, FP, GH, HC/HIT, IID, IVP, LGBT, OH, PHI, SDOH & V)
- Schools (AH, C, ECBP, EMC, FP, OH, SDOH & PREP)
- Transportation (EH, IVP, PA, SH & SU)
- Workplace (EH, ECBP, OSH, TU & V)

Social Determinants of Health
- Economic Stability (A, AH, NWS, OSH & SDOH)
- Education Access and Quality (AH, DH, ECBP, EMC & SDOH)
- Health Care Access and Quality (AH, AHS, C, DH, ECBP, EMC, FP, HC/HIT, HIV, HOSCD, MICH, OH, STI, SU & V)
- Neighborhood and Built Environment (AH, DH, ECBP, EH, HC/HIT, HOSCD, IVP, OH, PA, RD, SDOH & TU)
- Social and Community Context (AH, DH, EMC, HC/HIT, LGBT, NWS & SDOH)

Acronyms for the Types of Objectives in Each Topic
- A—Arthritis
- AH—Adolescent Health
- AHS—Access to Health Services
- BDBS—Blood Disorders and Blood Safety
- C—Cancer
- CKD—Chronic Kidney Disease
- CP—Chronic Pain
- DIA—Dementias
- D—Diabetes
- DH—Disability and Health
- ECBP—Educational and Community-Based Programs
- EH—Environmental Health
- EMC—Early and Middle Childhood
- FP—Family Planning
- FS—Food Safety
- GH—Global Health
- HAI—Healthcare-Associated Infections
- HC/HIT—Health Communication and Health Information Technology
- HDS—Heart Disease and Stroke
- HIV—Human Immunodeficiency Virus
- HOSCD—Hearing and Other Sensory or Communication Disorders
- IID—Immunization and Infectious Diseases
- IVP—Injury and Violence Prevention
- LGBT—Lesbian, Gay, Bisexual, and Transgender Health
- MHMD—Mental Health and Mental Disorders
- MICH—Maternal, Infant, and Child Health
- MPS—Medical Product Safety
- NWS—Nutrition and Weight Status
- O - Osteoporosis
- OA—Older Adults
- ***OH— Oral Health***
- OSH—Occupational Safety and Health
- PA—Physical Activity
- PHI—Public Health Infrastructure
- PREP - Preparedness
- RD—Respiratory Diseases
- SDOH—Social Determinants of Health
- SH—Sleep Health
- STI—Sexually Transmitted Infections
- SU—Substance Use
- TU—Tobacco Use
- V—Vision

(From Healthy People 2030. Rockville, MD: Office of Disease Prevention and Health Promotion. Available at: <https://health.gov/healthypeople/objectives-and-data/browse-objectives/>; [Accessed September 2020].)

the FIW,[9] and finalized by the FIW and Advisory Committee with input from public comments.[13] Compared with previous decades, the approach of *Healthy People 2030* objectives to improve health has included a greater focus on targeting reductions in adverse social and physical determinants of health.[8]

A smaller set of *Healthy People* objectives have been identified each decade as high-priority health issues and are known as the **leading health indicators** (LHI).[12] These LHIs do not represent all topic areas and are key measures for national population health improvement efforts.[12] Because they are based on current needs and priorities, they change from one decade to another. The 23 LHIs for this decade address the life span, and many focus on how people live their lives.[12] Shaped by the broad context of policies, systems, social structures, and economic forces in the nation,[12] they:

1. focus on upstream measures, like risk factors and behaviors, instead of disease outcomes,
2. speak to issues of national importance,
3. address high-priority public health issues that have a major impact on public health outcomes,
4. are modifiable in the short erm (through evidence-based interventions and strategies to motivate action at the national, state, local, and community levels),
5. focus on social determinants of health, health disparities, and health equity, and
6. help organizations, communities, and states "focus their resources and efforts to improve the health and well-being of all people."[12]

See Figure 4.2 for the *Healthy People 2030* LHI that represents the Oral Conditions topic area.[12] However, awareness of all LHIs is important in relation to interpreofessional collaborative practice.

During the last four decades, many states and localities have used the *Healthy People* framework, objectives, LHIs, tools, and resources to guide the development of state and community health improvement plans and performance standards.[8] Communities as small as neighborhoods and as large as municipalities, can adopt or alter the goals and objectives to meet their own needs and/or use them to set priorities for their region and population groups. Several resources based on the national health objectives have been developed to guide these planning initiatives (see Additional Resources at the end of this chapter and Chapters 3 and 5). Outcomes data will be available periodically during the decade to monitor progress in relation to the targets of the objectives and LHIs.

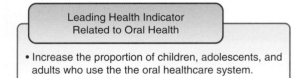

Fig 4.2 Leading health indicator representing the Oral Conditions topic area of *Healthy People 2030*. (From Healthy People 2030. Rockville, MD: Office of Disease Prevention and Health Promotion. Availalbe at: <https://health.gov/healthypeople>; [Accessed December 2020].)

National Oral Conditions Objectives

Oral Conditions is one of the 62 *Healthy People 2030* topics by which the objectives are organized.[12] The Oral Conditions objectives (see Table 4.1) define the nation's oral health agenda and serve as a road map of national oral health benchmarks.[12] Additionally, oral health is integrated into the following selected objectives in other *Healthy People 2030* topics:[12]

Cancer (C)
- Reduce the overall cancer death rate.

Environmental Health (EH)
- Increase the proportion of people whose water supply meets Safe Drinking Water Act regulations.

Tobacco Use (TU)
- Reduce current tobacco in adults.
- Increase the proportion of adults who get advice to quit smoking from a healthcare provider.
- Increase use of smoking cessation counseling and/or medication in adults who smoke.
- Reduce current tobacco use in adolescents (including smokeless tobacco and e-cigarettes).
- Reduce the proportion of adolescents exposed to tobacco marketing.

The *Healthy People 2030* Oral Conditions objectives and other objectives that relate to oral health are based on the latest oral health research and scientific evidence.[12] They combine current information with contemporary public health principles to benefit the largest number of people in the U.S. The Oral Conditions objectives are designed to be used in the following ways:[9]

- Inform decision-making and resource allocation by driving action at national, state, and local levels toward the achievement of common oral health improvement goals.
- Guide states, territories, tribes, and localities in forming health plans for oral health improvements.
- Shape the development and implementation of policies, interventions, programs, and practices tailored for specific population groups.
- Provide significant opportunities to improve oral health for all Americans by providing a focus for efforts in the public, private, and nonprofit sectors.
- Provide a framework for measuring oral health indicators and progress toward achievement of targets (see Opening Statement for a list of oral health indicators).

Additional information about measures used to monitor *Healthy People 2030* objectives related to oral health and the key data sources will be discussed throughout the rest of this chapter and in Chapter 5.

ORAL HEALTH SURVEILLANCE SYSTEMS

An effective public health **surveillance system** routinely collects data on health outcomes, risk factors, and intervention strategies for the whole population or representative samples of the population.[6] The CDC recommends surveillance of any health-related event that affects many people, requires large expenditures of resources, is largely preventable, and is of public health importance, including an oral disease or condition.[1]

TABLE 4.1 *Healthy People 2030* Oral Conditions Objectives

Number	Objective	Baseline	Target	Data Sources
OH-1	Reduce the proportion of children and adolescents with lifetime tooth decay experience in their primary or permanent teeth (ages 3–19 years)	48.4%	42.3%	National Health and Nutrition Examination Survey (NHANES), Centers for Disease Control and Prevention (CDC)/National Center for Health Statistics (NCHS)
OH-2	Reduce the proportion of children and adolescents with active and currently untreated tooth decay in their primary or permanent teeth (ages 3–19 years)	13.4%	10.2%	NHANES, CDC/NCHS
OH-3	Reduce the proportion of adults with active or currently untreated tooth decay (ages 20–74 years)	22.8%	17.3%	NHANES, CDC/NCHS
OH-4	Reduce the proportion of older adults with untreated root surface decay (ages ≥75 years)	29.1%	20.1%	NHANES, CDC/NCHS
OH-5	Reduce the proportion of adults who have lost all of their natural teeth (ages ≥45 years)	7.9%	5.4%	NHANES, CDC/NCHS
OH-6	Reduce the proportion of adults with moderate and severe periodontitis (≥45 years)	44.5%	39.3%	NHANES, CDC/NCHS
OH-7	Increase the proportion of oral and pharyngeal cancers detected at the earliest stage	29.5%	34.2%	Surveillance, Epidemiology, and End Results Program (SEER); National Institutes of Health (NIH)/National Cancer Institute (NCI)
OH-8[a]	Increase the proportion of children, adolescents, and adults who use the oral healthcare system	43.3%	45.0%	Medical Expenditure Panel Survey (MEPS), Agency for Healthcare Research and Quality (AHRQ)
OH-9[b]	Increase the proportion of low-income youth who have a preventive dental visit (ages 1–17 years)	78.8%	82.7%	National Survey of Children's Health (NSCH), Health Resources & Services Administration (HRSA)/Maternal and Child Health Bureau (MCHB)
OH-10	Increase the proportion of children and adolescents who have received dental sealants on one or more of their primary or permanent molar teeth (ages 3–19 years)	37.0%	42.5%	NHANES, CDC/NCHS
OH-11[b]	Increase the proportion of persons served by community systems with optimally fluoridated water	72.8%	77.1%	Water Fluoridation Reporting System (WFRS), CDC/National Center for Chronic Disease Prevention and Health Promotion (NCCDPHP)
OH-D01[c]	Increase the number of states and the District of Columbia that have an oral and craniofacial health surveillance system	N/A	N/A	N/A
AHS-02	Increase the proportion of persons with dental insurance	54.4%	59.8%	National Health Interview Survey (NHIS), CDC/NCHS
AHS-05	Reduce the proportion of persons who are unable to obtain or are delayed in obtaining necessary dental care	4.6%	4.1%	MEPS, AHRQ
NWS-10	Reduce the consumption of calories from added sugars (ages ≥2 years)	13.5%	11.5%	NHANES, CDC/NCHS

[a]Leading health indicator
[b]Relates to health equity
[c]Developmental objective (a high-priority public health issue that has evidence-based interventions to address it, but does not yet have reliable baseline data)
(From Healthy People 2030. Rockville, MD: Office of Disease Prevention and Health Promotion. Available at: <https://health.gov/healthypeople/objectives-and-data/browse-objectives/>; [Accessed December 2020].Secretary's Advisory Committee on National Health Promotion and Disease Prevention Objectives for 2030: Report #7: Assessment and Recommendations for Proposed Objectives for *Healthy People 2030*. Washington, DC: Secretary's Advisory Committee for Healthy People 2030. 2019 Apr. Available at: <https://www.healthypeople.gov/sites/default/files/Report%207_Reviewing%20Assessing%20Set%20of%20HP2030%20Objectives_Formatted%20EO_508_05.21.pdf>; [Accessed March 2020].)

Because of the oral-systemic link, oral health surveillance efforts build on overall health surveillance. A comprehensive public health surveillance system integrates oral health and is essential for programmatic activities to improve oral health.[2] This chapter concentrates on oral health surveillance, which is important for all vulnerable underserved population groups.[4,6] Surveillance is accomplished in relation to various common oral and craniofacial diseases and conditions (see Appendix E). Several agencies and national organizations have stressed the importance of oral health surveillance systems to routinely collect data on oral health outcomes, risk factors, and outcomes of intervention strategies for the population.[6,14]

In addition to the collection of oral health data, oral health surveillance also involves timely communication of oral health findings to responsible parties and the public.[1] Surveillance also encompasses using the data to initiate and evaluate public health measures to prevent and control oral diseases.[14]

Collaborative steps have been taken in the U.S. at the national, state, and local levels to formulate a systematic approach for oral health data collection and reporting.[6,14] Results of these actions include dissemination of procedures for collecting comparable data, expansion of indicators, development of standard ways to monitor the national objectives related to oral health, creation of an oral health needs assessment model, and documentation of uniform methods to measure community oral health.[6,14]

The ASTDD is a national nonprofit organization that represents state and territorial public health agency programs for oral health. The organization has developed and updated several resources that provide guidance on oral health surveillance, including a best-practices report that provides a review of oral health assessment measures, methods, and standards (Box 4.3).[6]

National Oral Health Surveillance System

Historically, the oral health surveillance system has been under the control of the federal government. The **National Oral Health Surveillance System** (NOHSS) is an important system of oral health data sources to track oral health surveillance indicators. It was established by and operates through a collaborative effort between the CDC Division of Oral Health and the ASTDD.[14] The NOHSS is designed to monitor the burden of oral disease, the use of the oral healthcare delivery system, and the status of community water fluoridation on both a national and state level.

The usefulness of the NOHSS is based on states having available data sources and the ability to collect data.[14] The NOHSS is under continual revision to provide the best data available for decision-making. A functioning state oral health surveillance system is central to enabling states to submit data for inclusion in the NOHSS.[6] At the same time, the submission of data by states is imperative to provide a complete national picture and to enable comparisons among states.[6,14] Even though a few states have collected data over the years, a comprehensive oral health surveillance system at the state level does not exist.[6,14]

The NOHSS was developed to track basic **oral health indicators,** which are a recommended standard set of minimal quantifiable characteristics of a population used by researchers to describe the oral health of the a population (see Opening Statement).[6,14] These oral health indicators are evaluated and revised as the need arises and line up with the current *Healthy People* Oral Conditions objectives.[14]

A major data source for assessment and surveillance data is the **National Health and Nutrition Examination Survey** (NHANES), an initiative of the CDC.[15] The NHANES is a program of studies designed to provide a comprehensive assessment of the health and nutritional status of adults and children in the U.S. The survey is unique in that it combines interviews and physical examinations (Figure 4.3). Oral health is a component of this survey, providing comprehensive data for surveillance, assessment for program planning, and research. Two other important national health surveillance surveys that include questions related to oral health are the **National Health Interview Survey** (NHIS) and the **Behavioral Risk Factor Surveillance System** (BRFSS).[16,17] The NHIS monitors health status and access to care in the population with personal household interviews on a broad range of health topics. The BRFSS is a state-specific telephone survey conducted with individuals and parents to assess their practice of behaviors that influence health status, including the use of health services.

These and other data sources presented in Table 4.1 and Appendix D will bring about an understanding of the breadth of available oral health-related data. These data sources are useful for surveillance purposes and to assess needs for program

---

BOX 4.3 Best Practice Criteria for a State-Based Oral Health Surveillance System, Association of State and Territorial Dental Directors

1. Impact/Effectiveness:
   - Contains a core set of measures that describe the status of important oral health conditions and behaviors and serve as benchmarks for assessing progress in achieving good oral health.
   - Communicates data and information to responsible parties and to the public in a timely manner.
   - Data and findings used for public health actions.
2. Efficiency:
   - Data collection managed on a periodic but regular schedule.
   - Cost-effective strategies used to collect, analyze, and communicate surveillance data.
3. Demonstrated Sustainability:
   - Several years of data and analysis of trends to demonstrate maturity.
4. Collaboration/Integration:
   - Partnerships established to leverage resources in data collection.
   - Use of data and findings to integrate oral health into other health programs.
5. Objectives/Rationale:
   - Clear purpose and objectives that specify how data will be used for public health action.

(From Best Practice Approach: State-Based Oral Health Surveillance System. Reno, NV: Association of State and Territorial Dental Directors; 2017 Jul. Available at: https://www.astdd.org/docs/BPASurveillanceSystem.pdf>; [Accessed December 2019].)

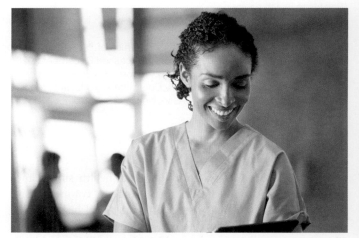

Fig 4.3 The National Health and Nutrition Examination Survey (NHANES) is unique in that it includes interviewing by an examiner in addition to an oral examination. (© iStock.com.)

planning (see Chapter 3). Data are available in various forms from these sources, including charts, graphs, and interactive web-based oral health maps, presented for the nation and by state and county. Several resources have been developed to provide guidance to national, state, territorial, tribal, and local oral health programs in planning and implementing oral health surveillance systems (see the Measurement of Infrastructure, Capacity, and Resources section later in this chapter and Additional Resources and References at the end of the chapter).

MEASURING ORAL HEALTH AND ITS DETERMINANTS IN POPULATIONS

This chapter focuses on measurements of oral health used in population-based oral health surveillance systems, oral health surveys, and research. Highlighted are common measures used to assess specific oral health indicators included in *Healthy People* and the NOHSS to monitor the oral health of the population. The chapter also provides an overview of clinical and nonclinical data collection measures of oral health and related factors. Measures and methods used to assess individual patients in clinical settings or in clinical studies and clinical trials are not emphasized in this chapter. (See Chapter 7 for measurement related to research studies.)

Selection of data collection methods and measures for community oral health assessment should be based on the following:

1. Information of interest (e.g., types of conditions, factors to be assessed).
2. Social and demographic factors of the population and community.
3. Purpose of the assessment (e.g., surveillance, needs assessment).

Common nonclinical measures include face-to-face personal interviews, telephone interviews, self-administered questionnaires, and computer-assisted personal interviews, although other nonclinical methods can be used to assess various factors influencing oral health (see Appendix D). Topics of oral health questions that can be used in oral health surveys for assessment and surveillance are outlined in Appendix E.

Basic screening and epidemiologic examination are clinical methods used for assessment and surveillance of various oral conditions and related factors (see Appendix E). **Basic screening** involves the use of direct observation to visually detect and identify gross dental and oral lesions in the oral cavity with a tongue blade, a dental mirror, and appropriate lighting.[18,19,20] However, an **epidemiologic examination** entails the use of detailed visual-tactile assessment of the oral cavity with dental instruments and a light source.[15] Basic screening and epidemiologic examination do not constitute a thorough clinical examination, and they do not involve making a clinical diagnosis that would result in a treatment plan.[15] Because dichotomous measures of the screening indicators (yes/no) are used, the basic screening approach is generally not appropriate for research; more precise measures are required for clinical trials (see Chapter 7).

Regardless of whether clinical or nonclinical data are required, community oral health assessment involves the use of surveys. Surveys are descriptive and cross-sectional. They allow for oral health determinants to be ascertained and oral health status to be estimated for a defined population at a point in time[21] (see Chapter 7 for more details about research methods).

TYPES OF MEASUREMENTS

This section describes specific dental indices and measurements used to assess the various diseases and conditions of interest, as well as specific factors that relate to oral health. The measurements described in this section are used to generate the data within the data sources used for oral health surveillance.

Examination Methods

Basic Screening. Designed to minimize the time required and resources necessary for scoring, the basic screening approach is used in several basic screening survey tools used for surveillance and assessment:

- **Basic Screening Survey: Preschool and School Children—** designed by ASTDD for state and local surveillance and assessment.[20]
- **Basic Screening Survey: Older Adults—** designed by ASTDD for state and local surveillance and assessment.[19]
- **Basic Oral Health Survey—** designed by the World Health Organization (WHO) for global surveillance.[18]

The Basic Screening Survey (BSS) tools are useful for screening in local oral health programs and in assessing needs for program planning, are in common use in the U.S., and are used in some state-level surveillance surveys. Recommended and optional variables called screening indicators (see Table 4.2) are measured via questionnaire, intraoral screening, or both.[19,20,22] The WHO survey tool is used by WHO member countries for global surveillance.[18]

For all age groups, observations of oral health status on BSS surveys are made by dentists, dental hygienists, or other appropriate healthcare workers in accordance with state law, and questionnaires can be administered by nondental personnel.[19,20] When the BSS is used with an older adult population that has limited cognitive function, the ASTDD suggests that data collection be limited to an in-mouth screening with an option to obtain some information from the resident, resident's guardian, or staff if in a residential facility.[19]

Epidemiologic Examinations. Frequently, a dental index is used for measurement during an epidemiologic examination. A **dental index** is an abbreviated measurement of the amount or condition of oral disease or related condition in a population.[23] An index is based on a graduated numeric scale with defined upper and lower limits. It is an aid in data collection, allowing for comparisons among population groups that are classified by the same criteria and methods. Thus, dental indexes, also called dental indices, can be used to assess oral diseases and conditions in oral health surveys and are frequently also used to measure variables in clinical trials (see Chapter 7).

When planning data collection with a dental index, it is critical to select an appropriate index[23] (Table 4.3). Appendix F is a resource of common dental indexes for use in epidemiologic examinations of clinical measures for assessment or research

TABLE 4.2	Screening Indicators on the Basic Screening Survey	
Preschool Children	**School Children**	**Older Adults**
Recommended Indicators		
• Untreated decay • Treated decay • Urgency of need for dental care	• Untreated decay • Treated decay • Dental sealants on permanent molars • Urgency of need for dental care	• Dentures and denture use • Number of natural teeth • Untreated decay (coronal and root) • Root fragments • Need for periodontal care • Suspicious soft tissue lesions • Urgency of need for dental care
Optional Indicators		
• Sealants on primary molars • Rampant decay (seven or more teeth with untreated and/or treated decay) • Potentially arrested decay • Number of quadrants with untreated decay	• Dental sealants on primary and permanent molars • Rampant decay • Potentially arrested decay • Number of quadrants with untreated decay	• Functonal posterior occlusal contacts • Substantial oral debris • Severe gingival inflammation • Obvious tooth mobility • Severe dry mouth

(From The Basic Screening Survey: A Tool for Oral Health Surveillance, not Research. Reno, NV: Association of State and Territorial Dental Directors; 2017 Jul. Available at: <https://www.astdd.org/docs/bss-surveillance-not-research-july-2017.pdf>; [Accessed December 2019]; Phipps K. The New & Improved Children's Basic Screening Survey (Webinar). Reno, NV: Association of State and Territorial Dental Directors; 2017. Available at: <https://www.astdd.org/docs/childrens-bss-webinar-ppt-10-12-2017.pdf>; [Accessed March 2020].)

TABLE 4.3	Attributes of an Effective Dental Index
Attribute	**Explanation**
Validity	Index accurately measures what is intended
Reliability	Index measures consistently at different times; results of measures are reproducible and stable
Utility	Criteria are clear, objective, easy to understand, simple to use and calculate, and require minimal equipment
Sensitivity	Small degrees of differences in the variable can be detected by the index
Specificity	Correctly identifies absence of the variable
Acceptability	Application of the index is not unnecessarily painful, time demanding, or demeaning to participants, and use of the index has minimal expense and hassle
Quantifiability	Statistics can be applied to data collected with the index
Clinical significance	Index criteria are clinically meaningful

(From Lo E. Caries Process and Prevention Strategies: Epidemiology, CE Course No. 368. Dentalcare.com; 2018. Available at: <https://www.dentalcare.com/en-us/professional-education/ce-courses/ce368>; [Accessed March 2020]; Wyche CJ. Indices and scoring methods. In: Boyd LD, Mallonee LF, Wyche CJ. Wilkins' Clinical Practice of the Dental Hygienist, 13th ed, pp 357-379. Burlington, MS: Jones & Bartlett Learning; 2021.)

purposes.[23] Dental indexes are also used also for surveillance, although currently the basic screening approach is used for surveillance in many cases.

Measurements of Dental Caries

Dental caries can occur in primary or permanent teeth, and general types of tooth decay include coronal and root caries.

Various measurement methods are used to assess dental caries in a population.

Coronal Dental Caries

In surveys of populations, coronal caries can be assessed by a systematic evaluation through epidemiologic examination or basic screening.[15] The best known and most widely used index to measure coronal caries is the *Decayed, Missing, Filled (DMF) Index*.[15] Recorded by an oral epidemiological examination, this index is used to measure past and present coronal caries experience of a population on permanent teeth (DMFT) or surfaces (DMFS), as well as on primary teeth or surfaces (dmf, df, or def). Each tooth space (T) or surface (S) is scored as sound, decayed, filled, or missing as a result of caries. The DMF is considered irreversible because it indicates the cumulative, lifetime caries experience. Refer to Appendix F for details and scoring criteria for the various variations of the DMF index. Examples of applying DMF results to decision-making in relation to program planning are described in Box 4.4.

The DMF index has been modified to the dmf, df, and def indexes for use with primary teeth in children.[23,24] The lower-case letters signify the use of the index on primary teeth, in contrast with the upper-case letters (e.g., DMFT) denoting the index for permanent teeth. In general, the dmf, df, and def are used and interpreted in the same way as the DMF. However, adjustments have been made in their scoring to compensate for the exfoliation of teeth in children.[23,24] The scoring criteria for the dmf, df, and def can also be found in Appendix F.

The BSS discussed earlier uses a basic screening approach to assess treated and untreated dental caries, scored on a per-person basis or by the number of quadrants or teeth exhibiting each caries indicator[19,20] (see Table 4.2 for the BSS screening indicators). Population measures are formulated

BOX 4.4　Application of Decayed, Missing, Filled Survey Results in Relation to Community Program Planning

Assessment

Decayed, missing, filled (DMF) survey results can be used to prioritize community programming needs by considering the total DMF score for the population in combination with the scores within each category. For example, a high DMF signifies a high level of caries experience, indicating a need to develop programs to prevent and control caries in the population. However, to determine which specific programs are priorities, the components must be analyzed. A high D demonstrates a need for dental treatment, and a high F indicates that the population is receiving treatment. A high M indicates the need for education and earlier intervention to avoid additional extractions in the future. A high D, M, or F indicates the need for prevention.

Program Evaluation

DMF scoring can be repeated for a comparison of outcomes data with baseline data, providing a measure of program success or failure. For example, a reduction of the D component along with an increase in the F component indicates that the population is benefiting from prevention and dental treatment. On the other hand, a marked increase in the D component indicates failure of caries prevention, even if the F component also increases.

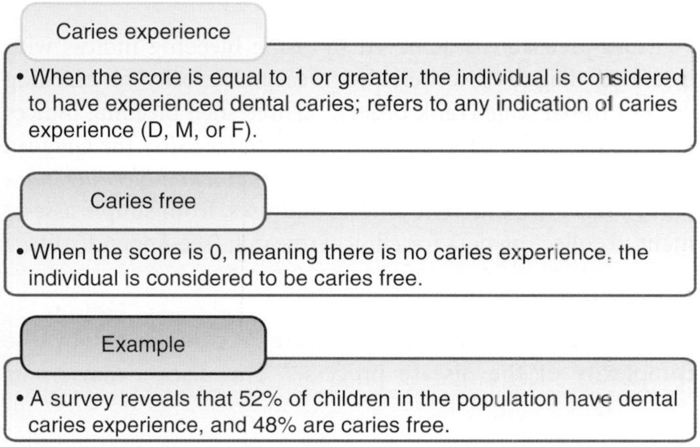

Caries experience

- When the score is equal to 1 or greater, the individual is considered to have experienced dental caries; refers to any indication of caries experience (D, M, or F).

Caries free

- When the score is 0, meaning there is no caries experience, the individual is considered to be caries free.

Example

- A survey reveals that 52% of children in the population have dental caries experience, and 48% are caries free.

Fig 4.4 Caries experience and caries-free. (From Basic Screening Surveys: An Approach to Monitoring Community Oral Health: Preschool & School Children. Reno, NV: Association of State and Territorial Dental Directors; 2008. Available at: <http://www.azdhs.gov/phs/owch/oral-health/documents/infant-youth/ASTDD-BSS-manual.pdf>; [Accessed March 2020].)

---

to indicate the proportion of the population that has *caries experience* versus being *caries-free*. These terms are used commonly to describe the dental caries status of population groups, which can be determined with the BSS or the DMF index (Figure 4.4).

Additional dental caries measures have been developed to reflect treatment needs and to demonstrate the severity of physical and biologic conditions that result from dental caries.[25] These complex indices have not been used for surveillance purposes on a regular basis.

Early Childhood Caries. Use of the *Early Childhood Caries (ECC) Classification* system will result in more detailed reporting of dental caries in preschool-age children. The ECC consists

of case definitions based on the number of dmf surfaces and the child's age [26] (see Appendix F for a detailed explanation and criteria). Assessment of ECC can be accomplished with an epidemiological examination or the basic screening approach, depending on the purpose and precision required.

Missing anterior teeth in preschool children can be a result of caries or traumatic injury. Therefore, the cause of missing anterior teeth should be identified by questioning the parent or guardian, if present during the screening. An alternative is to include a question on the consent form.[20]

Root Surface Caries

Basic screening and epidemiological examinations can be used to assess the occurrence of root surface caries in oral health surveys.[5,20] When using the BSS to screen older adults, root caries is considered along with coronal caries in the dichotomous scoring of untreated decay on a per-person basis[19] (Table 4.2). However, BSS scoring can be adapted to score root caries and coronal caries separately. A similar dichotomous scale for assessing root caries with an intraoral epidemiological examination was applied in the 2020 NHANES.[15] Similar to the BSS, with this approach the survey participant's whole mouth was scored by the examiner for the following variables:

- Root caries detected/root caries not detected/cannot be assessed
- Root restoration detected/root restoration not detected/cannot be assessed

The *Root Caries Index (RCI)* is a common index that can be used to score root caries with an epidemiologic examination when more precise data are required.[23] Cavitated or filled root carious lesions are scored on each surface (see Appendix F for details of scoring criteria). The measurement of root surface caries in populations with the RCI is generally based on the proportion of root surfaces that are decayed or filled, in relation to the number of surfaces that are present in the mouth and at risk for dental caries, including subgingival root surfaces.[23]

In addition to using clinical examinations to assess dental caries in the population, some surveillance surveys include questions that relate to factors associated with dental caries. For example, the 2020 NHANES questionnaire included questions about the age at which the individual started brushing and using toothpaste, and the use of fluorides.[27]

Future Directions for Assessing Dental Caries

Even though major improvements are shown in the oral health of the nation, concerns have continued regarding the prevalence and inequity of dental caries in vulnerable population groups. Thus, oral epidemiologists have suggested the use of improved evidence-based approaches to better measure dental caries for clinical research and population-based assessments.[28]

Because of the dichotomous scale of the commonly used dental caries measurements (presence or absence of caries), assessment of the severity of caries in oral health surveys has been limited generally to the number of teeth or surfaces involved. As patterns of dental caries change, technology develops, and the goals of oral health surveys shift, different approaches for the measurement of dental caries may emerge.[24,28]

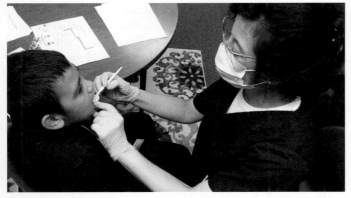

Fig 4.5 A young child is screened for sealants in a school-based oral health program. (Photograph courtesy Terri Patrick.)

Measurement of Dental Sealants

The presence of dental sealants is traditionally assessed in populations through a basic screening or epidemiologic examination procedure (Figure 4.5).[15,20] The criteria for scoring of sealants varies depending on the oral health surveillance survey. See Table 4.4 for a comparison of sealant scoring criteria on the BSS and NHANES. These survey protocols differ for the age of survey participants, selected teeth to be scored, the manner of sealant identification, and the data scoring method (per person or per tooth). A survey protocol will depend on the way the data will be used. For example, the NHANES is designed to provide data to track the current *Healthy People* dental sealant objectives regarding the use of sealants in different age groups.[15,29]

Another important measure of sealant use is the presence of school-based sealant programs in the various states. These programs are recommended by the CDC and ASTDD to increase sealant use among children, especially children of low-income families[30] (see Chapter 6). Using their annual survey of state oral health programs, the ASTDD assesses the number of school-based programs in each state.[31]

Measurement of Periodontal Disease

The term *periodontal disease* represents a group of closely related different diseases with similar presentation rather than a single disease entity.[21] Measurement of periodontal disease in the U.S. population involves assessment of gingivitis and mild to moderate periodontitis, based on the signs and symptoms of each disease. Gingival and periodontal indices have been used to assess periodontal status at the community level.

Gingivitis

The *Gingival Index (GI)* is a core dental index that can be used to assess swelling, color, consistency, and bleeding of the gingiva. The original GI has been adapted as the *Modified Gingival Index (MGI)*, eliminating the probing requirement to avoid potential trauma and to increase reliability.[21] The criteria for these indexes are described in Appendix F.

The BSS includes an optional indicator of severe gingival inflammation based on the GI.[19] It is scored on a dichotomous scale (yes/no) using the GI severe gingivitis category, which is defined as "marked redness and edema, ulceration, tendency to spontaneous bleeding."[19] In addition, population measurement of gingivitis has been accomplished on the NHANES in the past although it has not been included in recent NHANES surveys.[15]

More precision is achieved by using bleeding indices with extended diagnostic criteria to measure severity of bleeding on an ordinal scale (rank order).[23] Three such bleeding indices commonly used are the *Sulcus Bleeding Index (SBI)*, the *Gingival Bleeding Index (GBI)*, and the *Eastman Interdental Bleeding Index (EIBI)*. Each has different criteria and uses, from simple assessment to collecting data for clinical research (see Appendix F).

Periodontitis

Measurement of periodontal disease is complicated by the complexity of the disease process.[32] The disease may occur

TABLE 4.4 Scoring of Sealants for Surveillance

Basic Screening Survey (BSS)	National Health and Nutrition Examination Survey (NHANES)
Dichotomous measure (yes/no) of the presence of at least one dental sealant, scored on a per-person basis; some states elect to adapt this by counting the number of sealed molars in the mouth (per tooth basis)	Dichotomous measure of dental sealants present on the permanent maxillary lateral incisors, first and second premolars/primary molars, and first and second molars; scored on a per tooth basis on primary molars and lateral incisor and per surface basis on permanent molars
Scored on ages 1 year through 12th grade	Scored on ages 3–19 years
Scoring is based on permanent molars; scoring primary molars is optional	Scoring is required on specified teeth (see earlier in the table)
Scored as present whether or not the sealant covers all or part of the pits or fissures or is partially lost	Scored as present whether or not the sealant covers all or part of the pits or fissures or is partially lost
Visual examination with no instruments or air; can be augmented by using an adjunct such as a toothpick or a long-handled cotton tipped applicator to gently feel the surface	Visual examination including drying with air and examining with a surface reflecting mirror and a No. 23 explorer to feel the surface

(From Basic Screening Surveys: An Approach to Monitoring Community Oral Health: Preschool & School Children. Reno, NV: Association of State and Territorial Dental Directors; 2008. Available at: <https://azdhs.gov/documents/prevention/womens-childrens-health/oral-health/infant-youth/ASTDD-BSS-manual.pdf>; [Accessed March 2020]; Phipps K. The New & Improved Children's Basic Screening Survey. Reno, NV: Association of State and Territorial Dental Directors; 2017. Available at: <https://www.astdd.org/docs/childrens-bss-webinar-ppt-10-12-2017.pdf>; [Accessed December 2019]; National Health and Nutrition Examination Survey (NHANES) Oral Health Examiners Manual. Atlanta, GA: Centers for Disease Control; 2020. Available at: <https://wwwn.cdc.gov/nchs/data/nhanes/2019-2020/manuals/2020-Oral-Health-Examiners-Manual-508.pdf>; [Accessed May 2020].)

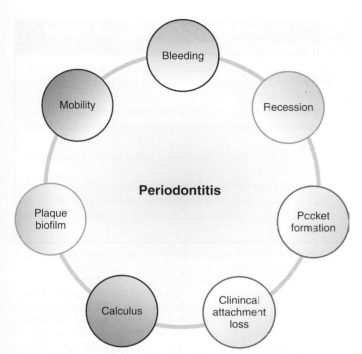

Fig 4.6 Markers of periodontitis. (From Tonetti, MS, Greenwell H, Kornman KS. Staging and grading of periodontitis: Framework and proposal of a new classification and case definition. J Periodontol 2018;89(Suppl1):S159-S172. Available at: <https://aap.onlinelibrary.wiley.com/doi/epdf/10.1002/JPER.18-0006>; [Accessed March 2020].)

differently around different teeth and around different sites of the periodontium surrounding the same tooth. Also, the different rates of disease progression, its varied pathophysiology, and its range of presentation add to the difficulty of accurate measurement.

Various scaled indexes have been used in the past to assess periodontitis, but these were *composite* indexes that scored gingivitis and periodontitis on the same scale. Composite indices are now considered invalid and thus have been discarded.[21] Contemporary measurements of the health of periodontal tissues in population-based surveys reflect current theories of the pathogenesis of periodontal diseases.[21]

The American Academy of Periodontology identifies various diagnostic markers for periodontitis, including a measure of past disease.[32] A disaggregated approach based on these markers is used to evaluate and record associated risk factors, current clinical signs, and destructive results of periodontitis (Figure 4.6). This disaggregated measurement method has been used in the NHANES to monitor status and trends and to track achievement of current *Healthy People* objectives related to periodontitis.[15] The WHO and BSS also use this manner of measuring periodontitis, allowing for program evaluation and comparison of the status and trends among populations.[18,19]

Historically, clinical periodontal examination has been included in the NHANES surveys in the U.S. and in the WHO surveys in other countries.[18,25] However, recent NHANES surveys have used patient self-report of periodontal status and related factors instead of clinical examination (see Box 4.5 for questions included on the 2020 NHANES).[15] Research has

demonstrated that such self-reported measures performed well in predicting periodontitis in U.S. adults.[33]

In the past, periodontitis has been measured in the population by using a sample of adults that did not include older adults.[25] This practice reflected the age range of the *Healthy People* objective related to periodontitis in adults at that time (35- to 44-year-olds). Epidemiologists were concerned that this practice led to underestimating the prevalence of periodontal disease.[21] Therefore, current periodontal disease objectives focus on a more representative age range of adults (ages 45 and older), and recent NHANES surveys have been adjusted to assess periodontitis in this same age group.[15]

The *Community Periodontal Index (CPI)* was developed by the WHO to assess periodontal status and was included in their *Oral Health Surveys: Basic Methods* manual.[18] Used for community surveillance, the CPI assesses selected markers of periodontitis. It allows for a rapid assessment of a population according to various grades of periodontal health (see Appendix F).

Sometimes, to increase efficiency, lower cost, and decrease time spent on the epidemiological examination, partial-mouth periodontal scoring is used to assess periodontal status.[18] For example, the CPI identifies different teeth to be scored in different age groups,[23] although it can be applied to whole mouth scoring as well. Also, the NHANES has used partial-mouth scoring in past clinical assessments.[34] Historically, the *Periodontal Disease Index (PDI)* included specific teeth to be measured (see Appendix F), which presumably represented the whole mouth; these teeth are referred to as the "Ramfjord teeth," named after Dr. Ramfjord, who created the index.[21] Although the index is no longer useful because it does not reflect contemporary theories of periodontal disease, the validity of continuing to use the Ramfjord teeth for partial-mouth scoring of dental indices and disease measures in assessment, surveillance, and clinical research studies has been demonstrated.[21,35]

Future Directions for Assessing Periodontal Disease

Future surveillance measures will be affected by several challenges. First, there is greater emphasis in health care on the oral-systemic link.[36] With stronger evidence of the potential of periodontitis to influence systemic disease, and considering the inflammatory burden as a modifiable contributor, there is greater concern regarding the prevalence and incidence of periodontal disease, especially in vulnerable population groups who have limited access to care.[36] Therefore, epidemiologists and researchers are challenged to apply an interprofessional approach to the measurement of periodontal disease for surveillance, research, and clinical application.

Oral epidemiologists have explored ways to improve periodontal disease surveillance, utilizing case definitions that must be applied across all contexts, namely patient care, epidemiologic surveys, and research on disease mechanisms or therapeutic outcomes.[32] Further challenging this endeavor is the incorporation of the new American Academy of Periodontology (AAP) Periodontal classification. A new focus is on stratification of risk factors such as smoking, uncontrolled type II diabetes, clinical evidence of disease diagnosis and progression at an early age, and severity of bone loss relative to patient age. These risk factors will need to be added to surveillance criteria.[32]

Measurement of Tooth Loss

Complete tooth loss, also referred to as *edentulism*, reflects no remaining teeth regardless of the cause of the loss.[18,19] An individual with at least one natural tooth is considered *dentate*. *Tooth retention* is the presence of a tooth in the mouth; the term is used to refer to the retention of some or all teeth.[18] For example, if 10 teeth are lost, 22 teeth are retained, and the individual is dentate.

Tooth retention and complete or partial tooth loss can be measured in oral health surveys. The number and types of teeth retained by the individual are assessed clinically by scoring each tooth space as present or absent.[15,18] These data can be used to indicate tooth loss at the tooth, arch, or individual level in population studies.

Assessment of tooth loss can be made in the primary or permanent dentition. However, a missing primary tooth should be scored only in an age group in which tooth absence would not be a result of normal exfoliation. Missing teeth can be assessed also according to cause of loss (e.g., caries, periodontal disease, trauma, congenital absence, or orthodontia).[18] Because of the difficulty of correctly distinguishing between teeth extracted because of caries and those extracted for periodontal reasons, in the 2020 NHANES no attempt was made at the time of the examination to differentiate between caries and periodontal disease as the cause of tooth loss.[15] However, if it was determined that teeth were missing for reasons other than caries or periodontal disease, the tooth was not indicated as extracted.[15]

It is recommended that tooth loss be measured in older adults using a basic screening approach.[18,19] The BSS for older adults includes assessment of edentulism on a per-person basis. In addition, the BSS criteria describe a simple count of the number of teeth present in each arch to determine partial tooth loss (Table 4.2).[19]

> ### BOX 4.6   Self-Report Surveillance Survey Questions: Tooth Loss
>
> - Not including teeth lost for injury or orthodontics, how many of your permanent teeth have been removed because of tooth decay or gum disease? (2019–2020 NHANES)
> - Not including teeth lost for injury or orthodontics, how many of your[a] permanent teeth have been removed because of tooth decay or gum disease? (2018 BRFSS)
> - Have you[a] lost all of your[a] upper and lower natural (permanent) teeth? (2018 NHIS; 2017 MEPS)
> - How many of your[a] permanent teeth have been removed because of tooth decay or gum disease? Include teeth lost to infection, but do not include teeth lost for other reasons, such as injury or orthodontics. (BSS Older Adult)

[a] Questions were/can be adapted as needed when asked of a parent, guardian, or care provider.
(From NHANES Questionnaire Instruments: Sample Person Questionnaire: Oral Health: 2019. Hyattsville, MD: National Center for Health Statistics; 2020 Feb 21. Available at: <https://wwwn.cdc.gov/nchs/data/nhanes/2019-2020/questionnaires/OHQ_K.pdf>; [Accessed March 2020]; 2018 BRFSS Questionnaire; 2018 Jan 18. Available at: <https://www.cdc.gov/brfss/questionnaires/pdf-ques/2019_BRFSS_English_Questionnaire-508.pdf>; [Accessed March 2020]; National Health Interview Survey: Adult: 2018. Atlanta, GA: Centers for Disease Control and Prevention; 2019 May 6. Available at: <https://www.cdc.gov/nchs/nhis/nhis_questionnaires.htm>; [Accessed March 2020]; Medical Expenditure Panel Survey Questionnaire: 2017: Additional Health Care. Rockville, MD: Agency for Healthcare Research and Quality; 2019 Nov 18. Available at: <https://www.meps.ahrq.gov/mepsweb/survey_comp/survey.jsp>; [Accessed March 2020]; Basic Screening Surveys: An Approach to Monitoring Community Oral Health: Older Adults. Association of State and Territorial Dental Directors; 2010. Available at: <http://www.prevmed.org/wp-content/uploads/2013/11/BSS-SeniorsManual.pdf>; [Accessed March 2020].)

In the U.S., tooth loss has been assessed also by self-report with personal and telephone interviews.[16,17,37] Questions related to tooth loss have been included on national oral health surveys, and the BSS for older adults also includes a question (see Box 4.6). A combination of BSS screening and interview questions is considered adequate to track progress of partial and complete tooth loss in relation to the associated *Healthy People* objectives and NOHSS oral health indicators.[19]

Measurement of Oral and Pharyngeal Cancer

Surveillance is important for oral and pharyngeal cancer (OPC), which includes cancers of the lip, tongue, buccal mucosa, floor of the mouth, pharynx, parotid gland, tonsil, nasal cavity, and sinus.[38] Together the CDC National Program of Cancer Registries and the NIH National Cancer Institute's **Surveillance, Epidemiology and End Results Program** (SEER) collect population data on OPC occurrence, including the type, extent, and location of the cancer.[39,40] Specific factors related to population groups (e.g., age, gender, race, or ethnicity) are also often identified in OPC assessments in populations.[40]

NHANES developed a human papillomavirus (HPV) oral rinse to provide estimates of the proportion of the population with oral HPV infection.[15] These data along with information concurrently collected in other research studies on the natural history of oral HPV infection may provide additional information about those at risk for HPV-positive oral squamous cell carcinoma.[15] This evidence will inform HPV-prophylactic-vaccine policy to prevent potential oral cancer.

National surveillance survey questionnaires are also used to assess for OPC prevalence (see Box 4.7). This national coverage enables researchers, clinicians, policymakers, public health professionals, and members of the public to monitor the burden of OPC, evaluate the success of programs, and identify additional needs for OPC prevention and control efforts at national, state, and local levels and with priority populations.[39]

Data to measure the number of deaths resulting from OPC are obtained from death certificates collected through the National Vital Statistics System within the CDC National Center for Health Statistics (NCHS);[40] such data are available at the state and local levels.[41] This measure is based on the number of deaths resulting from OPC per 100,000 people attributed to cancers that are classified in the 11th edition of the *International Classification of Diseases* (ICD-11), sponsored by the WHO.[38] The ICD-11 is used to define the measurement of OPC for the *Healthy People 2030* Cancer topic objective to reduce the overall cancer death rate, which includes deaths resulting from OPC. Also tracked is the proportion of OPC lesions diagnosed at the earliest stage (Stage 1, localized),[38] which is associated with an increased survival rate.[42] (See https://www.cancer.net/cancer-types/oral-and-oropharyngeal-cancer/stages-and-grades for information on staging of cancer.) One of the *Healthy People 2030* Oral Conditions objectives is to increase the proportion of OPC detected at the earliest stage.[12] The stage of diagnosis is collected through state cancer registries and SEER.[40]

A strategy to increase the diagnosis of OPC at the earliest stage is to increase the occurrence of routine oral cancer screening by oral health professionals to detect OPC.[29] Determining the prevalence and frequency of this professional practice has been achieved with self-report on national surveillance survey questionnaires (see Box 4.7).

Use of Tobacco in Relation to Oral and Pharyngeal Cancer

The use of tobacco in all forms is the biggest risk factor for OPC, placing extreme importance on efforts to reduce the use of tobacco products.[43] Several national surveys include questions to track the use of smoking and other tobacco products in the nation, including e-cigarettes and flavored tobacco products (see Box 4.7). An important approach to achieve reduction of tobacco use is the provision of tobacco counseling by health professionals.[43] Surveillance survey questions are also used to track the provision of this important service (see Box 4.7)

Having a strong tobacco surveillance system enables a country to build an effective program that can address tobacco issues and reduce the use of tobacco significantly.[44] To assist other countries with these efforts, the CDC collaborated with the WHO and the Canadian Public Health Association to develop the Global Tobacco Surveillance System (GTSS) for the WHO Tobacco Free Initiative.[44] Through this surveillance system, the WHO is collecting data on the prevalence of tobacco use and related factors, which are made available globally. The GTSS also supports the tobacco surveillance efforts of other countries by making available questionnaires that can be used by countries and communities for tobacco surveillance, to which they can add their own country- or community-specific questions. Also available are resources for tobacco prevention and control programs. The intended result of these efforts is to enhance the capacity of countries to design, implement, and evaluate their national comprehensive tobacco action plans and to monitor their efforts related to tobacco control.[44] Box 4.8 presents a

---

> ### BOX 4.7 Self-Report Surveillance Survey Questions: Oral and Pharyngeal Cancer and Related Factors
>
> **Prevalence of Oral and Pharyngeal Cancer**
> - Have you[a] ever been told by a doctor or other health professional that you[a] had cancer or a malignancy of any kind? If yes, what kind of cancer? (tongue/mouth/lip was an option to select), how old were you[a] when it was first diagnosed, and how long have you[a] had cancer? (2018 NHIS)
>
> **Provision of Oral Cancer Examinations**
> - In the past 12 months, have you[a] had an examination for oral cancer in which the doctor or dentist pulls on your[a] tongue, sometimes with gauze wrapped around it, and feels under the tongue and inside the cheeks? (2019–2020 NHANES)
> - Have you[a] ever had a check for oral cancer in which the doctor or dentist pulls on your tongue, sometimes with gauze wrapped around it, and feels under the tongue and inside the cheeks? If yes: When did you[a] have your most recent oral cancer exam? (BSS Older Adult)
> - What type of healthcare professional performed your[a] most recent oral cancer exam? (2017–2018 NHANES)
>
> **Prevalence of Tobacco Use**
> - Have you ever used an e-cigarette or other electronic vaping product, even just one time, in your entire life? (2018 BRFSS)
> - Do you[a] now smoke cigarettes every day, some days or not at all? (2018 MEPS)
>
> **Provision of Tobacco Cessation Counseling**
> - In the past 12 months, did a dentist, hygienist or other dental professional have a direct conversation with you[a] about the benefits of giving up cigarettes or other types of tobacco to improve your[a] dental health? (2019–2020 NHANES)
>
> [a] Questions were adapted as needed when asked of a parent, guardian, or care provider.
> (From National Health Interview Survey: Adult: 2018. Atlanta, GA: Centers for Disease Control and Prevention; 2019 May 6. Available at: <https://www.cdc.gov/nchs/nhis/nhis_questionnaires.htm>; [Accessed March 2020]; NHANES Questionnaire Instruments: Sample Person Questionnaires: Oral Health: 2017 & 2019. Hyattsville, MD: National Center for Health Statistics; 2020 Feb 21. Available at: <https://wwwn.cdc.gov/nchs/data/nhanes/2019-2020/questionnaires/OHQ_K.pdf>; [Accessed March 2020]; Basic Screening Surveys: An Approach to Monitoring Community Oral Health: Older Adults. Association of State and Territorial Dental Directors; 2010. Available at: <http://www.prevmed.org/wp-content/uploads/2013/11/BSS-SeniorsManual.pdf>; [Accessed March 2020]; 2018 BRFSS Questionnaire; 2018 Jan 18. Available at: <https://www.cdc.gov/brfss/questionnaires/pdf-ques/2019_BRFSS_English_Questionnaire-508.pdf>; [Accessed March 2020]; Medical Expenditure Panel Survey Questionnaire: 2018: Additional Health Care. Rockville, MD: Agency for Healthcare Research and Quality; 2019 Nov 18. Available at: <https://www.meps.ahrq.gov/mepsweb/survey_comp/survey.jsp>; [Accessed March 2020].)

BOX 4.8   Components of the World Health Organization Global Tobacco Surveillance System

- Global Youth Tobacco Survey (GYTS)—survey for youth aged 13–15 years conducted in schools
  - 56 core questions designed to gather data on the following seven domains:
    - Knowledge and attitudes of young people toward cigarette smoking
    - Prevalence of cigarette smoking and other tobacco use among young people
    - Role of the media and advertising in young people's use of cigarettes
    - Access to cigarettes
    - Tobacco-related school curriculum
    - Environmental tobacco smoke
    - Cessation of cigarette smoking
- Global School Professionals Survey (GSPS)—survey for teachers and administrators from the same schools that participate in the GYTS
  - Collects information on tobacco use
  - Determines school personnel knowledge of and attitudes toward tobacco
  - Evaluates existence and effectiveness of tobacco control policies in schools
  - Provides training and materials to implement tobacco prevention and control interventions
- Global Health Professions Students Survey (GHPSS)—survey for use with third-year students pursuing degrees in dentistry, medicine, nursing, and pharmacology
  - Core questions over the following:
    - Demographics
    - Prevalence of cigarette smoking and other tobacco use
    - Knowledge and attitudes about tobacco use
    - Exposure to second-hand tobacco smoke
    - Willingness to stop smoking
    - Training received regarding patient counseling on smoking cessation techniques
- Global Adult Tobacco Survey (GATS)—a household survey to monitor tobacco use among adults (15 years and older)
  - Has been implemented in more than 19 low- and middle-income countries with the highest burden of tobacco use
  - Topics included in GATS questions:
    - Tobacco use prevalence (smoking and smokeless tobacco products)
    - Second-hand tobacco smoke exposure and policies
    - Tobacco cessation
    - Knowledge, attitudes, and perceptions
    - Exposure to media
    - Economics
  - Example subset of key questions from the GATS:
    - Current Smokeless Tobacco Use: Do you currently use smokeless tobacco on a daily basis, less than daily, or not at all?
    - Past Daily Smokeless Tobacco Use: Have you used smokeless tobacco daily in the past? (yes, no, or don't know)
    - Past Smokeless Tobacco Use: In the past, have you used smokeless tobacco on a daily basis, less than daily, or not at all?

(From About GTSS. Atlanta, GA: Centers for Disease Control and Prevention; 2018 Feb 12. Available at: <https://www.cdc.gov/tobacco/global/gtss/index.htm>; [Accessed March 2020].)

description of tobacco surveillance questionnaires that are part of the GTSS. To successfully impact the prevalence and incidence of OPC, surveillance efforts related to OPC and tobacco use need to have a strong interprofessional collaborative focus among the healthcare professions.

Measurement of Other Oral and Craniofacial Diseases, Conditions, and Injuries

Some oral diseases and conditions are not routinely represented in oral health surveillance, the *Healthy People* objectives, or the NOHSS oral health indicators. Even so, conditions such as orofacial clefts, malocclusion, orofacial pain and temporomandibular disorders, orofacial injuries and tooth trauma, xerostomia, and tooth wear can adversely affect oral health and overall health and thus impact quality of life.[45] In addition, failure or inability to use dentures when indicated can be detrimental to health and quality of life. These conditions have been measured by NHANES, BSS, WHO, and other surveys at various times. This section will provide an overview of the measurement of some of these conditions in relation to oral health surveillance.

Craniofacial Anomalies

Orofacial clefts (see Chapter 5) have a significant impact on the healthcare system and are candidates for public health surveillance.[46] In the U.S., craniofacial anomalies (including cleft lip and palate) are usually expressed as a proportion or rate based on their recordings on birth certificates.[46] However, recording these anomalies is not universal. This inadequacy of surveillance has been addressed by establishing a *Healthy People 2030* Oral Conditions developmental objective to increase the number of states and D.C. that have an oral and craniofacial health surveillance system.[12] These data are reported through the Annual Synopses of State and Territorial Dental Public Health Programs routinely prepared by the ASTDD.[31]

Malocclusion

Malocclusion can be assessed during a population-based oral health survey through evaluation of occlusal characteristics. The BSS includes the measurement of posterior functional contacts as an optional indicator on the older adult survey to determine whether teeth oppose each other and can function properly while the individual is eating.[19] A dichotomous measure (yes/no) is used to indicate if any functional contacts exist on each side of the mouth.

Dry Mouth

With the increasing average age of the U.S. population and the greater use of medications that produce xerostomia, there has been interest in tracking dry mouth in the population. The older adult BSS includes severe dry mouth as an optional indicator on the oral examination.[19] It also includes the following interview questions that can be used to assess the prevalence of dry mouth in a population:

- Do you[a] sip liquids to aid in swallowing any foods?
- Does the amount of saliva in your mouth[a] seem to be too little, too much, or do you[a] not notice it?

---

[a]Questions can be adapted as needed when asked of a parent, guardian, or care provider.

- Do you[a] have difficulties swallowing any foods?
- Does your mouth feel dry when you[a] eat a meal?

Denture Use

The use of dentures can be assessed in epidemiologic surveys with interview questions regarding denture wear. NHANES, including the 2020 survey, has routinely included questions about the use of partial and full dentures during the last 14 years.[15] In addition, the 2020 NHANES included a clinical assessment of the presence of full and partial dentures and their condition in relation to a need for referral.[15] The BSS includes a question asked of participants during screening about whether they have an upper and/or a lower denture and whether or not they wear their dentures while they eat.[19]

Orofacial Injuries and Tooth Trauma

Measurement of orofacial injuries and tooth trauma can be incorporated into oral health surveillance. Tooth trauma has been assessed in specific-aged children and adults on past NHANES by questioning individuals in the sample about a history of tooth trauma and by examining the eight permanent incisors.[47]

Orofacial Pain and Temporomandibular Disorders

General oral pain and temporomandibular joint (TMJ) assessment is included in the WHO basic oral health survey guide.[18]The assessment of general oral pain is included in the NHANES and linked to the measurement of oral health-related quality of life (see later in chapter).[15]

Tooth Wear and Erosion

The NHANES has included a measurement of dental tooth wear and erosion in the past to assess the prevalence of the condition across the lifespan among varied population groups.[34] The purpose was to discern if health disparities existed in relation to tooth wear and erosion.

Measurement of Dental Fluorosis

Dean's Fluorosis Index (DFI), also known as the *Community Fluorosis Index (CFI)*, was developed and is still used today to measure the prevalence and severity of dental fluorosis in the population.[23] It is one of the most universally accepted classifications for dental fluorosis, and other fluorosis indices are based on it.[21] Although less sensitive than other fluorosis indexes,[23] it is still recommended for use in community studies.

The DFI scores fluorosis on a 0 to 4 scale to represent categories of normal, questionable, very mild, mild, moderate, and severe fluorosis. Criteria for scoring and a comparison to other fluorosis indices can be found in Appendix F. Community levels of fluorosis are indicated by the proportion of survey participants that receive scores in each category.[23] Dean's CFI is included in the WHO basic oral health survey methods for global surveillance.[18] It has also been used on the NHANES to establish the prevalence and trend of fluorosis in the U.S.[48]

NHANES surveys have also included the recording of nonfluoride opacities as part of the fluorosis scoring.[49] Differentiation of mild fluorosis from nonfluoride opacities is difficult to distinguish, possibly leading to fluorosis misclassification, which can result in inflation of fluorosis prevalence.[50] The greater awareness of fluorosis issues and the sensitive political nature of water fluoridation could increase such a measurement error.[21] Scoring nonfluoride opacities can help control for fluorosis measurement error. Table 4.5 describes how to differentiate mild fluorosis from nonfluoride opacities.

On the 2013–2014 and 2015–2016 NHANES surveys, digital imaging of teeth was accomplished, and, to score fluorosis, these images were read and analyzed remotely by experts.[51,52] Reading digital images instead of clinical examination to score fluorosis was implemented to increase the sensitivity of fluorosis scoring and avoid the problems of clinical examination.[52] Advantages and disadvantages have been reported for the scoring of fluorosis from digital images versus a clinical examination (see Table 4.6).[53]

TABLE 4.5 Enamel Opacities: Differential Diagnosis

Characteristic	Milder Forms of Fluorosis	Nonfluoride Enamel Opacities
Area affected	Usually seen on or near cusp tips or incisal edges	Usually centered in smooth surface; may affect entire crown
Shape of lesion	Resembles line shading in a pencil sketch; lines follow incremental lines in enamel, form irregular caps on cusps	Often round or oval
Demarcation	Shades off imperceptibly into surrounding enamel	Clearly differentiated from adjacent normal enamel
Color	Slightly more opaque than normal enamel; "paper-white" areas; incisal edges and tips of cusps may have frosted appearance; does not show stain at time of eruption (in milder degrees, rarely at any time)	Usually pigmented at time of eruption; often creamy-yellow to dark reddish orange
Teeth affected	Most frequently affects teeth that calcify slowly (cuspids, bicuspids, second and third molars); rare on lower incisors; usually seen on six or eight homologous teeth; extremely rare in deciduous teeth	Any tooth affected; frequent on labial surfaces of lower incisors, usually one to three teeth affected; may occur singly; common in deciduous teeth
Gross hypoplasia	None; no pitting in milder forms; enamel surface may have a glazed appearance; smooth to point of explorer	Absent to severe; enamel surface etched and rough to explorer
Detection	Often invisible under strong light; most easily detected by line of sight tangential to tooth surface	Seen most easily under strong light on line of sight perpendicular to tooth surface

(From National Health and Nutrition Examination Survey (NHANES) Oral Health Examiners Procedures Manual, 2016. Atlanta, GA: Centers for Disease Control and Prevention; 2016 Jan. Available at: <https://wwwn.cdc.gov/nchs/data/nhanes/2015-2016/manuals/2016_Oral_Health_Examiners_Procedures_Manual.pdf>; [Accessed March 2020]; Chattopadhyay A. Oral Health Epidemiology: Principles and Practice. Sudbury, MA: Jones and Bartlett; 2011.0

TABLE 4.6 Advantages and Disadvantages of Digital Imaging and Clinical Examination to Score Fluorosis

Clinical Examination	Digital Imaging
Advantages	**Advantages**
• Fast	• Provides permanent record
• Easy	• Can archive images to allow repeated scoring by multiple examiners
• Cost-effective	
• Ability to examine all surfaces	• Can be kept for longitudinal assessment, research to compare indices, and training of examiners
• Ability to perform tactile examination	
• Dependence on subject cooperation	• Allows blinding of examiners to minimize bias
Disadvantages	**Disadvantages**
• Method of examination	• More costly
• Lighting conditions	• Technique sensitive
• Potential for examiner bias	• Possible image variation introduced by technique, camera equipment, and/or quality of image
• Lack of examiner reliability	• Appearance of reflections from the ring flash used for lighting can mimic appearance of white spot lesions, resulting in over reporting of fluorosis
	• Poor photographic access to posterior teeth can result in under reporting in a whole mouth examination

(From Nor NAM. Methods and indices in measuring fluorosis: A review. Arch Orofac Sci 2017;12(2):77-85. Available at <http://aos.usm.my/docs/Vol_12/aos-article-0280.pdf>; [Accessed March 2020].)

BOX 4.9 Self-Report Surveillance Survey Questions: Use of Fluorides, National Health and Nutrition Examination Survey (NHANES) 2019–2020

- At what age did you[a] start brushing your[a] teeth?
- At what age did you[a] start using toothpaste?
- On average, how much toothpaste do you[a] use when brushing your[a] teeth?
- Have you[a] ever received prescription fluoride drops or fluoride tablets?
- If yes, how old in months or years were you[a] when you[a] started and stopped taking prescription fluoride drops or fluoride tablets?

[a] Questions were adapted as needed when asked of a parent, guardian, or care provider.
(From NHANES Questionnaire Instruments: Sample Person Questionnaire: Oral Health: 2019. Hyattsville, MD: National Center for Health Statistics; 2020 Feb 21. Available at: <https://wwwn.cdc.gov/nchs/data/nhanes/2019-2020/questionnaires/OHQ_K.pdf>; [Accessed March 2020].)

The use of fluorides has also been monitored, not only because of its effect on caries reduction, but also because of its relationship to the development of fluorosis.[52] This has been achieved by including questions about fluoride use on the NHANES (see Box 4.9).

According to the DHHS, the need to continue surveillance of fluorosis continues, especially to monitor the effect of the new optimal fluoride level recommendation for water fluoridation that went into effect in 2015.[54] Epidemiologists and researchers agree, partially in light of the surprisingly high level of fluorosis found by the 2013–2014 NHANES and the need to verify or nullify the validity of these results (see Chapter 5).[48,55]

Measurement of Oral Health Treatment Needs

Summary assessments that record overall need for oral health care (e.g., treatment urgency) are used in oral health surveys. For example, as previously explained, the BSS measures the status of specific disease indicators, including the *urgency of need for dental care*. The urgency criterion especially indicates the need for treatment as it is defined and linked to the need for **referral** for oral health care (see Table 4.7).[19,20] This referral is a necessary component of assessment and screening and is an ethical obligation when the need for dental care is observed. The NHANES also classifies the urgency of treatment needed by each survey participant for referral purposes.[15]

The WHO basic screening method used in international population-based surveillance surveys is designed to predict the oral health treatment needs of different countries for prioritization purposes.[18] This survey method includes an appraisal of status on several major oral diseases and conditions along with an evaluation of the need for intervention or treatment. Assessment categories include the following:[18]

- Dentition status: basic screening
- Periodontal status: CPI (see Appendix F)
- Loss of attachment: CPI
- Enamel fluorosis: DFI (see Appendix F)
- Dental erosion
- Traumatic dental injuries
- Oral mucosal lesions
- Denture status
- Intervention urgency

For each person examined, the clinical examination includes an assessment of evident dental caries, periodontal disease, and abnormalities of the tissues of the head and neck, with a determination of treatment urgency based on this assessment.

The treatment need classification systems of the BSS, NHANES, and WHO differ in the number of categories and have slight variations in definitions.[15,18,19,20] They are contrasted in Table 4.7 to provide better understanding of how these various systems classify treatment needs.

Measurement of Access to Water Fluoridation

Community water fluoridation is measured by the percentage of people served by public water systems that are optimally fluoridated.[29] Surveillance data about the fluoridation status of public water systems can be obtained from the **Water Fluoridation Reporting System** (WFRS), a voluntary, interactive, Internet-based monitoring and surveillance program developed by the CDC in partnership with the ASTDD.[56] State and tribal fluoridation managers enter data into the WFRS to monitor fluoridation quality, including average fluoride concentrations, results of daily testing, and dates of facility inspections and operator

TABLE 4.7 Comparison of Treatment Urgency Classification: Basic Screening Survey, World Health Organization, National Health and Nutrition Examination Survey

Basic Screening Survey (BSS)	World Health Organization (WHO)	National Health and Nutrition Examination Survey (NHANES)
• Urgent need for dental care—To be seen as soon as possible, signs or symptoms include pain, infection, or swelling	0—No treatment needed	1—Should see a dentist immediately
	1—Preventive or routine treatment needed	2—Should see a dentist within 2 weeks
• Early dental care needed—To be seen within several weeks; Caries without accompanying signs or symptoms or individuals with other oral health problems requiring care before their next routine dental visit	2—Prompt treatment including scaling needed	3—Should see a dentist at earliest convenience
	3—Immediate (urgent) treatment needed because of pain or infection of dental or oral origin	4—Should continue with regular routine dental care
• No obvious problems—To be seen at next regular check-up; any patient without previously mentioned problems	4—Referred for comprehensive evaluation of medical/dental treatment (systemic conditions)	

(From Basic Screening Surveys: An Approach to Monitoring Community Oral Health: Preschool & School Children. Association of State and Territorial Dental Directors; 2008. Available at: <https://azdhs.gov/documents/prevention/womens-childrens-health/oral-health/infant-youth/ASTDD-BSS-manual.pdf>; [Accessed March 2020]; Basic Screening Surveys: An Approach to Monitoring Community Oral Health: Older Adults. Reno, NV: Association of State and Territorial Dental Directors; 2010. Available at: <http://www.prevmed.org/wp-content/uploads/2013/11/BSS-SeniorsManual.pdf>; [Accessed March 2020]; Oral Health Surveys: Basic Methods, 5th ed. Geneva, Switzerland: World Health Organization; 2013. Available at: <http://apps.who.int/iris/bitstream/10665/97035/1/9789241548649_eng.pdf>; [Accessed March 2020]; National Health and Nutrition Examination Survey (NHANES) Oral Health Examiners Manual, 2020. Atlanta, GA: Centers for Disease Control and Prevention; 2020 Jan. Available at: <https://wwwn.cdc.gov/nchs/data/nhanes/2019-2020/manuals/2020-Oral-Health-Examiners-Manual-508.pdf>; [Accessed March 2020].)

training. These WFRS surveillance data are available for various purposes, including the following:[56]

• Updating water fluoridation maps maintained by the CDC in Oral Health Maps, a web-based interactive-mapping application that shows the percentage of people receiving fluoridated water at the state and local levels.

• Preparation of national surveillance reports that describe the percentage of the U.S. population on community water systems who receive optimally fluoridated drinking water.

• Generation of reports by state and tribal fluoridation managers for use in assuring program quality.

My Water's Fluoride (see Resources at the end of this chapter) is a source of surveillance information available to the public.[57] Approximately 40 states share their fluoridation status and data via this CDC data application. In states that participate, professionals and consumers can learn basic information about their community water system, including the number of people served and the fluoride level.

Measurement of Access to the Oral Healthcare System

Many facets comprise access to the oral healthcare system, referred to more simply as **access to oral health care**, including availability, accessibility, accommodation, affordability, and acceptability.[58] Multiple factors have been assessed to explain the use of clinical oral healthcare services. These factors have been summarized as epidemiological, social, demographic, personal, and psychological, as well as characteristics of the oral healthcare system.[4] Some specific examples include language, literacy level, oral health literacy, fear and anxiety, transportation, dental office staff attitudes toward disadvantaged groups, and medical and mental health issues, including substance abuse.[58]

A common measure of access to and use of the oral healthcare system is having a dental visit in the past year, sometimes referred to as dental *attendance* (see Figure 4.7). This is a *Healthy People 2030* Oral Conditions objective (see OH-8 in Table 4.1) and one of the LHIs (Figure 4.2). Other *Healthy People 2030* objectives in the topics Oral Conditions, Health Insurance, and Health Care Access and Quality address access to oral health care, including the need to increase the proportion of persons with dental insurance, to reduce the proportion of people who

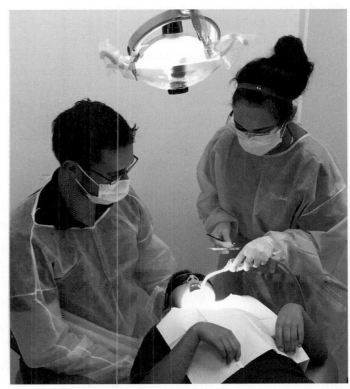

Fig 4.7 A young child patient has a routine dental examination in a safety-net clinic.

can't get the dental care they need when they need it, to increase the proportion of low-income youth who have a preventive dental visit, and to increase the proportion of the U.S. population served by community systems with optimally fluoridated water systems (see Table 4.1 and the National Oral Conditions Objectives section earlier in this chapter).[12]

Important factors associated with access to oral health care have been measured in various national, state, and local surveillance surveys by including questions to assess the following:[15,17,18,19,37,59]

- Dental attendance for routine check-ups or cleanings
- Dental insurance coverage
- Self-reported oral health
- Time since last dental visit/frequency of dental visits
- Access to oral health care

The **Medical Expenditure Panel Survey** (MEPS) collects information from healthcare providers and employers on the cost and use of health care and health insurance coverage, including the number and nature of annual dental visits for various population groups, type of dental care provider, services provided, and dental insurance.[37] This survey and other previously described national and state surveys (NHANES, NHIS, BRFSS, BSS) have included questions that measure the factors associated with access to care to evaluate progress on these *Healthy People* objectives (see Box 4.10). These validated questions can be included in questionnaires and interviews conducted by states and local communities for needs assessment and surveillance.

The CDC conducts the biennial National Study of Long-Term Care Providers (NSLTCP) in which data are collected from administrators of residential care communities and directors of adult day services centers relative to various services provided for clients, including dental care.[60] One of the purposes of the NSLTCP is to offer reliable, accurate, relevant, and timely statistical information to support and inform long-term care services policies, research, and practice, which could impact the future of dental care provision for this vulnerable population.[60] In 2018, both questionnaires used for this study, the Residential Care Community Provider Questionnaire and the Adult Day Services Centers Questionnaire, included questions about the provision of, arrangement for, referral for, and/or transportation to routine and emergency dental services by a licensed dentist.[61]

Measurement of Oral Health-Related Quality of Life

The construct of **oral health-related quality of life** (OHRQOL) builds on the concepts of *quality of life (QOL)* and *health-related quality of life* (HRQOL).[62] Thus, to comprehend OHRQOL, one must first understand QOL and HRQOL because they are interrelated. Table 4.8 presents six broad domains, various facets within the domains, and a general umbrella category of subjective overall QOL and general health to describe the multidimensional core aspects of QOL.[63]

Health-Related Quality of Life

HRQOL reflects QOL in relation to health and disease.[64] HRQOL is integral to the WHO definition of health presented

---

BOX 4.10   Self-Report Surveillance Survey Questions: Access to and Use of the Oral Healthcare System

- About how long has it been since you[a] last visited a dentist (or clinic; for any reason)? Include all types of dentists such as orthodontists, oral surgeons, and all other dental specialists, as well as dental hygienists. (2019–2020 NHIS, 2018 BRFSS, BSS Older Adult, BSS Child)
- On average, how often do you[a] receive a dental check-up? (2017 MEPS)
- What types of dental care providers did you[a] see at your[a] last dental visit? (2018 MEPS)
- What services did you[a] have done at your last dental visit? (2018 MEPS)
- What was the total charge for your[a] last dental visit, and if paid by insurance, what was the co-pay? (2017 MEPS)
- What was the main reason you[a] last visited the dentist? (2019–2020 NHANES, BSS Older Adult, BSS Child)
- During the past 12 months, was there a time when you[a] needed dental care but could not get it at that time (or delayed it)? (2019–2020 NHANES, 2018 MEPS, BSS Older Adult, BSS Child)
- What were the reasons that you[a] could not get the dental care needed? (worry about the cost, inability to afford it, and lack of insurance were optional responses; 2019–2020 NHANES, 2018 MEPS, 2018 NHIS, BSS Older Adult, BSS Child)
- Is there a particular dentist or dental clinic that you[a] usually go to if you need dental care or dental advice? (BSS Older Adult)
- During the past 3 years, have you[a] been (and how often) to the dentist for routine check-ups or cleanings? (BSS Older Adult)
- What is the main reason (barrier) you[a] have not visited the dentist in the past year? (BSS Older Adult)
- Do you[a] have any kind of insurance coverage (including dental insurance, prepaid plans such as HMOs, or government plans such as Medicaid) that pays for some or all of your routine dental care, including cleaning, x-rays, and examinations? (BSS Older Adult, BSS Child)
- Do you[a] currently have any healthcare bills (including dental) that are being paid off over time? (2018 BRFSS)

[a] Questions were/can be adapted as needed when asked of a parent, guardian, or care provider.
(From NHANES Questionnaire Instruments: Sample Person Questionnaire: Oral Health: 2019. Hyattsville, MD: National Center for Health Statistics; 2020 Feb 21. Available at: <https://wwwn.cdc.gov/nchs/data/nhanes/2019-2020/questionnaires/OHQ_K.pdf>; [Accessed March 2020]; Medical Expenditure Panel Survey Questionnaires: 2018 Access to Care, 2018: Dental Care, 2017: Charge Payment, 2017: Alternative/Preventive Care. Rockville, MD: Agency for Healthcare Research and Quality; 2019 Nov 18. Available at: <https://www.meps.ahrq.gov/mepsweb/survey_comp/survey.jsp>; [Accessed March 2020]; National Health Interview Survey: Adult: 2018. Atlanta, GA: Centers for Disease Control and Prevention; 2019 May 6. Available at: <https://www.cdc.gov/nchs/nhis/nhis_questonnaires.htm>; [Accessed March 2020]; 2018 Behavioral Risk Factor Surveillance System (BRFSS) Questionnaire. Atlanta, GA: Centers for Disease Control and Prevention; 2018. Available at: <https://www.cdc.gov/brfss/questionnaires/pdf-ques/2019_BRFSS_English_Questionnaire-508.pdf>; [Accessed March 2020]; Basic Screening Survey: An Approach to Monitoring Community Oral Health: Older Adults. Association of State and Territorial Dental Directors; 2010. Available at: <http://www.prevmed.org/wp-content/uploads/2013/11/BSS-SeniorsManual.pdf>; [Accessed March 2020]; Basic Screening Surveys: An Approach to Monitoring Oral Health: Preschool & School Children. Reno, NV: Association of State and Territorial Dental Directors; Available at: <https://azdhs.gov/documents/prevention/womens-childrens-health/oral-health/infant-youth/ASTDD-BSS-manual.pdf> [Accessed March 2020].)

TABLE 4.8	Domains of Quality of Life and Facets of Each Domain
Umbrella	• Overall quality of life (QOL) and general health
Physical Health	• Energy and fatigue • Pain and discomfort • Sleep and rest
Psychological	• Body image and appearance • Negative feelings • Positive feelings • Self-esteem • Thinking, learning, memory, and concentration
Level of Independence	• Mobility • Activities of daily living • Dependence on medicinal substances and medical aids • Work capacity
Social Relations	• Personal relationships • Social support • Sexual activity
Environment	• Financial resources • Freedom, physical safety and security • Health and social care: accessibility and quality • Home environment • Opportunities to acquire new information and skills • Participation in and opportunities for recreation/leisure • Physical environment (pollution/noise/traffic/climate) • Transportation
Spirituality/Religion/Personal beliefs	• Meaning of life

(Modified from WHOQOL: Measuring Quality of Life. Geneva, Switzerland: World Health Organization. Available at: <https://www.who.int/healthinfo/survey/whoqol-qualityoflife/en/index4.html>; [Accessed March 2020].)

in Chapter 1 (a state of complete physical, mental, and social well-being and not merely the absence of disease). The concept of well-being in this definition is the connection to QOL. Well-being refers to the positive aspects of a person's life, such as positive emotions and satisfaction with life.[64] Well-being occurs when supportive environments are used to make the most of one's physical, mental, and social functioning to produce a full, satisfying, and productive life.[64]

HRQOL is supported by the five overarching goals of *Healthy People 2030* presented in Box 4.1. Even so, measuring HRQOL is subjective, more difficult than measuring health outcomes, and based on the individual's self-report of perceptions of health.[64] Three complementary and related domains provide a means to measure HRQOL[64]:

- Self-rated physical and mental health, including fatigue, pain, emotional distress, and social activities
- Overall well-being
  - Physical—relates to vigor and vitality, feeling very healthy and full of energy

- Mental—includes satisfaction with one's life, balancing positive and negative emotions, accepting one's self, finding purpose and meaning in one's life, believing one's life and circumstances are under one's control, generally experiencing optimism, and seeking personal growth, autonomy, and competence
- Social—involves providing and receiving quality support from family, friends, and others
- Participation in society—education, employment, family role participation, and civic, social, and leisure activities

Oral Health-Related Quality of Life

It is now recognized that QOL relates to nearly every area of health, including oral health, according to the **FDI World Dental Federation** (FDI).[65] The elements of QOL and HRQOL are shared by OHRQOL.[62] In addition, OHRQOL impacts HRQOL, which in turn affects QOL.[66] Examination of the definitions of oral health and OHRQOL makes this clear. The FDI has defined oral health as "multifaceted and includes the ability to speak, smile, smell, taste, touch, chew, swallow and convey a range of emotions through facial expressions with confidence and without pain, discomfort and disease of the craniofacial complex"[67] and OHRQOL as "a multidimensional construct that reflects (among other things) people's comfort when eating, sleeping, and engaging in social interaction; their self-esteem; and their satisfaction with respect to their oral health."[65] People's satisfaction with oral health depends in part on their perspectives of the ways in which oral diseases, conditions, and treatments affect their lives.[56] Dimensions of OHRQOL are presented in Figure 4.8.

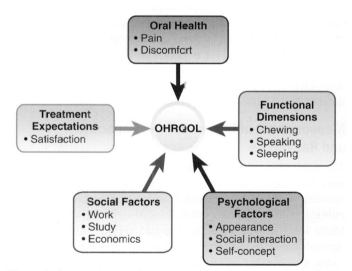

Fig 4.8 Dimensions of oral health-related quality of life (*OHRQOL*). (Modified from Sischo L, Broder HL. Oral health-related quality of life: What, why, how, and future implications. J Dent Res 2011;90(11):1264-1270. Available at: <http://www.ncbi.nlm.nih.gov/pmc/articles/PMC3318061/>; [Accessed April 2020]; Alzoubi EE, Hariri R, Attard NJ. Oral health related quality of life impact in dentistry. J Dent Health Oral Disord Ther 2017;6(6):183-188. Available at: <http://dx.doi.org/10.15406/jdhodt.2017.06.00221>; [Accessed March 2020].)

The measurement of OHRQOL is based on measuring the impact of the various physical, psychological, and social dimensions with questionnaires.[62,66] Although specific instruments have been developed to measure OHRQOL, the FDI policy on OHRQOL includes the following recommendations related to its measurement:[65]

- OHRQOL should be combined with clinical and behavioral indicators in assessments of oral healthcare needs of populations to provide a comprehensive and holistic approach to planning oral health services and setting strategic targets for improvement of oral health.
- All national oral health surveys should include a validated OHRQOL measure to provide a profile of the impacts of oral diseases on people's daily life.
- OHRQOL measures are essential outcomes to determine the cost-effectiveness of oral care/treatments and public health interventions.

For these purposes, oral health surveillance questionnaires in the U.S. and internationally include questions to assess OHRQOL (see Box 4.11), providing a basis to prioritize groups for health promotion and disease prevention efforts.[21] These validated questions are also used for state and local assessment.[19,20]

Future Directions for Assessing Oral Health-Related Quality of Life

Formal measurement of OHRQOL outcomes has not been applied routinely in regular clinical practice. It has been suggested that such application has the potential to improve quality of care, patient satisfaction, quality of research, and public health practice.[21]

To enhance decision-making, relevant information about OHRQOL is of practical significance for various entities in the health sector such as health policymakers, health services researchers, epidemiologists, and health program evaluators. However, the profession is challenged not to substitute evaluation of OHRQOL for evaluation of clinical outcomes; rather they should complement each other as applied to decisions concerning the improvement of oral health and the OHRQOL of the nation.[65,68]

Measurement of Infrastructure, Capacity, and Resources

The work of dental public health is achieved through various state, territorial, federal, regional, tribal, county, and local government oral health programs.[69] Included are territorial dental public health programs operated by American Indian nations. Many local programs, activities, and services are supported through the state and territorial dental public health programs. These government programs are situated within government structures to develop partnerships and resources that provide leadership for oral health initiatives. These and other dental safety-net programs make up the infrastructure for delivering oral health services and activities.[70]

Throughout this section, the term dental public health program, or oral public health program, is used to refer to large-scale programs operated by a government entity such as these, not to be confused with the common use of the same terms to denote a local initiative such as a fluoride varnish program

---

BOX 4.11 Self-Report Surveillance Survey Questions: Oral Health-Related Quality of Life

- During the past 12 months, did your[a] teeth or mouth cause any pain or discomfort? (World Health Organization [WHO][b], Basic Screening Survey [BSS] Older Adult) How often? (2019–2020 NHANES)
- During the past 6 months, did your[a] child have a toothache more than once, when biting or chewing? (BSS Child)
- How often during the last year have you[a] had difficulty doing your[a] usual jobs or attending school because of problems with your[a] teeth, mouth or dentures? (2019–2020 NHANES)
- How often during the last year have you[a] been self-conscious or embarrassed because of your[a] teeth, mouth or dentures? (2017–2018 NHANES)
- How often during the last year have you[a] avoided particular foods because of problems with your[a] teeth, mouth or dentures? (BSS Older Adult)
- Because of the state of your[a] teeth or mouth, how often have you[a] experienced any of the following problems during the past 12 months? (WHO)
  - Difficulty biting foods
  - Difficulty chewing foods
  - Difficulty with speech/trouble pronouncing words
  - Dry mouth
  - Embarrassment because of appearance of teeth
  - Feeling tense because of problems with teeth or mouth
  - Avoiding smiling because of teeth
  - Sleep that is often interrupted
  - Having to take days off work
  - Difficulty doing usual activities
  - Feeling less tolerant of spouse or people who are close to you
  - Reduced participation in social activities
- Overall, how would you[a] rate the health of your[a] teeth and gums? (2019-2020 NHANES)
- How would you[a] describe the condition of your mouth and teeth, including false teeth or dentures? (BSS Older Adult)

[a] Questions were/can be adapted as needed when asked of a parent, guardian, or care provider.
(From Oral Health Surveys: Basic Methods. 5th ed. Geneva, Switzerland: World Health Organization; 2013. Available at: <http://apps.who.int/iris/bitstream/10665/97035/1/9789241548649_eng.pdf>; [Accessed March 2020]; Basic Screening Survey: An Approach to Monitoring Community Oral Health: Older Adults. Association of State and Territorial Dental Directors; 2010. Available at: <http://www.prevmed.org/wp-content/uploads/2013/11/BSS-SeniorsManual.pdf>; [Accessed March 2020]; NHANES Questionnaire Instruments: Sample Person Questionnaire: Oral Health: 2017 & 2019. Hyattsville, MD: National Center for Health Statistics; 2020 Feb 21. Available at: <https://wwwn.cdc.gov/nchs/data/nhanes/2019-2020/questionnaires/OHQ_K.pdf>; [Accessed March 2020]; Basic Screening Surveys: An Approach to Monitoring Oral Health: Preschool & School Children. Reno, NV: Association of State and Territorial Dental Directors; Available at: <https://azdhs.gov/documents/prevention/womens-childrens-health/oral-health/infant-youth/ASTDD-BSS-manual.pdf>; [Accessed March 2020].)

---

operated by a local dental hygiene society or a school-based dental sealant program operated by a faith-based community health center. In addition, the term **state oral health program** (SOHP) is used to refer to a state dental public health program, as used by ASTDD, although other government programs have similarities to SOHPs.[71] SOHPs are also referred to as departments or divisions because they are organized within state health departments.

Infrastructure

- Systems, people, relationships, and resources that enable federal, state, and local agencies to perform public health functions and address oral health problems.
- Includes assessment, surveillance, information systems, planning, policy development, applied research, training, standards development, quality management, coordination, and systems of care.

Capacity

- The ability of the oral healthcare system to implement public health strategies, deliver oral health services, and develop oral health literacy of the public.
- Increased by sound infrastructure enabling basic programs to become strong, robust, and resilient, and requiring high levels of investment, expertise, and political will.

Resources

- Include personnel and their expertise, financial capital, available time, and collaborative relationships among the agencies within the overall public health system and with partner groups and local communities.

Fig 4.9 Infrastructure, capacity, and resources

Strong and vibrant government oral health programs at all levels are essential to achieving optimal oral health for all people.[71] **Infrastructure** and **capacity** are key elements by which states and localities can effectively address oral health problems[71] and are impacted by community resources (Figure 4.9).[69,71,72]

Strong infrastructure and adequate capacity at the federal, state, and local levels are necessary to be able to sustain effective dental public health programs that can have an impact over time.[69] Assessment of the infrastructure and capacity of the oral healthcare system is achieved by examining their components such as funding, workforce, other resources, program structure, public health activities, and interprofessional and other collaborative relationships.[69,71] A solid dental public health infrastructure that possesses successful capacity and access to adequate resources is critical to ensure that agencies are able to effectively and efficiently meet the oral health needs of the populations they serve. As a resource, the pubic health and personal health workforce must have the necessary capacity and expertise to effectively address oral health problems and issues.[69]

The three core public health functions and 10 essential public health services, both described in the Role of Government in Public Health section of Chapter 1, provide the foundation of public health programs to ensure adequate infrastructure and capacity. The core functions and essential services have been adapted by various agencies to support the infrastructure for developing and evaluating public health programs. For example, ASTDD and CDC provide resources, and ASTDD provides technical assistance to states to help build and enhance the infrastructure and capacity of dental public health programs.[71,73]

Role of the Association of State and Territorial Dental Directors

The mission of the ASTDD is to "promote and support a governmental oral health presence in each state and territory, increase

awareness of oral health as an important and integral part of overall health, address oral health equity, promote evidence-based oral health policies and practices, and assist in the development of initiatives to prevent and control oral diseases."[74] To this end, the ASTDD has published and revised guidelines, best practices, and competencies for SOHPs since the 1980s. The purpose of these efforts is to assist health agency officials and public health administrators in developing and operating strong SOHPs by helping them strengthen the infrastructure and build the capacity of the programs.[71] These documents are useful resources for development, enhancement, and evaluation of SOHPs.

The ASTDD SOHP guidelines have been framed around the core public health functions and 10 essential public health services to promote health and oral health.[71] The various revisions have reflected changes in national public health guidelines, best practice models, and advances in the field. The *Guidelines for State and Territorial Health Programs* consists of two parts. Part I is an overview of oral health disparities and strategies for prevention that describes the diversity and uniqueness of oral health programs and successful efforts to increase infrastructure and capacity.[72] Part II is a matrix of state oral health program roles for each of the 10 essential public health services, including examples of specific activities for each role and selected resources to help states accomplish the activities.[75] The aim of these guidelines is to ensure that SOHPs reflect the necessary infrastructure and capacity to adequately meet the needs of the populations served.

Based on its best practice approach (see Chapter 6), ASTDD also developed a best practice document related to workforce capacity.[76] In addition, the ASTDD *Competencies for State Oral Health Programs* is a companion tool to the guidelines that outlines skill sets that represent the core public health functions and essential services categorized under seven domains (see Box 4.12).[69] Criteria and levels to score the skill sets of each domain are included, making it possible to use the document to assess the effectiveness of a public health program.[69]

The infrastructure and capacity principles, standards, best-practices criteria, activities, and skills in these documents represent key factors associated with success and are used to increase program sustainability.[71] They can be used by SOHPs for self-assessment. A SOHP can also request technical assistance from ASTDD to conduct a self-study to determine progress or areas for improvement, have a comprehensive onsite program review by a consulting team, or follow up on an onsite review, all for the purpose of strengthening the program.[77]

These ASTDD SOHP guidelines, best practices, and competencies can be adapted for use by territorial, federal, regional, tribal, county, and local oral health programs.[69] Many of them can also be applied to small local programs.

Methods of Evaluation

Well-established dental public health programs are critical to the oral health of the public, and it is essential to strengthen these programs through systematic oral health surveillance linked with planning, implementation, and evaluation of effective measures.[72] In addition, instruments and methods are needed to assess the current status, best practices, and future development of infrastructure, capacity, and resources that

---

BOX 4.12   Competency Domains for Strong State Oral Health Programs

Build Support
Establish strong working relationships with stakeholders to build support for oral health through promotion, disease prevention, and control.

Plan and Evaluate Programs
Develop and implement evidence-based interventions and conduct evaluations to ensure ongoing feedback and program effectiveness.

Influence Policies and Systems Change
Promote and implement strategies to inform, enhance, or change the health-related policies of organizations or governmental entities capable of affecting the health of populations.

Manage People
Oversee and support the optimal performance and growth of team members.

Manage Programs and Resources
Ensure the administrative, financial, and staff support necessary to sustain activities and to build opportunities.

Use Public Health Science
Gather, analyze, interpret, and disseminate data and research findings to assure that oral disease prevention and control approaches are evidence-based.

Lead Strategically
Create strategic vision, serve as a catalyst for change and demonstrate program accomplishments.

(From Competencies for State Oral Health Programs. Reno, NV: Association of State and Territorial Dental Directors; 2020. Available at: <https://www.astdd.org/docs/competencies-and-levels-for-state-oral-health-programs-2020.pdf>; [Accessed May 2020].)

---

are necessary to improve oral health at state and local levels.[69] States and localities that evaluate these key elements will be better prepared to maintain fully effective essential public oral health services to achieve their oral health objectives and contribute to the *Healthy People 2030* Oral Conditions objectives.[69]

ASTDD annually surveys SOHPs to collect and report data on best-practice parameters and status of the programs. This serves as an evaluation mechanism to monitor the infrastructure and capacity of SOHPs across the nation as a measure of their effectiveness in meeting the needs of the populations served.[31] Also, each decade outcomes of *Healthy People* Oral Conditions objectives are compared with targets to determine if infrastructure and capacity objectives have been met.[29]

FUTURE CONSIDERATIONS FOR ORAL HEALTH SURVEILLANCE

A core foundation of successful planning in dental public health is information collected through oral health surveillance systems about the epidemiology of oral diseases and factors that could be targets for prevention.[6,69,72] Assessment of key oral health indicators is central to effective public health planning that tailors oral health policies, programs, and practices based on oral health status and trends among population groups.[6,69,72] Oral health surveillance and assessment methods should evolve

as oral disease patterns and population demographics change.[6] These changes demand new techniques and the development of skills by dental public health professionals.

Public health surveillance is being transformed by various influences. Public health information and preparedness are emerging as national security issues, resulting in the demand for timely access to high-quality data. Yet, security demands sometimes divert attention from oral health surveillance efforts to lethal events such as the COVID-19 pandemic.[6]

New information technologies such as electronic health records have the potential to improve public health surveillance systems, but their impact on oral health surveillance is currently limited.[6] A potential for improvement in this area is the use of diagnostic codes in dentistry. As pressure from insurance providers makes diagnostic coding standard practice, dental claims data can be used to monitor disease trends, access to care, and the cost effectiveness of various services and interventions.[6]

With the advent of healthcare reform based on the Patient Protection and Affordable Care Act, many states have built and established a database of claims and cost data from both private and public insurers. This provides states new opportunities to more fully understand healthcare delivery, measure quality of health care, and report on population health.[6] In addition, some states have begun collecting oral health workforce data through their licensing boards. These data allow states to better measure the capacity, distribution, and age of the current workforce and plan for the future workforce.[6]

Major challenges for state oral health surveillance moving forward are limited infrastructure, insufficient resources, public health workforce shortages, and frequent staff turnover. Thus, future considerations should focus on the challenges faced by federal, state, and local agencies to ensure the availability of sufficient resources such as staffing and funding. These issues must be addressed to assure that oral health surveillance systems can be maintained, continue to mature, and be linked at the national, state, and local levels. A workforce of adequate size and consistency that has dental public health knowledge and skills is required to ensure high-quality oral health surveillance.[6,72]

Oral health surveillance depends mainly on federal funding. As government budgets are stressed by multiple priorities and changes in political agendas, oral health surveillance can be overshadowed by other critical public health needs.[6] Identifying cost-efficient methods of oral health surveillance is a priority.[6] This challenge can be addressed partially by coordinating various oral health surveillance programs. For example, states and localities have reported success by linking to existing surveillance systems for oral health data such as the CDC/BRFSS and adding new self-report oral health questions to existing surveys or surveillance systems such as NHANES and NHIS.[33]

Even so, substantial resources are still needed to collect primary oral health data through open-mouth screenings. Although the unit cost of a survey screening using the BSS tool is more cost-efficient compared with an epidemiological survey that uses the DMFT index,[20] states and local agencies still require ongoing resources to regularly and periodically collect oral health status data through screening surveys.[6] In addition, repetition of these costly screening surveys is necessary to monitor trends over time and to collect data for different population groups (e.g., preschool children, school-age children, adults, older adults, and special needs individuals).

These oral screenings for the purposes of surveillance of oral and dental diseases and conditions have typically been completed by dentists. The use of dental hygienists to measure clinical indicators such as dental caries, sealants, and probing depths has been attempted in recent NHANES survey periods,[78] which can be more cost effective when conducting open-mouth screenings. Reliability analyses of outcomes data from these NHANES periods indicated an acceptable

level of data quality and similar examiner performance by dental hygienists compared with the use of dentists as examiners.[78]

Substantial progress has been made in state oral health surveillance in the past 2 decades.[6,72] An increasing, although not universal, number of states collect information on a host of oral health indicators. An expansion of the definition of an oral health surveillance system to include an oral health surveillance plan, evaluation plan, and data dissemination will make surveillance systems more powerful and allow them to use data to protect and promote the oral health of the population.[6]

SUMMARY

This chapter describes the *Healthy People* initiative and presents the Oral Conditions objectives of *Healthy People 2030;* these benchmarks provide an important basis for the assessment of oral health in the U.S. during the remainder of this decade. Furthermore, the chapter focuses on oral health surveillance as the ongoing and systematic collection, analysis, and interpretation of oral health indicators for use in planning, implementing, and evaluating dental public health practice. The chapter describes how assessments are important to monitor changes in oral health and disease patterns; the use of oral health services;

social, demographic, and economic factors that influence oral health; and workforce- and service-system capacity with the public, private, and nonprofit sectors.

Specific measures used in assessing oral health and related factors in populations are examined. Examples of oral health surveys are presented, and the importance of using standardized measurements to assess oral health trends is highlighted. Also discussed is the need to strengthen surveillance measures for future planning, implementation, and evaluation of dental public health practice.

APPLYING YOUR KNOWLEDGE

1. Select three *Healthy People 2030* Oral Conditions objectives. For each one, identify and describe data sources you could use to retrieve existing data for your local area population. Retrieve data on each one, and share the results with your class.
2. Select a population for whom to design an oral health program. Research *Healthy People 2030* leading health indicators that relate to that population and design an interprofessional collaborative activity that involves other members of the healthcare team.
3. As a member of the board of your state dental hygiene association, you are appointed to a task force to partner with the state dental association to explore ways to strengthen the oral health program in your state. What principles of infrastructure and capacity will guide your efforts on this initiative? What information about the infrastructure and capacity of the current state oral health program do you need, and where can you find the information? What sources, resources, and contacts would help you find information to aid you in meeting the objectives of the task force?
4. Your local community water supply has been fluoridated for over 25 years. The city council is reconsidering water fluoridation for the community. As a dental hygienist practicing in the community, you would like to meet with city council members to provide current, evidence-based information to help them make the decision to continue fluoridating the community water supply because the natural fluoride level is well below the optimal level. Describe how you would

prepare to meet with them. What information would you need? Where could you get the information? How else could you assist the city council with this important decision?
5. As a local practicing dental hygienist, you serve on the board of a community-based dental clinic that provides oral healthcare services and school-based primary preventive initiatives in the Title I schools of the local school district. You and another board member collaborate to write a grant to help support the school-based prevention programs. What *Healthy People 2030* objectives would you be targeting with the grant? What data would be required to demonstrate a need for funding for sealant and fluoride varnish programs for schoolchildren in your community? What resources would be useful to find data to help with the grant proposal? (See References and Additional Resources for ideas.)
6. Your mother lives in a residential facility for older adults in your community. The director of the facility asks for your assistance as a dental hygienist to develop a comprehensive oral health program for the residents of the facility. What general information about access to oral health care and oral health-related quality of life specific to this population in our nation would you need to learn? What resources could you use to acquire this information? What steps could you take to identify the oral health needs and the oral health-related quality of life of the residents of the facility? How could you find out what resources are available for oral health care for this population in your community? Who could you contact?

LEARNING OBJECTIVES AND COMPETENCIES

This chapter addresses the following community oral health learning objectives and competencies for dental hygienists that are presented in the revised May 2015-2016 *ADEA Compendium of Curriculum Guidelines for Allied Dental Education Programs:*

Learning Objectives:
• Perform a needs assessment of the target population.

• Identify possible evaluation tools for the program.
• Describe and define the goals of various dental indices.

Competencies
• Assessing, planning, implementing and evaluating community-based oral health programs.

COMMUNITY CASE

In your position as the State Dental Director, you have received a request from the State Health Officer for the State Department of Public Health that the State Health Surveillance System be reorganized and updated based on the *Healthy People 2030* health objectives. You are asked to develop a plan to integrate an updated oral health component for this State Health Surveillance System.

1. Which of the following resources would be the LEAST useful to review during the early planning of the oral health component for the State Health Surveillance System?
   a. *Healthy People 2030* Oral Conditions objectives
   b. National Oral Health Surveillance System (NOHSS)
   c. Association of State and Territorial Dental Directors (ASTDD) report *Best Practice Approach: State-Based Oral Health Surveillance System*
   d. Results of the most recent ASTDD annual survey
2. What measure would be most useful to provide information about untreated tooth decay?
   a. Percentage of persons with a CPI score of 1 or more
   b. Percentage of persons with 1 or more dft or DMFT
   c. Percentage of persons with 1 or more dt or DT
   d. Percentage of edentulous adults

3. In designing a survey to evaluate access to dental care, all of the following EXCEPT one is most often collected with the use of a questionnaire. Which is the EXCEPTION?
   a. Last oral and pharyngeal cancer examination
   b. Usual source of dental care
   c. Annual dental visit
   d. Reason for not having a dental visit in the past year
4. Which is the best survey method to replicate in order to assess the presence of dental sealants among third-grade students?
   a. National Health Interview Survey (NHIS)
   b. Association for State and Territorial Dental Directors (ASTDD) Basic Screening Survey (BSS)
   c. Behavioral Risk Factor Surveillance System (BRFSS)
   d. National Vital Statistics System
5. All of the following factors EXCEPT one are important to include in the State Oral Health Surveillance System to track oral health disparities. Which is the EXCEPTION?
   a. Geographic location
   b. Age
   c. Occupation
   d. Racial and ethnic background

REFERENCES

1. Introduction to Public Health Surveillance. Public Health 101 Series. Atlanta, GA: Centers for Disease Control and Prevention; 2018 Nov 5. Available at: <https://www.cdc.gov/publichealth101/surveillance.html>; [Accessed March 2020].
2. Public Health Surveillance. Geneva, Switzerland: World Health Organization. Available at: <http://www.who.int/topics/public_health_surveillance/en/>; [Accessed December 2019].
3. Overview of Midcourse Progress and Health Disparities. Revised Chapter III of *Healthy People 2020* Midcourse Review. Hyattsville, MD: National Center for Health Statistics; 2017 Apr 20. Available at: <https://www.cdc.gov/nchs/data/hpdata2020/HP2020M-CR-B03-Overview.pdf>;[Accessed September 2019].
4. 2000 Surgeon General's Report on Oral Health in America : Bethesda, MD: National Institute of Dental and Craniofacial Research; 2019 Jan. Available at: <https://www.nidcr.nih.gov/research/data-statistics/surgeon-general>; [Accessed December 2019].
5. Rozier RG, White BA, Slade GD. Trends in oral diseases in the U.S. population. J Dent Educ 2017;81(8):eS97–eS109. Available at: <https://doi.org/10.21815/JDE.017.016>; [Accessed March 2020].

6. Best Practice Approach: State-Based Oral Health Surveillance System. Reno, NV: Association of State and Territorial Dental Directors; 2017 Jul. Available at: <https://www.astdd.org/docs/BPASurveillanceSystem.pdf>; [Accessed December 2019].
7. National Center for Chronic Disease Prevention and Health Promotion. About the Center. Atlanta, GA: Centers for Disease Control and Prevention; 2020 Jan 20. Available at: <https://www.cdc.gov/chronicdisease/center/index.htm>; [Accessed March 2020].
8. Healthy People 2030 Framework. What is the Healthy People 2030 Framework? Rockville, MD: Office of Disease Prevention and Health Promotion; 2020. Available at: <https://www.healthypeople.gov/2020/About-Healthy-People/Development-Healthy-People-2030/Framework>; [Accessed March 2020].
9. Secretary's Advisory Committee on National Health Promotion and Disease Prevention Objectives for 2030 Report #7: Assessment and Recommendations for Proposed Objectives for Healthy People 2030. Washington, DC: Secretary's Advisory Committee for Healthy People 2030; 2019. Available at: <https://www.healthypeople.gov/sites/default/files/Report%207_Reviewing%20Assessing%20Set%20of%20HP2030%20Objectives_Formatted%20EO_508_05.21.pdf>; [Accessed March 2020].

10. Progress Reviews. Hyattsville, MD: National Center for Health Statistics; 2019. Available at: <https://www.cdc.gov/nchs/healthy_people/hp2020/hp2020_progress_reviews.htm>; [Accessed December 2019].

11. Secretary's Advisory Committee on National Health Promotion and Disease Prevention Objectives for 2030 Report #2: Recommendations for Developing Objectives, Setting Priorities, Identifying Data Needs, and Involving Stakeholders for Healthy People 2030. Washington, DC: Secretary's Advisory Committee for Healthy People 2030; 2017. Available at: <https://www.healthypeople.gov/sites/default/files/Advisory_Committee_Objectives_for_HP2030_Report.pdf>; [Accessed March 2020].

12. Healthy People 2030. Rockville, MD: Office of Disease Prevention and Health Promotion. Available at: <https://health.gov/healthypeople>; [Accessed December 2020].

13. The Secretary's Advisory Committee on National Health Promotion and Disease Prevention Objectives for 2030, Report #8. Recommendations for Implementation and the Framework Graphic for Healthy People 2030. Washington, DC: Secretary's Advisory Committee for Healthy People 2030; 2019. Available at: <https://www.healthypeople.gov/sites/default/files/Report%208_Implementation%20and%20Graphic_Formatted_%20EO_508c-final_0.pdf>; [Accessed March 2020].

14. National Oral Health Surveillance System (NOHSS). Atlanta, GA: Centers for Disease Control and Prevention; 2015. Available at: <https://www.cdc.gov/oralhealthdata/overview/nohss.html>; [Accessed December 2019].

15. National Health and Nutrition Examination Survey (NHANES) Oral Health Examiners Manual, 2020. Atlanta, GA: Centers for Disease Control and Prevention; 2020 Jan. Available at: <https://www.cdc.gov/nchs/data/nhanes/2019-2020/manuals/2020-Oral-Health-Examiners-Manual-508.pdf>; [Accessed March 2020].

16. National Health Interview Survey: Adult: 2018. Hyattsville, MD: National Center for Health Statistics; 2018. From Centers for Disease Control and Prevention; 2019 May 6. Available at: <https://www.cdc.gov/nchs/nhis/nhis_questionnaires.htm>; [Accessed February 2020].

17. Behavioral Risk Factor Surveillance System (BRFSS). Atlanta, GA: Centers for Disease Control and Prevention; 2018. Available at: <https://www.cdc.gov/brfss/index.html>; [Accessed February 2020].

18. Oral Health Surveys: Basic Methods. 5th ed. Geneva, Switzerland: World Health Organization; 2013. Available at: <http://apps.who.int/iris/bitstream/10665/97035/1/9789241548649_eng.pdf>; [Accessed March 2020].

19. Basic Screening Surveys: An Approach to Monitoring Community Oral Health: Older Adults. Reno, NV: Association of State and Territorial Dental Directors; 2010. Available at: <http://www.prevmed.org/wp-content/uploads/2013/11/BSS-SeniorsManual.pdf>; [Accessed March 2020].

20. Basic Screening Surveys: An Approach to Monitoring Oral Health: Preschool & School Children. Reno, NV: Association of State and Territorial Dental Directors. Available at: <https://azdhs.gov/documents/prevention/womens-childrens-health/oral-health/infant-youth/ASTDD-BSS-manual.pdf>; [Accessed March 2020].

21. Chattopadhyay A. Oral Health Epidemiology: Principles and Practice. Sudbury, MA: Jones and Bartlett; 2011.

22. Phipps K. The New & Improved Children's Basic Screening Survey. Reno, NV: Association of State and Territorial Dental Directors; 2017. Available at: <https://www.astdd.org/docs/childrens-bss-webinar-ppt-10-12-2017.pdf>; [Accessed December 2019].

23. Wyche CJ. Indices and scoring methods. In: Boyd LD, Mallonee LF, Wyche CJ, editors. Wilkins' Clinical Practice of the Dental Hygienist. 13th ed. Burlington, MS: Jones & Bartlett Learning; 2021. p. 357–79.

24. Lo E. Caries Process and Prevention Strategies: Epidemiology: The DMF Index, Course No. 368. Cincinnati, OH; Proctor & Gamble Dentalcare.com; 2019. Available at: <https://www.dentalcare.com/en-us/professional-education/ce-courses/ce368/epidemiology-the-dmf-index>; [Accessed January 2020].

25. Drury TF, Winn DM, Snowden CB, et al. An overview of the oral health component of the 1988-1991 National Health and Nutrition Examination Survey (NHANES III, Phase 1). J Dent Res 1996;75(special issue):620–30. Available at: <https://www.ncbi.nlm.nih.gov/pubmed/8594086>; [Accessed March 2020].

26. Early Childhood Oral Health. Reno, NV: Association of State and Territorial Dental Directors; 2017. Available at: <http://www.astdd.org/early-childhood-oral-health-committee/>; [Accessed February 2020].

27. NHANES Questionnaire Instruments: Sample Person Questionnaire: Oral Health: 2019. Hyattsville, MD: National Center for Health Statistics; 2020 Feb 21. Available at: <https://wwwn.cdc.gov/nchs/data/nhanes/2019-2020/questionnaires/OHQ_K.pdf>; [Accessed March 2020].

28. Castro ALS, Vianna MIP, Mendes CMC. Comparison of caries lesion detection methods in epidemiological surveys: CAST, ICDAS and DMF. BMC Oral Health 2018;18:e122. Available at: <https://bmcoralhealth.biomedcentral.com/articles/10.1186/s12903-018-0583-6>; [Accessed March 2020].

29. Healthy People 2020 Midcourse Review. Hyattsville, MD: National Center for Health Statistics; 2018 Jun 5. Available at: <https://www.cdc.gov/nchs/healthy_people/hp2020/hp2020_midcourse_review.htm>; [Accessed March 2000].

30. Best Practice Approach: School-based Dental Sealant Programs. Reno, NV: Association of State and Territorial Dental Directors; 2017 Nov. Available at: <http://www.astdd.org/docs/sealant-bpar-update-11-2017-final.pdf>; [Accessed March 2020].

31. Summary Report: 2019 Synopses of State Dental Public Health Programs: Data for FY 2017-2013. Reno, NV: Association of State and Territorial Dental Directors; 2019. Available at: <https://www.astdd.org/docs/synopses-summary-report-2019.pdf>; [Accessed October 2019].

32. Tonetti MS, Greenwell H, Kornman KS. Staging and grading of periodontitis: Framework and proposal of a new classification and case definition. J Periodontol 2018;89(Suppl 1):S159–72. Available at: <https://aap.onlinelibrary.wiley.com/doi/epdf/10.1002/JPER.18-0006>; [Accessed March 2020].

33. Eke PI, Dye FA, Wei L, et al. Self-reported measures for surveillance of periodontitis. J Dent Res 2013;92:1041–7. Available at: <https://journals.sagepub.com/doi/10.1177/0022034513505621>; [Accessed March 2020].

34. Dye BA, Afful J, Thornton-Evans G, Iafolla T. Overview and quality assurance for the oral health component of the National Health and Nutrition Examination Survey (NHANES), 2011-2014. BMC Oral Health 2019;19:95. Available at: <https://www.ncbi.nlm.nih.gov/pmc/articles/PMC6542072/>; [Accessed March 2020].

35. Ali OH, Mazin H. The benefit of Ramfjord teeth to represent the full-mouth clinical attachment level in epidemiological study. J Bagh Coll Dent 2014;26(2):122–4. Available at: <https://pdfs.semanticscholar.org/0cfd/b629cc198d53133ec80042becb986417033f.pdf?_ga=2.161638140.1963827071.1584369097-129317003.1584369097>; [Accessed March 2020].

36. Oral-Systemic Health. Chicago, IL: American Dental Association Center for Scientific Information; 2019 Sep 23. Available at: <https://www.ada.org/en/member-center/oral-health-topics/oral-systemic-health>; [Accessed March 2020].

37. Medical Expenditure Panel Survey: Survey Background. Rockville, MD: Agency for Healthcare Research and Quality; 2019 Apr 22. Available at: <https://www.meps.ahrq.gov/mepsweb/about_meps/survey_back.jsp>; [Accessed March 2020].

38. International Classification of Diseases (ICD-11). Geneva, Switzerland: World Health Organization; 2018 Jun 18. Available at: <https://www.who.int/classifications/icd/en/>; [Accessed March 2020].

39. National Program of Cancer Registries (NPCR): About the Program. Atlanta, GA: Centers for Disease Control and Prevention; 2019. Available at: <http://www.cdc.gov/cancer/npcr/about.htm>; [Accessed March 2020].

40. About the SEER Program. Bethesda, MD: National Cancer Institute, Surveillance, Epidemiology, and End Results Program; 2020. Available at: <https://seer.cancer.gov/>; [Accessed March 2020].

41. Cancer Data and Statistics. Atlanta, GA: Centers for Disease Control and Prevention; 2019 Jul 9. Available at: <https://www.cdc.gov/cancer/dcpc/data/>; [Accessed March 2020].

42. Early Detection, Diagnosis, and Staging. Atlanta, GA: American Cancer Society; 2020. Available at: <https://www.cancer.org/cancer/oral-cavity-and-oropharyngeal-cancer/detection-diagnosis-staging.html>; [Accessed March 2020].

43. Risk Factors for Oral Cavity and Oropharyngeal Cancers. Atlanta, GA: American Cancer Society; 2020. Available at: <https://www.cancer.org/cancer/oral-cavity-and-oropharyngeal-cancer/causes-risks-prevention/risk-factors.html>; [Accessed March 2020].

44. About GTSS: Smoking and Tobacco Use. Atlanta, GA: Centers for Disease Control and Prevention; 2018. Available at: <https://www.cdc.gov/tobacco/global/gtss/index.htm>; [Accessed March 2020].

45. Best Practice Approach Report: Oral Health in the Older Adult Population (Age 65 and older). Reno, NV: Association of State and Territorial Dental Directors; 2018 May. Available at: <https://www.astdd.org/bestpractices/bpar-oral-health-in-the-older-adult-population-age-65-and-older.pdf>; [Accessed March 2020].

46. Facts About Cleft Lip and Cleft Palate, Birth Defects. Atlanta, GA: Centers for Disease Control and Prevention; 2019 Dec 5. Available at: <https://www.cdc.gov/ncbddd/birthdefects/CleftLip.html>; [Accessed March 2020].

47. Kaste LM, Gift HC, Bhat M. Prevalence of incisor trauma in persons 5 to 50 years of age: United States, 1988-1991. J Dent Res 1996;75(2):696–705. Available at: <https://www.researchgate.net/publication/14606644_Prevalence_of_incisor_trauma_in_persons_6-50_years_of_age_United_States_1988-1991>; [Accessed March 2020].

48. Data quality evaluation of the dental fluorosis clinical assessment data from the National Health and Nutrition Examination Survey, 1999-2004 and 2011-2016. Hyattsville, MD: National Center for Health Statistics. Vital Health Stat 2019 Apr;2(183). Available at: <https://www.cdc.gov/nchs/data/series/sr_02/sr02_183-508.pdf>; [Accessed March 2020].

49. National Health and Nutrition Examination Survey 2015-2016 Data Documentation, Codebook, and Frequencies, Fluorosis - Clinical. Atlanta, GA: Centers for Disease Control and Prevention; April 2019. Available at: <https://wwwn.cdc.gov/Nchs/Nhanes/2015-2016/FLXCLN_I.htm>; [Accessed March 2020].

50. Sabokseir A, Golkari A, Sheiham A. Distinguishing between enamel fluorosis and other enamel defects in permanent teeth of children. Peer J 2016;4(2):e1745. Available at: <https://peerj.com/articles/1745/>; [Accessed March 2020].

51. National Health and Nutrition Examination Survey (NHANES) Oral Health Examiners Procedures Manual, 2013. Atlanta, GA: Centers for Disease Control and Prevention; 2013 May. Available at: <https://wwwn.cdc.gov/nchs/data/nhanes/2013-2014/manuals/Oral_Health_Examiners.pdf>; [Accessed March 2020].

52. National Health and Nutrition Examination Survey (NHANES) Oral Health Examiners Procedures Manual, 2016. Atlanta, GA: Centers for Disease Control and Prevention; 2016 Jan. Available at: <https://wwwn.cdc.gov/nchs/data/nhanes/2015-2016/manuals/2016_Oral_Health_Examiners_Procedures_Manual.pdf>; [Accessed March 2020].

53. Nor NAM. Methods and indices in measuring fluorosis: A review. Arch Orofac Sci 2017;12(2):77–85. Available at: <http://aos.usm.my/docs/Vol_12/aos-article-0280.pdf>; [Accessed March 2020].

54. Department of Health and Human Services Federal Panel on Community Water Fluoridation. U.S. Public Health Service recommendation for fluoride concentration in drinking water for the prevention of dental caries. Public Health Rep 2015; 130(July–August):14p/e. Available at: <https://www.ncbi.nlm.nih.gov/pmc/articles/PMC4547570/>; [Accessed March 2020].

55. Ajiboye S. AADR Response to New NCHS Evaluation of Dental Fluorosis Clinical Assessment Data from NHANES Over Time. Government Affairs & Science Policy Blog. Washington, DC: American Association for Dental Research; 2019 Apr 22. Available at: <http://ga.dentalresearchblog.org/?p=3344>; [Accessed March 2020].

56. Water Fluoridation Reporting System. Healthy People.gov; 2020 Mar 13. Available at: <https://www.healthypeople.gov/2020/datasource/water-fluoridation-reporting-system>; [Accessed March 2020].

57. My Water's Fluoride. Atlanta, GA: Centers for Disease Control and Prevention. Available at: <https://nccd.cdc.gov/DOH_MWF/Default/AboutMWF.aspx>; [Accessed March 2020].

58. Horst, K. Barriers to Accessing Oral Health Care: A report for the Waterloo Region Oral Health Coalition. Kitchener Downtown Community Health Centre; 2017. Available at: <http://kdchc.org/wp-content/uploads/2018/03/Barriers-to-Accessing-Oral-Health-Care-in-Waterloo-Region.pdf>; [Accessed March 2020].

59. Detailed Outline of Topics in the Redesigned National Health Interview Survey (NHIS): Sample Adult Questionnaire Version: March 2019. Hyattsville, MD: National Center for Health Statistics; 2019. Available at: <https://www.cdc.gov/nchs/data/nhis/AdultNHISRedesignTopics201903.pdf>; [Accessed March 2020].

60. National Study of Long-Term Care Providers. Atlanta, GA: Centers for Disease Control and Prevention; 2019 Oct 2. Available at: <https://www.cdc.gov/nchs/nsltcp/index.htm>; [Accessed March 2020].

61. Questionnaires, Datasets, and Related Documentation. National Study of Long-Term Care Providers; 2018. Hyattsville, MD: National Center for Health Statistics. Available at: <https://www.cdc.gov/nchs/nsltcp/nsltcp_questionnaires.htm>; [Accessed March 2020].

62. Zucoloto ML, Maroco J, Campos JADB. Impact of oral health on health-related quality of life: a cross-sectional study. BMC Oral Health 2016;16(55). Available at: <https://doi.org/10.1186/s12903-016-0211-2>; [Accessed March 2020].

63. WHOQOL: Measuring Quality of Life. Geneva, Switzerland: World Health Organization. Available at: <https://www.who.int/healthinfo/survey/whoqol-qualityoflife/en/index4.html>; [Accessed March 2020].

64. Health-Related Quality of Life & Well-Being. Healthy People 2020. Rockville, MD: Office of Disease Prevention and Health Promotion; 2020 Mar 13. Available at: <http://www.healthy-people.gov/2020/topics-objectives/topic/health-related-quality-of-life-well-being>; [Accessed March 2020].

65. Oral Health and Quality of Life (Policy Statement). Geneva, Switzerland: FDI World Dental Federation; 2015 Sep. Available at: <https://www.fdiworlddental.org/resources/policy-statements-and-resolutions/oral-health-and-quality-of-life>; [Accessed March 2020].

66. Alzoubi EE, Hariri R, Attard NJ. Oral health related quality of life impact in dentistry. J Dent Health Oral Disord Ther 2017;6(6):183–8. Available at: <http://dx.doi.org/10.15406/jd-hodt.2017.06.00221>; [Accessed March 2020].

67. FDI's Definition of Oral Health. Geneva, Switzerland: FDI World Dental Federation. Available at: <https://www.fdiworlddental.org/oral-health/fdi-definition-of-oral-health>; [Accessed March 2020].

68. de la Fuente Hernández J, del Carmen Aguilar Díaz F, del Carmen Villanueva Vilchis M. Oral health related quality of life. In: Virdi MS, editor. Emerging Trends in Oral Health Sciences and Dentistry. Rijeka, Croatia: InTech Europe; 2015. Available at: <http://dx.doi.org/10.5772/59262>; [Accessed March 2020].

69. Competencies for State Oral Health Programs. Reno, NV: Association of State and Territorial Dental Directors; 2020. Available at: <https://www.astdd.org/docs/competencies-and-levels-for-state-oral-health-programs-2020.pdf>; [Accessed May 2020].

70. Contreras, OA, Steward, D, Valachovic, RW. Examining America's Dental Safety Net (ADEA's Data Brief). Washington, DC: American Dental Education Association; 2018 Apr. Available at: < file:///C:/Users/Admin/AppData/Local/Temp/ADEA_Data-Brief_SafetyNet_April2018_WEB%20(1).pdf >; [Accessed February 2020].

71. State Oral Health Program Infrastructure. Reno, NV: Association of State and Territorial Dental Directors; 2018. Available at: <https://www.astdd.org/state-oral-health-program-structure/>; [Accessed November 2019].

72. Guidelines for State and Territorial Oral Health Programs Part I. Reno, NV: Association of State and Territorial Dental Directors; 2015 Dec. Available at: <https://www.astdd.org/docs/astdd-guidelines-part-I-2015-update-january-2016.pdf>; [Accessed October 2019].

73. Oral Health Programs. Atlanta, GA: Centers for Disease Control and Prevention; 2019 Dec 19. Available at: <https://www.cdc.gov/oral-health/funded_programs/index.htm>; [Accessed December 2019].

74. Association of State and Territorial Dental Directors Strategic Map 2019-2021. Reno, NV: Association of State and Territorial Dental Directors; 2019 Jun 10. Available at: <https://www.astdd.org/docs/astdd-strategic-map-2019-2021.pdf>; [Accessed May 2020].

75. Guidelines for State and Territorial Oral Health Programs Part II. Reno, NV: Association of State and Territorial Dental Directors; 2018 Jan. Available at: <https://www.astdd.org/docs/astdd-guidelines-section-II-matrix-for-state-roles-examples-and-resources-1-2018-revisions.pdf>; [Accessed October 2019].

76. Best Practice Approach: Developing Workforce Capacity in State Oral Health Programs. Reno, NV: Association of State and Territorial Dental Directors; 2016 Jan. Available at: <https://www.astdd.org/bestpractices/bpa-developing-workforce-capacity-2016-01.pdf>; [Accessed November 2019].

77. Program Support. Reno, NV: Association of State and Territorial Dental Directors. Available at: <https://www.astdd.org/program-support/>; [Accessed November 2019].

78. Dye BA, Li X, Lewis BG, et al. Overview and quality assurance for the oral health component of the National Health and Nutrition Examination Survey (NHANES), 2009-2010. J Public Health Dent 2014;74:248–56. Available at: <https://www.ncbi.nlm.nih.gov/pmc/articles/PMC6542072/>; [Accessed May 2020].

ADDITIONAL RESOURCES

CDC Surveillance Resource Center
http://www.cdc.gov/surveillancepractice/index.html
Healthy People 2030
https://health.gov/healthypeople
Introduction to Public Health Surveillance (CDC PowerPoint)
https://www.cdc.gov/publichealth101/surveillance.html
My Water's Fluoride
https://nccd.cdc.gov/doh_mwf/Default/Default.aspx
National Maternal & Child Oral Health Resource Center
https://www.mchoralhealth.org/
NIDCR/CDC Dental, Oral and Craniofacial Data Resource Data Center
https://www.nidcr.nih.gov/research
Oral Health for Independent Older Adults (ADEA Resource Guide)
https://www.adea.org/publications/Pages/OralHealthforIndependent
    OlderAdults.aspx
The State of Aging and Health in America
http://www.cdc.gov/aging/pdf/state-aging-health-in-america-2013.pdf

Population Health

Amanda M. Hinson-Enslin and Christine French Beatty

OBJECTIVES

1. Describe the burden of oral disease globally and in the United States (U.S.).
2. Describe the social effects of oral disease.
3. Discuss the oral health status and trends in the U.S.
4. Explain the oral health disparities and inequities among population groups.
5. Describe dental care financing mechanisms in the U.S. and related issues that enhance or diminish oral health care.
6. Explain the issues related to the adequacy of the oral health workforce in the U.S., as well as the future outlook and recommendations.
7. Describe the infrastructure and capacity of dental public health programs in the U.S. and the future outlook.
8. Describe how teledentistry can enhance workforce capacity and improve access to oral health care.
9. Discuss the factors that influence oral health in the U.S. and future changes recommended to improve access.

OPENING STATEMENT: Fast Facts About Oral Conditions in the U.S.

- Although oral health has been improving in most of the population, many subgroups experience disparities and are not faring well.[1]
- Mexican American and black, non-Hispanic children 2–4 and 6–8 years old experience the greatest racial and ethnic disparities in dental caries experience.[1]
- Nearly 50% of children aged 9–11 years have at least one dental sealant on a permanent tooth, whereas only 31% of children aged 6–8 years have one.[2]
- Over 25% of adults have untreated dental caries.[3]
- Nearly 73% of the population are served by optimally fluoridated community water systems.[4]
- Nearly 45% of adults have periodontitis.[5]
- Approximately 17% of adults aged 65 years and older are edentulous.[6]

PART ONE: ORAL HEALTH STATUS AND TRENDS

Global Burden of Oral Diseases

Oral health problems persist in countries around the globe despite great improvements in the oral health of some populations. Significant oral disease burdens exist among different age groups, in people with lower incomes and educational levels, and among certain racial and ethnic groups in developing and developed countries.[7] Seven oral diseases and conditions account for most of the global oral disease burden: dental caries, periodontal diseases, oral cancers, oral manifestations of human immunodeficiency virus (HIV), oro-dental trauma, cleft lip (CL) and cleft palate (CP), and noma (see Box 5.1

for noma).[7] The following relates to selected oral conditions worldwide:

- Untreated dental caries is the most prevalent oral condition: nearly 2.4 billion people have caries in permanent teeth, and nearly half a million children have caries in primary teeth.[7]
- About 20% of people experience oro-dental trauma.[7]
- The annual cleft-lip-and-palate **rate** is 1 case per 1000 newborns.[7]
- Severe periodontitis is the 11th most prevalent disease.[7]
- Oral cancer **incidence** is 4 cases per 100,000 people yearly,[7] with over 400,000 new cases of lip, oral, and salivary gland cancer each year.[8]
- Between 30% and 80% of individuals with HIV experience oral manifestations such as bacterial, fungal, and/or viral infections.[7]

The inadequate alignment of oral health professionals remains a core issue globally. This leads to the absence of concentrated prevention, treatment, and advocacy in many nations, especially for vulnerable and disadvantaged groups in developing countries.[7]

The important role of behavioral, social, cultural, and environmental factors in oral health and disease has been shown in epidemiological surveys and data systems supported by the **World Health Organization** (WHO) Global Oral Health Program.[9,10] To address this, the WHO Oral Health Country/Area Profile Programme was developed to organize and present data for various countries and regions to be able to describe oral health status and services on the web.[9,11] Also, the WHO Global Oral Health Database was developed as part of the WHO Global InfoBase to track oral health indicators for

BOX 5.1   Noma

Noma, also known as cancrum oris and gangrenous stomatitis, is a painful, devastating, and disfiguring form of gangrene that destroys orofacial tissues.[1] Affecting the world's poorest citizens,[2] noma primarily occurs in young children 2–6 years old who are malnourished, have had another illness such as measles, malaria, or an immunodeficiency, and live in extreme poverty.[1,3] However, it can be seen in older children and adults.[2] It is more common in underdeveloped nations such as in sub-Saharan Africa.[2] The survival rate is only 15% worldwide because of lack of care.[3] The World Health Organization (WHO) estimates 140,000 new cases annually.[3] However, the exact incidence and **prevalence** is unknown because of the high mortality rate; difficulty registering, treating, and managing the disease owing to nomadic cultures; and the isolation of affected individuals because of the stigma associated with the disease.

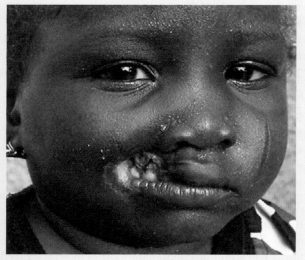

(From Baratti-Mayer D, Pittet B, Montandon D, et al. Geneva Study Group on Noma. Noma: an infectious disease of unknown aetiology. Lancet Infect Dis 2003;3:419–431.)

Research suggests that the possible cause is a fusospirochetal bacterium, but the pathogenesis is not clear.[1,2] Noma causes tissue destruction of the gingiva, lips, buccal mucosa, cheeks, and even muscle tissue.[1–3] The infection can lead to the development of draining ulcers, results in tissue death, and if left untreated, ends in an agonizing death.[2,3] Noma is treated with a regimen of antibiotics, debridement, and proper nutrition.[2] In cases of disfigurement, plastic surgery is necessary to remove dead tissue and reconstruct facial tissues to improve function of the mouth and jaw and to improve appearance.[3] Noma may heal without treatment, but it can still cause extreme disfigurement.[3] Proper nutrition, cleanliness, and sanitation are used for prevention and treatment.[3]

In the 19th century noma occurred in the U.S. in areas of poverty, malnutrition, and unsanitary conditions as the pioneers migrated west.[3] As public health measures improved, environmental conditions and oral cleanliness became more the norm. Thus, noma virtually disappeared from developed countries during the 20th century.[3] However, a case of noma was reported recently in the U.S. in an older adult who was malnourished and immunocompromised.[2]

1. Enwonwu, C. Noma (cancrum oris). UpToDate; 2019. Available at: <https://www.uptodate.com/contents/noma-cancrum-oris>; [Accessed December 2019].
2. Maley A, Desai M, Parker S. Noma: A disease of poverty presenting at an urban hospital in the United States. JAAD Case Rep 2015 Jan 1;1(1):18-20. Available at: <https://www.ncbi.nlm.nih.gov/pmc/articles/PMC4802558/>; [Accessed December 2019].
3. Srour ML, Marck K, Baratti-Mayer D. Noma: overview of a neglected disease and human rights violation. Am J Trop Med Hyg; 2017 Feb 8;96(2):268-274. Available at: <https://www.ncbi.nlm.nih.gov/pmc/articles/PMC5303022/>; [Accessed December 2019].

priority population groups worldwide.[12] The *Oral Health Atlas* maps oral health globally, describing oral health **status** and key factors influencing **trends** in oral diseases.[13] The United Nations has recognized that oral diseases are a major health burden for several countries and recommended global coordination of national dental public health promotion and prevention efforts.[14]

U.S. national oral health indicators are included in the global and regional oral health **surveillance systems**. The Pan American Health Organization (PAHO) is the WHO Regional Office for the Americas. The PAHO leads the oral health surveillance effort to track selected oral health indicators in the U.S. and 39 other nations in North, Central, and South America.[15]

Burden of Oral Diseases in the U.S.

Progress has been made to reduce the extent and severity of common oral diseases in the U.S.[1] During the last half of the 20th century and since the beginning of the 21st century, major strides in oral health have been seen nationally, yet oral diseases remain common and widespread.[1] Oral diseases and conditions afflict most people at some time in their lives.[1] For example, dental caries is considered one of the most common and preventable chronic diseases of children.[16]

As explained in Chapter 4, *Healthy People* tracks progress of oral health indicators each decade. A midcourse report published in 2017 indicated the progress made toward the *Healthy People 2020* benchmarks.[17] At that time, 16 oral health subobjectives had met or exceeded their targets, 3 had improved toward the targets, 5 had little to no movement toward the targets, 1 regressed by moving away from the baseline, and 8 could not be assessed because of a lack of sufficient data.[17] These data reinforced that improvements have been made in addressing oral health needs, yet more effort is needed to reduce oral diseases and oral health disparities. A full evaluation of the outcomes of *Healthy People 2020* is anticipated in the near future.

Despite improvements, profound oral **health disparities** remain in specific population groups, with striking magnitude in some cases.[1] Multiple demographic, social, and environmental characteristics and personal behaviors contribute to oral health disparities (see Chapter 3 Determinants of Health section). Thus, the burden of oral diseases is spread unevenly throughout the population.[18,19] People who experience the poorest oral health are found among the poor of all ages, especially children and older adults living in poverty. Members of racial and ethnic minorities and individuals who are medically compromised or have disabilities also experience oral health disparities.[1,19,20]

Social Impact of Oral Diseases

Oral diseases are progressive, cumulative, and become more complex over time.[18] These diseases can have various effects that jeopardize physical growth, development, self-concept, and the capacity to learn.[18,20] (Box 5.2). Poor oral health-related quality of life, partially resulting from the burden of oral diseases, can affect economic productivity and compromise a person's ability to work at home and on the job, as well as their school performance.[20] **Socioeconomic status** (SES) is associated with oral diseases, and individuals in poverty experience more serious consequences of oral disease because they lack the resources

BOX 5.2 Social Impact of Oral Diseases and Conditions on Children and Adults

Children
- Experience delayed growth and development
- Have poor self-esteem
- Avoid talking
- Have poor school performance
- Miss school
- Avoid smiling
- Experience difficulty eating and drinking

Adults
- Experience impaired oral functions
- Suffer disfigurement
- Have poor work performance
- Lose work hours
- Have difficulty speaking
- Have poor self-esteem
- Are affected by poor nutrition
- Endure stress within the work-family relationship

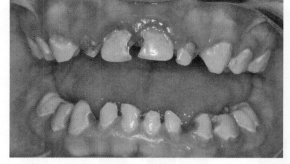

Fig 5.1 Early childhood caries. (Courtesy Dr. Frank Hodges.)

for preventive care, have less access to care, and have lower oral health literacy.[19] Poor oral health can also result in premature death when oral diseases are left untreated.[7]

The National Health and Nutrition Examination Survey (NHANES) has included survey questions that measure oral health-related quality of life (see Measurement of Oral Health–Related Quality of Life section in Chapter 4). The following results are from the 2017–2018 NHANES:[21]

- Experiencing oral pain within the last year: nearly 48% never, 28% hardly ever, 17% occasionally, 4% fairly often, and 4% very often
- Having difficulty attending or completing tasks at school or work within the last year because of problems with teeth, mouth, or dentures: about 86% never, 8% hardly ever, 3% occasionally, 1% fairly often, and 1% very often
- Being embarrassed because of their teeth, mouth, or dentures within the last year: 7% very often, 4% fairly often, 8% occasionally, 11% hardly ever, and 69% never

STATUS AND TRENDS OF SPECIFIC ORAL CONDITIONS IN THE U.S.

As described in Chapter 4, national surveys and surveillance systems are used to track oral health indicators, monitor attainment of national oral health objectives, and reveal national trends. This chapter provides a broad overview of the status and trends associated with oral health established with the various assessment and data collection methods described in Chapters 3 and 4. In recent years, lack of funding has limited reporting, but additional reports are expected soon, such as the *Healthy People 2020* final reports and the 2020 Surgeon General's Report on Oral Health.[20] However, the release of some of these reports has been delayed because of the need to refocus priorities and redistribute resources to address the COVID-19 pandemic.

Dental Caries

Although lower than in other countries, the U.S. has a high rate of treated and untreated dental caries. Untreated caries can lead to pain, abscesses, extensive dental treatment, extraction of teeth, costly dental care, compromising of existing medical conditions, and sometimes even death.

Children and Adolescents

Despite a tremendous decline in dental caries in children since the 1950s, it remains the most common chronic disease of children and has been reported to be four times more common than asthma among adolescents 14–17 years old.[16] The prevalence of **early childhood caries** (ECC) is also significant, especially in children from low-income families[22] (Figure 5.1). According to the American Academy of Pediatric Dentistry, the total ECC experience (treated and untreated caries combined) is unchanged in recent surveys, but the number of filled carious lesions has increased, indicating the provision of more treatment to preschool children.[22] However, outcomes data for *Healthy People 2020* indicate a decrease in the prevalence of caries in 3–5-year-old children when examined over a longer period, from 33.3% in 1999–2004 to 27.9% in 2011–2012 and 2013–2016.[23]

A general decline of caries prevalence in children since the 1980s is the result of various preventive measures such as community water fluoridation, increased use of other fluorides, and application of dental sealants.[16,24] Nevertheless, the prevalence of total caries is staggering. Nearly 50% of children 2–19 years old have caries experience, 13% have untreated caries, and both rates increase as children get older (Figure 5.2). The prevalence of caries experience decreases as family income increases[25] (Figure 5.3). Although the overall prevalence of caries experience in 2–19-year-old children declined from 2011 to 2016, the decline was not statistically significant.[25] However, the prevalence of untreated dental caries markedly increased from 2011 to 2014 and then decreased slightly in 2015–2016.[25]

These data show a somewhat promising indication of some improvement in the rates of caries experience and untreated caries of children and adolescents when compared to *Healthy People 2020* baseline data and other tracking sources. This may relate to the increasing numbers of children getting preventive dental care at younger ages as a result of the **Patient Protection and Affordable Care Act** (Affordable Care Act; ACA), and the **Medicaid** expansion in 2010[26] (see later in this chapter).

Young and Older Adults

Even though the magnitude of dental caries has decreased since the 1960s, the vast majority of people, including adults, have

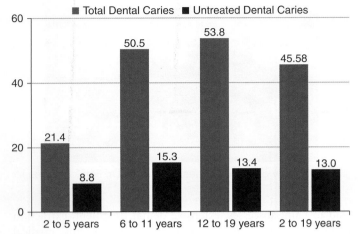

Fig 5.2 Percentage of dental caries among children and adolescents in the U.S., 2015–2016. (From Fleming E, Afful J. Prevalence of total and untreated dental caries among youth: United States, 2015–2016. NCHS Data Brief, no. 307. Hyattsville, MD: National Center for Health Statistics; 2018. Available at: <https://www.cdc.gov/nchs/products/databriefs/db307.htm>; [Accessed December 2019].)

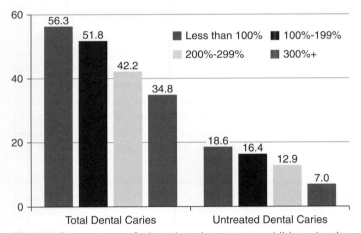

Fig 5.3 Percentage of dental caries among children in the U.S. by poverty levels, 2015–2016. (From Fleming E, Afful J. Prevalence of total and untreated dental caries among youth: United States, 2015–2016. NCHS Data Brief, no. 307. Hyattsville, MD: National Center for Health Statistics; 2018. Available at: <https://www.cdc.gov/nchs/products/databriefs/db307.htm>; [Accessed December 2019].)

TABLE 5.1 Prevalence of Dental Caries Among Adults Aged 20 to >75, 2011–2016		
Age Group	Percent Caries Experience	Percent Untreated Caries
20–34	82.0	29.3
35–49	92.5	26.4
50–64	96.4	21.5
65–74	96.4	15.4
≥75	96.0	16.5
20–64	89.9	26.1
≥65	96.2	15.9

(From Centers for Disease Control and Prevention. Oral Health Surveillance Report: Trends in Dental Caries and Sealants, Tooth Retention, and Edentulism, United States, 1999–2004 to 2011–2016. Atlanta, GA: Centers for Disease Control and Prevention; 2019. Available at: <https://www.cdc.gov/oralhealth/publications/OHSR-2019-index.html>; [Accessed April 2020].)

caries experience, and disparities still exist.[6] The Oral Health Surveillance Report indicated that in 2011–2016 nearly 90% of 20–64-year-olds who were sampled had experienced dental caries, and 26.1% had untreated dental caries[3] (Table 5.1). However, over 96% of 65-year-old and older adults had experienced dental caries, and nearly 16% had untreated dental caries[3] (Table 5.1). According to *Healthy People 2020* outcomes, even though it was reduced, the prevalence of untreated root surface caries in older adults aged 75 years and older was still a significant 29.1% in 2015–2016.[23] Disparities in dental caries were apparent in the Oral Health Surveillance Report for younger and older adults, especially for untreated dental caries.[3]

Non-Hispanic white adults had considerably higher dental caries experience and noticeably less untreated dental caries compared with Hispanic adults and non-Hispanic black adults in both age groups.[3]

Community Preventive Services

Dental Sealants

Although dental sealants are very effective in preventing pit-and-fissure caries, they are underutilized,[3] and most states do not adequately meet the need for school-based sealant programs (SBSPs) in high-need schools.[24] In addition, public knowledge of their effectiveness is still low and is associated with their underutilization. The most recent data pertaining to sealants are as follows:

- Sealant prevalence in primary molars among children aged 3–5 years increased from 1.4% in 1999–2004 to 4.3% in 2011–2012.[17]
- Sealant prevalence among children aged 6–9 years increased from 31% in 1999–2004 to 41% 2011–2016.[3]
- In 1999–2004, approximately 3 in 10 children aged 6–11 years had sealants on permanent teeth; this increased in 2011–2016 to approximately 4 in 10.[3]
- Sealant prevalence among adolescents aged 12–19 years increased from 38% in 1999–2004 to 48% in 2011–2016.[3]

These results indicate an increase in sealant use in these age groups and across several sociodemographic characteristics. Even so, all age groups from families living in poverty had no increase, and disparities existed for SES and racial groups in both age groups (Figure 5.4). In the 3–5-year-old group, children from low-income families had a higher rate of sealants in primary teeth, likely because of the higher caries risk and increase in Medicaid coverage in this population.[17]

Community Water Fluoridation

Community water fluoridation is a cornerstone of dental caries prevention in the U.S.[27] In contrast to other fluoride delivery modes, fluoridation benefits Americans of all ages and SES

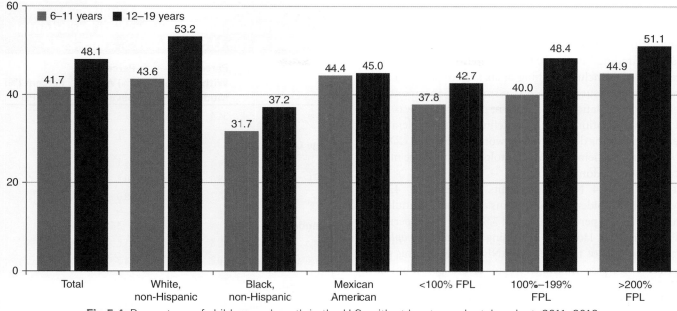

Fig 5.4 Percentage of children and youth in the U.S. with at least one dental sealant. 2011–2016. *FPL,* Federal poverty level. (From Centers for Disease Control and Prevention. Ora Health Surveillance Report: Trends in Dental Caries and Sealants, Tooth Retention, and Edentulism, United States, 1999–2004 to 2011–2016. Atlanta, GA: Centers for Disease Control and Prevention, US Dept of Health and Human Services; 2019.Available at: <https://www.cdc.gov/oralhealth/pdfs_and_other_files/Oral-Health-Surveillance-Report-2019-h.pdf>; [Accessed December 2019].)

in a passive vehicle, making it easily accessible and helping to reduce oral health disparities at the community level.[27] (See Chapter 6 Community Water Fluoridation section.) Water fluoridation has been a national health objective since the beginning of the *Healthy People* initiative. The *Healthy People 2030* goal is to increase to 77.1% by 2030 the **proportion** of people served by community water systems that are optimally fluoridated.[28]

The Centers for Disease Control and Prevention (CDC) analysis of 1992–2014 fluoridation data from the 50 states and the District of Columbia (D.C.) revealed a steady increase in the proportion of the population served by optimally fluoridated community water systems, from 62% in 1992 to 65% in 2000 to 69% in 2006 to 72.4% in 2008 to 74.6% in 2012, and a slight drop to 74.4% in 2014.[4] However, the *Healthy People 2020* target of 79.6% was not reached nationally.[17] Also, by 2014, less than one-third of the states and D.C. had reached this national *Healthy People 2020* target for community water fluoridation.[4]

In 2016, the proportion of the population with access to a fluoridated community water supply was 72.8%.[4] According to the CDC, the drop in 2016 was due to a methodology change in data analysis introduced that year because the previous methodology overestimated fluoridation status.[4] Thus, the 2016 data for fluoridated community water systems are not directly comparable with data from previous years, but they were used to establish the target for *Healthy People 2030*.[4,28] An additional 11.3 million people had access to community water systems with natural fluoride at or above optimum level in 2016.[4]

The number of states and D.C. with various proportions of the population having access to fluoridated community water supplies in 2016 is presented in Table 5.2. These percentages

TABLE 5.2   Number of States and D.C. With Various Proportions of the Population Having Access to Community Water Fluoridation, 2016

Percent (%) of Population	Number of States	Percent (%) of States
<25.0	3	5.9
25.0–49.9	5	9.8
50.0–74.9	15	29.4
≥75.0	28	54.9

(From 2016 Fluoridation Statistics. Atlanta, GA: Centers for Disease Control and Prevention; 2020 Jan 23. Available at: <https://www.cdc.gov/fluoridation/statistics/2016stats.htm>; [Accessed August 2020].)

varied substantially by state.[4] In three states—Hawaii, New Jersey, and Oregon—less than 25% of the population had access to a fluoridated community water supply.[4]

Of the 30 largest cities, only one is not fluoridated: Portland, Oregon.[29] Public health officials, policymakers, and stakeholders in states and major cities with lower rates of residents receiving water fluoridation should expand their efforts to promote fluoridation of community water systems.[27] In addition, since the optimal recommended concentration of fluoride in the water was reduced to 0.7 ppm, major cities have begun evaluating their fluoridation status.[30] From 2013 to 2018, 72 cities voted to stop fluoridating.[30] The American Dental Association (ADA) and public health officials have recommended that communities be alert to the potential for antifluoridationists to use this opportunity to gain ground for their cause.[27]

Periodontal Diseases

In the NHANES studies before 2009, partial-mouth scoring of periodontitis was used to assess the periodontal status because of lack of funding.[5] In the 2009–2014 NHANES, the protocols were updated to include probing of six sites on all teeth except third molars to ensure accurate assessments of periodontal diseases in the population.[5] In addition, periodontitis was classified in the population using case definitions of moderate and severe periodontitis developed by a workgroup of the CDC and the American Academy of Periodontology to minimize misclassification of periodontitis.[5]

The 2009–2014 NHANES results revealed that 42% of 30-year-old and older civilian noninstitutionalized adults that were sampled had periodontitis, and 7.8% had severe periodontitis[5] (Figure 5.5). However, according to *Healthy People 2020* outcomes, results of the three NHANES surveys in this period revealed a decrease in moderate to severe periodontitis in 2013–2014 compared with 2009–2010 and 2011–2012.[23] Using the newer self-report method of data collection for periodontitis (see Chapter 4 Periodontitis section), in the 2017–2018 NHANES, 19% of respondents stated they thought they had periodontal disease ("swollen gums, receding gums, sore or infected gums or loose teeth").[21]

The 2009–2014 NHANES clinical data revealed a greater prevalence of total periodontitis among men, Mexican American individuals, adults below 100% of the **federal poverty level** (FPL), current smokers, and those who self-reported diabetes.[5] Severe periodontitis was highest among adults aged 65 years and older, Mexican American and non-Hispanic black individuals, and smokers.[5] Groups with the lowest prevalence of periodontitis were 30–44-year-old non-Hispanic white individuals, nonsmokers, and those who were 400% above the FPL.[5] Moderate periodontitis increased significantly with age while mild and severe periodontitis increased only slightly with age.[5] Details of analysis of the distribution of periodontitis by demographic factors and smoking status are presented in Table 5.3.

Gingivitis only (without periodontitis) was not reported in the most recent NHANES that included a clinical assessment because of failure to assess specific signs of gingivitis (bleeding

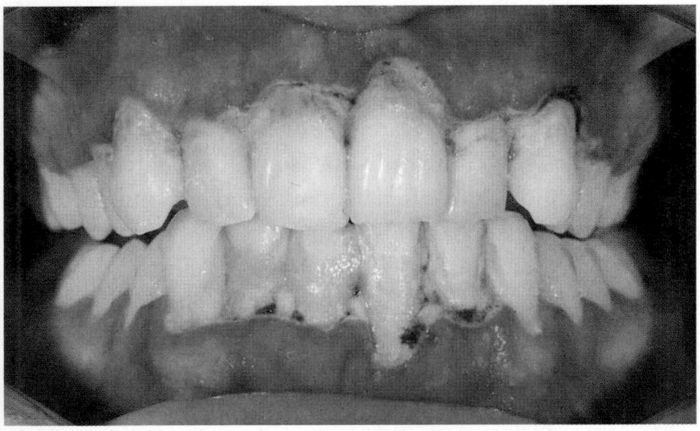

Fig 5.5 Severe periodontitis. (From Battani K, Horowitz AM. Pregnancy and oral health. In: Bowen DM, Pieren JA. Darby and Walsh: Dental Hygiene Theory and Practice, 5th ed. Maryland Heights, MO: Elsevier; 2020.)

TABLE 5.3   Percentage of Civilian Noninstitutionalized Adults With Periodontal Disease in the U.S., NHANES, 2009–2014

	Percent (%) With Mild or Moderate PD	Percent (%) With Severe PD	Percent (%) With PD
Total	34.4	7.8	42.2
Age Groups (Years)			
30–44	25.3	4.1	29.5
45–64	35.6	10.4	46.0
65+	50.7	9.0	59.8
Gender			
Male	38.8	11.5	50.2
Female	30.2	4.3	34.6
Race/Ethnicity			
Mexican American	46.4	12.4	59.7
Other Hispanic	40.7	7.8	48.5
Non-Hispanic White	31.1	5.9	37.0
Non-Hispanic Black	42.0	14.7	56.6
Other race including multiracial	36.9	9.3	46.2
Poverty Level			
<100%	46.5	13.9	60.4
100–199% FPL	41.5	12.1	53.6
200–399% FPL	37.4	7.2	44.6
>400% FPL	24.6	4.0	28.6
Smoking Status			
Current Smoker	45.5	16.9	62.4
Former Smoker	37.7	8.0	45.8
Nonsmoker	29.5	4.9	34.4

FPL, Federal poverty level; *PD*, periodontal disease; *NHANES*, National Health and Nutrition Examination Survey.
(From Eke PI, Thornton-Evans GO, Wei L, Borgnakke WS, Dye BA, Genco RJ. Periodontitis in US adults: National health and nutrition examination survey 2009-2014. J Am Dent Assoc 2018;149(7):576-588. Available at: <https://jada.ada.org/article/S0002-8177(18)30276-9/fulltext>; [Accessed November 2019].)

and coloration).[5] The most recent clinical gingivitis data are from the NHANES III in 1988–1994, which indicated that nearly half (48%) of adults 35–44 years of age had gingivitis.[31] This represented an increase from the 41% of young adults with gingivitis in the 1985–1986 NHANES.[32]

Tooth Loss

The American College of Prosthodontists (ACP) reports that the consequences of missing teeth include significant nutritional changes, obesity, diabetes, coronary artery disease, and some forms of cancer.[33] Fewer adults lose teeth due to dental caries or periodontal disease than in the past,[33] and the percentage of

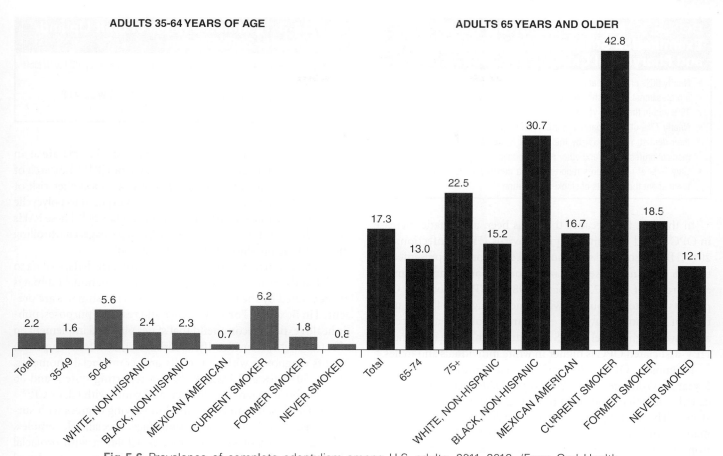

Fig 5.6 Prevalence of complete edentulism among U.S. adults, 2011–2016. (From Oral Health Surveillance Report, 2019. Oral Health. Atlanta, GA: Centers for Disease Control and Prevention; 2019. Available at: <https://www.cdc.gov/oralhealth/publications/OHSR-2019-index.html>; [Accessed December 2019].)

people with complete tooth loss has declined since the 1960s.[6] Even so, the ACP anticipates tooth loss and the need for denture care to increase in upcoming decades because of the increasing numbers of older adults.[33] In the 2017–2018 NHANES survey, 1.03% of all adults examined received a recommendation for care in relation to a full or partial denture.[21]

The Oral Health Surveillance Report provides the most recent status of tooth loss during 2011–2016 (see Figure 5.6).[3] The following are highlights of the data:[3]

- The prevalence of complete edentulism in adults 65 years and older was 17.3% (Figure 5.6), a decrease from 27.2% in 1999–2004.
- The prevalence of edentulism during 2011–2016 was nearly twice as high among adults 75 years and older (23%) compared with adults 65–74 years old (13%).
- Only 1.6% of adults 35–49 years of age and 5.6% of adults 50–64 years of age were completely edentulous (Figure 5.6), a decrease from 2.7% and 10.3% respectively in 1999–2004.

The telephone survey Behavioral Risk Factor Surveillance System (BRFSS) includes a question about how many permanent teeth participants have lost in their lifetime because of caries and/or "gum disease."[34] Results from the 2018 BRFSS were the following:[34]

- 29% reported 1–5 teeth removed.
- 11.8% reported 6 or more but not all teeth removed.

- 6.73% reported all teeth removed.
- 50% reported no teeth removed.

Oral and Pharyngeal Cancer

Oral and pharyngeal cancers (OPC) include different malignant tumors that affect the oral cavity and pharynx, most of which are squamous cell carcinomas.[35,36] OPC include cancers of the lip, tongue, floor of the mouth, palate, gingival and alveolar mucosa, buccal mucosa, and oropharynx, with the most common intraoral sites being the tongue, tonsils, oropharynx, gingiva, and floor of the mouth.[36] In advanced stages, OPC metastasize to the lymph nodes of the neck and then to more distant sites.[37] The Surveillance, Epidemiology, and End Results (SEER) Program of the National Cancer Institute estimated the incidence of OPC in 2020 was approximately 53,260 new cases or 2.9% of all new cancer cases. This proportion of OPC cases is less than other cancers such as breast, lung, and prostate cancers.[38] The estimated number of deaths from OPC in 2020 was 10,750, which is only 1.8% of all cancer deaths.[38] The relative 5-year survival rate of OPC was 66.2% during 2010–2016;[38] data suggest that survival varies based on the location of the OPC.[39]

Significant disparities exist in some population groups; minority men especially experience a higher incidence of OPC and higher death rates.[40] Also, OPC are significantly more common in men compared with women.[40]

BOX 5.3   **National Health and Nutrition Examination Survey Data Related to Oral and Pharyngeal Cancer, 2017–2018**

- Nearly 60% of participants reported having an oral cancer examination by a professional within the past year, 22% within the past 1 to 3 years, and 18% within the past 3 years.
- Nearly 77% of participants reported having an oral cancer examination by their dentist, nearly 15% by their dental hygienist, and less than 8% by medical professionals and other professionals.
- Only 11% of respondents reported that a dental professional spoke with them about the benefits of smoking cessation.

BOX 5.4   **Estimated Rates of Cleft Lip and Cleft Palate, 2010–2014**

- Approximately 1 in every 1,600 babies is born with cleft lip (CL) with cleft palate (CP).
- Approximately 1 in every 2,800 babies is born with CL without CP.
- About 1 in every 1,700 babies is born with CP.

In the past few decades there has been a dramatic increase in OPC linked to human papillomavirus (HPV) infection.[41] In 2019, HPV-associated squamous cell carcinomas represented up to 90% of all new cases of cancers of the tongue and pharynx, an increase of over 225% since 1988.[42] HPV-associated OPC patients tend to be younger with a median age of 54 years at the time of diagnosis, have less exposure to tobacco and alcohol, and have a higher level of SES and education.[42] The incidence of HPV-associated OPC is higher in white individuals and males.[42]

Diagnosing OPC at the earliest stage significantly increases 5-year survival rates.[38] *Healthy People 2020* outcomes data indicate that less than one-third of OPC are detected at the earliest stage.[23] The goal of early detection makes the routine performance of oral cancer examinations critical. Box 5.3 presents data from the 2017–2018 NHANES related to this important service being performed by a professional.[21] Box 5.3 also presents data related to the provision of tobacco education and smoking cessation counseling by oral health professionals, which is critical for the prevention of OPC.[21]

Other Oral Conditions
Cleft Lip and Cleft Palate

Cleft lip (CL) and cleft palate (CP) are the most common birth defects[43] (Figure 5.7). Their **occurrence** can be isolated with a genetic origin, part of an inherited disease or syndrome, or a result of fetal exposure to other factors during pregnancy.[43,44] Women who smoke or overconsume alcoholic beverages while pregnant, have diabetes prior to pregnancy, are in poor health during pregnancy, and/or use certain epilepsy medicines

(topiramate or valproic acid) during the first trimester are at an increased risk of the fetus developing a CL or CP.[43,44] Research of working environments has also demonstrated a higher risk of CL and CP in the fetus when the mother is exposed to polycyclic aromatic hydrocarbons (PAHs) during pregnancy.[45] These PAHs are produced by burning coal, oil, gas, and garbage, charbroiling meat, and the presence of second-hand smoke.

There is no national surveillance of orofacial clefts, so data to track trends are unavailable. In their absence, national estimates are generated by the CDC.[44] The most recent estimates are presented in Box 5.4.[44] For surveillance and research purposes, public health experts recommend that states plan and implement an effective method to identify, record, refer, and follow up with infants diagnosed with oral clefts and craniofacial anomalies. Of the 50 states and D.C., 39 have a reporting system and 36 have a referral system for children and youth with CL or CP.[23]

Orofacial clefts can be repaired to varying degrees with surgery. Treatment is long-term, multistage, specialized, complex, and may consist of several surgeries. Children with orofacial clefts frequently suffer from self-esteem issues, are burdened with accompanying medical and dental problems, and experience discomfort from long-term treatment.[44] Care by a multidisciplinary team has been shown to be an effective approach to provide services across the lifespan for individuals with craniofacial anomalies.[43] Thus, continued access to an integrated healthcare system is essential for them to be able to receive necessary dental and healthcare services.

One study estimated a mean cost of $7,564–$8,393 in 2009 for each hospitalization to correct a CL or CP, including primary and additional revision surgeries.[46] The lifetime cost of children born each year with CL or CP is estimated to be close to $697 million.[43] For these reasons, researchers are working to understand the developmental processes that lead to orofacial clefts and how to prevent and more effectively treat them.

Malocclusion

Current national data are unavailable for malocclusion. The latest data were the results of the NHANES III published in the 1990s.[47] According to the American Association of Orthodontists, in 2014, approximately 7.5 million people received orthodontic treatment, and one in five patients were adults, with many ranging in age from 50–90 years.[48]

Craniofacial Injuries

Injuries to the head, face, and teeth are common, usually caused by accidents, sports-related injuries, and individuals falling.[49] Approximately one-third are sports related,[50] the majority of which affect the upper lip, maxilla, and maxillary incisors, with 50–90% involving the maxillary incisors.[50] Dentoalveolar trauma from an injury can result in significant lifetime costs

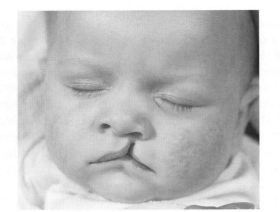

Fig 5.7 Cleft lip. (From Regezi JA, Sciubba JA, Jordan CK. Oral Pathology: Clinical Pathologic Correlations, 7th ed. St Louis, MO: Elsevier; 2017.)

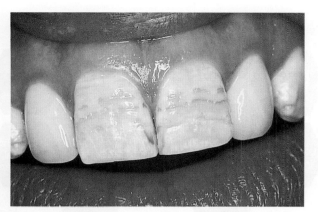

Fig 5.8 Dental fluorosis. (From: Robinson D, Bird D. Torres and Erhlich Modern Dental Assisting, 9th ed. St. Louis: Saunders: 2009.)

for restorative, endodontic, prosthodontic, implant, or surgical treatment as well as indirect costs, including time lost from school or work.[50] These consequences are especially significant for lower income and uninsured individuals.[50]

The latest national data for craniofacial injuries were collected in 6–19-year-olds by the NHANES during 1999–2004, with a focus on incisal trauma (traumatic injury affecting either an upper or lower permanent incisor).[51] These results indicated

higher prevalence of incisal trauma in males than females and the highest rate in 12–15-year-olds compared with other age groups.[51]

More widespread use of effective population-based interventions could help reduce the **morbidity**, **mortality**, and economic burden associated with craniofacial injuries. Community-based interventions, professional practices, and personal behaviors that increase the use of passenger restraints, air bags, helmets, protective gear, and mouth guards are recommended, especially during organized sports.[50]

Dental Fluorosis

Most of the current research focuses on fluorosis in the adolescent population to evaluate the effects of a lifetime of increased exposure to fluorides by this population. An analysis that compared 2001–2002 and 2011–2012 NHANES fluorosis data for 16–17-year-olds noted the following rates:[52]

- In 2001–2002, percentage prevalence was 49.8% normal, 20.5% questionable, and 29.7% very mild and above.
- In 2011–2012 percentage prevalence was 31.2% normal, 7.5% questionable, and 61.3% very mild and above.
- The prevalence of very mild and greater severity fluorosis increased by 31.6% from 2001–2002 to 2011–2012.

The results of the 2011–2014 NHANES regarding the prevalence of fluorosis in ages 6–19 years sparked debate and a call to action (Figures 5.8 and 5.9). One report revealed a "dramatic"

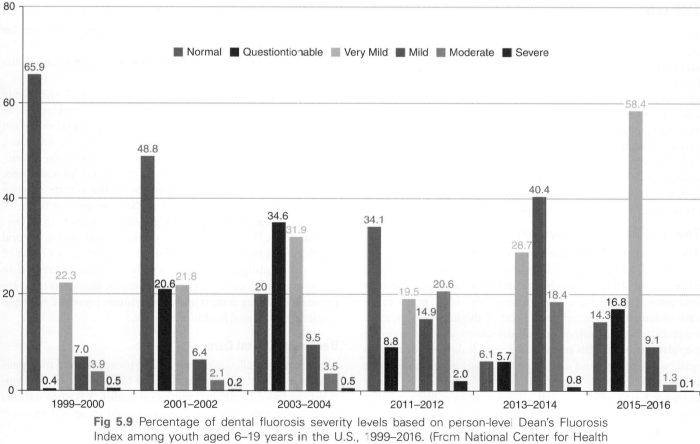

Fig 5.9 Percentage of dental fluorosis severity levels based on person-level Dean's Fluorosis Index among youth aged 6–19 years in the U.S., 1999–2016. (From National Center for Health Statistics, National Center for Chronic Disease Prevention and Health Promotion. Data quality evaluation of the dental fluorosis clinical assessment data from the National Health and Nutrition Examination Survey, 1999–2004 and 2011–2016. Hyattsville, MD: National Center for Health Statistics. Vital Health Stat 2(183); 2019. Available at: <https://www.cdc.gov/nchs/data/series/sr_02/sr02_183-508.pdf>; [Accessed December 2019].)

increase of dental fluorosis from 1986 to 2012 with speculation that the extent of the increase could be overestimated because of research methodology issues.[53] After further analysis of the data, the CDC National Center for Health Statistics (NCHS) suggested that the increase in prevalence between the 2001–2004 and 2011–2014 periods was not biologically plausible and agreed a measurement error might have occurred.[54]

Because of the increase in fluorosis cases and the debate between the findings of different studies, the American Association for Dental Research urged dental professionals to review dental fluorosis evaluation methods to achieve accurate diagnosis.[55] Researchers reinforced previous recommendations to control the overuse of fluorides that contributes to the development of fluorosis, noting that the optimal level of fluoride in community water fluoridation had already been adjusted for this purpose.[52,53] (See Community Water Fluoridation and Prevention of Fluorosis sections and Box 6.14 in Chapter 6). To help monitor the use of fluoride products, the NHANES gathers data on the use of fluoride drops and tablets. In the 2017–2018 NHANES, about 11% of parents of 3–15-year-old children and youth stated they received a prescription for fluoride drops or tablets.[21]

PART TWO: ACCESS TO ORAL HEALTH CARE AND DENTAL PUBLIC HEALTH SYSTEMS IN THE U.S.

The ability of the oral healthcare system to meet the population's oral healthcare needs is largely dependent on its **infrastructure** and **capacity** (see Measurement of Infrastructure, Capacity, and Resources section of Chapter 4). Assessment of the infrastructure and capacity of the oral healthcare system is achieved by examining the components of these concepts such as funding of programs, financing of care, availability and education of workforce, administrative placement of dental public health within public health, and interprofessional and other collaborative relationships. These and other concepts related to infrastructure and capacity affect **access to care** and will be discussed in this section of the chapter.

The Oral Healthcare System

The current oral healthcare system is complex, needs reform, and should address external and internal barriers, oral health literacy, and strategies to change attitudes, beliefs, and behaviors among individuals and groups.[19] An ideal oral healthcare system should integrate the rest of the healthcare system, emphasize health promotion and disease prevention, monitor population oral health status and needs, link with continuous quality assessment and assurance, empower communities and individuals to create conditions conducive to health, and be evidence based, effective, cost effective, sustainable, equitable, universal, comprehensive, ethical, and culturally competent.[19,56]

Leaders from various groups of the healthcare system have called for greater prevention of oral diseases, elimination of oral health disparities, and changes to ensure access to oral health services for individuals. Much of this has been prompted by the need to increase access to oral health care for specific potentially

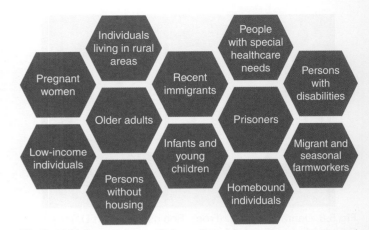

Fig 5.10 Vulnerable populations that often lack access to oral health care.

vulnerable populations[18,19,56,57] (see Figure 5.10). Changes needed to improve oral healthcare access include the following:[19,56,57]
- Expansion of the oral healthcare workforce
- Increasing the number of oral healthcare professionals in the public sector
- Regulatory changes for allied oral healthcare providers
- Greater collaboration between oral healthcare and other healthcare professionals
- More dental insurance coverage for individuals who are uninsured or underinsured
- Increased funding and grants to support initiatives
- Comprehensive education focused on oral health prevention coordinated at the national level

Some of these transformations are beginning to occur as discussed in Chapters 1, 2, 6, 9, and 11.

The current primary model for oral health care is the private practice delivery model with a **safety net** that provides care to people with no or limited insurance.[18,19] The dental safety net is a patchwork of organizations and oral healthcare providers, is not uniform among all communities, has dissimilar financing options, and has no continuity of services provided (see Chapter 2, Public Health section). With the private practice model, dentists are located in areas that can support them;[18,19] thus, more dentists practice in high-income areas than in low-income areas.[57,58] This practice pattern limits access to oral health care to those who can afford it. In general, as a result of these culminating factors, only certain populations are able to access oral health care.[18,19] The goal of recent changes is to evolve the oral healthcare system into a continuous, proactive model to enable access to oral health care for all.

Barriers to Dental Care

Many people of all ages do not receive preventive and therapeutic dental care that is essential for their healthy growth, development, and well-being, including oral health. A host of barriers to accessing this care have been identified in several reports[59] (see Box 5.5).

Regular Dental Visits and Use of Oral Health Services

The number of children, adolescents, and adults who used the oral healthcare system in the previous year was a leading health

BOX 5.5 Key Barriers to Accessing Oral Health Care

Internal

- Not having a **dental home**
- Financial cost
- Lack of dental insurance
- Lack of awareness of the importance of oral health
- Lack of awareness of the need for regular dental care on the part of individuals or health professionals
- Cultural values and beliefs
- Fear of dental care
- Age
- Language
- Habits
- Lack of education
- Lack of perceived susceptibility
- Lack of perceived severity
- Lack of access
- Attitudes
- Lack of faith in treatment and/or belief that treatment is unsafe
- Denial of diagnosis
- Illiteracy
- Low health literacy

External

- Lack of availability of providers
- Narrow scope of dental hygiene practice
- Cultural values and beliefs
- Environmental barriers
- Prohibitive costs
- Lack of interdisciplinary collaboration
- Complexity and inadequacy of the oral healthcare system
- Inconvenience of treatment
- Lack of transportation
- Provider conflicts
- Culturally insensitive providers
- Dental hygiene supervision requirements

BOX 5.6 Dental Attendance of Children, Adolescents, and Adults, National Health Interview Survey, 1997–2017

- In 2017, 84.9% of children aged 2–17 years visited a dentist within the past year, a 12.2% increase since 1997.
- In 2017, 64% of adults aged 18–64 years visited a dentist within the past year, a 0.1% decrease since 1997.
- In 2017, 65.6% of adults 65 and older visited a dentist within the past year, a 10.8% increase since 1997.

(From Health United States, 2018 Data Finder, Dental visit in the past year, by selected characteristics: United States, selected years 1997-2017. Available at: <https://www.cdc.gov/nchs/hus/contents2018.htm#Table_037>; [Accessed November 2019].)

and consistent regular dental visits also vary significantly for other social and demographic factors.[18,60] Utilization rates are greater in white individuals and those with higher education levels and are lower for individuals from families with family members who have various physical, mental, and medical disabilities.[60] Thus, despite overall increases in dental attendance, the *Healthy People 2030* objectives still emphasize increasing the proportion of low-income youth who have preventive dental visits and increasing the proportion of all children, adolescents, and adults who use the oral healthcare system, which is also one of the leading health indicators.[28]

Unmet Dental Needs

People's perception of their unmet oral healthcare needs is also an important indicator of access to oral health care. Females, those without a high school or general education development (GED) diploma, those with low incomes, those who are uninsured, and those who are disabled are less likely to receive needed dental care due to cost.[60] Nearly 20% of participants in the 2017–2018 NHANES reported they were unable to obtain needed dental care during the previous year.[21] The same survey revealed the following data concerning the participants' current need to visit a dentist for treatment: 5% immediately or within the next 2 weeks, 29% at their earliest convenience, and 66% on routine schedule to continue with regular care.[21]

Various factors can explain a decrease in financial barriers to dental care from 1997 to 2016, including economic recovery, flattening of dental fees, and increases in public dental insurance coverage.[60] The CDC NCHS noted the following data pertaining to individuals not receiving needed dental care within the year because of cost:[60]

- Decrease from 6.0% in 1997 to 4.6% in 2017 among children 18 years and younger
- Decrease from 6.0% in 1997 to 4.5% in 2017 among children and youth <19 years old
- Increase from 10.6% in 1997 to 17.3% in 2010 and then decrease to 11.5% in 2017 among adults aged 18–64 years
- Increase from 3.5% in 1997 to 7.7% in 2017 among adults aged 65 and older

The increase in utilization of dental care has resulted in fewer unmet dental needs. Both have been attributed to a decrease in the cost of dental care as a barrier to access.

indicator for *Healthy People 2020*. According to *Healthy People 2020* outcomes, this measure of *dental attendance* or *dental utilization* as an indication of access to care increased slightly from 41.8% in 2011 to 43.3% in 2016.[23] More significantly, the proportion of low-income children and adolescents who received any preventive dental service within the past year increased from 33.3% in 2011 to 38.7% in 2016,[23] and dental attendance increased among very young children during the last decade owing to the emphasis on improving preventive dental care delivery to children.[26]

The 2018 BRFSS reported the following dental attendance data for respondents aged 18 years and older, by how long it had been since their last visit to a dentist or clinic:[34]

- 67.68% visited within the past year.
- 10.64% visited within the past 2 years.
- 8.86% visited within the past 5 years.
- 11.18% had not visited within the past 5 years.
- Less than 1% had never visited a dentist or clinic.

Box 5.6 presents results of the 2017 National Health Interview Survey regarding frequency of dental visits by age.[60] Timely

TABLE 5.4   Types of Dental Insurance

Insurance Type	Persons Eligible	Coverage of Plan	Funding
Private (or commercial)	• 90% obtain coverage through employer-sponsored group plans • Occasionally obtained through private purchase	Dental coverage and cost vary depending on plan and provider	Privately funded by employers or individuals
Medicaid	• 49 states and D.C. cover children with incomes up to at least 200% of FPL through Medicaid and CHIP; 19 states cover children with incomes at or above 300% of FPL • 34 states and D.C. cover pregnant women through Medicaid and CHIP; states vary based on FPL status • 32 states and D.C. cover parents and other adults at up to 138% of FPL under ACA Medicaid expansion; 14 states have not adopted Medicaid expansion	• Relief of pain and infections • Restoration of teeth • Preventive services (e.g., prophylaxis, fluoride, sealants) • Dental treatment benefit is a required competent of EPSDT for ages ≤21 years • In some states, dental services are available to adults; may be limited to emergency services • Each state is required to develop a dental periodicity schedule in consultation with recognized dental organizations involved in child health	Federal and state funded; percentage of each varies by state
CHIP	• For uninsured children ages 0–19 years • Coverage provided by 46 states and D.C. for up to or above 200% of FPL, with 24 of these states offering coverage at 250% of FPL or greater • States may get CHIP enhanced match for coverage up to 300% of FPL	• Required to include coverage for dental services needed to prevent disease and promote oral health, restore oral structures to health and function, and treat emergency conditions • States with Medicaid expansion must provide children and adolescents EPSDT services • States are required to post a listing of all participating Medicaid and CHIP dental providers and benefit packages	Federal and state funded, percentage of each varies by state

ACA, Affordable Care Act; *CHIP*, Children's Health Insurance Program; *EPSDT*, Early and Periodic Screening, Diagnostic, and Treatment; *FPL*, federal poverty level.
(From Beatty CF. Community Oral Health Planning and Practice. In: Blue CM, ed. Darby's Comprehensive Review of Dental Hygiene, 9th ed. Maryland Heights MO: Elsevier; 2021.)

Dental Care Financing

Dental insurance coverage (also called **third-party payment**) is an important factor that influences access to oral health services. A complex combination of private and public insurance is utilized by our **pluralistic** system of oral healthcare delivery (Table 5.4). While highly criticized, a pluralistic healthcare system is valued by societies, can be an asset, and can enhance efficiency if designed and managed properly. The proportion of the total population with dental insurance coverage has increased from 57% in 2006 to 77% in 2016.[61] About two-thirds of those who are insured have private dental insurance, 90% of which is acquired through an employment group plan and the rest of which is purchased by individuals.[61,62] About one-third receive benefits through public programs such as Medicaid, the **Children's Health Insurance Program** (CHIP), Medicare Advantage, and Indian Health Services.[61] Figure 5.11 compares the percentage of dental insurance coverage by age group in 2015. People without dental insurance pay out of pocket on a **fee-for-service** basis.[61]

In general, fewer people have dental insurance than overall healthcare coverage.[62] Private dental insurance differs from private health insurance in that dental-plan premiums cost less than health-plan premiums.[62,63] However, dental-plan enrollees must pay greater out-of-pocket individual contributions for the cost of services compared to health plans.[6,63] Dental care fees are usually charged by procedure and traditionally have been paid on a fee-for-service basis[63] (Figure 5.12).

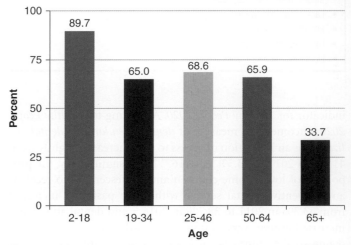

Fig 5.11 Percentage of dental insurance coverage in different age groups in the U.S., 2015. (From Health Policy Institute. Dental Benefits Coverage in the US; 2017. Available at: <https://www.ada.org/~/media/ADA/Science%20and%20Research/HPI/Files/HPIgraphic_1117_3.pdf?la=en>; [Accessed November 2019].)

The differences between health and dental coverage are attributable to different assumptions about risk underlying each type of plan and how the risk is shared among plan enrollees.[62] The risk-sharing propositions of the different types of plans have been shown to have an impact on utilization and premium rates with differences in costs and cost sharing by

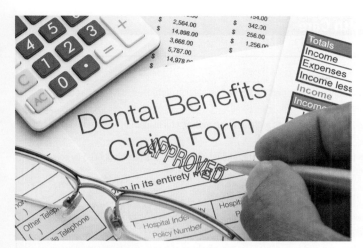

Fig 5.12 Dental insurance benefits and procedures vary for different types of insurance. (@ iStock.com/courtneyk)

beneficiaries.[63,64] Because of the low level of dental insurance coverage and the structure of dental benefits, out-of-pocket cost sharing of expenses (deductibles, copayments, co-insurance, and maximum annual benefits) account for a much larger percentage of total dental care spending for individuals in comparison to out-of-pocket costs for general healthcare spending.[62,63]

Public programs covering dental care include Medicaid and CHIP.[65] **Medicare** is a source of health coverage for older adults but not a current source of dental coverage, only paying for limited hospital-based oral surgery needed in conjunction with medical treatment, such as organ transplantation.[66,67] Primary and secondary services are modestly covered by a few Medicare Advantage plans.[66]

Financing of dental care is further complicated by the varied types of dental benefits plans (Table 5.5), some of which are fee-for-service, while others have various **managed care**

TABLE 5.5 Dental Insurance (Benefits) Plans

Type of Plan	Provider	Description
Fee-for-Service		
Indemnity dental benefits plan	For-profit, commercial insurance companies	Traditional plan; patient can visit any provider (freedom of choice) and provider is free to set fees; includes deductible, co-insurance, and maximums; company reimburses patient or provider based on usual, customary, and reasonable (UCR) fee (see Table 5.6); patient is responsible for difference between benefit paid and fee charged; may include a prepayment review and require preauthorization; most expensive form of insurance
Direct reimbursement	Employers	Not a true insurance plan; self-funded plan that reimburses patients according to dollars spent rather than type of treatment; administrator (can be employer) pays patient percentage of actual treatments received, saving the cost of the middleman; allows freedom of choice and autonomy of decision-making about treatment; may eliminate claim forms and administrative processing by dental offices
Managed Care		
Preferred provider organization (PPO)	Health service and dental service corporations (not for profit), commercial insurance companies (for profit)	Regular indemnity insurance combined with a network of dentists under contract to the insurance company to provide services for set fees below the average; patient can visit a dentist outside the PPO and pay the difference (amount above the discounted fee); includes co-insurance, deductible, and maximum coverage; insurance company reimburses patient or dentist accepts payment directly from insurance company; less costly than traditional indemnity plan
Exclusive provider organization (EPO)	Same as PPO	A closed panel variation of a PPO; does not cover out-of-network care; can severely limit access to care
Dental health maintenance organization (DHMO; prepaid plan)	Health service and dental service corporations; commercial insurance companies; prepaid, large group practices	Patients must use one dentist or facility (plan does not pay if they go outside the HMO); includes copayment and possibly maximums but no deductibles; uses capitation (see Table 5.6); usually lowest-cost program; uncommon for dental benefits; dentists frequently limit number of HMO patients to offset loss of income
Point of service plan	Same as DHMO	Variation of DHMO; patient may go out of network and be reimbursed based on a low table of allowances that reflects reduced benefits
Dental discount plan	Employers, provider organizations; organization of corporate clinics	Providers join the plan by paying a fee and agreeing to offer discounted fees (see Table 5.6), then are listed as a member provider (way of recruiting patients); patients join the plan by paying a fee, receive a list of providers who are on the plan and a card to present to the member provider, and pay deeply discounted fees to member providers; not "true" insurance; no deductibles, no annual limits, no copayments, no paperwork for the patient or dentist for reimbursement, and no prequalifications; more employers are providing this type of plan
Table or schedule of allowances plan	Same as PPO	Indemnity plan that pays a set dollar amount for each procedure and patient pays the difference; may also be a variation of a PPO that limits contracted dentists to a maximum allowable charge
Individual practice association (IPA)	Association of independent dental providers	More of a business arrangement than a dental benefits plan; organization contracts with independent dentists to provide services to DHMO patients for discounted fees or through capitation arrangement

(From Beatty CF. Community oral health planning and practice. In: Blue CM, ed. Darby's Comprehensive Review of Dental Hygiene, 9th ed. Maryland Heights MO: Elsevier; 2021.)

TABLE 5.6 Mechanisms of Payment for Oral Health Care

Mechanism	Description
Individual Payment Methods	
Fee-for-service	Traditional two-party arrangement in which fee is set for a service and patient is charged for service performed; declining method of payment as third-party payment becomes more prevalent
Barter system	The provider and patient negotiate payment by exchanging goods or services without using money; still evident in some rural areas and developing countries
Encounter fee	A set fee each time a patient has a treatment encounter (comes in for treatment), regardless of the services provided; used by community programs as a discounted fee for patients with no dental insurance
Third-Party Reimbursement Methods	
Usual, customary, and reasonable (UCR) fee	Third-party payment generally based on an average of fees for the area; varies by geographic area and population size, and from carrier to carrier; most commonly used payment method in dentistry
Discounted fee	Third-party system in which fees lower than the area UCR are agreed to by a provider for members of a specifically identified group (e.g., students, older adults) or participants in a prepaid group; becoming more common in dentistry
Fee schedule	List of charges set by the third-party payer and agreed to by the provider who enrolls as a provider; provider is reimbursed by the third-party payer and cannot charge more; system used by Medicaid/Children's Health Insurance Program (CHIP)
Table of allowances	List of covered services with an assigned dollar amount set by the third-party payer; providers are reimbursed by the third-party payer and can charge patients the difference between their fees and the fees set by the table of allowances
Capitation	A form of contracted care in which a provider receives a fixed payment from a third-party payer in exchange for all or most care needed by a group of patients during the contract period; method used by health maintenance organizations (HMOs); designed to increase preventive care; payment is made to the provider regardless of use by enrollees; effectiveness is in question; not typically used in dentistry
Direct reimbursement	Beneficiaries (patients) are reimbursed by the employer or benefits administrator (e.g., insurance company) for a specified percentage of dental expenses on presentation of evidence of expenses
Methods Used to Minimize Costs	
Copayment	Patient pays a fixed amount at each visit, and the remainder of the fee is covered by the third party; the purpose is to discourage overuse
Co-insurance	Similar to copayment, but it is a percentage rather than a fixed amount; used by most dental insurance plans
Deductible	Patient must pay a required amount as an out-of-pocket expense before the insurance plan will pay
Pre-existing conditions	Coverage is restricted for dental conditions that are present before enrollment in the plan
Annual limits (maximum coverage)	Insurance plan will pay only up to a specific dollar limit each year, can be based on individual or family maximums
Waiting period	Patient must wait a specified length of time before coverage begins
Use of UCR	There is no universally accepted method for determining the UCR fee schedule; may vary a great deal among plans, even when the plans operate in the same area

(From Beatty CF. Community Oral Health Planning and Practice. In: Blue CM, ed. Darby's Comprehensive Review of Dental Hygiene, 9th ed. Maryland Heights, MO: Elsevier; 2021.)

characteristics and its numerous payment mechanisms (Table 5.6). (See Chapter 6 Financing Programs section for information on dental public health program funding.)

Expenditures

The substantial national total of dental expenditures was steady for several years, but dental expenditures increased notably in 2015 and 2016.[68] Box 5.7 presents the financial burden for dental expenditures, explaining why many are unable to access dental care.

Dental care expenditures vary by state of residence. In 2014, the **per capita** expenditures for all publicly (Medicaid and CHIP) and privately (private insurance) funded dental services ranged from $253 in Mississippi to $542 in Alaska.[69] The national average was $354, and 25 states and D.C. were above the national average.[69]

BOX 5.7 National Dental Care Expenditures in the U.S., 2016

- About $124 billion in 2016; a 3.3% increase from 2015
- Accounted for 3.7% of all healthcare expenditures
- A per capita average of $384; a 2.4% increase from 2015
- Increased for all sources of financing: private insurance, out-of-pocket, Medicaid, and Children's Health Insurance Program (CHIP)

(From U.S. Dental Expenditures: 2017 Update. Chicago, IL: ADA Health Policy Institute; 2017 Available at: <https://www.ada.org/~/media/ADA/Science%20and%20Research/HPI/Files/HPIBrief_1217_1.pdf?la=en>; [Accessed November 2019].)

Dental Insurance Coverage: Children and Adolescents

Children receive dental coverage from private insurance, Medicaid, and CHIP. As represented in Figure 5.11, the number of uninsured children 18 years old and younger declined from 15.8% in 2010 to 10.3% in 2015.[70] This is an all-time low and is attributed to the increase in children's dental coverage resulting from the ACA.[70]

Dental Coverage: Younger and Older Adults

Dental insurance coverage among adults varies by age (Figure 5.11), family income, race and ethnicity, and education. In 2015, estimates were that 28% of adults had no dental coverage.[70] The Health Policy Institute reported that 59% of adults had private benefits and 7.4% had Medicaid/CHIP benefits.[70] In 2014, 29.4% of adults 19–65 years of age had no dental benefits, and 58.1% had private dental insurance.[71] Also, in 2014, more that half of the 12.5% of people who had public insurance had no accompanying dental benefits.[71] The dearth of dental coverage for adults aged 65 and older is staggering. In 2014, only 27.9% of them had private dental insurance, 10.1% had public insurance, and 62% were uninsured.[71]

The overall coverage of adults has increased since the implementation of the ACA, but it did not impact the older adult population.[72] When older adults retire, they potentially lose their employer-based dental benefits, which is not addressed by the ACA and restricts their access to dental care.[73] However, since the ACA, there has been an increase in coverage of young adults 19–26 years old by their parents' private dental insurance[72] and of low- and moderate-income adults through the expansion of Medicaid[74] (Figure 5.13).

Publicly Funded Health Insurance Programs

The cost of dental care can be a significant burden for low-income Americans. Thus, dental care in the private sector is often inaccessible for many Americans. Medicaid and CHIP are sources of dental benefits for individuals who qualify for these programs.

Medicaid. Medicaid, or Title XIX, is a joint state-federal financed program that is administered by the states to provide comprehensive medical and dental coverage for children of low-income families and some adults. Dental coverage is required for all child enrollees as part of a comprehensive set of **Early and Periodic Screening, Diagnostic and Treatment** (EPSDT) benefits[75] (see Table 5.4). The minimum benefits must cover relief of pain and infections, tooth restoration, and dental health maintenance.[75]

In 2019, more than 65 million people were enrolled in Medicaid and 6 million in CHIP.[75] With the passage of the ACA, some states expanded Medicaid coverage for children through their state CHIP program.[75] Every child enrolled in Medicaid or CHIP has dental coverage, and the rates of not being covered by dental insurance are at the lowest they have ever been due to the expansion.[70,75]

Federal law requires states to offer Medicaid to all people 21 years and younger in explicit groups and according to specified income thresholds[75] (Table 5.4). For example, in 2020 a family of four earning up to $34,846 a year might qualify.[76] Also, states have broad authority to expand Medicaid beyond these federal minimum standards, and they have done so to varying degrees. Additionally, the state programs work with children's dental health organizations to develop a periodicity schedule for pediatric dental services and with pediatric primary care providers to determine a dental referral system.[75] In many states the Medicaid program has ventured into the managed care health arena for both medical and dental services to reduce healthcare expenditures and maximize preventive health measures.

Although state Medicaid programs are required by federal rules to cover comprehensive oral health services for children, coverage for adult dental services is considered optional except for a select few (see Table 5.4). States have the flexibility to determine what dental benefits are provided to adult Medicaid enrollees.[75] Most states (47 states and D.C.) provide at least emergency dental services for adults, only 35 states then cover services beyond emergency care, and only 19 states provide extensive dental services for adults enrolled in Medicaid.[77] As of now, only North Dakota provides the same dental benefits package to the base Medicaid and expanded Medicaid populations.[77]

Children's Health Insurance Program. CHIP is a joint state-federal funded program to finance comprehensive health insurance coverage, including dental, for children who are not eligible for Medicaid, do not have other health insurance, and meet the family income eligibility requirements[75] (see Table 5.4). For example, in 2020 a family of four earning up to $52,662 a year may qualify.[76] In January 2018, after a 114-day lapse in CHIP funding and a government shutdown, Congress extended funding for 6 years. Continuation of CHIP was approved through fiscal year 2027, with $159.7 billion allotted through 2023 and additional sums available as needed for years 2024–2027.[78]

As the nation's safety net health insurance programs, Medicaid and CHIP are a major source of dental coverage for children.[79] The rate of children covered by Medicaid has increased from 27% in 2008 to 39% in 2017.[80] In contrast, the rate of uninsured children has declined from 10% in 2008 to 5% in 2017.[80] The ACA expansion of Medicaid and CHIP enables more children to be eligible for dental benefits.[79] As of August 2019, 65 million individuals were enrolled in Medicaid, and 6.6 million were enrolled in CHIP. Nearly 49.3% of the 71 million enrolled in Medicaid and CHIP were children.[81]

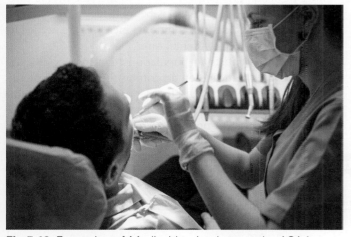

Fig 5.13 Expansion of Medicaid to implement the ACA has resulted in increased access to care for certain adult population groups. (@ iStock.com.)

Medicare. According to Title XVIII of the Social Security Act, Medicare is a federal health insurance program enacted in 1965 and administered by the Social Security Administration to provide health care for adults ages 65 and older.[82] In 2018, nearly 60 million older adults were enrolled in Medicare.[83] Although traditionally Medicare has not been a source of dental coverage, a bill was introduced to the House in 2019 aimed at increasing Medicare benefits to include dental and other services.[84] (See Oral Health Services for Older Adults section of Chapter 6.)

Vouchers for Dental Care

Some community programs that serve vulnerable populations in the community provide **dental care vouchers** to clients who qualify based on being uninsured or underinsured and in need of urgent care for an acute dental problem. Organizations partner with schools and other groups to identify low income families, children, adults, and seniors who urgently need dental care and have no financial resources to access it. They also partner with local dental providers for a referral base.

Dental voucher programs can help to reduce the number of people who seek emergency room care for acute dental problems. They can also serve as a means of establishing a future dental home, especially for children.

Future Considerations for Financing Dental Care

The expansion of dental coverage has improved since the implementation of ACA; however, many individuals are still uninsured and face financial barriers accessing care. Although an opportunity to assure universal access to dental coverage was lost, these efforts continue, especially in relation to older adults.

Dental public health professionals will be called on to foster linkages for adults to access dental care in communities across the country. Also, programs will be required to provide services to individuals that currently still lack dental care.[19,73] Financing the oral healthcare needs of a growing number of adults and older adults, especially among vulnerable population groups, will be a challenge for communities.[85]

Oral Health Workforce

Supply of Oral Health Professionals

The current dental workforce is unable to meet present day **need** and **demand** for dental care because of inadequate supply of dental workforce. This inadequacy is expected to increase, based on future dental workforce projections and an expected increase in the need and demand for dental care produced partially by changing population trends and increased public dental insurance coverage. The nation needs to advocate for a

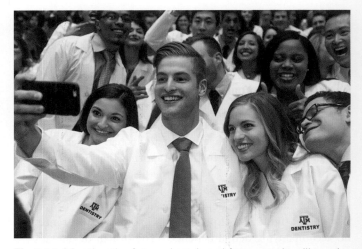

Fig 5.14 Meeting the future dental workforce needs will require innovative solutions and collaboration of dental schools and dental education and other relevant organizations. (Courtesy Texas A&M College of Dentistry.)

vital and sufficient oral healthcare workforce to allow universal access to oral health care (Figure 5.14).

Dentists. In 2015, the Department of Health and Human Services (DHHS), proposed that the dental graduation rate will not keep up with the increasing demand.[86] The number of practicing dentists was 190,900 in 2012, and it was projected to increase by 6% by 2025, whereas the estimated demand for dentists was expected to increase by 10%.[86] Additionally, the U.S. Bureau of Labor Statistics projects a 7% increase in the employment of dentists from 2018 to 2028, which is faster than the average.[87] Based on these data, the DHHS projects a significant shortage of dentists in 2025[86] (Table 5.7).

There were 6305 dental school graduates in 2018 and 3780 graduates of advanced dental education programs in 2018–2019[88] (Figure 5.15). There is debate about how many dental graduates are needed to meet the demand for dental services. One report suggests there will be a surplus of dentists based on current graduation rates.[89] However, to meet population demands for dental care in 2037, based on the anticipated number of graduates in 2022, another report proposes that the number of dental graduates will need to increase by 1% each year following.[90] While progress is being made to increase the number of dental graduates, additional increases are needed to meet the growing need for dental care.[90]

The **ratio** of dentists to population (dentists per 100,000 people) provides a means of describing the adequacy of the workforce.[91] In previous years the dentist-to-population ratio has remained consistent at approximately 60 to 100,000, and the estimated dentist-to-population ratio in 2018 was 60.97 to

TABLE 5.7	Projections of the Number of Dentists and Dental Hygienists by 2025			
	Estimated Number, 2012	**Projected Number, 2025**	**Projected Demand, 2025**	**Projected Shortage or Surplus, 2025**
Dentists	190,800	202,600	218,200	Shortage of 15,600
Dental Hygienists	153,600	197,200	169,100	Surplus of 28,100

(From National and State-Level Projections of Dentists and Dental Hygienists in the U.S., 2012–2025. Rockville, MD: Health Resources and Services Administration, National Center for Health Workforce Analysis; 2015. Available at: <http://bhpr.hrsa.gov/healthworkforce/supplydemand/dentistry/nationalstatelevelprojectionsdentists.pdf>; [Accessed April 2020].)

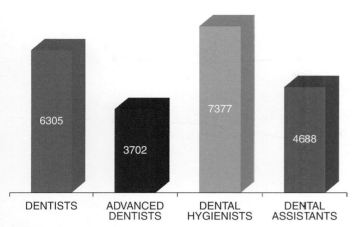

Fig 5.15 Number of oral health workforce graduates in the U.S., 2018. (From Dental Education. Survey of Dental Education Series Report 1: Academic Programs, Enrollment and Graduates, 2018–2019; Survey of Advanced Dental Education, 2017–2018; Survey of Allied Dental Education Report 1: Dental Hygiene Education Programs, 2018–2019 and Report 2: Dental Assisting Education Program, 2018–2019. Chicago, IL: American Dental Association Health Policy Institute; 2020. Available at: <https://www.ada.org/en/science-research/health-policy-institute/data-center/dental-education>; [Accessed June 2020].)

100,000.[91] The ratio has been predicted to decline in the future because of the growth of the population.[91] Other estimates suggest that the expected economic environment and the trend of dental graduates will lead to a dentist-to-population ratio of 63.7 to 100,000 in 2037, which will still be insufficient based on an expected increase in demand for dental care.[90]

Of the nation's professionally active dentists, the majority provide dental care in the private sector; however, more dentists are practicing in corporate dental groups rather than solo in private practice.[92] Furthermore, few dentists practice in public health settings, and the number has declined, from 1004 in 2005 to 835 in 2018,[91] thus stressing the dental safety net.[18] Greater numbers of dentists, especially general, pediatric, and public health dentists, are needed in the public sector because

of the increasing use of the dental safety net.[18] According to the American Dental Education Association, approximately 80% of all dentists practice general dentistry, and the remaining 20% practice in one of the nine recognized specialty areas.[91]

Dental Hygienists. In 2018, there were about 219,900 dental hygienists in the workforce,[87] with 7377 new graduates that year[88] (Figure 5.15). Dental hygiene has an expected employment growth of 11% through 2028 and is among the fastest growing occupations in the nation.[87] Potential reasons for this are the increasing demand for dental services as the population ages,[93] the move toward interprofessional practice,[19] and increased awareness of the need to take up the challenge of medical-dental collaboration to address the link of oral health to overall health.[56] It is also expected that the number of dental hygienists employed in community settings will increase because of changes in the healthcare delivery system.[94]

In the late 1980s there were more dental graduates than dental hygiene graduates, a trend that changed in 1991.[95] Since then, more dental hygienists than dentists have graduated, with an increasingly greater difference each year through 2012[95] (Figure 5.16) and a projected surplus through 2025 (Table 5.7). However, data from 2013–2018 indicate a lessening of this difference (Figure 5.17). In 2018, there were 7377 dental hygiene graduates and 6305 dental graduates.[88] Of particular importance to the projected need for dental hygienists are the recent and anticipated future regulatory changes in the practice of dental hygiene described in Chapter 2, which can produce more employment opportunities for dental hygienists, utilize the surplus of dental hygienists, and compensate for the shortage of dentists to expand access to oral health care.

Dental Assistants. About 346,000 dental assistants were in the U.S. workforce in 2018,[87] with 4688 new graduates from accredited dental assisting programs in 2018[88] (Figure 5.15). The number of dental assistants graduating from accredited programs decreased gradually each year from 2010 to 2018, with close to a 36% decrease during the period.[88] This is in line with the 8% decrease in the number of accredited dental assisting programs from 2014 to 2019.[88] Even so, dental assisting has an

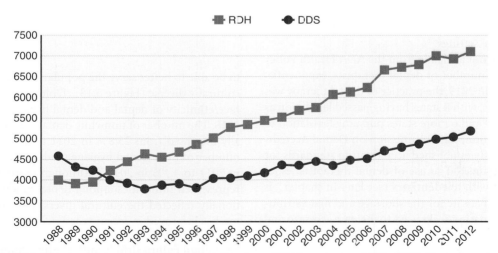

Fig 5.16 Number of dental (*DDS*) and dental hygiene (*RDH*) graduates, 1988–2012. (From American Dental Hygienists' Association. Dental Hygiene Education: Curricula, Program, Enrollment and Graduate Information; 2014. Available at: <https://www.adha.org/resources-docs/72611_Dental_Hygiene_Education_Fact_Sheet.pdf>; [Accessed December 2019].)

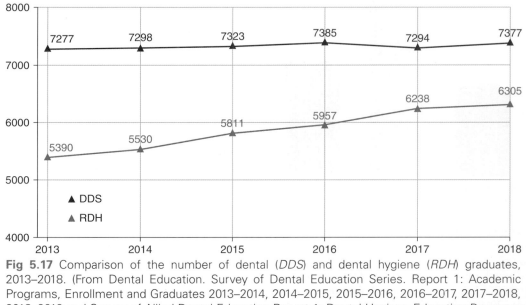

Fig 5.17 Comparison of the number of dental (*DDS*) and dental hygiene (*RDH*) graduates, 2013–2018. (From Dental Education. Survey of Dental Education Series. Report 1: Academic Programs, Enrollment and Graduates 2013–2014, 2014–2015, 2015–2016, 2016–2017, 2017–2018, 2018–2019 and Survey of Allied Dental Education Report 1: Dental Hygiene Education Programs 2013–2014, 2014–2015, 2015–2016, 2016–2017, 2017–2018, 2018–2019. Chicago, IL: American Dental Association Health Policy Institute; 2020. Available at: <https://www.ada.org/en/science-research/health-policy-institute/data-center/dental-education>; [Accessed June 2020].)

expected growth of 11% through 2028 and is among the fastest growing occupations in the U.S.[87] These data seem to indicate an increase in the number of dental assistants trained in dental offices and nonaccredited programs.

Dental Therapists. The introduction of dental therapy has expanded the capacity of dentistry to meet the needs of underserved populations (see Dental Therapist section in Chapter 2).[96] Dental therapists have been practicing alongside dentistry in the U.S. since 2005 when the first dental therapy students graduated in Alaska.[96] This innovative practice model has grown significantly since then, in spite of dentistry's opposition.[97] In 2019, dental therapists could practice statewide in eight states and serve Alaska Native and American Indian populations in five other states.[98] In addition, proposed dental therapy legislation was pending in six additional states in 2019.[98] Dental therapists practice primarily in public health settings, although as the practice model has grown, more are practicing in private practice and corporate settings.[96]

Although data are not available from the ADA Health Policy Institute for the total number of dental therapists, exponential growth is expected.[96] In 2019, the practice of dental therapy was authorized in 11 states, with 8 states having passed legislation as recently as 2017–2019 and 6 more states pursuing legislation to authorize it.[98] In addition, the Commission on Dental Accreditation (CODA) recently established accreditation standards for dental therapy programs.[99] The use of dental therapists, especially in conjunction with **teledentistry** (see later in chapter), is expected to help compensate for the shortage and maldistribution of dentists as the nation seeks ways to increase access to and decrease costs of dental care.[96]

Diversity of the Oral Health Workforce

Though strides have been made to increase the cultural diversity of the oral health workforce, continued efforts are needed

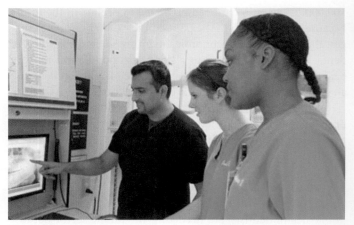

Fig 5.18 Efforts to increase the cultural diversity of the oral health workforce must continue, to meet the needs of an increasingly culturally diverse population. (Courtesy Faizan Kabani and Charlene Dickinson.)

to be able to better serve the population that is becoming more culturally diverse (Figure 5.18). Table 5.8 shows the gender and race/ethnicity of dental and dental hygiene graduates in 2017–2018. The number of nonwhite dental hygiene graduates gradually increased from 23.8% in 2011 to 31.8% in 2018, and the number of male dental hygiene graduates increased from 2.8% in 2011 to 4.4% in 2018.[88] Although representation by underrepresented minorities among dental graduates has not traditionally reflected the cultural diversity of the population, this too has improved in recent years[88] (see Figure 5.19).

Educating Future Oral Health Professionals

Each year academic dental institutions, including dental, postdoctoral, and advanced dental and allied dental education programs, graduate new oral health professionals. At these private

TABLE 5.8   Number of Dental and Dental Hygiene Graduates by Race and Gender, 2017–2018

Characteristic	Male	Percent (%) of Males	Female	Percent (%) of Females	Total	Total Percent (%)
Dental Graduates						
Hispanic/Latino (any race)	204	6.8	303	11.1	507	8.9
White	1872	62.4	1370	50.2	3242	56.6
Black or African American	120	4.0	175	6.4	295	5.2
American Indian/Alaska Native	11	0.4	11	0.4	22	0.4
Asian	686	22.9	810	29.7	1496	26.1
Hawaiian/Other Pacific Islander	5	0.2	10	0.4	15	0.3
Two or more races (not Hispanic)	69	2.3	62	2.3	131	2.3
Unknown	99	3.3	97	3.6	196	3.4
Nonresident Alien	139	4.6	192	7.0	331	5.8
Unknown or other gender or race/ethnicity	N/A	—	N/A	—	7	0.1
Total	**3001**	**100**	**2727**	**100**	**5728**	**100**
Dental Hygiene Graduates						
Hispanic/Latino (any race)	81	23.3	949	13.7	1030	14.1
White	137	39.4	4772	69.0	4909	67.3
Black or African American	29	8.3	264	3.8	293	4.0
American Indian/Alaska Native	3	0.9	38	0.5	41	0.6
Asian	68	19.5	490	7.1	558	7.7
Hawaiian/Other Pacific Islander	7	2.0	41	0.6	48	0.7
Two or more races (not Hispanic)	7	2.0	141	2.0	148	2.0
Unknown	14	4.0	215	3.1	229	3.1
Nonresident Alien	2	0.6	7	0.1	9	0.1
Race/ethnicity and gender not available	N/A	—	N/A	—	29	0.4
Total	**348**	**100**	**6917**	**100**	**7294**	**100**

(From Survey of Dental Education Series Report 1: Academic Programs, Enrollment and Graduates 2017–2018; Survey of Allied Dental Education Report 1: Dental Hygiene Education Programs 2017–2018. Chicago, IL: ADA Health Policy Institute. Available at: <https://www.ada.org/en/science-research/health-policy-institute/data-center/dental-education>. [Accessed November 2019].)

and public educational institutions, future oral health practitioners and researchers gain knowledge, conduct the majority of dental research, and provide significant oral health care in on-site and community-based clinical settings.

The number of accredited dental schools in the U.S. has increased from 56 in 1990[100] to 66 in 2018[88] with 768 advanced dental education programs in 2019.[88] The number of accredited dental hygiene programs has increased dramatically from 202 in 1990[95] to 327 in 2018.[83] In 2018, there were 251 accredited dental assisting programs compared to 279 in 2010.[88] Three dental therapy education programs exist in the U.S.[96] However, although CODA adopted standards for dental therapy education programs in 2015,[99] as of 2019, none of the programs is listed yet as accredited on the CODA website.[101]

Distribution of Dental Professionals

National reports have discussed how the geographic maldistribution of dentists influences the ability to meet the oral health needs of the population.[18] Even when the number of dentists is adequate, maldistribution remains a major challenge, compromising the ability of the oral healthcare system to provide access to oral healthcare services for many people.[18] This reinforces the

need to develop workforce solutions to address oral healthcare needs in underserved areas.

Maldistribution of dental professionals contributes to poor access to dental care in many areas, especially rural and inner-city areas, as local programs struggle to meet the oral healthcare needs within their communities.[18] The dentist-to-population ratio can be compared from one area to another to examine the distribution of dentists. Currently, the dentist-to-population ratio varies by state and even by county, which contributes to oral health disparities in areas with a low ratio. For example, in 2018, Alabama had a dentist-to-population ratio of 41.78 to 100,000, whereas D.C. had a ratio of 102.78 to 100,000.[91] Data indicate that an overwhelming majority of dental professionals are located in urban areas; thus, people in rural areas have less access to dental care.[18] The allied oral health workforce, including new workforce models, are central to meeting the increasing needs and demands for dental care, especially in rural and other underserved areas.[85] (See the Future Trends for Dental Hygienists in Public Health section in Chapter 2.)

Health Professional Shortage Areas. A **dental health professional shortage area** (dental HPSA) is one type of HPSA identified by the **Health Resources and Services Administration** (HRSA).[102] A HPSA "is a geographic area, population,

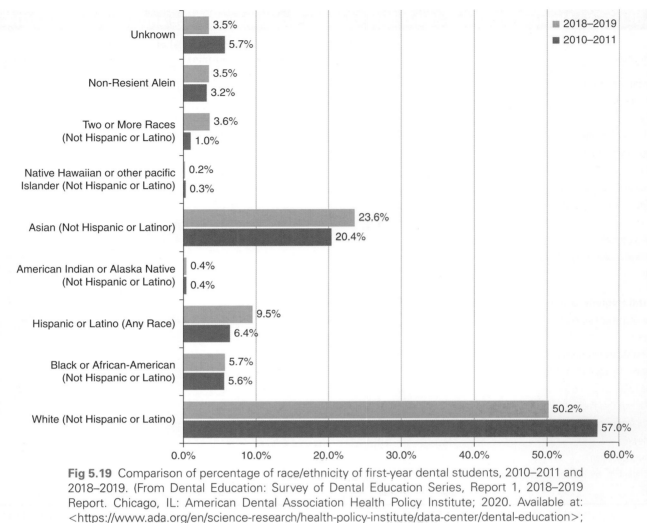

Fig 5.19 Comparison of percentage of race/ethnicity of first-year dental students, 2010–2011 and 2018–2019. (From Dental Education: Survey of Dental Education Series, Report 1, 2018–2019 Report. Chicago, IL: American Dental Association Health Policy Institute; 2020. Available at: <https://www.ada.org/en/science-research/health-policy-institute/data-center/dental-education>; [Accessed July 2020].)

or facility with a shortage of primary care, dental, or mental health providers and services."[102] The shortages may be based on geographic, population, or facility-based factors.[103] A geographic area shortage is an inadequate number of providers for the population within a specific area.[103] Population-group designation indicates a shortage within a specific population group, such as low-income or migrant farmworkers. Federal stipulations dictate that a HPSA designation occurs when the population-to-provider ratio is higher than a certain threshold, which is 5,000:1 for the dental workforce.[104]

In some cases, facilities may be designated as HPSAs, which applies to public or nonprofit facilities, correctional facilities, and state mental hospitals.[103] Some facilities are designated as HPSAs automatically, for example, federally qualified health centers (FQHC), FQHC look-a-likes, Indian Health Service facilities, and federally recognized community and rural health centers (see Box 6.20 in Chapter 6).[103] Public and nonprofit private facilities located outside designated HPSAs may receive facility HPSA designation if they are accessible to and serving a designated geographic area or population group HPSA.[103]

Dental HPSA designation is used for a variety of purposes, including evaluation of the eligibility of a given area or population for a number of federal and state programs to expand the oral health workforce.[18] These programs include the National Health Service Corps, federal and state loan repayment programs, and community health center programs.[105] The criteria for HPSA designation are established by HRSA and are discipline specific.[102] The dental HPSA designation is made by HRSA in collaboration with local communities and state health departments.[102] HRSA scores the area or population on a scale of 0 to 26 based on established criteria, with a higher score indicating greater need[102] (see Figure 5.20).

The number and location of dental HPSAs indicate the severity of the dental workforce shortage and maldistribution.[104] The number of dental HPSAs designated by HRSA has grown exponentially from 792 in 1993, to 3527 in 2006, to 4230 in 2009, to 4900 in 2014, and to 6782 in 2019.[104,106] Based on this and the current number of dentists, additional dental and allied oral healthcare workforce are needed nationwide.[104] The need for dental health professionals to remove current dental HPSA designations varies by state and territory. For example, Florida needs 1,230 dentists to remove all their HPSA designations whereas Vermont needs only 2 dentists.[104]

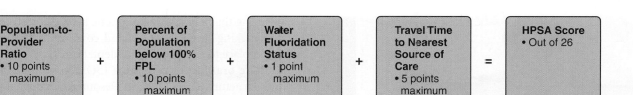

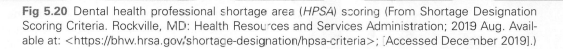

Fig 5.20 Dental health professional shortage area (*HPSA*) scoring (From Shortage Designation Scoring Criteria. Rockville, MD: Health Resources and Services Administration; 2019 Aug. Available at: <https://bhw.hrsa.gov/shortage-designation/hpsa-criteria>; [Accessed December 2019].)

Innovative strategies are needed to recruit and retain oral health professionals who will seek careers in both private and public health settings.[19] As demands for oral health services increase both nationally and by programs serving specific vulnerable population groups, collaboration is essential among state and local oral health programs and key stakeholders to enhance workforce development and expansion.

Other Workforce Issues

Two other workforce issues weaken the infrastructure and capacity of the oral healthcare system in relation to providing maximum access to care. First is the number of oral healthcare professionals available to provide oral healthcare services to individuals with Medicaid or CHIP benefits. In 2018, about 39% of dentists accepted Medicaid or CHIP for child dental services.[107] However, some private practices in states that authorize dental therapists to practice employ them to serve the Medicaid population.[108] In addition, only 18 states allowed direct Medicaid reimbursement to dental hygienists in 2020, limiting their ability to provide care through collaborative agreements with dentists, even in some states where the state statute allows direct

access of the dental hygienist to the public with no or limited dental supervision.[109] Greater numbers of Medicaid providers are needed to serve the needs of the population.[108]

Another relevant workforce issue is the recommendation that for maximum success, the dental public health infrastructure requires legal authority to use personnel efficiently and cost-effectively.[85,110,111] This is reflected in government recommendations to increase the use of dental therapists, expand dental hygienists' and dental therapists' scope of practice, relax dental hygienists' supervision requirements, and allow for their direct reimbursement and license portability.[85]

Population Trends and Future Dental Workforce

Changing demographics will have a long-term impact on the future oral healthcare system (see Figure 5.21). The number of older adults (ages ≥65) in the population is expected to almost double during 2016–2060, from 49.2 million (15%) to 94.7 million (23%),[93] and to outnumber children by 2034.[93] Furthermore, racial diversity is expected to increase. The non-Hispanic white population is expected to decrease to 44.3% by 2060, accompanied by growth of minority and mixed-race groups.[93]

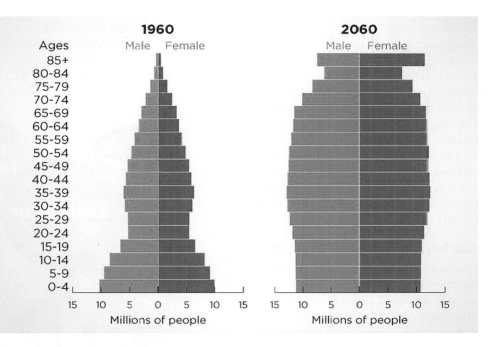

Fig 5.21 A century of projected change in the age distribution of the United States population. The continuing change in demographics will influence the demand for dentists. (From U.S. Census Bureau. National Population Projections; 2017. Available at: <https://www.census.gov/library/visualizations/2018/comm/century-of-change.html>; [Accessed October 2020].)

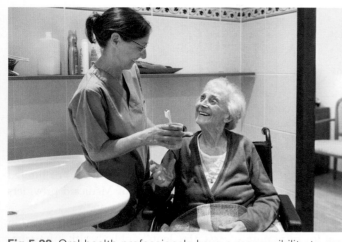

Fig 5.22 Oral health professionals have a responsibility to provide access to effective oral health services for underserved, vulnerable populations such as older adults. (© iStock.com/FredFroese.)

Additionally, it has been projected that the increasing diversity will result in fewer than 50% of children under age 18 years being non-Hispanic white in 2020 and about 72% being white, regardless of Hispanic origin.[93] The Pew Research Center has estimated that immigrants and their children may account for 88% of the population growth from 2015 to 2065.[112] Because immigration currently occurs primarily from Asian and Latin American countries and foreign-born women give birth to more children than native-born women, immigration will greatly impact the challenges of diversity of the population.[93]

These population trends will have far-reaching effects not only for the oral healthcare system but also for patients and oral healthcare providers. More programs for older adults will be needed (Figure 5.22; see Chapter 6 Oral Health Services for Older Adults section). Also, with the growth of minority groups, strategies are required to ensure that the dental workforce is culturally competent to provide oral health services to an increasingly diverse population[19] (see Chapter 10). Moreover, oral health professionals will need to provide leadership locally and at the state and national levels to ensure universal access to care in spite of these significant changes in population demographics (see Chapter 9). These professionals will have leadership opportunities to contribute to improvements in oral health outcomes of individuals and communities by shaping policies, programs, and practices that will influence the future development of an integrated system of quality health services including oral health care (Figure 5.23).

Dental Public Health Infrastructure and Capacity

The burden of oral diseases and the needs of populations are in transition, and oral health systems and scientific knowledge are changing rapidly. Even with improved access to dental care as a result of the ACA, oral health needs of many adults, children, and vulnerable population groups continue to be unmet.[19,85] Economic fluctuations stress families and challenge their abilities to access oral health care.[19] The infrastructure and capacity of many dental public health programs at the national, state, and local levels are limited and stretched.[113] Challenges include

ensuring that a viable dental public health infrastructure exists and making sure that state- and community-based programs are in place to ensure access to dental care.[19,113,114,115]

State oral health programs (SOHPs; see Measurement of Infrastructure, Capacity, and Resources section of Chapter 4 and State Level section of Chapter 6) and similar agencies at the national, state, and local levels are running at full capacity because their programs are part of the critical dental safety net.[18,19] At the same time, the structures of public health agencies are undergoing significant changes.[113,116] These agencies and related oral public health programs at all levels vary in size, structure, staffing, and funding.[117,118]

Current Status of Infrastructure and Capacity of State Oral Health Programs

With each new version of the SOHP guidelines, best practices, and competencies described in Chapter 4, the Association of State and Territorial Dental Directors (ASTDD) evaluates the overall status of SOHPs nationwide and makes recommendations for future direction.[113] In 2012, the ASTDD, funded by the CDC, published an assessment of SOHP infrastructure from 2000–2010 titled *State Oral Health Infrastructure and Capacity: Reflecting on Progress and Charting the Future.*[119] The aim was to assist state agency staff, policymakers, coalitions, funders, and other organizations in gaining a better understanding of ways to achieve positive oral health outcomes by building, expanding, and sustaining current SOHPs. In general, the outcomes of this evaluation demonstrated the need to strengthen the infrastructure and capacity of SOHPs.[119] Many states did not have a strong SOHP; numbers, training, and longevity of the dental public health workforce were inadequate; and funding was limited.[119]

Since then, numerous agencies, including HRSA, CDC, National Institute of Dental and Craniofacial Research, and ASTDD, have focused on building the infrastructure and capacity of SOHPs to be able to positively impact the oral health of the nation. The ASTDD has continued to conduct annual assessments of SOHPs since 2012 to evaluate their current

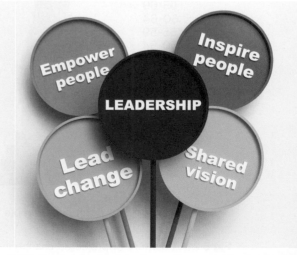

Fig 5.23 Dental hygienists have the opportunity to provide leadership to improve oral health in the nation. (© iStock.com/matdesign24)

infrastructure and capacity. The most recent results are discussed here in relation to structure, staffing, services, and funding.[118]

Structure. All reporting states and D.C. (four states did not report) had an oral health program in service areas with populations over 250,000.[118] All reporting states also had multiple local programs, totaling 194 programs.

Most SOHPs were located within a health department, FQHC, or a broader department of human services.[113] Whatever the designation, most states placed dental public health programs or functions under a broader organizational umbrella such as maternal and child health, family health, rural health, primary care, chronic disease and disease prevention, or health promotion. This practice reduces the effectiveness of a SOHP.[113] According to the ASTDD, SOHPs should be placed at a high and visible enough level to be able to provide overall agency coordination and leadership, develop and carry out specific program initiatives, represent the agency to outside organizations, and allow the director of the oral health program to communicate readily with state health officials or with directors responsible for preventive health services.[113]

Staffing. Staffing patterns for SOHPs varied substantially in terms of numbers of personnel, job categories, responsibilities, level and type of education, lines of supervision, employee versus contractor status, and job location.[113] A total of 44 states and D.C. reported having a full-time dental director, four reported having a part-time director, and three did not report or had no director.[118] The number of states with full-time dental directors increased during the previous decade; however, nearly 75% of them also served as advisor to other programs or agencies, committing up to 30% of their time to this outside activity, which significantly limited their effectiveness as director of the oral health program.[118]

Only 31 of the 42 states and D.C. reported having a dental director with dental public health training.[118] In addition, Table 5.9 shows the still limited number of large state and local programs that have a dental public health professional as the SOHP director. These results are significant in light of ASTDD's recommendations that a state dental director should be full-time and have a dental background and public health experience.[113] This is key to functioning effectively in the public health environment and to the sustainability of a strong SOHP.[113]

It is also significant that in 32 of the 48 states, the dental director had less than 5 years of service.[118] This can reduce the effectiveness of a SOHP. Vacancies and repeated turnovers in directors and staff of SOHPs interfere with program development, long-term strategic planning and evaluation, and breadth and continuity of programming.[113]

In addition to state dental directors, SOHPs employ regional dental directors, public health educators, and clinical dentists, dental hygienists, and dental assistants who provide oral health services to underserved populations and conduct oral health promotion programs.[118] Most staff who work in the state office have nonclinical roles such as managers, coordinators, regional consultants, public health educators, program planners, and evaluators.

Many SOHPs are small. In 2017–2018, 22 out of 48 states and D.C. had four or fewer full-time-equivalent (FTE) employees and contractors working for or funded by the state.[118] Some programs may also hire, contract with, or share specialized staff with other state programs.[113] Higher numbers of employees are likely to reflect states that administer programs that provide services directly.[113] These programs often employ clinical, clerical, and administrative staff for programs such as school-based sealant and fluoride programs, community clinics, and mobile clinics. In some states, grants are offered for initiatives and programs to increase access to oral health care locally, for which oral health professionals are hired but may not be state employees.[113]

Services. The ultimate goal of SOHPs is to provide services that meet the needs of the population served.[115] The infrastructure and capacity of a SOHP will determine its ability to deliver programs to meet this need for services. These programs and activities are described in Chapter 6. Included there in Table 6.1 is a summary of oral health services offered by SOHPs.

The Pew Charitable Trusts has also evaluated the performance of SOHPs regarding their oral health policies and programs.[120] Two recent examples of Pew assessments are presented in Box 5.8. The first is an assessment of the SOPHs of 50 states and D.C. conducted in 2011 in relation to their implementation of eight recommended cost-effective preventive strategies and promising policy approaches to improve access to oral health services for children (called benchmarks in Box 5.8).[120] The results indicated that most states were experiencing barriers to enacting some significant oral health initiatives. The majority did not have key policies in place. No state met all policy benchmarks, and half or less of the benchmarks were met by 23 states.

The second example is a Pew assessment of SOHPs conducted in 2014 in relation to their sealant programs.[24] Evidence-based benchmarks were used to assess the reach, efficiency, and effectiveness of the states' sealant programs (see Box 5.8). Results of this Pew assessment revealed that more than 75% of states had dental hygiene-supervision regulations that interfered with

TABLE 5.9 Percentage of Large[a] State and Local Dental Public Health Programs Managed by a Dental Public Health Professional, 2017–2018[b]

Percent (%) of Programs	Number of States	Percent (%) of States
0.0	19	37.3
1.0–24.9	4	7.8
25–49.9	7	13.7
50–74.9	3	5.9
>75	9	17.6
Not reported or applicable	9	17.6

[a]Serving a population >250,000
[b]Includes all states and D.C.
(From Summary Report: 2019 Synopses of State Dental Public Health Programs: Data for FY 2017–2018. Reno, NV: Association of State and Territorial Dental Directors; 2019. Available at: <https://www.astdd.org/docs/synopses-summary-report-2019.pdf>; [Accessed May 2020].)

BOX 5.8 PEW Evaluations of State Oral Health Programs (SOHPs)

Key Policy Benchmarks Used to Evaluate SOHPs, 2011

1. Having sealant programs in at least 25% of high-risk schools
2. Allowing a hygienist to place sealants in a school-based program without requiring a dentist's examination
3. Providing optimally fluoridated water to at least 75% of residents who are served by community water systems
4. Meeting or exceeding the 2007 national average (38.1%) of Medicaid-enrolled children aged 1–18 years who are receiving dental services
5. Paying dentists who serve Medicaid-enrolled children at least the 2008 national average (60.5%) of dentists' median retail fees
6. Reimbursing medical care providers through its state Medicaid program for preventive dental services
7. Authorizing a new type of primary care dental provider
8. Submitting basic screening data to the national surveillance database

Evaluation Benchmarks for SOHP Sealant Programs, 2014

1. The extent to which sealant programs are serving high-need schools
2. Hygienists' authorization to place sealants in school programs without a dentist's prior examination
3. Whether the state collects data and participates in a national database
4. The proportion of students receiving sealants across the state

(From The State of Children's Dental Health: Making Coverage Matter. Pew Children's Dental Campaign. Philadelphia, PA: Pew Charitable Trusts; 2011. Available at: <http://www.pewtrusts.org/~/media/legacy/uploadedfiles/wwwpewtrustsorg/reports/state_policy/ChildrensDental50StateReport2011pdf.pdf>; [Accessed March 2020]; States Stalled on Dental Sealant Programs. Pew Children's Dental Campaign. Pew Charitable Trusts; 2015 Apr 23. Available at: <https://www.pewtrusts.org/en/research-and-analysis/reports/2015/04/states-stalled-on-dental-sealant-programs>; [Accessed March 2020].)

BOX 5.9 Sources of Funding of State Oral Health Program (SOHP) Initiatives

- School sealant programs, community water fluoridation, oral health surveillance, and medical-dental integration are funded by Centers for Disease Control and Prevention (CDC).
- Association of State and Territorial Dental Directors (ASTDD) is funded by CDC to provide SOHPs technical assistance and capacity-building resources in funded states and to conduct state oral health program assessments of all states.
- Community-based dental clinics are funded through a variety of sources, including Health Resources and Services Administration (HRSA) Bureau of Primary Health Care.
- Efforts to promote oral health activities for children with special healthcare needs are funded by HRSA/Maternal and Child Health Bureau.
- Programs to promote the oral health of Head Start children and their families, including children with disabilities, are funded by the Office of Head Start.
- Oral health outreach-related programs and teledentistry networks focused in rural areas are funded by HRSA Office of Rural Health.

(From CDC-Funded States. Atlanta, GA: Centers for Disease Control and Prevention; 2019 Sep 27. Available at: <https://www.cdc.gov/oralhealth/state_programs/cooperative_agreements/index.htm>; [Accessed November 2019]; Dental Clinics. Reno, NV: Association of State and Territorial Dental Directors. Available at: <https://www.astdd.org/dental-clinics/>; [Accessed November 2019]; Children with Special Health Care Needs. Reno, NV: Association of State and Territorial Dental Directors. Available at: <https://www.astdd.org/children-with-special-health-care-needs/>; [Accessed November 2019]; Head Start Program Performance Standards Related to Oral Health. Administration for Children and Families; 2018 Aug 31. Available at: <https://eclkc.ohs.acf.hhs.gov/oral-health/article/head-start-program-performance-standards-related-oral-health>; [Accessed November 2019]; Improving Oral Health Care Services in Rural America. National Advisory Committee on Rural Health and Human Services; 2018 Dec. Available at: <https://www.hrsa.gov/sites/default/files/hrsa/advisory-committees/rural/publications/2018-Oral-Health-Policy-Brief.pdf>; [Accessed November 2019].)

---

conducting SBSPs and provided SBSPs to less than half the high-need schools in the state. In addition, 72% of states failed to meet the existing *Healthy People* sealant objectives.[24]

Funding. Consistently funded SOHPs have shown evidence of positive outcomes in building and maintaining infrastructure and capacity.[113] They are able to provide programs and resources to decrease oral diseases and promote oral health by establishing systems that foster oral disease surveillance, coalition-building, and partnerships. States then leverage support for increased promotion and coordination of effective public health preventive interventions such as SBSPs.[113]

SOHPs are funded by a variety of means, including state general revenues, foundations, and federal grants, primarily through the Maternal and Child Health Bureau and other HRSA agencies, CDC, and Medicaid.[113,118] The reported sources of funding of SOHP initiatives presented in Box 5.9 reflect the ASTDD guideline for diversified funding to maintain fully effective dental public health programs and to increase program sustainability.[113,115,121]

To effectively meet the challenges of addressing the dental public health needs of the nation, public health administrators, stakeholders, and decision makers must collaborate to work with policy makers to assure sufficient levels of funding for dental public health programs.[19,122] These are required to be able to assess and monitor health needs, implement intervention strategies, and design policy options appropriate for various unique circumstances to improve the performance of the public and private oral healthcare systems.

The *Healthy People* initiative has also addressed the need to strengthen the infrastructure and increase the capacity of SOHPs. The outcomes of related objectives for *Healthy People 2010* and *Healthy People 2020* are presented in Table 5.10. Although there have been some gains in the size and strength of SOHPs, these programs generally remain small, understaffed, and underfunded with great variation in capacity to meet oral health needs.[113] Because of the continuing need to strengthen the oral healthcare system, infrastructure and capacity of the system have been integrated into *Healthy People 2030* and oral health surveillance (see Chapter 4).[28, 113–115]

Community Health Centers

For more than 50 years government-funded health centers have provided comprehensive, culturally competent, and quality primary healthcare services to underserved communities and vulnerable populations[123] (Figure 5.24). Health centers are community-based and patient-directed organizations that serve

TABLE 5.10 *Healthy People* Emphasis on Infrastructure and Capacity of the Oral Healthcare System

Healthy People (HP) Objective	Decade	Outcomes Data
Increase the proportion of school-based health centers with an oral health component that includes dental sealants	HP 2010 HP 2020	100% increase[1] 42.7% increase[2]
Increase the proportion of school-based health centers with an oral health component that includes dental care	HP 2010 HP 2020	11.1% increase[1] 42.2% increase[2]
Increase the proportion of school-based health centers with an oral health component that includes topical fluoride	HP 2020	60.7% increase[2]
Increase the proportion of federally qualified health centers (FQHCs) that have an oral healthcare program	HP 2010 HP 2020	44% increase[1] 4.8% decrease[2]
Increase the proportion of local health departments that have oral health prevention or care programs	HP 2020	25.8% in 2008[a]
Increase the proportion of patients who receive oral health services at FQHCs each year	HP 2020	9.4% increase[2]
Increase the number of health agencies that have a dental public health program directed by a dental professional with public health training		
• In local health agencies serving jurisdictions of >250,000 persons	HP 2020	168% increase[3]
• In Indian Health Service Areas and Tribal Health Programs serving jurisdictions of >30,000 persons	HP 2020	11 in 2010[a]
Increase the proportion of dentists with geriatric certification to strengthen the capacity of the dental workforce in relation to treating this growing vulnerable population.	HP 2020	50% decrease[2]
Increase surveillance systems:		
• Increase the number of states with a recording system for cleft lips and cleft palates	HP 2020	11.4% increase[2]
• Increase the number of states with a referral system for cleft lips and cleft palates	HP 2020	16.1% increase[2]
• Increase the number of states with oral and craniofacial state-based surveillance systems	HP 2020	32 in 2009[a]

[a]Baseline data provided; no comparison data available

1. Healthy People 2010 Final Review. Hyattsville, MD: National Center for Health Statistics; 2012. Available at: <http://www.cdc.gov/nchs/data/hpdata2010/hp2010_final_review.pdf>; [Accessed November 2019].
2. Healthy People 2020 Midcourse Review. Hyattsville, MD: National Center for Health Statistics; January 11, 2017. Available at: <https://www.cdc.gov/nchs/healthy_people/hp2020/hp2020_midcourse_review.htm>; [Accessed November 2019].
3. Summary Report: 2019 Synopses of State Dental Public Health Programs Data for FY 2017-2018. Reno, NV: Association of State and Territorial Dental Directors; 2019. Available at: <https://www.astdd.org/docs/synopses-summary-report-2019.pdf>; [Accessed October 2019].

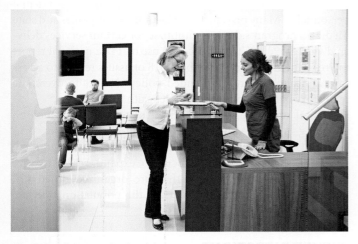

Fig 5.24 Community health centers have the potential to serve diverse populations to improve oral health conditions, but this component of the safety net is strained and unable to meet the demands for oral healthcare services. (@ Stock.com/Dean Mitchell)

28 million of the nation's vulnerable individuals and families, including 8 million children and 355,000 veterans.[123] People experiencing homelessness, low-income populations, the uninsured, those with limited English proficiency, migrant and seasonal farm workers, and residents of public housing are served by community health centers.[123] With bipartisan support, these health centers address the nation's changing healthcare needs (e.g., the increasing older adult population) and respond to public health crises (e.g., the opioid epidemic, flu outbreaks, natural disasters, and the COVID-19 pandemic).[123]

Nearly 1400 health centers operate in about 12,000 service delivery sites in every state, D.C., Puerto Rico, the Virgin Islands, and the Pacific Basin, providing one of the largest safety-net systems of oral health care.[123] Currently, 1 in 12 people rely on federally-funded health centers for care.[123] In 2018, health centers were funded over $5 billion with HRSA and other federal grants and nearly $3 billion with state, local, and foundation grants and contracts.[123]

Nationwide, in 2018, health centers employed the following FTE dental personnel: 5099 dentists, 2682 dental hygienists, 37 dental therapists, and 10,895 other dental personnel.[124] Nearly 13.6% of the total financial cost of clinical services was spent on oral health services.[123] (See Chapter 6 Financing Programs section for more financial information about community health centers.)

In 2018, 64 million patients in community health centers received oral health care during 16.5 million visits.[123] This reflected a greater than 106% increase in the number of patients and a greater than 126% increase in the number of visits compared with the previous decade.[123] Even so, less than 25% of health center patients receive oral health services because not all community health centers have an oral health component.[125]

Teledentistry: Improving Population Health Through Technology

Even with the variety of options available in the safety net described earlier, the oral healthcare needs of many are unmet.[18,19] Thus, new models of care are emerging that are designed to meet the needs of vulnerable, underserved, and rural communities.[126] Teledentistry (TD) is one of those models that can expand the inadequate capacity of SOHPs and community health centers by providing a remote workforce. An important consideration with the use of TD is the comparable quality of care and success rates of treating patients through telehealth.[127] Some examples of the application of TD are presented in Box 5.10.

TD makes it possible to take oral healthcare services to underserved communities where barriers interfere with the delivery of dental and dental hygiene care.[127] With TD oral health care can be provided in hard-to-reach areas where there are no dentists by using nondentists such as dental hygienists, dental therapists, and other mid-level providers. These providers can consult with remote dentists to increase the available workforce in underserved communities, alternative practice settings, and safety-net facilities[128,129,130] (see Figure 5.25). TD has also increased access to specialty services in dental HPSAs.

TD has the capacity to impact oral health care in other ways as well, for example, increasing interprofessional collaboration that will improve the integration of oral health care into the overall healthcare delivery system, enhancing early diagnosis and treatment of oral diseases, improving oral health, reducing costs, reducing patient anxiety, increasing appointment compliance, reducing appointment wait times, and removing barriers to dental care utilization.[127,128,130] Benefits of the use of TD in combination with community-based preventive programs are a

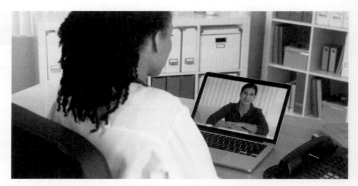

Fig 5.25 Teledentistry facilitates the provision of services to underserved populations and expands the reach of oral health care beyond the dental office or community clinic to improve access to oral health care for some populations. (Courtesy American Teledentistry Association.)

continuous presence of the program in communities; verification of oral health onsite to avoid unnecessary, costly referral of healthy patients; and integration of dentists into the program to provide full dental services despite dental team members being in different locations.[130]

TD is becoming more common, but barriers still exist. Current Dental Terminology codes were created in 2018 by the ADA for insurance reimbursement for services that involve the use of TD,[131] yet reimbursement can be problematic. States vary in the laws and policies on the use of telehealth, payment for telehealth-facilitated services, requirements for in-state licensure of oral health personnel providing services, and requirements related to informed consent for TD services.[132] The use of TD is also limited by the varying scope-of-practice state laws that regulate the practice of oral health professionals, especially allied dental personnel.[132] Many private dental insurance companies and state Medicaid programs do not reimburse for certain services delivered via TD.[129,130,132] To enhance the use of TD, a national report to President Trump in December 2018 on issues related to access to oral health care recommended policy changes to overcome regulatory barriers to the use of telehealth technologies.[85]

Several states are at the forefront of telehealth technology, including Alaska, Minnesota, and California.[129,133] Box 5.11 highlights three programs that depend on TD. Although these programs share a common focus to expand access to care for underserved populations, they are organized differently, provide care for diverse segments of the population, and use various workforce models.

FUTURE DIRECTIONS

As discussed in Chapter 1, various foundational reports beginning with the Surgeon General's report on oral health in 2000 have provided focus and direction for the improvement of the oral health of the U.S. population. The second Surgeon General's report on oral health originally scheduled to release in 2020 is expected to offer additional focus and direction for the future.[20] The ACA has offered opportunities to increase access to dental care, expand dental public health capacity and

---

BOX 5.10   Examples of Teledentistry in Action

- A patient that is admitted to the emergency room requires a teledentistry consult with a dentist to assess the situation and make clinical recommendations to the attending physician.
- A patient at home initiates an unscheduled video conferencing session for dental infection and possible antibiotic prescription.
- A patient uses a high-resolution camera to take an image of a fractured tooth and electronically sends it to a prosthodontist for consultation.
- A parent initiates video conferencing from home to consult with an orthodontist on the appropriateness of treatment for their child who is diagnosed with autism spectrum disorder.
- An orthodontist uses Store and Forward records to diagnose and treat patients via Doctor Direct who are undergoing at-home clear aligner therapy.
- A dental therapist consults with the supervising dentist concerning dental treatment being provided for a patient in a rural setting.

(From Teledental Practice and Teledental Encounters: An American Association of Teledentistry Position Paper. Boston, MA: American TeleDentistry Association; 2018. Available at: <https://www.americanteledentistry.org/>; [Accessed October 2019].)

BOX 5.11 Examples of Successful Teledentistry-Based Programs

Alaska Tribal Health System, Alaska

Alaska Dental Health Aide Therapists (DHATs) provide dental services to the residents of the most isolated rural regions of Alaska, where there are no dentists. Since 2004, they have functioned as part of an integrated team of dental care providers, through village health clinics of the Alaska Tribal Health System (ATHS) that serve the Alaskan native people. The ATHS uses teledentistry for DHATs to collaborate and communicate with geographically distant ATHS dentists to provide preventive and restorative services within a defined scope of practice regulated by the Alaska tribal government. During the first 10 years of the DHAT program, the ATHS established access to regular preventive and restorative oral health care for 45,000 Alaska native citizens in remote rural communities, which resulted in savings of $40,000 a year in patient travel costs. (See Chapter 2 Innovative Workforce Models section for additional information on DHATs.)

Apple Tree Dental, Minnesota

Apple Tree Dental is a nonprofit dental practice that operates eight regional dental centers in urban and rural areas of Minnesota. The organization also operates mobile programs in community settings such as schools, Head Start centers, group homes, assisted-living centers, nursing facilities, and other community locations that serve individuals with physical, financial, and geographic barriers to dental care. Dental hygienists, advanced dental therapists, and dental assistants provide oral health services in collaboration with Apple Tree dentists or existing dental homes via teledentistry. Apple Tree provided community-based teledentistry services for 7 years until 2010 when a change in Minnesota Medicaid policy prohibited reimbursement for teledentistry services. Apple Tree was able to restore the community-based teledentistry program in 2016 when Minnesota law reinstated insurance reimbursement for teledentistry services.

Virtual Dental Home, California

The Virtual Dental Home links dental hygienists and expanded function dental assistants who provide community-based diagnostic, preventive, and early intervention services with dental offices and clinics. This approach enhances the provision of dental care to underserved populations in the community through schools, nursing homes, community centers, and Head Start centers. Onsite allied oral health personnel collaborate with geographically distant dentists to provide triage, case management, preventive procedures, and early intervention therapeutic services. Via telehealth technology, the dentist can review a medical history and dental images, create a treatment plan, and provide a patient referral to a local dentist when more complex treatment is required.

(From Lenaker D. The dental health aide therapist program in Alaska: An example for the 21st century. Am J Public Health 2017 Jun;107(Suppl 1):S24-S25. Available at: <https://www.ncbi.nlm.nih.gov/pmc/articles/PMC5497887/>; [Accessed December 2019]; Case Studies of 6 Teledentistry Programs: Strategies to Increase Access to General and Specialty Dental Services. State University of New York, University of Albany, School of Public Health, Center for Health Workforce Studies; 2016 Dec. Available at: <http://www.oralhealthworkforce.org/wp-content/uploads/2017/02/OHWRC_Case_Studies_of_6_Teledentistry_Programs_2016.pdf>; [Accessed October 2019]; Howatt G. 'Teledentistry' expands preventive care to more Minnesota families. Minneapolis, MN: Star Tribune; 2018 Oct 8. Available at: <http://www.startribune.com/teledentistry-expands-preventive-care-to-more-minnesota-families/496043791/>; [Accessed October 2019]; Apple Tree Dental; 2020. Available at: <https://www.appletreedental.org/>; [Accessed October 2020].)

infrastructure, and improve integration of oral health care and primary health care.[122,134,135] Other initiatives of various entities highlighted in Chapter 1 have also contributed to improved oral health of the population. Together, these reports and initiatives provide the framework for potential future oral health improvements.

With the current oral health disparities and expected population growth, creative measures are crucial to further improve the oral health of the population and increase quality dental care for vulnerable population groups.[19,85,94] Various current dental public health issues are likely to influence the dynamics of the oral healthcare system as changes in the organization and financing of health services occur in the coming decades. Developments are needed in education, research, health promotion, and expanded clinical care within the private, public, and nonprofit sectors.[19,85,94]

The oral healthcare system depends on the size, composition, characteristics, and distribution of the oral health workforce.[18,19] Furthermore, provider participation in public insurance programs impacts the capacity of the workforce to serve the population, especially vulnerable groups.[18,19,111] The public health competence and diversity of the oral health workforce also affect its ability to serve an increasingly culturally diverse population.[113] The following factors are expected to impact future changes in the composition, size, and capacity of the oral health workforce:[18,19,90,94,96]

- Decline or growth in the number of dentists

- Number and location of retiring dentists
- Growth in the number of dental hygienists
- Growth in the number of dental therapists
- Expanded scope of practice for dental hygienists and dental therapists
- Relaxation of supervision and increase in direct access for dental hygienists
- Increase in direct reimbursement for dental hygienists
- The increasing use of telehealth in dentistry
- Increasing interprofessional collaborative practice settings and opportunities
- Demographic shifts among graduates of academic dental and allied dental institutions
- Shifts in population and demographic trends
- Changing oral disease patterns
- Barriers to dental care faced by underserved population groups

Some oral health indicators show promise of improvement. National oral health objectives each decade outline oral health benchmarks, and *Healthy People 2030* Oral Conditions objectives provide the road map for this decade.[28] Political will is critical at all government levels for improved oral health outcomes to come to fruition. Future national, state, and local dental public health programs need certain key elements to be better prepared to achieve the *Healthy People 2030* Oral Conditions objectives to improve the oral health of the public (see Guiding Principles).

GUIDING PRINCIPLES

Key Elements Necessary to Achieve Improved Oral Health in the Future Decades

- Innovative strategies to increase access to oral health care and improve oral health status
- Health systems interventions that ensure access to oral health care for all
- A culturally diverse, educated, competent, and skilled dental public health workforce that has the capacity to support programs
- Innovative solutions for workforce development and reduction of workforce regulations to maximize the provision of cost-effective oral health services
- Legal authority to use personnel in an effective and cost-efficient manner in relation to scope of practice, direct access, and supervision
- Reduction of regulations of state licensing boards and state practice acts that limit access to care such as limitations on the use of telehealth, direct reimbursement, and mobility
- Sufficient administrative presence with skilled staff and leadership from full-time oral health program directors with a dental background and public health training at the international, national, state, and local levels
- Robust and sustainable partnerships with private and local, state, federal, and international public agencies
- Collaborative evidence-based public oral health planning and implementation
- Empowerment of local communities to become actively involved in oral public health efforts
- Support of informed policymakers to change and promote policies that will enhance access to oral health care

- Ability to obtain and leverage sufficient, diversified, and sustained financial resources for programs at the state and local levels
- Infrastructure and capacity that are necessary to plan, implement, evaluate, and sustain oral health policies, practices, and programs
- Evidence-based, population-based interventions to prevent oral diseases in communities, including implementation of dental sealant and fluoride programs and coordination and monitoring of community water fluoridation
- Choice and competition in relation to patient selection of a provider, purchase of dental insurance, and expansion of health savings accounts and other healthcare reimbursement arrangements
- Flexibility of states to create policies that fit the various demands of consumers
- Clarity of price and quality so people can make well-informed oral healthcare decisions
- Interprofessional collaborative approach to practice and education
- Prioritization of the following specific public health focus areas:
  - Conducting surveillance of oral diseases and conditions
  - Reporting changes in the burden of oral disease
  - Facilitating the development and implementation of oral health coalitions
  - Careful and far-sighted planning of oral health initiatives
  - Focus on comprehensive, evidence-based oral health education aimed at improving preventive oral health behaviors
  - Increasing oral health literacy

(From Reforming America's Healthcare System Through Choice and Competition. Washington, DC: Department of Health and Human Services, Department of the Treasury, Department of Labor; 2018. Available at: <https://www.hhs.gov/sites/default/files/Reforming-Americas-Healthcare-System-Through-Choice-and-Competition.pdf>; [Accessed September 2019]; Guidelines for State and Territorial Oral Health Programs Part I. Reno, NV: Association of State and Territorial Dental Directors; 2015. Available at: <https://www.astdd.org/docs/astdd-guidelines-part-I-2015-update-january-2016.pdf>; [Accessed October 2019]; Competencies for State Oral Health Programs. Reno, NV: Association of State and Territorial Dental Directors; 2020. Available at: <https://www.astdd.org/docs/competencies-and-levels-for-state-oral-health-programs-2020.pdf>; [Accessed May 2020].)

SUMMARY

This chapter describes the burdens of oral disease globally and nationally. Also described and discussed are the current status and trends of oral health and access to oral health services used as key indicators in the U.S. In addition, important oral health disparities among population groups based on race and ethnicity, family income, education level, gender, age, geographic location, and disability are highlighted in the chapter. SOHPs are discussed in relation to the infrastructure and capacity of the oral healthcare system, and teledentistry is presented as a means of expanding access to oral health care. Finally, critical issues are discussed that must be considered in the future to further improve the oral health of the nation.

APPLYING YOUR KNOWLEDGE

1. Select an oral health indicator such as dental caries or periodontal disease. For the oral health indicator that you selected, find information on the current status, past trends, and disparities among population groups. Use information presented in the chapter, websites listed in the appendices, library resources, and the Internet for updated information now available to describe the oral health status of the selected indicator. Present the information in class.

2. Prepare a presentation to make in class describing how you would use the information found on the selected oral health indicator to plan, implement, and evaluate an oral health program in your role as one of the following:
   a. State Dental Director
   b. County Oral Health Director
   c. Dental Director of a Community Health Center

3. Develop a dental public health strategy for a specific population that will increase access to oral healthcare services for the underrepresented public using teledentistry as an emerging model of patient care. Present your plan in class.

4. Go to the *Healthy People 2030* website (www.health.gov/healthypeople) to review the current Oral Conditions overview, objectives, and their summaries, baseline data, and data measurement. Share the information in class.

5. Review the trends and baseline data for specific Oral Conditions objectives on the *Healthy People 2030* website (www.health.gov/healthypeople). Then on the *FDI Data Hub for Global Oral Health* review the data and trends for Oral Conditions in other countries that match the *Healthy People 2030* objectives. Prepare a presentation on the differences and similarities to share in class.

LEARNING OBJECTIVES AND COMPETENCIES

This chapter addresses the following community oral health learning objectives and competencies for dental hygienists that are presented in the revised May 2015 to 2016 *ADEA Compendium of Curriculum Guidelines for Allied Dental Education Programs:*

Learning Objectives

- Describe the state of oral health in the U.S.
- Describe the dental care delivery system in the U.S.
- Evaluate the dental hygienist employment opportunity ratio.
- Describe dental labor force in relation to utilization and access to dental care.
- Analyze need, supply, demand and use of dental care as it pertains to utilization.
- Critique current methods of payment for dental care.
- Define and apply terminology associated with financing dental care.

- List the different insurance coverage options available for dental care.
- Evaluate the role of the government in financing dental care.
- List and define the international professional organizations involving dental public health.
- List barriers to obtaining and delivering dental hygiene care.
- Describe various government-related opportunities for dental public health programs.

Competencies

- Providing dental hygiene services in a variety of settings, including offices, hospitals, clinics, extended care facilities, community programs and schools.
- Evaluating reimbursement mechanisms and their impact on the patient's access to dental care.
- Assessing, planning, implementing and evaluating community-based oral health programs.

COMMUNITY CASE

As the State Dental Director, you are working with a state oral health coalition to develop a statewide oral health plan for the state. You review the current status of key oral health indicators represented in data from state and regional surveys (Table A and Figure B) and the most recent national data in *Healthy People 2030*. Your state is represented as State E on Table A. Census data indicate that approximately 33% of children and adolescents in the state are in families that live at or below 133% of the FPL, and nearly 24% of the population lives in rural areas. There are 70 community-based clinics in the state, but less than a third of them have an oral health component.

1. Which oral health program has the lowest priority for this state?
   a. A statewide school-based dental sealant program
   b. A statewide school-based fluoride varnish program
   c. A statewide school-based dental treatment program
   d. Brushing and flossing presentations at schools across the state

2. Where are you most likely to find information on how the oral health status and trends of this state compare to that of the nation?
   a. 2020 Surgeon General's Report on Oral Health
   b. *Healthy People 2030*
   c. NHANES
   d. NOHSS

3. Which is the most likely mechanism for payment of dental services for this population?
   a. CHIP and Medicaid
   b. Head Start
   c. Medicare
   d. Private insurance

4. Which of the following statements is true when comparing the state-level oral health data with *Healthy People 2030* data for the Oral Conditions objectives?

TABLE A	Percentage of Third-Grade Students With Untreated Tooth Decay in the Regional States	
State	School Year	Percent (%) with Untreated Tooth Decay
A	2016–2019	29.5
B	2016–2019	28.7
C	2018–2021	25.4
D	2018–2021	41.3
E	2017–2020	43.1
F	2017–2020	34.5
G	2018–2021	33.2
H	2016–2019	29.4

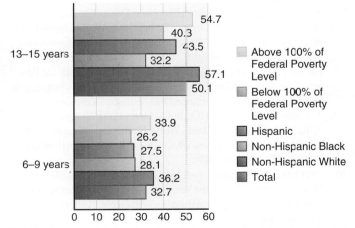

Fig B Percentage of at least one dental sealant in a permanent tooth among children and adolescents in the state, 2017–2018 school year.

Statement 1: The state has a higher rate of untreated dental caries among children and adolescents compared with the national average.

Statement 2: *Healthy People 2030* data can be used to support the need for a sealant program in the state.

a. The first statement is true, and the second statement is false.
b. The first statement is false, and the second statement is true.
c. Both statements are true.
d. Both statements are false.

5. Which of the following initiatives related to workforce capacity and infrastructure would be the lowest priority for this state?
   a. Advocate for a mid-level workforce model
   b. Increase the number of community-based clinics with an oral health component
   c. Increase the number of community-based clinics
   d. Seek funding for a statewide teledentistry program

REFERENCES

1. Disparities in Oral Health. Atlanta, GA: Centers for Disease Control and Prevention; 2016 May 17. Available at: <https://www.cdc.gov/oralhealth/oral_health_disparities/index.htm>; [Accessed December 2019].

2. Dental Caries and Sealant Prevalence in Children and Adolescents in the United States, 2011-2012 (Key Findings). Hyattsville, MD: CDC National Center for Health Statistics; 2015 Nov 6. Available at: <https://www.cdc.gov/nchs/products/databriefs/db191.htm>; [Accessed December 2019].

3. Oral Health Surveillance Report, 2019: Trends in Dental Caries and Sealants, Tooth Retention, and Edentulism, United States, 1999-2004 to 2011-2016. Atlanta, GA: Centers for Disease Control and Prevention; 2019. Available at: <https://www.cdc.gov/oralhealth/publications/OHSR-2019-index.html>; [Accessed December 2019].

4. Fluoridation Statistics. Atlanta, GA: Centers for Disease Control and Prevention; 2020 Jan 13. Available at: <https://www.cdc.gov/fluoridation/statistics/reference_stats.htm>; [Accessed August 2020].

5. Eke PI, Thornton-Evans GO, Wei L, Borgnakke WS, Dye BA, Genco RJ. Periodontitis in US adults: National health and nutrition examination survey 2009-2014. J Am Dent Assoc 2018 Jul 1;149(7):576-588. Available at: <https://www.sciencedirect.com/science/article/pii/S0002817718302769?via%3Dihub>; [Accessed December 2019].

6. Dye BA, Thornton-Evans G, Li X, Iafolla TJ. Dental caries and tooth loss in adults in the United States, 2011-2012. NCHS data brief, no 197. Hyattsville, MD: CDC National Center for Health Statistics; 2015. Available at: <https://www.cdc.gov/nchs/products/databriefs/db197.htm>; [Accessed December 2019].

7. Oral Health: Key Facts. Geneva, Switzerland: World Health Organization; 2019. Available at: <https://www.who.int/news-room/fact-sheets/detail/oral-health>; [Accessed December 2019].

8. Cancer Fact Sheets. Lyon, France: International Agency for Research on Cancer: Cancer Today; 2019. Available at: <https://gco.iarc.fr/today/fact-sheets-cancers>; [Accessed December 2019].

9. The objectives of the WHO Global Oral Health Programme (ORH). Geneva, Switzerland: World Health Organization; 2019. Available at: <https://www.who.int/oral_health/objectives/en/>; [Accessed December 2019].

10. Oral health information systems. Geneva, Switzerland: World Health Organization; 2019. Available at: <https://www.who.int/oral_health/action/information/surveillance/en/index1.html>; [Accessed December 2019].

11. Oral Health Databases. Geneva, Switzerland: World Health Organization; 2019. Available at: <https://www.who.int/oral_health/databases/en/>; [Accessed December 2019].

12. WHO Global InfoBase. Geneva, Switzerland: World Health Organization; 2019. Available at: <https://www.who.int/ncd_surveillance/infobase/en>; [Accessed December 2019].

13. Oral Health Atlas. Geneva, Switzerland: FDI World Dental Federation; 2019. Available at: <https://www.fdiworlddental.org/resources/publications/oral-health-atlas/oral-health-atlas-2015>; [Accessed December 2019].

14. Oral Health and the UN Political Declaration on NCDs. Geneva, Switzerland: FDI World Dental Federation; 2019. Available at: <https://www.fdiworlddental.org/what-we-do/advocacy/declarations/oral-health-and-the-un-political-declaration-on-ncds>; [Accessed December 2019].

15. About the Pan American Health Organization (PAHO). Washington, DC: Pan American Health Organization. Available at: <https://www.paho.org/hq/index.php?option=com_content&view=article&id=91:about-paho&Itemid=220&lang=en>; [Accessed February 2020].

16. Hygiene-related Diseases. Atlanta, GA: Centers for Disease Control and Prevention; 2016 Sep 22. Available at: <https://www.cdc.gov/healthywater/hygiene/disease/dental_caries.html>; [Accessed April 2020].

17. Healthy People 2020 Midcourse Review. Hyattsville, MD: CDC National Center for Health Statistics; 2017 Jan 11. Available at: <https://www.cdc.gov/nchs/healthy_people/hp2020/hp2020_midcourse_review.htm>; [Accessed November 2019].

18. Institute of Medicine of the National Academies. Advancing Oral Health in America. Washington, DC: The National Academies Press; 2011. Available at: <http://www.hrsa.gov/publichealth/clinical/oralhealth/advancingoralhealth.pdf>; [Accessed December 2019].

19. Bersell CH. Access to oral health care: A national crisis and call for reform. J Dent Hyg 2017;91(1):6-14. Available at: <https://jdh.adha.org/content/jdenthyg/91/1/6.full.pdf>; [Accessed December 2019].

20. Surgeon General Priority: Oral Health. Washington, DC: Office of the Surgeon General; 2019 May 14. Available at: <https://www.hhs.gov/surgeongeneral/priorities/oral-health/index.html>; [Accessed December 2019].

21. NHANES 2017-2018. Atlanta, GA: Centers for Disease Control and Prevention. Available at: <https://wwwn.cdc.gov/nchs/nhanes/continuousnhanes/default.aspx?BeginYear=2017>; [Accessed May 2020].

22. Policy on Early Childhood Caries (ECC): Classifications, Consequences, and Preventive Strategies, 2016. In Reference Manual of Pediatric Dentistry, 2019-2020, pp 71-73. Chicago, IL: American Academy of Pediatric Dentistry. Available at: <https://www.aapd.org/research/oral-health-policies--recommendations/early-childhood-caries-classifications-consequences-and-preventive-strategies/>; [Accessed March 2020].

23. DATA2020 Search. Healthy People 2020. Rockville, MD: Office of Disease Prevention and Health Promotion; 2020 Jul 14. Available at: <https://www.healthypeople.gov/2020/data-search/>; [Accessed July 2020].

24. States Stalled on Dental Sealant Programs. Pew Children's Dental Campaign. Philadelphia, PA: Pew Charitable Trusts; 2015 Apr 23. Available at: <https://www.pewtrusts.org/en/research-and-analysis/reports/2015/04/states-stalled-on-dental-sealant-programs>; [Accessed November 2019].

25. Fleming E, Afful J. Prevalence of total and untreated dental caries among youth: United States, 2015-2016. NCHS Data Brief, no 307. Hyattsville, MD: CDC National Center for Health Statistics; 2018. Available at: <https://www.cdc.gov/nchs/products/data-briefs/db307.htm>; [Accessed December 2019].

26. Children's Oral Health. National Conference of State Legislatures; 2018 Feb 2. Available at: <https://www.ncsl.org/research/health/childrens-oral-health-policy-issues-overview.aspx>; [Accessed March 2020].

27. Fluoridation Facts. Chicago, IL: American Dental Association; 2018. Available at: <https://ebooks.ada.org/fluoridationfacts/>; [Accessed March 2020].

28. Healthy People 2030. Rockville, MD: Office of Disease Prevention and Health Promotion. Available at: <https://health.gov/healthypeople/objectives-and-data/browse-objectives/>; [Accessed August 2020].

29. My Water's Fluoride. Atlanta, GA: Centers for Disease Control and Prevention. Available at: <https://nccd.cdc.gov/doh_mwf/Default/Default.aspx>; [Accessed March 2020].

30. Chuck E. Science says fluoride in water is good for kids. NBC News; 2018 Oct 17. Available at: <https://www.nbcnews.com/news/us-news/science-says-fluoride-water-good-kids-so-why-are-these-n920851>; [Accessed December 2019].

31. Healthy People 2010 Data: What is Data 2010? Atlanta, GA: Centers for Disease Control and Prevention; 2011. Available at: <http://www.cdc.gov/nchs/healthy_people/hp2010/data2010.htm>; [Accessed December 2019].

32. Healthy People 2000 Final Review. Hyattsville, MD: CDC National Center for Health Statistics; 2001. Available at: <http://www.cdc.gov/nchs/data/hp2000/hp2k01.pdf>; [Accessed December 2019].

33. Facts & Figures. Chicago, IL: American College of Prosthodontists; 2019. Available at: <https://www.gotoapro.org/facts-figures>; [Accessed December 2019].

34. LLCP 2018 Codebook Report: Behavioral Risk Factor Surveillance System. Atlanta, GA: Centers for Disease Control and Prevention; 2019. Available at: <https://www.cdc.gov/brfss/annual_data/2018/pdf/codebook18_llcp-v2-508.pdf>; [Accessed May 2020].

35. Key Statistics for Oral Cavity and Oropharyngeal Cancers. Atlanta, GA: American Cancer Society; 2019. Available at: <https://www.cancer.org/cancer/oral-cavity-and-oropharyngeal-cancer/about/key-statistics.html>; [Accessed December 2019].

36. Oral and Oropharyngeal Cancer: Introduction. Alexandria, VA: American Society of Clinical Oncology; 2019. Available at: <https://www.cancer.net/cancer-types/oral-and-oropharyngeal-cancer/introduction>; [Accessed December 2019].

37. Metastasis. Oral Cancer Foundation; 2019. Available at: <https://oralcancerfoundation.org/facts/metastasis/>; [Accessed December 2019].

38. Cancer Stat Facts: Oral Cavity and Pharynx Cancer. Bethesda, MD: National Cancer Institute, Surveillance, Epidemiology, and End Results Program. Available at: <https://seer.cancer.gov/statfacts/html/oralcav.html>; [Accessed December 2019].

39. SEER Cancer Statistics Review 1975-2015; National Cancer Institute. Available at: <https://seer.cancer.gov/archive/csr/1975_2015/results_merged/sect_20_oral_cavity_pharynx.pdf>; [Accessed April 2020].

40. Oral Cancer Incidence (New Cases) by Age, Race, and Gender. Bethesda, MD: National Institute of Dental and Craniofacial Research. Available at: <https://www.nidcr.nih.gov/research/data-statistics/oral-cancer/incidence>; [Accessed December 2019].

41. About Oral Cavity and Oropharyngeal Cancer. Atlanta, GA: American Cancer Society; 2018. Available at: <https://www.cancer.org/content/dam/cancer-org/cancer-control/en/cancer-types/oral-cavity-oropharyngeal-cancer-complete.pdf/>; [Accessed December 2019].

42. You EL, Henry M, Zeitouni AG. Human papillomavirus–associated oropharyngeal cancer: review of current evidence and management. Curr Oncol 2019;26(2):119-123. Available at: <https://www.ncbi.nlm.nih.gov/pmc/articles/PMC6476447/>; [Accessed March 2020].

43. Cleft Lip & Palate, Health Info. Bethesda, MD: National Institute of Dental and Craniofacial Research. Available at: <https://www.nidcr.nih.gov/health-info/cleft-lip-palate?_ga=2.187524074.372015400.1574088946-528209316.1570742253>; [Accessed December 2019].

44. Facts about Cleft Lip and Cleft Palate, Birth Defects. Atlanta, GA: Centers for Disease Control and Prevention; 2019 Dec 5. Available at: <https://www.cdc.gov/ncbddd/birthdefects/CleftLip.html>; [Accessed December 2019].

45. National Birth Defects Prevention Study (NBDPS), Birth Defects. Atlanta, GA: Centers for Disease Control and Prevention; 2019 Dec 5. Available at: <https://www.cdc.gov/ncbddd/birthdefects/nbdps.html>; [Accessed December 2019].

46. Thompson JA, Heaton PC, Kelton CM, Sitzman TJ. National estimates of and risk factors for inpatient revision surgeries for orofacial clefts. Cleft Palate-Craniofac J 2017;54(1):60-69. Available at: <http://dx.doi.org/10.1597/15-206>; [Accessed February 2020].

47. Proffit W, Jackson T, Turvey T. Changes in the pattern of patients receiving surgical-orthodontic treatment. Am J Orthod Dentofacial Orthop [online] 2013;143(6):793-798. Available at: <https://www.ncbi.nlm.nih.gov/pmc/articles/PMC4034071/>; [Accessed March 2020].

48. American Association of Orthodontists; 2019. Available at: <https://www.aaoinfo.org/>; [Accessed March 2020].

49. Traumatic Dental Injuries. Chicago, IL: American Association of Endodontists; 2019. Available at: <https://www.aae.org/specialty/clinical-resources/treatment-planning/traumatic-dental-injuries/>; [Accessed December 2019].

50. American Academy of Pediatric Dentistry. Policy on Prevention of Sports-related Orofacial Injuries. The Reference Manual of Pediatric Dentistry pp. 97-103; 2018. Available at: <https://www.aapd.org/media/policies_guidelines/p_sports.pdf>; [Accessed December 2019].

51. Dye BA, Tan S, Smith V, Lewis BD, Barker LK, Thorton-Evans GO, et al. Trends in Oral Health Status, United States, 1988-1994 and 1999-2004. Hyattsville, MD: CDC National Center for Health Statistics 2007 April;11(248):1-92. Available at: <https://www.ncbi.nlm.nih.gov/pubmed/17633507>; [Accessed March 2020].

52. Neurath C, Limeback H, Osmunson B, Connett M, Kanter V, Wells CR. Dental fluorosis trends in US oral health surveys:

1986 to 2012. JDR Clin Trans Res 2019;4(4):298-308. doi: 10.1177/2380084419830957 Available at: <http://fluoridealert. org/wp-content/uploads/neurath.2019-1.pdf>; [Accessed February 2020].

53. National Center for Chronic Disease Prevention and Health Promotion. Data quality evaluation of the dental fluorosis clinical assessment data from the National Health and Nutrition Examination Survey, 1999-2004 and 2011-2016. Hyattsville, MD: National Center for Health Statistics. Vital Health Stat 2(183); 2019. Available at: <https://www.cdc.gov/nchs/data/series/sr_02/ sr02_183-508.pdf>; [Accessed December 2019].

54. Wiener RC, Shen C, Findley P, Tan X, Sambamoorthi U. Dental fluorosis over time: A comparison of national health and nutrition examination survey data from 2001-2002 and 2011-2012. J Dent Hyg 2018;92(1):23-29. Available at: <https://www.ncbi. nlm.nih.gov/pmc/articles/PMC5929463/>; [Accessed December 2019].

55. Ajiboye S. AADR Response to New NCHS Evaluation of Dental Fluorosis Clinical Assessment Data from NHANES Over Time. Government Affairs & Science Policy Blog. Washington, DC: American Association for Dental Research; 2019 Apr 22. Available at: <http://ga.dentalresearchblog.org/?p=3344>; [Accessed December 2019].

56. Atchison, KA, Rozier, G, Weintraub JA. Integration of Oral Health and Primary Care: Communication, Coordination and Referral. Washington, DC: National Academy of Medicine, National Academy of Sciences; 2019. Available at: <https://nam. edu/integration-of-oral-health-and-primary-care-communication-coordination-and-referral/>; [Accessed December 2019].

57. Patterson, DG, Andrilla, HA, Schwartz, MR, Hager, L, Skillman, SM. Assessing the Impact of Washington State's Oral Health Workforce on Patient Access to Care. Seattle, WA: University of Washington Center for Health Workforce Studies; 2017. Available at: <http://depts.washington.edu/fammed/chws/wp-content/ uploads/sites/5/2017/11/Washington_State_Oral_Health_ Workforce_FR_Nov_2017_Patterson.pdf>; [Accessed December 2019].

58. ASTDD Orientation Module: Dental Public Health 101. Reno, NV: Association of State and Territorial Dental Directors; 2016. Available at: <https://www.astdd.org/docs/dph-101-with-slide-notes-04-06-2016.pptx>; [Accessed March 2019].

59. Gupta N, Vujicic M. Main Barriers to Getting Needed Dental Care All Relate to Affordability. Chicago IL: American Dental Association Health Policy Institute; 2019. Available at: <http:// www.ada.org/~/media/ADA/Science%20and%20Research/HPI/ Files/HPIBrief_0419_1.pdf>;[Accessed December 2019].

60. Health, United States, 2018. Hyattsville, MD: CDC National Center for Health Statistics; 2019 Oct 30. Available at: <https:// www.cdc.gov/nchs/hus/index.htm>; [Accessed December 2019].

61. Who Has Dental Benefits Today? Dallas, TX: National Association of Dental Plans; 2019. Available at: <https://www.nadp.org/ Dental_Benefits_Basics/Dental_BB_1.aspx>; [Accessed March 2020].

62. Mertz EA. The dental–medical divide. Health Affairs; 2016 Dec 1;35(12):2168-2175. Available at: <https://www.healthaffairs. org/doi/10.1377/hlthaff.2016.0886>; [Accessed December 2019].

63. Guide to Dental Benefit Plans. Chicago, IL: American Association of Endodontists; 2017. Available at: <https://www.aae.org/ specialty/wp-content/uploads/sites/2/2017/07/Guide-to-Dental-Benefits-Plan.pdf?_ga=2.198353967.1481632447.1554661016-55010317.1543596731>; [Accessed November 2019].

64. Artiga S, Ubri P, Zur J. The Effects of Premiums and Cost Sharing on Low-Income Populations: Updated Review of Research Findings (Issue Brief). San Francisco, CA: Kaiser Family Foundation; 2017 Jun 1. Available at: <https://www.kff.org/medicaid/ issue-brief/the-effects-of-premiums-and-cost-sharing-on-low-income-populations-updated-review-of-research-findings/view/ print/>; [Accessed November 2019].

65. Dental Care. Woodlawn, MD: Centers for Medicare and Medicaid Services. Available at: <https://www.medicaid.gov/medicaid/ benefits/dental/index.html>; [Accessed December 2019].

66. Freed M, Neuman T, Jacobson G. Drilling down on dental coverage and costs for Medicare beneficiaries. San Francisco, CA: Kaiser Family Foundation; 2019 Mar 13. Available at: <https://www.kff. org/medicare/issue-brief/drilling-down-on-dental-coverage-and-costs-for-medicare-beneficiaries/>; [Accessed December 2019].

67. Dental Services. Woodlawn, MD: Centers for Medicare and Medicaid Services. Available at: <https://www.medicare.gov/ coverage/dental-services>; [Accessed November 2019].

68. U.S. Dental Expenditures: 2017 Update. Chicago, IL: American Dental Association Health Policy Institute. Available at: https:// www.ada.org/~/media/ADA/Science%20and%20Research/HPI/ Files/HPIBrief_1217_1.pdf?la=en>; [Accessed November 2019].

69. Health Care Expenditures Per Capita by Service by State of Residence. San Francisco, CA: Kaiser Family Foundation; 2014. Available at: <https://www.kff.org/other/state-indicator/health-spending-per-capita-by-service/?currentTimeframe=0&selectedDistributions=dental-services&sortModel=%7B%22colId%22:%22Dental%20Services%22,%22sort%22:%22desc%22%7D>; [Accessed November 2019].

70. Dental Benefits Coverage in the US. Chicago, IL: American Dental Association Health Policy Institute; 2017. Available at: <https://www.ada.org/~/media/ADA/Science%20and%20 Research/HPI/Files/HPIgraphic_1117_3.pdf?la=en>; [Accessed November 2019].

71. Nasseh K, Vujicic M. Early impact of the Affordable Care Act's Medicaid expansion on dental care use. Health Serv Res 2017;52(6):2256-2268. Available at: <https://onlinelibrary.wiley. com/doi/full/10.1111/1475-6773.12606>; [Accessed December 2019].

72. Vujicic M. Obamacare, Trumpcare, and your mouth. Health Affairs Blog; 2017 Jan 13. Available at: <https://www.healthaffairs.org/do/10.1377/hblog20170113.058329/full/>; [Accessed December 2019].

73. Medicaid enrollment changes following the ACA. Washington, DC: Medicaid and CHIP Payment and Access Commission; 2019. Available at: <https://www.macpac.gov/subtopic/medicaid-enrollment-changes-following-the-aca/>; [Accessed July 2020].

74. Nasseh K, Vujicic M. Dental benefits coverage increased for working-age adults in 2014. Chicago, IL: American Dental Association Health Policy Institute; 2016. Available at: <http://www. ada.org/~/media/ADA/Science%20and%20Research/HPI/Files/ HPIBrief_1016_2.pdf>; [Accessed November 2019].

75. CHIP and Children's Medicaid. Texas Health and Human Services; 2020. Available at: <https://yourtexasbenefits.hhsc.texas. gov/programs/health/child/childrens-medicaid>; [Accessed July 2020].

76. Medicaid. Woodlawn, MD: Centers for Medicare & Medicaid Services; 2019. Available at: <https://www.medicaid.gov/medicaid/index.html>; [Accessed October 2019].

77. Medicaid Adult Benefits: An Overview (Fact Sheet). Center for Health Care Strategies, Inc; 2019 Sep. Available at: <https://www.

chcs.org/media/Adult-Oral-Health-Fact-Sheet_091519.pdf>; [Accessed February 2020].

78. Healthy Kids and Access Acts: Summary of Key Provisions Impacting Children. Washington, DC: Georgetown University Health Policy Institute, Center for Children and Families; 2018. Available at: <https://ccf.georgetown.edu/wp-content/uploads/2018/03/Healthy-Kids-Access-Acts-FINAL-1.pdf>; [Accessed October 2019].

79. Contreras OA, Stewart D, Valachovic RW. Examining America's Dental Safety Net. Washington, DC: American Dental Education Association; 2018 Apr. Available at: <https://www.adea.org/policy/white-papers/Dental-Safety-Net.aspx>; [Accessed February 2020].

80. Health Insurance Coverage of Children 0-18, 2009-2018. San Francisco, CA: Kaiser Family Foundation. Available at: <https://www.kff.org/other/state-indicator/children-0-18/?activeTab=graph&currentTimeframe=0&startTimeframe=9&selectedDistributions=medicaid&sortModel=%7B%22colId%22:%22Location%22,%22sort%22:%22asc%22%7D>; [Accessed November 2019].

81. August 2019 Medicaid & CHIP Enrollment Data Highlights. Woodlawn, MD: Centers for Medicare and Medicaid Services; 2019. Available at: <https://www.medicaid.gov/medicaid/program-information/medicaid-and-chip-enrollment-data/report-highlights/index.html>; [Accessed November 2019].

82. Medicare Law of 1965. Washington, DC: U.S. Government Publishing Office. Available at: <https://www.govinfo.gov/features/medicare-law>; [Accessed November 2019].

83. Total Number of Medicare Beneficiaries. San Francisco, CA: Kaiser Family Foundation; 2019. Available at: <https://www.kff.org/medicare/state-indicator/total-medicare-beneficiaries/?currentTimeframe=0&sortModel=%7B%22colId%22:%22Location%22,%22sort%22:%22asc%22%7D>; [Accessed November 2019].

84. O'Brien S. Medicare would cover dental and vision if these bills pass Congress. CNBC; 2019 Oct 28. Available at: <https://www.cnbc.com/2019/10/28/medicare-would-cover-dental-and-vision-if-these-bills-pass-congress.html>; [Accessed July 2020].

85. Reforming America's Healthcare System Through Choice and Competition. Washington, DC: Department of Health and Human Services, Department of the Treasury, Department of Labor; 2018 Dec. Available at: <https://www.hhs.gov/sites/default/files/Reforming-Americas-Healthcare-System-Through-Choice-and-Competition.pdf>; [Accessed September 2019].

86. National and State-Level Projections of Dentists and Dental Hygienists in the U.S., 2012-2025. Rockville, MD: Health Resources and Services Administration, National Center for Health Workforce Analysis; 2015. Available at: <https://bhw.hrsa.gov/sites/default/files/bhw/nchwa/projections/nationalstatelevelprojectionsdentists.pdfhttp://bhpr.hrsa.gov/healthworkforce/supplydemand/dentistry/nationalstatelevelprojectionsdentists.pdf>; [Accessed November 2019].

87. Occupational Outlook Handbook. Washington, DC: U.S. Bureau of Labor Statistics; 2019 Sep 4. Available at: <https://www.bls.gov/ooh/>; [Accessed March 2020].

88. Dental Education. Survey of Dental Education Series: Report 1: Academic Programs, Enrollment, and Graduates; Survey of Advanced Dental Education; Survey of Allied Dental Education: Report 1: Dental Hygiene Education Programs 2018-2019 and Report 2: Dental Assisting Education Programs 2018-2019. Chicago, IL: American Dental Association Health Policy Institute. Available at: <https://www.ada.org/en/science-research/health-policy-institute/data-center/dental-education>; [Accessed June 2020].

89. Eklund SA, Bailit HL. Estimating the number of dentists needed in 2040. J Dent Educ 2017;81(8):eS146-152. Available at: <http://www.jdentaled.org/content/81/8/eS146.long>; [Accessed December 2019].

90. Munson B, Vujicic M. Supply of full-time equivalent dentists in the U.S. expected to increase steadily (Research Brief). Chicago, IL: American Dental Association Health Policy Institute; 2018 Jul. Available at: <http://www.ada.org/~/media/ADA/Science%20and%20Research/HPI/Files/HPIBrief_0718_1.pdf>; [Accessed December 2019].

91. Supply of Dentists in the U.S.: 2001-2018. Chicago, IL: American Dental Association Health Policy Institute; 2019 Feb. Available at: <https://www.ada.org/en/science-research/health-policy-institute/data-center/supply-and-profile-of-dentists>; [Accessed November 2019].

92. HPI: Fewer dentists are practicing solo. Chicago, IL: American Dental Association Health Policy Institute; 2018 Oct 10. Available at: <https://www.ada.org/en/publications/ada-news/2018-archive/october/hpi-fewer-dentists-are-practicing-solo>; [Accessed November 2019].

93. Vespa J, Medina L, Armstrong DM. Demographic Turning Points for the United States: Population Projections for 2020 to 2060: Population Estimates and Projections: Current Population Reports. U.S. Census Bureau; 2020. Available at: <https://www.census.gov/content/dam/Census/library/publications/2020/demo/p25-1144.pdf>; [Accessed March 2020].

94. Fried JL, Maxey HL, Battani K, Gurenlian JR, Byrd TO, Brunick A. Preparing the future dental hygiene workforce: Knowledge, skills, and reform. J Dent Educ 2017; 81(9)eS45-52. Available at: <http://www.jdentaled.org/content/81/9/eS45.long>; [Accessed September 2019].

95. Dental Hygiene Education: Curricula, Program, Enrollment and Graduate Information. Chicago, IL: American Dental Hygienists' Association; 2014. Available at: <https://www.adha.org/resources-docs/72611_Dental_Hygiene_Education_Fact_Sheet.pdf>; [Accessed November 2019].

96. Brickle CM, Self KD. Dental therapists as new oral health practitioners: increasing access for underserved populations. J Dent Educ 2017; 81(9)eS65-72. Available at: <https://doi.org/10.21815/JDE.017.036>; [Accessed November 2019].

97. Minjarez J, Nuzzo S. Dental Therapists: Sinking Our Teeth into Innovative Reform. Tallahassee, FL: James Madison Institute; 2019. Available at: <https://www.jamesmadison.org/wp-content/uploads/2019/01/PolicyBrief_DentalTherapy_2019_v01.pdf>; [Accessed November 2019].

98. Expanding Access to Care through Dental Therapy. Chicago, IL: American Dental Hygienists' Association; 2019 Jul. Available at: <https://www.adha.org/resources-docs/Expanding_Access_to_Dental_Therapy.pdf>; [Accessed October 2019].

99. Accreditation Standards for Dental Therapy Education Programs. Chicago, IL: Commission on Dental Accreditation; 2015. Available at: <https://www.ada.org/~/media/CODA/Files/dental_therapy_standards.pdf?la=en>; [Accessed July 2020].

100. Trends in U.S. Dental Schools. Chicago, IL: ADA Health Policy Institute. Available at: <http://www.ada.org/~/media/ADA/Science%20and%20Research/HPI/Files/HPIgraphic_0416_1.pdf?la=en>; [Accessed July 2020].

101. Search for Dental Programs. Chicago, IL: Commission on Dental Accreditation; 2019. Available at: <https://www.ada.org/en/coda/find-a-program/search-dental-programs#t=us&sort=%40codastatecitysort%20ascending>; [Accessed July 2020].

102. Shortage Designation Scoring Criteria. Rockville, MD: Health Resources and Services Administration; 2019 Aug. Available at: <https://bhw.hrsa.gov/shortage-designation/hpsa-criteria>; [Accessed November 2019].

103. Health Professional Shortage Areas (HPSAs). Rockville, MD: Health Resources and Services Administration; 2019 May. Available at: <https://bhw.hrsa.gov/shortage-designation/hpsas>; [Accessed November 2019].

104. Dental Care Health Professionals Shortage Areas (HPSAs). San Francisco, CA: Kaiser Family Foundation; 2019 Sep 30. Available at: <https://www.kff.org/other/state-indicator/dental-care-health-professional-shortage-areas-hpsas/?currentTimeframe=0&sortModel=%7B%22colId%22:%22Total%20Dental%20Care%20HPSA%20Designations%22,%22sort%22:%22desc%22%7D>; [Accessed November 2019].

105. What is a shortage designation? Rockville, MD: Health Resources and Services Administration, Health Workforce; 2019 Aug. Available at: <https://bhw.hrsa.gov/shortage-designation/what-is-shortage-designation>; [Accessed November 2019].

106. Swift JQ. Statement of the American Dental Education Association (ADEA), Presented before the U.S. Senate Committee on Health Education Labor and Pensions Hearing "Addressing Health Care Workforce Issues." Washington, DC: American Dental Education Association; 2008. Available at: <https://www.help.senate.gov/imo/media/doc/Swift.pdf>; [Accessed November 2019].

107. 39 percent of U.S. dentists participate in Medicaid or CHIP for child dental services. ADA News; 2018 Mar 14. ADA Health Policy Institute. Available at: <https://www.ada.org/en/publications/ada-news/2018-archive/march/more-than-a-third-of-all-us-dentists-participate-in-medicaid-or-chip-for-child-dental-services>; [Accessed March 2020].

108. Koppelman J, Singer-Cohen R. A workforce strategy for reducing oral health disparities: Dental therapists. Am J Public Health; 2017;107(S1):S13-17. Available at: <https://www.ncbi.nlm.nih.gov/pmc/articles/PMC5497880/>; [Accessed December 2019].

109. Reimbursement. Chicago, IL: American Dental Hygienists' Association. Available at: <https://www.adha.org/reimbursement>; [Accessed November 2019].

110. State Oral Health Program Infrastructure and Capacity Policy Statement. Reno, NV: Association of State and Territorial Dental Directors; 2013 May 17. Available at: <https://www.astdd.org/docs/sohp-infrastructure-and-capacity-policy-statement-may-17-2013.pdf>; [Accessed November 2019].

111. Development of a New Dental Hygiene Professional Practice Index by State. Oral Health Workforce Research Center; 2016. Available at: <http://www.oralhealthworkforce.org/wp-content/uploads/2018/02/OHWRC_Dental_Hygiene_Scope_of_Practice_2016.pdf>; [Accessed December 2019].

112. Modern Immigration Wave Brings 59 Million to U.S., Driving Population Growth and Change Through 2065. Washington, DC: Pew Research Center; 2015 Sep 28. Available at: <https://www.pewresearch.org/hispanic/2015/09/28/modern-immigration-wave-brings-59-million-to-u-s-driving-population-growth-and-change-through-2065/>; [Accessed December 2019].

113. Guidelines for State and Territorial Oral Health Programs Part I. Reno, NV: Association of State and Territorial Dental Directors; 2015 Dec. Available at: <https://www.astdd.org/docs/astdd-guidelines-part-I-2015-update-january-2016.pdf>; [Accessed October 2019].

114. Guidelines for State and Territorial Oral Health Programs Part II. Reno, NV: Association of State and Territorial Dental Directors; 2018 Jan. Available at: <https://www.astdd.org/docs/astdd-guidelines-section-II-matrix-for-state-roles-examples-and-resources-1-2018-revisions.pdf>; [Accessed October 2019].

115. Competencies for State Oral Health Programs. Reno, NV: Association of State and Territorial Dental Directors; 2020. Available at: <https://www.astdd.org/docs/competencies-and-levels-for-state-oral-health-programs-2020.pdf>; [Accessed May 2020].

116. Public Health Agency Structure, Organization and Accreditation. The Network for Public Health Law. Available at: <https://www.networkforphl.org/resources/topics__resources/public_health_agency_structure_organization_and_accreditation/>; [Accessed October 2019].

117. State Oral Health Programs. Reno, NV: Association of State and Territorial Dental Directors. Available at: <https://www.astdd.org/state-programs>; [Accessed November 2019].

118. Summary Report: 2019 Synopses of State Dental Public Health Programs: Data for FY 2017-2018. Reno, NV: Association of State and Territorial Dental Directors; 2019. Available at: <https://www.astdd.org/docs/synopses-summary-report-2019.pdf>; [Accessed October 2019].

119. State Oral Health Infrastructure and Capacity: Reflecting on Progress and Charting the Future: State Oral Health Program (SOHP) Infrastructure Elements. Reno, NV: Association of State and Territorial Dental Directors; 2012. Available at: <http://www.astdd.org/docs/infrastructure-enhancement-project-feb-2012.pdf>; [Accessed December 2019].

120. The State of Children's Dental Health: Making Coverage Matter. Pew Children's Dental Campaign. Philadelphia, PA: Pew Charitable Trusts; 2011. Available at: <http://www.pewtrusts.org/~/media/legacy/uploadedfiles/wwwpewtrustsorg/reports/state_policy/ChildrensDental50StateReport2011pdf.pdf>; [Accessed November 2019].

121. Best Practice Approach: Developing Workforce Capacity in State Oral Health Programs. Reno, NV: Association of State and Territorial Dental Directors; 2016 Jan. Available at: <https://www.astdd.org/bestpractices/bpa-developing-workforce-capacity-2016-01.pdf>; [Accessed November 2019].

122. Department of Health and Human Services Oral Health Coordinating Committee. U.S. Department of Health and Human Services Oral Health Strategic Framework, 2014-2017. Public Health Rep 2016;131(2):242-257. Available at: <https://www.ncbi.nlm.nih.gov/pmc/articles/PMC4765973/>; [Accessed November 2019].

123. Health Center Program. Rockville, MD: Health and Resources Administration, Bureau of Primary Health Care. Available at: <https://bphc.hrsa.gov/>; [Accessed November 2019].

124. Start-Up Resources Toolkit. Denver, CO: National Network for Oral Health Access; 2016 Mar 1. Available at: <http://www.nnoha.org/nnoha-content/uploads/2016/03/NNOHA-OH-Start-Up-Resources-Toolkit-revised-3-2016.pdf>; [Accessed November 2016].

125. Crall JJ, Pourat N, Inkelas M, Lampron C, Scoville R. Improving the oral health care capacity of federally qualified health centers. Health Aff 2016; 35(12)e. Available at: <https://www.healthaffairs.org/doi/10.1377/hlthaff.2016.0880>; [Accessed November 2019].

126. National Advisory Committee on Rural Health and Human Services. Improving Oral Health Care Services in Rural America. Washington, DC: Department of Health and Human Services; 2018 Dec. Available at: <https://www.hrsa.gov/sites/default/files/hrsa/advisory-committees/rural/publications/2018-Oral-Health-Policy-Brief.pdf>; [Accessed October 2019].

127. Facts About Teledentistry. Boston, MA: American TeleDentistry Association; 2019. Available at: <https://www.americanteledentistry.org/>; [Accessed October 2019].

128. Moore TA, Rover J. Advantages of teledentistry technologies. Decisions in Dent e;2017 Nov 8. Available at: <https://decisionsindentistry.com/article/advantages-teledentistry-technologies/>; [Accessed October 2019].

129. White Paper Teledentistry: How Technology Can Facilitate Access to Care. Reno, NV: Association of State and Territorial Dental Directors; 2019 Mar. Available at: <https://www.astdd.org/docs/teledentistry-how-technology-can-facilitate-access-to-care-3-4-19.pdf>; [Accessed October 2019].

130. Case Studies of 6 Teledentistry Programs: Strategies to Increase Access to General and Specialty Dental Services. Rensselaer, NY: State University of New York, University of Albany, School of Public Health, Center for Health Workforce Studies; 2016 Dec. Available at: <http://www.oralhealthworkforce.org/wp-content/uploads/2017/02/OHWRC_Case_Studies_of_6_Teledentistry_Programs_2016.pdf>; [Accessed October 2019].

131. D9995 and D9996 – ADA Guide to Understanding and Documenting Teledentistry Events – Version 2. Chicago, IL: American Dental Association; 2020 Mar 27. Available at: <https://www.ada.org/~/media/ADA/Publications/Files/CDT_D9995D9996-GuideTo_v1_2017Jul17.pdf?la=en>; [Accessed July 2020].

132. Glassman P. Expanding Oral Health: Teledentistry. San Francisco, CA: University of the Pacific; 2019 Aug. Available at: <https://www.dentaquestpartnership.org/system/files/DQ_Whitepaper_Teledentistry%20%289.19%29.pdf>; [Accessed November 2019].

133. Howatt G. 'Teledentistry' expands preventive care to more Minnesota families. Minneapolis, MN: Star Tribune; 2018 Oct 8. Available at: <http://www.startribune.com/teledentistry-expands-preventive-care-to-more-minnesota-families/496043791/>; [Accessed October 2019].

134. Chait N, Glied S. Promoting prevention under the Affordable Care Act. Annu Rev Public Health 2018 Apr 1;39:507-524. Available at: <https://www.annualreviews.org/doi/10.1146/annurev-publhealth-040617-013534>; [Accessed November 2019].

135. How the Affordable Care Act moved oral health forward. Teeth Matter Blog. Washington, DC: Children's Dental Health Project; 2018 Mar 23. Available at: <https://www.cdhp.org/blog/502-how-the-affordable-care-act-moved-oral-health-forward>; [Accessed November 2019].

ADDITIONAL RESOURCES

Centers for Disease Control and Prevention (Oral Health)
https://www.cdc.gov/oralhealth/index.html
Data Hub, World Dental Federation
https://www.fdiworlddental.org/oral-health/statistics/data-hub
Oral Health Programs, CDC
https://www.cdc.gov/oralhealth/funded_programs/index.htm
PEW Project Dental Campaign
https://www.pewtrusts.org/en/projects/dental-campaign
State Oral Health Infrastructure, ASTDD
https://www.astdd.org/state-oral-health-program-structure/
The Dental Safety Net and Access to Oral Health (Webinar), American Dental Education Association (YouTube video)
https://www.youtube.com/watch?v=FWLxRsJEqEI

6

Oral Health Programs in the Community

Charlene B. Dickinson, Christine French Beatty, Amanda M. Hinson-Enslin

OBJECTIVES

1. Describe oral health programs at the national, state, and local levels that have the purpose of improving oral health in the community.
2. Describe the five steps of the community program planning process that are necessary to organize an effective community oral health program.
3. Explain how program goals and objectives are used in program planning, implementation, and evaluation; develop specific, measurable objectives for community oral health programs using SMART + C objectives.
4. Explain water fluoridation in terms of its history, effectiveness, mechanisms of action, safety, recommendations, cost, optimal level, and approaches recommended for a fluoridation campaign to be able to defeat antifluoridationists.

5. Discuss the benefits of primary prevention programs, including various fluoride modalities, sealants, and oral health education, and recommendations for conducting these programs.
6. Describe the goals, mission, and oral health component of Head Start (HS), and explain the potential for the dental hygienist in a HS program.
7. Discuss secondary and tertiary preventive oral health programs.
8. Identify the various funding streams, programs, initiatives, and structures to finance oral health services through public health systems.

OPENING STATEMENTS

- Dental caries is a chronic transmissible disease that can be prevented.
- School-based dental sealant programs have been shown to reduce dental caries by up to 60%.
- Fluoride varnish applied every 6 months is effective in preventing dental caries in primary and permanent teeth of children and adolescents who are at moderate to high risk for caries.
- Integrating oral health into school-based health programs increases access to care for this population.
- Water fluoridation decreases tooth decay by about 27%.
- HS programs provide the opportunity for oral health programs and establishment of dental homes for young children.
- By 2050 there will be 89 million older adults in America, requiring greater coordination of oral health services and programs for this population.
- The increasing complexity of public financing of oral health care is enhancing opportunities for community oral health programs.

IMPROVING ORAL HEALTH IN THE COMMUNITY

The mission of public health is accomplished through oral health programs in the community. The social impact of oral diseases in specific population groups is substantial and can present a significant financial burden.[1] Results of untreated oral diseases include lost productivity, loss of wages, increased healthcare

costs, decreased quality of life, and decreased learning among school-age children because of oral health–related absences and inability to attend to learning. In some cases, even death can stem from untreated oral diseases such as tooth decay.[1]

Community oral health programs extend the dental hygienist's role from the traditional private practice to the community as a whole. This chapter discusses community oral health programs as opportunities to address the prevention of oral diseases and problems of access to oral health care for various population groups. Community oral health programs should emphasize current *Healthy People* national health objectives and leading health indicators (see Chapter 4) and reflect the **best practice approach**[2,3] (Box 6.1).

NATIONAL, STATE, AND LOCAL PROGRAMS: ROLE OF THE HEALTH DEPARTMENT

National Level

National, state, and local dental public health programs in the U.S. have similar roles but widely varying organizational schemes. Several federal government programs are involved in oral health promotion and disease prevention (see Figure 1.2 and Box 1.2 in Chapter 1). As the largest grant-making agency in the federal government for health and human service programs,

BOX 6.1 Definition and Rationale for the Best Practice Approach

Definition: "a public health strategy that is supported by evidence for its impact and effectiveness. Evidence includes research, expert opinion, field lessons, and theoretical rationale."

- Applied to oral health programs by the Association of State and Territorial Dental Directors, Centers for Disease Control and Prevention, and other public health organizations and agencies.
- Promotes health equity and quality of life and improves opportunities to eliminate oral health disparities and achieve improved oral health and overall health for the population.
- Increases the chances of accomplishing health goals such as *Healthy People* objectives and other national recommendations such as those presented in Chapter 1.

(From Best Practice Approaches. Association of State and Territorial Dental Directors. Available at: <https://www.astdd.org/best-practices/>; [Accessed November 2019].)

the Department of Health and Human Services (DHHS) works with state and local governments to fund services at the local level through state or county agencies, nonprofit organizations, educational institutions, and private sector grantees.[4] The DHHS also provides regulatory oversight and monitoring of the grantees' expenditures.[4] The President's 2020 budget proposed $87.1 billion in discretionary funds and $1.2 trillion in mandatory funding for DHHS to support their mission to improve American health care and healthcare issues.[4]

State Level

State oral health programs (SOHPs) exist in all states as a major source of planning, funding, implementing, and coordinating of oral health promotion programs for the states' residents.[5] SOHPs vary in their scope of services, programs, and organization across the U.S.[5] Table 6.1 provides information on the percent of SOHPs that offered specific oral health services during 2017–2018. These programs are operated in a variety of settings such as public and private schools; Head Start centers; **Women, Infants, and Children Special Supplemental Nutrition Program (WIC)** programs; county and city health departments; and community-based, faith-based, and civic organizations.[5] Programs are frequently provided in partnership with other agencies and organizations such as dental and dental hygiene schools and non-profit organizations.

SOHPs are funded by state general revenues and national sources of funding from various DHHS operating divisions and offices. Detailed information on federal initiatives that fund SOHPs and other community programs is presented later in this chapter. SOHPs make an essential contribution to public health and must be continued and enhanced.[5] (Refer to Chapters 4 and 5 for additional information about SOHPs.)

TABLE 6.1 Percent of State Oral Health Programs That Offer Specific Oral Health Services, 2017–2018[a]

Program	Has Program	No Program	Not Reported or No State Oral Health Program
Access to Care Program	54.9%	39.2%	5.9%
Dental Screening Program	64.7%	29.4%	5.9%
Fluoride Mouthrinse Program	23.5%	70.6%	5.9%
Fluoride Varnish Program	72.5%	21.6%	5.9%
Silver Diamine Fluoride Program	3.9%	90.2%	5.9%
Oral Health Literacy/Education Program	68.6%	25.5%	5.9%
Basic Screening Surveys			
Head Start	23.5%	70.6%	5.9%
Kindergarten	13.7%	80.4%	5.9%
Third Grade	41.2%	52.9%	5.9%
Older Adults	15.7%	78.4%	5.9%
Programs for Preschool Children	49.0%	45.1%	5.9%
Programs for Elementary School Children	58.8%	33.3%	7.8%
Programs for Adolescents	39.2%	54.9%	5.9%
Programs for Pregnant Women	52.9%	37.3%	9.8%
Programs for Adults 18–64 Years	13.7%	80.4%	5.9%
Programs for Older Adults	25.5%	68.6%	5.9%
Programs for Children with Special Healthcare Needs	31.4%	62.7%	5.9%
Craniofacial Recording System	74.5%	17.6%	7.8%
Craniofacial Referral System	60.8%	31.4%	7.8%

[a]Includes all states and the District of Columbia.

(From Summary Report: 2019 Synopses of State Dental Public Health Programs: Data for FY 2017–2018. Association of State and Territorial Dental Directors; 2019. Available at: <https://www.astdd.org/docs/synopses-summary-report-2019.pdf>; [Accessed October 2019].)

- Smile Survey—surveillance system of statewide screenings for children every 5 years to assess their oral health status and identify gaps in access to oral health care
- Development of preventive programs such as school-based sealants, fluoride varnish, and oral health education based on ongoing assessment results
- Development of the *Washington State Collaborative Oral Health Improvement Plan 2009-2014* with comprehensive input from key partners and stakeholders, the public, and all health professions, which established guiding principles and defined strategic areas, goals, and objectives to reflect *Healthy People* oral health objectives
- Publication of *Assessing the Impact of Washington State's Oral Health Workforce on Patient Access to Care* in 2017 to report results of state's oral health workforce and patient access to oral care study; describes challenges and potential opportunities to improve access

(From Washington State Oral Health Data. Washington State Department of Health. Available at: <https://www.doh.wa.gov/DataandStatisticalReports/DiseasesandChronicConditions/OralHealth>; [Accessed November 2019].)

Role of Essential Public Health Services to Promote Oral Health

As discussed in Chapter 1, the core public health functions and essential public health services to promote oral health developed by the Association of State and Territorial Dental Directors (ASTDD; see Box 1.5 and Table 1.3) shape the basic practice of dental public health.[6] The ASTDD has also identified roles of and competencies for SOHPs in line with the essential services that serve as guidelines in carrying out SOHP activities to meet the essential services, and has provided examples of activities for the various roles.[6] See the References and Additional Resources at the end of this chapter and Chapter 4 for these and other resources to assist with these activities.

Many states have developed programs that include the essential services for oral health. Some examples for the state of Washington are provided in Box 6.2 to assist the reader with understanding the role of SOHPs in the dental public health arena.

Role of Oral Health Coalitions

According to the ASTDD *State Oral Health Coalitions and Collaborative Partnerships* best-practice-approach report, SOHPs depend on oral health **coalitions** and community advocates to implement and promote comprehensive oral health services in the state and local communities.[2] See Box 6.3 for the important role of coalitions in the work of a SOHP. An effective SOHP collaborates with one or more broad-based coalitions that include partners with fiscal and political clout.[5]

An example is the Wisconsin Oral Health Coalition (WOHC) developed through the Children's Health Alliance of Wisconsin.[7] The WOHC is a collaboration of more than 200 diverse individuals, organizations, and agencies addressing oral health access issues and working to improve oral health statewide.[7] Programs operated by the WOHC are presented in Box 6.4.

- Provide an avenue for recruiting participants from diverse constituencies, such as political, business, human services, social and religious groups; grassroots groups; and individuals.
- Exploit new resources in changing situations to expand the potential scope and range of services that can be achieved.
- Demonstrate and develop widespread public support for issues, actions, or unmet needs.
- Maximize the power of individuals and groups through joint action, increasing the "critical mass" behind a community effort, providing a comprehensive approach to programming, and enhancing competence and clout in advocacy and resource development.
- Enable organizations to become involved in new and broader issues without having the sole responsibility for managing or developing those issues.
- Minimize duplication of services and fill gaps in service delivery while improving trust and communication among groups that would normally compete with one another.
- Mobilize more talents, resources, and approaches to accomplish what single members cannot.

(Modified from State Oral Health Coalitions and Collaborative Partnerships. Best Practice Approaches for State and Community Oral Health Programs. Reno, NV: Association of State and Territorial Dental Directors; May 2011. Available at: <http://www.astdd.org/bestpractices-opastatecoalitions.pdf>; [Accessed November 2019].)

Seal-A-Smile Program
- A collaborative effort between the Children's Health Alliance of Wisconsin, Wisconsin Department of Health Services, and Delta Dental of Wisconsin.
- Program mission: to improve the oral health of Wisconsin children by providing school-based dental sealants.
- Grantees include dentists, dental hygienists, schools, hospitals, local health departments, community health centers, nonprofit agencies, and free clinics.

Healthy Smiles for Mom and Baby
- Funded in part by the Health Resources and Services Administration.
- Statewide program to integrate oral health into prenatal and pediatric healthcare systems.
- Provides online oral health training for professionals working with pregnant women, infants, and toddlers that combines oral health information with conversation techniques for effective family-centered oral health discussions.

Wisconsin Medical Dental Integration Project
- An interprofessional collaboration funded in part by Advancing a Healthier Wisconsin at the Medical College of Wisconsin and the Delta Dental of Wisconsin Foundation.
- Focus on integrating dental hygienists into medical teams to increase the utilization of dental services for children ages birth to 5 years.

(From Wisconsin Oral Health Coalition. Children's Health Alliance of Wisconsin. Available at <https://www.chawisconsin.org/initiatives/oral-health/wisconsin-medical-dental-integration/>; [Accessed October 2019].)

The ASTDD best-practice-approach report emphasizes the importance of coalitions as a public health approach, has assessed their effectiveness, and has provided examples of coalition practices to illustrate successful, innovative implementation

TABLE 6.2   Percentage of States with Local Health Departments Offering Preventive Oral Health, Restorative Dental Services, and Oral Health Education Programs[a]

Program	States With Program	States Without Program	States Not Reporting
Preventive (e.g., sealants, fluoride)	53%	29%	18%
Restorative	51%	33%	16%
Education Only	33%	49%	18%

[a]Includes all states and the District of Columbia

(From Summary Report: 2019 Synopses of State Dental Public Health Programs: Data for FY 2017–2018. Association of State and Territorial Dental Directors; 2019. Available at <https://www.astdd.org/docs/synopses-summary-report-2019.pdf>; [Accessed October 2019].)

of coalition strategies.[2] This report can be used by oral health professionals to enhance the work of oral health coalitions. (See the Collaboration in Public Health Practice section of Chapter 3 for information on the formation of a coalition.)

Local Level

Local programs also carry out public health activities reflected in the core public health functions and essential public health services, with assistance from SOHPs through consultation and funding. ASTDD guidelines and other resources also serve to guide local programs[6,8]

Individual county and city health departments across the nation have recognized the need within their communities to provide oral health services to various members of their populations. These services can be offered at local clinics or through school-based or mobile programs. Presented in Table 6.2 is the percentage of states with local health departments offering oral health education, preventive services, and restorative dental services programs. It is noteworthy that in many states no preventive or restorative services programs are offered by local health departments, and in a similar number of states only oral health education programs are offered by local health departments.

Many local health department dental clinics are federally funded, offering services on a sliding scale fee schedule and accepting clients who receive public assistance through Medicaid. Hours of clinic operation are tailored to best meet the needs of the population they serve. The clinics provide diagnostic, preventive, and restorative oral health services to older adults, the indigent population, and the working poor. In addition, some of these clinics operate sealant, oral health education, and other preventive programs in local schools.

Nonprofit and faith-based organizations also establish community-based clinics that are funded through a variety of sources, including government, United Way, and foundation grants; local community organizations; donations; sale of goods and services; special events; fundraisers; and other sources. These clinics employ oral health professionals and sometimes have supplemental clinical coverage provided by local volunteer dental professionals. Such community-based dental clinics can be part of a comprehensive health center or free-standing community oral health program. Two examples are described here.

Future Smiles of Northern Nevada

An example of a local program is Future Smiles of Northern Nevada (FSNN), a nonprofit school-based oral health program that serves an underserved, vulnerable population. The program is funded by grants and donations and is supported by various community organizations, including county alliances, local federally qualified health centers, a community-based health and wellness hub, the nearby dental hygiene program, and two county school districts. With start-up grant funding in 2017, FSNN was able to purchase mobile equipment and hire two part-time staff.[9]

FSNN provides oral health education, disease prevention, preventive services, and follow-up case management to families.[9] In the first year of operation, the FSNN team provided over $35,000 in dental hygiene primary preventive services. Oral health education was provided to 4106 students, and 635 sealants and 249 fluoride varnish treatments were applied.[9]

Nevada ranks among the last in the nation with respect to oral health, and one mission of the program is to "bring critical preventive services to children who need it the most."[9] FSNN is operating in two counties, including one rural county classified as a 100% dental health professional shortage area.[9] The program is serving all grade levels at 10 high-risk schools within an 85-mile radius. Schools participating in this program have 56% to 88% of students receiving free or reduced-cost lunches through the **National School Lunch Program**.[9] The number of children in a school that qualify for this program is a standard criterion used to target schools for school-based oral health programs. To be eligible for the school lunch program, children must be from families with incomes at or below 130% of the **federal poverty level** (FPL) for free lunches and between 130% and 185% of the FPL for reduced-price lunches.[10]

Dental Health Arlington

Another example of a local program is Dental Health Arlington (DHA), a nonprofit organization that has operated a dental clinic since 1993, providing dental access for low-income residents of the county.[11] The need for accessible, affordable dental care is addressed by staff and volunteer dentists, dental hygienists, and dental assistants; dental hygiene, dental assisting, dental, and predental students from local programs; and college students providing community service. Routine preventive and comprehensive restorative services are delivered in the clinic at a reduced fee, including dental examinations, x-rays, cleanings, extractions, restorations, and a limited number of dentures, root canals, and crowns. A pro-bono or reduced-fee dental referral program is available for more complex services.

In addition, DHA operates a mobile school-based program in local Title 1 schools, providing oral health education to children in grades 1 through 3, as well as screenings and preventive services to second- and third-grade children.[11] During the 2016–2017 school year, 9941 children in 40 schools were served with classroom oral health education, 3394 children were screened and received fluoride varnish application, and 5558 sealants were placed on 1868 children, for a total value of over $506,000. Children whose screening reveals severe decay and who do not have a dental home are scheduled for treatment in the DHA clinic and then referred to an outside provider if they qualify for Medicaid or the Children's Health Insurance Program (CHIP).[11]

DHA is funded through a variety of sources, including grants from the United Way; Delta Dental; a national faith-based, nonprofit health system; a community development block grant; the local hospital district; the area Agency on Aging; local foundations and philanthropic organizations; in-kind donations from local businesses; individual donations; and fund-raising events such as a casino night and dental continuing education seminars. DHA has received numerous federal, regional, and local awards including the President's Service Award from Points of Light in Washington, DC and recognition from the Pew Partnership, American Dental Association (ADA), the state dental association and oral health coalition, and the local school district.[11]

Local Coalitions

The ASTDD best-practice-approach report also describes the function of coalitions at the regional or community level.[2] These coalitions can be developed through local jurisdictions, hospitals, or other local organizations, and they collaborate with a state coalition to address and support local issues and programs. An example is the Children's Oral Health Coalition (COHC) of Tarrant County, Texas, developed and supported by the Cook Children's Health Care System of Fort Worth Community Health Outreach Department.[12] The COHC collaborates with various community partners to improve the oral health of underserved children in the county.[12] Activities include train-the-trainer programs for community professionals, such as social workers and community workers, that work with underserved pregnant women and parents of young children birth to age 8 years (Figure 6.1); distribution of oral health/oral hygiene kits to low-income children and families through community partners; targeted oral health education programs through local schools that serve children from low-income families; and legislative advocacy for children's oral health issues, including access to care.

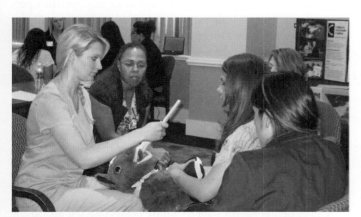

Fig 6.1 A volunteer dental hygienist teaches oral health basics to community professionals who work with underserved pregnant women and mothers of young children. (Courtesy Lisa Englehart.)

Some local coalitions are formed in association with a state coalition to provide focused, community-driven solutions across the state. In Oregon, there are currently 10 established local coalitions, and more are being developed. Expanding the network of local oral health coalitions across the state is one of the Oregon Oral Health Coalition's (OrOHC) strategic goals and was a major focus of 2018.[13] The OrOHC has a Coalition Building Toolkit that can be used by local communities and others interested in developing a coalition.[13]

Another example is a network of local coalitions in Wisconsin under the umbrella of the Midwest Collaborative Initiative and funded by the DentaQuest Foundation.[14] In Nevada, the Northern Nevada Dental Coalition for Underserved Populations works in tandem with its southern Nevada partner, the Community Coalition for Oral Health. Together, they support the State Advisory Committee for Oral Health, which is charged with advising and making recommendations to the Nevada Division of Public and Behavioral Health.[15]

PROGRAM PLANNING PROCESS

With increased emphasis on improving public access to oral health care, the responsibilities of the dental hygienist to promote oral health in communities takes on renewed importance. An organized program planning process is critical to effective community oral health programs.[3,16] Even small programs operated by volunteers and through local dental hygiene societies should have the program planning process applied. Therefore, it is important that the dental hygienist understand the basic concepts and steps involved in planning and conducting oral health programs in communities.

The **program planning process** is a basic model commonly used in public health practice.[17] The model provides a continuous cycle of basic steps to assess, plan, implement, and evaluate a community program, which was expanded as the Community Health Program Planning Process (CHPPP) in Figure 3.7 in Chapter 3. Examining how the steps used in planning and conducting community oral health programs parallels the steps involved in the dental hygiene process of care[18] can facilitate understanding. Although the CHPPP has five steps and the dental hygiene process of care has six steps, they correspond to each other as illustrated in Table 6.3. For example, the community survey conducted to identify the community's primary health issues is comparable to the patient's examination and interview for assessment. In this step, reviewing secondary data in the community setting can be compared with reviewing data previously recorded in a patient's chart or prior radiographs. Critically analyzing community data in this step is similar to using decision-making skills to analyze patient data and reach conclusions about the patient's treatment needs in forming a diagnosis. Developing program goals and objectives and selecting and planning interventions for the community are akin to establishing goals for the patient's treatment outcomes and planning treatment interventions. Implementing the program is equivalent to completing the patient's treatment. Evaluation and review of the program can be compared with evaluating the patient's treatment. A formal report of the program outcomes in the evaluation step of the CHPPP is similar to documentation of patient care and outcomes.

Five Steps of Community Health Program Planning Process	Six Steps of Dental Hygiene (DH) Process of Care
Community Is the Patient	**Individual Is the Patient**
1. Identify the Primary Health Issues	**1. Assessment**
Example: Collection of data via community survey and review of existing data (secondary data previously collected); critical analysis of data to conclude that high rates of tooth decay exist in the community and to identify associated risk factors	Example: Collection of data via review of dental history and previous dental records, patient interview, clinical examination, and radiographs
	2. DH Diagnosis
	Example: Critical analysis of data to conclude an indication for dental hygiene treatment
2. Develop a Measurable Process and Outcome Objectives to Assess Progress in Addressing the Health Issues	**3. Planning**
Example: Precise, measurable objectives set such as: Program will improve oral health; decay rates will be reduced by 20% in 2 years	Example: Establishment of realistic overall patient goals for behavioral outcomes, oral health, and overall health while planning DH interventions to move the patient toward oral health
3. Select and Plan Effective Health Interventions to Achieve Objectives	
Example: Determination that a fluoride varnish program and comprehensive parent education combined are the best interventions for this population group and these specific circumstances	
4. Implement the Selected Health Interventions	**4. Implementation**
Example: Fluoride varnish program and a parent education program conducted for 5 years	Example: Completion of the treatment plan
5. Evaluate the Selected Interventions Based on the Objectives and Use the Information to Improve the Program	**5. Evaluation**
Example: Evaluation of outcome objectives to determine a change in tooth decay rates and risk behaviors addressed in education program; formal report developed to share with stakeholders, including program description, processes, outcomes, and recommendations regarding continuation of the program	Example: Evaluation of treatment processes and outcomes by collecting and evaluating data to modify treatment as needed and to determine follow-up
	6. Documentation
	Example: Recording of assessment findings, treatment planned and delivered, patient communication, treatment outcomes, and recommendations

TABLE 6.3 Comparison of the Community Health Program Planning Process to the Dental Hygiene Process of Care for Individual Patients

Identify the Primary Health Issues

A community is comprised of numerous people, each with a unique personality, personal issues, values, beliefs, and health status. Even so, communities have similar health conditions that are caused by similar factors in the community such as social norms, culture, beliefs, and access to oral health care.[3,16] Systematically analyzing these factors and information leads to identifying the primary oral health issues of the specific community and the causes of any existing oral health inequities. This is accomplished through **assessment**, which is an organized and systematic approach to defining and describing a priority group, determining the extent and severity of oral health needs present, identifying the factors present in the community that are associated with the oral health status, and prioritizing the needs that are identified.

Assessing the relative importance of needs can be a complex process and leads to the establishment of priorities. Key questions are used to establish health priorities (see Guiding Principles). The assessment process is explained in more detail in Chapter 3.

GUIDING PRINCIPLES
Establishing Health Priorities

- What is the magnitude of the problem (does it cause death or disability)?
- How many people are affected (single person, small community, or entire country)?
- What types of resources are available (personnel, money, facilities, and technology)?
- What has already been done in the community?
- What are the prevailing attitudes toward the problem?
- Which groups are expressing the most interest in the problem?
- What are the legal constraints?

Compounding the problem of prioritizing health needs is the fact that each community is unique, with its own values and beliefs. If a community's basic needs for food and security are not being met, dental needs become a low priority. An issue that often arises is the belief that if a community's perception of needs is adhered to exclusively, actual clinical health problems may go untreated because the people are not knowledgeable about many areas of health care. The solution to this dilemma involves striking a delicate balance between negligence and overzealousness. Although it is unethical to impose one's perceptions on a community, it is the professional's responsibility to inform others of existing problems and their consequences.[3,16]

A community needs assessment can identify problems related to oral health status, and access to and utilization of dental care. The assessment also provides information about the community itself and the **priority populations** within the community. During the needs assessment, it is essential to involve the community and to form collaborations with community partners (see Chapter 3) to gain support from the community and maximize the use of community resources. The data collected can be used to develop a **community profile** that will assist in identifying appropriate solutions (see Chapter 3).

Use of dental survey data that have been collected previously by other organizations (secondary data) can make the assessment process easier. For example, dental surveys are conducted

BOX 6.5 Goals and Objectives for Program Planning

Goals

- Broadly based ambitious statements of the impact of an intervention, from which specific objectives are developed.
- Example: Improve the oral health of school-age children in the community.

Objectives

- Describe in a specific, measurable way the desired end results of program activities, aligned with overarching program goals.
- Clearly communicate expected outcomes of a program, achieved by careful construction.
- Can be constructed by using a format such as SMART or the expanded version of **SMART + C objectives** (see Box 6.6 for common characteristics and Box 6.7 for examples that illustrate the characteristics).
- Must have action verbs that communicate specific, measurable activities and outcomes (Box 6.8); verbs such as *understand, value,* or *learn* broadly describe outcomes and do not represent actions that can be measured, resulting in nonspecific, unmeasurable objectives.
- Must be both achievable and challenging, accomplished by basing them on baseline data.

Levels of Objectives

Process objectives: Actionable statements that describe activities, services, and strategies that will be delivered as part of implementing a program; usually short-term.

Outcome objectives: Statements of specific intended effects of a program or the priority population; the end result of a program; focused on a change in the priority population(s) such as a change in health status, knowledge, or ability as a result of the program or activity; can be short-term, intermediate, or long-term, thus expected to be measured after the program is or has been in place.

See Figure 6.2 for an illustration of the different levels of objectives.

Categories of Outcome Objectives

Learning objectives (also called instructional objectives): Explain what program participants will learn as a result of an educational program; communicate what the learner should be able to *do* to successfully demonstrate achievement of the objective, indicating that learning has occurred; can address the different learning domains (cognitive, psychomotor, and affective) while focusing on expected changes in the learner's awareness, knowledge, attitudes, and skills.

Behavioral objectives: Describe what actions program participants will take to improve or resolve the health issue; reflect changes in health behaviors

Environmental objectives: Explain how emotional, physical, and social surroundings of a community will change after a program is implemented

See Figure 6.2 for an illustration of the categories of outcome objectives.

Examples of Different Time Frames of Objectives

- *Short-term:* Two weeks following the completion of the infrastructure at the water treatment plant, the water fluoride (F) level will consistently be 0.7 mg F per liter of water
- *Intermediate-term:* Nine months after the school campaign, 50% of parents will report supplying their children with tap water rather than bottled water.
- *Long-term:* Three years after the seminar, 20% of parent-teacher association members will be able to identify three mechanisms of action of fluoride in relation to water fluoridation.

(From Community Tool Box. Work Group for Community Health and Development, University of Kansas; 2019. Available at: <https://ctb.ku.edu/en>; Accessed October 2019; McKenzie JF, Neiger BL, Thackeray R. Planning, Implementing & Evaluating: Health Promotion Programs: A Primer, 7th ed. Glenview, IL: Pearson Education; 2017; Developing Program Goals and Measurable Objectives. Centers for Disease Control and Prevention. Available at: <https://www.cdc.gov/std/Program/pupestd/Developing%20Program%20Goals%20and%20Objectives.pdf>; [Accessed August 2019]; ISD: Writing Performance Objectives. U.S. Department of Agriculture. Available at: <https://www.nrcs.usda.gov/wps/portal/nrcs/detail/national/nedc/?cid=stelprdb1185746>; [Accessed August 2019].)

by professionals at dental schools, local and state health departments, and community health centers. Collaboration with other agencies and organizations to learn what data are available can prevent duplication of services.[3,16] Data can be obtained and analyzed by various methods. (See Chapter 3 and Appendixes C and D for further information about needs assessment.)

Develop a Measurable Process and Outcome Objectives to Assess Progress in Addressing the Health Issues

After the needs are assessed and prioritized, the **planning** of oral health programs can begin. Planning is an organized response to the community's needs to reduce or eliminate one or more problems identified during the assessment. The first step of planning is to develop appropriate **goals** and **objectives**.[5,16] Formulating program goals and objectives offers specific proposals for changes to be made in the community. These changes address the specific problems identified in the needs assessment. Just like with assessment, it is essential to have community involvement and participation during this step.[3,16]

Goals and Objectives

Developing goals and objectives is critical in effective community program planning. Goals and objectives clarify the desired outcomes of a community health program. Without them, it

BOX 6.6 Characteristics of a SMART + C Objective

- **S**pecific, telling *how much* (e.g., 40%) of *what* is to be achieved (e.g., what behavior or outcome) by *whom* (e.g., individuals that will achieve it), *where* it will be achieved (e.g., community or priority group), and by *when* (e.g., 2022).
- **M**easurable, meaning that information concerning the objective potentially can be collected, detected, or obtained from records.
- **A**chievable in the sense that the objective is possible and the organization, agency, community, or priority group is capable of attaining it.
- **R**elevant to the overall vision and mission of the organization, program, community, or priority group.
- **T**ime-bound, indicated by a target date or timeframe by which the objective will be achieved.
- **C**hallenging, meaning it stretches the group to focus on a significant improvement that is important for the community.

is difficult to plan health interventions and activities that can result in desired outcomes. Also, proceeding without goals and objectives makes measurement of program success impossible. It is important to be able to measure success to justify continuation of a program. See Boxes 6.5, 6.6, 6.7, and 6.8 and Figure 6.2 for definitions, explanations, and examples of goals and objectives, the levels and categories of objectives, and instructions for developing effective objectives.

BOX 6.7   Examples of SMART + C Objectives

Goal:
To promote the use of fluoride mouthrinses

Objective 1:
Upon completion of today's six-step demonstration, 75% of the adolescent participants will demonstrate the six steps without error (compared with 20% baseline before the program) by rinsing at a sink in the classroom.

Action Verb:
Demonstrate

SMART + C Characteristics:
- **Specific:** The specifics are *who* will be evaluated (the adolescent participants), *what* will be evaluated (demonstrating the six steps), *how well* they must perform the action to demonstrate achievement (75% will perform the skill without error), *where* they will perform the action (at the sink in the classroom), and *when* they must perform it (after the demonstration and practice).
- **Measurable:** 75% of the participants will have to successfully demonstrate all six steps without error; there are baseline data available for comparison.
- **Achievable:** There is a margin of error in that 25% can make errors, and it is based on the activity that will teach them the procedure.
- **Realistic:** It is realistic because it aligns with the goal, reflects a realistic number of participants to complete the task compared with the baseline, and the participants have the necessary foundational abilities and maturity to perform the skill.
- **Time oriented:** It will be measured after the demonstration on the same day.
- **Challenging:** Given that only 20% of the participants were familiar with the correct process of rinsing before the program, it provides a challenge for 75% of them to demonstrate all six steps without error.

Objective 2:
One week following implementation of the program, 30% of adolescent participants will self-report that they are rinsing twice a day at home (compared with 10% doing so before the program) with a fluoride mouthrinse that will be provided to them.

Action Verb:
Will self-report

SMART + C Characteristics:
- **Specific:** It is specific *who* will provide the self-report (adolescent participants), *what* will be evaluated (self-report of using a fluoride mouthrinse), *how much* they must perform the expected action (twice a day rinsing), *where* they will perform it (rinse at home), and *when* it will be evaluated (1 week following the program).
- **Measurable:** 30% of the adolescent participants will report that they are using a mouthrinse two times a day, and there are baseline data available for comparison.
- **Achievable:** Participants have the skills and supplies to comply based on the program.
- **Realistic:** Although it reflects an increase in compliance, not all participants are expected to comply; it reflects a realistic number of participants achieving the objective.
- **Time oriented:** It is time oriented because the program objective will be achieved by measuring compliance 1 week following completion of the program.
- **Challenging:** Given that the participants are adolescents, it might be a challenge to increase their compliance of using mouthrinse two times a day from 10% to 30%.

BOX 6.8   Sample Performance Verbs Appropriate for Writing Objectives

Adjust	Describe	Interpret	Rank
Adopt	Design	Integrate	Rate
Analyze	Develop	Invent	Recognize
Apply	Diagnose	Join	Record
Arrange	Differentiate	Keep	Reduce
Assemble	Discuss	Label	Repeat
Attempt	Distinguish	List	Report
Brush	Estimate	Locate	Scale
Calculate	Examine	Map	Schedule
Categorize	Explain	Match	Select
Characterize	Express	Measure	Show
Choose	Find	Modify	Solve
Classify	Floss	Observe	Sort
Compare	Follow	Organize	Spell
Conclude	Form	Palpate	State
Contrast	Gather	Perform	Summarize
Copy	Group	Plan	Support
Count	Hypothesize	Practice	Test
Create	Identify	Predict	Try
Debate	Illustrate	Prepare	Unite
Define	Implement	Produce	Weigh
Demonstrate	Increase	Prove	Write

Select and Plan Effective Health Interventions to Achieve Objectives

Planning is a crucial element to a successful program. A community oral health program that is well planned, with specific evidence-based interventions, strategies, and activities, and consideration given to resources and constraints, is more likely to be successfully implemented and result in desired program outcomes. When the primary oral health issues have been identified

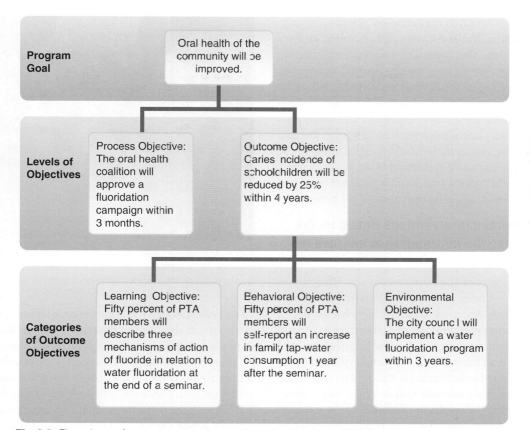

Fig 6.2 Flowchart of program planning goals and objectives. *PTA*, Parent-teacher association.

and program goals and objectives have been established with a description of the desired program outcomes, the next step is to select and plan interventions to bring about the desired results.[3,16]

This area of program planning describes how the objectives will be accomplished. An intervention or activity is selected based on best practices, established by scientific evidence of effectiveness. (Review the best-practice-approach discussion earlier in this chapter and Chapter 7 for a discussion of scientific evidence.) Community involvement and participation are also essential during this step.[3,16]

In planning these program activities, one must carefully consider the types of resources available, as well as program constraints. For example, in planning a school-based fluoride varnish program, available resources might include (1) the site at which the program will be conducted, (2) supportive personnel at the site, (3) supplies on hand, and (4) an industry sales representative willing to donate supplies. Constraints might include (1) need for dental personnel to conduct screenings and apply fluoride varnish, (2) negative attitudes of some parents, (3) the amount of time children are out of the classroom, or (4) lack of funding for additional costs. Additional information and details on the development of strategies for oral health programs and for oral health promotion are presented later in this chapter and in Chapters 8 and 11.

Implement the Selected Health Interventions

The **implementation** phase of a program includes the ongoing process of putting the plan into action and monitoring the plan's activities, personnel, equipment, resources, and supplies.[3,16] An

implementation strategy should be developed that answers the questions in Box 6.9.[3,16]

Feedback from personnel and participants, as well as ongoing evaluation mechanisms, should be included during the implementation to ensure effectiveness of program processes. **Formative evaluation** (sometimes referred to as process evaluation), is the type of evaluation that provides an internal assessment of a program and examines the processes, procedures, or activities of a program as they are taking place either before or early during the implementation of the program.[3] The purpose of formative evaluation is to identify problems and solutions to

---

BOX 6.9   Questions to Be Answered During Implementation Strategy Development

Question: Why?
What is the potential effect of the initiative on the oral health problem?

Question: What?
What activities are required to achieve the objective?

Question: Who?
Who is responsible for each action step of an activity or initiative?

Question: When?
What is the necessary chronological sequence of action steps?

Question: How?
What materials, media, methods, techniques, etc., are needed?

Question: How much?
What is the cost estimate of materials and time?

assist in revising the program as needed, even as it is being conducted. Implementation, like assessment and planning, involves individuals, agencies, and the community working together.

For ease in addressing these questions, many community oral health programs begin on a small scale. Using a smaller population with the intent to expand later is called **pilot testing**. For example, a pilot test for a school-based dental sealant program could involve only one school the first year with the goal of expanding the program to include additional schools in the future. This allows for formative evaluation of the program operation, makes it easier to control and monitor program activities, and enables decision-making about the future of the program.[3]

Evaluate the Selected Interventions Based on the Objectives and Use the Information to Improve the Program

Evaluation is a judgment of the effectiveness and efficiency of the program after it has been in operation. Referred to as **summative evaluation,** it is designed to determine whether a fully operational program has met the goals and objectives developed during the early planning stages.[3,16] Review of program outcomes is necessary for all programs. Even a small volunteer program should be evaluated to determine if it should be continued, modified, or replaced with another initiative. Because evaluation involves measuring the results or outcomes of the program against the objectives, the first step is to review the program goals and objectives. Summative evaluation can be referred to as outcome evaluation when it focuses on the changes in comprehension, attitudes, behaviors, and practices that result from program activities. It can also be referred to as impact evaluation when the focus is on long-term, sustained changes as a result of program activities. Also, program evaluation occurs at various times in relation to program operation according to the time frame of the objectives (short term, intermediate, or long term).

To evaluate the effectiveness of health interventions, specific measurement instruments must be set up to collect data related to attaining each program objective.[3,16] These data relative to *measurable outcomes* are compared with baseline data to determine the success of the program. In this way, the process of program evaluation is an example of applied research. Each objective should be reviewed to determine how well it was achieved. The bottom line in evaluation is accountability—to consumers, providers, involved agencies, and all other stakeholders. Through evaluation it can be determined whether the program accomplishes what it was designed to accomplish, in other words, were the objectives of the program successfully met, and if not, why not? Summarizing what went well and what did not, or drawing conclusions based on intuition, is not adequate; the objectives themselves must be specifically addressed, and data-driven outcomes must be analyzed.[3,16]

Upon completion of the evaluation, the results should be reported to the advisory committee, stakeholders, and/or the community at large. This can take the form of a journal article, written summary, or oral presentation. Reporting evaluation results to the community and stakeholders can increase community support and assist in gaining future funding and support from other organizations to be able to continue the program[3,16] (see Figure 6.3). According to the American Dental Hygienists'

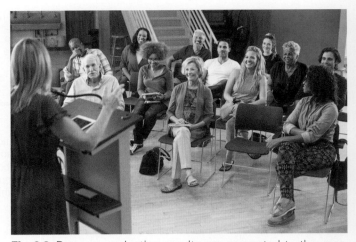

Fig 6.3 Program evaluation results are presented to the community and stakeholders to increase program support and sustainability. (@ iStock.com/monkeybusinessimages.)

Association (ADHA), sharing the results with other professionals is important also to meet the ethical responsibility to contribute "knowledge that is valid and useful to our clients and society."[19]

Inherent in program evaluation is the possibility of attaining a negative outcome, that is, concluding that the objectives have not been met. However, this does not mean that the program has been a failure. If a program is evaluated properly so negative outcomes become learning experiences and indicators of future programming and research needs, then in some sense it has been a success.[3,16] Formative evaluation during implementation can point out problems and identify opportunities to correct program deficiencies early on. With ongoing evaluation and adjustment, the end result may in fact indicate that a program was successful even if it had initial problems or flaws.[3,16]

Dental hygienists play a role in assessing the community, identifying the primary health issues, and planning, implementing, evaluating, and reporting community oral health program outcomes. Those who have chosen careers as state dental directors, public health educators and promoters, or advocates have played an important role in advancing dental public health, but there is more that can be accomplished by the dental hygiene profession. Many dental hygienists implement community oral health programs as volunteers in their own communities or as ADHA local component society members. By knowing how to organize an effective community oral health program, becoming involved in its implementation, and sharing the results, dental hygienists can impact the goal of optimal oral health care for all people. Additional Resources at the end of this chapter and Chapters 8 and 11 can assist with the steps of the Community Health Program Planning Process.

PRIMARY PREVENTION PROGRAMS: FLUORIDES, SEALANTS, ORAL HEALTH EDUCATION

Primary prevention is a major focus of community oral health programs. Multiple, varied primary prevention programs, based on established needs, are required to achieve the long-term outcome of optimal oral health in a population. Local evidence-based programs such as dental sealants and fluorides targeted to high-risk populations are essential. Although an essential component of any program, local programming that is limited to oral health education has not resulted in improving children's oral health.[8]

Community Water Fluoridation

Community water fluoridation is the addition of a controlled amount of fluoride to the public water supply to bring it to an optimal level to prevent dental caries in the population. It is recognized as one of the top 10 public health measures of the 20th century.[20] At the beginning of the 20th century, most Americans could expect to lose their teeth by middle age. That began to change with the introduction of water fluoridation and other uses of fluoride for dental caries prevention.[20]

In the early 1900s, Dr. Frederick McKay first noticed that many of his patients in Colorado had intrinsic brown stains on their teeth but few if any decayed teeth. He surveyed his practice area to establish the prevalence of this Colorado brown stain, later called mottled enamel and eventually called fluorosis. Dr. McKay determined that it was only present in long-term residents and most prevalent where deep artesian wells were the source of drinking water. By the 1920s, Dr. McKay reached the conclusion that the etiological agent had to be a constituent of some community water supplies.[20]

By the 1930s, new methods of spectrographic chemical analysis of water had developed, making it possible to identify fluoride as the common constituent of the water samples from areas with high rates of Colorado brown stain or mottled enamel. Dr. H. Trendley Dean was appointed to the newly established National Institutes of Health Dental Hygiene Unit (now the National Institute of Dental and Craniofacial Research) to conduct research on fluorosis and dental caries. Through epidemiological studies he determined the prevalence of fluorosis nationwide and demonstrated the relationships among fluorosis, water fluoride concentration, and dental caries rates. Additionally, he established a minimum level of naturally occurring fluoride that resulted in dental caries reduction.[20]

Fluoride is the 13th most abundant natural element; it is found in rocks, soil, fresh water, ocean water, and virtually all plants and animals. Therefore, trace amounts of fluoride are found in all natural-water sources. Many community water supplies are reservoirs of collected surface water and do not have adequate levels of fluoride. Even so, as a result of the general availability of these public water sources to most people, the adjustment of the natural fluoride content found in the water to optimal levels has proven to be a successful public health measure. This approach provides fluoride to the population in a passive vehicle for the consumer.[20] Fluoridation has been upheld in numerous studies over the years to be effective, safe, and cost effective.[20]

Benefits of Water Fluoridation

The first city in the U.S. to adjust the fluoride content of the drinking water was Grand Rapids, Michigan, in the 1940s. Subsequent studies of adjusted fluoridation demonstrated a 40% to 60% reduction of dental caries in the permanent teeth of children.[20] To illustrate this marked caries preventive effect, Figure 6.4 shows the relationship between the percentage of the population residing in areas with fluoridated community water systems in the U.S. and the mean number of decayed, missing, and filled teeth (DMFT) among children aged 12 years in the U.S. from 1967 to 1992. The graph shows the steady decline of DMFT from 1967 to 1992 as water fluoridation increased during the same period.

Today caries reduction rates in fluoridated communities are approximately 25% for all age groups.[20] Although the benefits of water fluoridation are lower today because of the multiple other sources of fluoride available to the population, it is still recommended as the most practical, cost-effective, equitable, and safe population-based means of preventing dental caries and improving oral health.[20] Furthermore, it is consistently effective across all ages and socioeconomic strata, thus reducing disparities.[20]

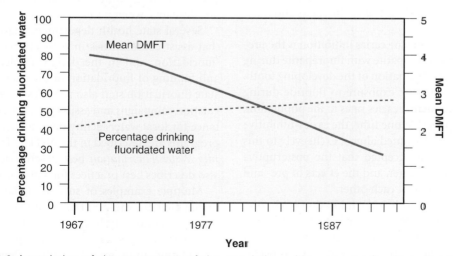

Fig 6.4 Association of the percentage of the population with access to fluoridated water and the mean decayed, missing, and filled teeth (DMFT) among children 12 years old, 1967 to 1992. *DMFT,* Decayed, missing, or filled teeth. (From Centers for Disease Control and Prevention Fluoridation Census, 1993; National Health and Nutrition Examination Survey, 1988 to 1994; National Center for Health Statistics, 1974 and 1981; and National Institute of Dental Research, 1989.)

Research also has shown a diffusion or halo effect of fluoridation. Individuals living in nonfluoridated communities in states that are highly fluoridated receive partial benefits of fluoridation from eating foods and drinking beverages processed in fluoridated communities. This halo effect can result in up to 25% fewer decayed, missing, and filled surfaces (DMFS) per year in children.[20] The high geographic mobility of our society also expands the benefit of water fluoridation to people not living in fluoridated communities. It is not unusual for them to benefit from access to fluoridated water during a significant part of their day while at work, school, or daycare.[20]

Over the years, water fluoridation has resulted in improved overall oral health. As decay rates decreased, tooth loss and iatrogenic causes of periodontal problems also declined. Water fluoridation has also resulted in lower expenditures for dental restorative procedures.[20] Likewise, absences from school and work due to oral pain are fewer in fluoridated communities, with subsequent increases in learning and productivity.[20]

The benefits and safety of fluoride are well documented and have been reevaluated frequently and reviewed comprehensively by several scientific organizations. No credible evidence supports an association between fluoridation and any potential adverse health effect or systemic disorder such as increased risk for cancer, Down syndrome, heart disease, osteoporosis and bone fracture, immune disorders, low intelligence, renal disorders, Alzheimer's disease, or allergic reactions.[20]

Mechanisms of Action of Fluoride

The primary mechanism of action of fluoride in caries inhibition is posteruptive.[20] Systemic fluoride is excreted partially via the saliva, thus making it available for absorption by plaque and in frequent contact with tooth surfaces for continual uptake and remineralization of the enamel. Because small quantities of fluoride are consumed throughout the day through water and foods that absorb fluoridated water during irrigation or while cooking, fluoridated water provides a continual source of topical fluoride to the teeth.[20] This posteruptive effect explains how fluoridation reduces coronal and root caries in adults and older adults.[21]

A secondary effect of fluoride for caries inhibition is the preeruptive replacement of hydroxyapatite with fluorapatite during the enamel crystalline matrix formation of the developing tooth. Current evidence is that systemic exposure to fluoride during tooth development reduces dental caries rates in the population, especially in pits and fissures.[20] At one time, the caries-inhibitive properties of fluoride were attributed almost exclusively to this preeruptive effect. Today, it is accepted that the posteruptive effect on caries prevention is greater, and the effects of pre- and posteruptive fluoride complement each other.[20]

Another topical effect of fluoride is the inhibition of glycolysis in microorganisms, thereby hindering the ability of bacteria to metabolize carbohydrates and produce acid.[20] The continual presence of fluoride in plaque is also important to this process.

Because the posteruptive effect is the primary benefit, the benefits of water fluoridation depend on consumption of the tap water daily (Figure 6.5) and continue throughout life as long as consumption of fluoridated water continues. If individuals

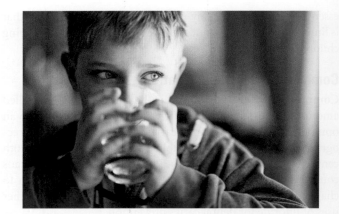

Fig 6.5 People require encouragement to consume fluoridated water regularly. (@ iStock.com/Imgorthand.)

do not consume tap water and if fluoridation is discontinued or a city changes to a nonfluoridated water source, the posteruptive caries reduction benefits are lost and caries rates will increase.[20]

Fluoridated Communities

In the 1950s and 1960s, many states and cities in the U.S. were quick to implement community water fluoridation. Over the years this trend began to level off. Fluoridation decisions are currently left to states and frequently to local governments and city councils. Therefore, the expansion of fluoridation is not easily accomplished and requires decisions at various levels. Increases in community water fluoridation in the last few decades can be attributed to the emphasis on its importance in caries prevention as discussed in the various national reports and as promoted by public health policymakers.[20,22]

Nearly all developed countries practice fluoridation. However, water fluoridation is not feasible in many other countries where community water supplies do not exist.[20] According to the Centers for Disease Control and Prevention (CDC),[22] the World Health Organization recommends water fluoridation where feasible and the use of salt or milk to deliver fluoride as an alternative when necessary.

Several state health departments have fluoridation projects that assist communities in their efforts to assess the need for fluoridation, and in the design, implementation, evaluation, and funding of fluoridation of their public water systems. The state fluoridation staff also provides consultation for local fluoridation campaigns and assists with training and technical assistance for local water facility operators. These state fluoridation programs are described in the ASTDD *Use of Fluoride: Community Water Fluoridation* best-practice-approach report, which also describes best practices for state fluoridation programs.[2]

Multiple examples of successful state fluoridation projects highlighted by the ASTDD at https://www.astdd.org/use-of-fluoride-community-water-fluoridation/ can serve as models for others. Certain key elements impact the success of a state fluoridation program (Box 6.10). Dental hygienists provide important contributions to these successes by fulfilling the roles of health educators, advocates, researchers, and administrators (see Chapter 2). See Chapter 5 for current data on fluoridated communities in the U.S.

BOX 6.10 Key Elements of a Successful State Fluoridation Program

- Assessment of community needs and feasibility studies to provide data for effective program planning
- Cooperative efforts of professionals, city officials, community leaders, citizens, and other government agencies in the voluntary adoption and implementation of fluoridation
- Funding from a variety of sustainable sources
- Provision by the state oral health department of training and technical assistance to schools, owners, and operators who fluoridate public water supplies
- Ongoing surveillance by the SOHP to monitor fluoride levels in the community drinking water
- Ongoing surveillance of dental caries rates by the SOHP to evaluate program success
- Ongoing provision of fluoridation information to citizens and communities
- Continuing efforts of dedicated professionals to support and assure continuation of the state program

(From Best Practice Approach Reports: Use of Fluoride: Community Water Fluoridation. Association of State and Territorial Dental Directors: 2015–2017. Available at: <http://www.astdd.org/use-of-fluoride-community-water-fluoridation/>; [Accessed August 2019].)

Cost of Water Fluoridation

The cost of water fluoridation varies with the size of the community because of the various types of equipment and chemicals required by different size water systems.[22] Cost figures from a 1992 evaluation and adjustments for inflation to estimate current costs are presented in Table 6.4.

The return on investment is a more important factor in determining the cost effectiveness of community water fluoridation. This also varies with the size of the community, increasing as the size increases. Nevertheless, fluoridation is cost-saving even for small communities. A recent economic analysis demonstrated that savings were greater than program costs, with an average 20:1 return on investment (annual savings of $20 per dollar invested). The same study estimated an average annual savings of $32 realized by each person living in a fluoridated

community and annual national savings of almost $6.5 billion as a result of fluoridation.[20]

With the escalating cost of health care, community water fluoridation remains a preventive measure of minimal cost that saves far more than it costs. In determining the economic impact of fluoridation, it is important to remember that the cost of treating dental disease is paid not only by affected individuals. Public funding of dental treatment must be considered also, for example through health departments, health insurance premiums, federally supported programs such as Medicaid and CHIP, and publicly supported community-based clinics.

Optimal Level of Fluoride

In 1962 the DHHS recommended fluoride (F) levels for water fluoridation ranging from 0.7 to 1.2 ppm F (equivalent to 0.7–1.2 mg F per liter of water [mg/L]), depending on the average daily temperature for the area. The range was based on the hypothesis that water consumption increased with increasing climatic temperature.[20] This recommendation remained in place until 2015, when the Public Health Service issued the final recommendation that the **optimal fluoride level** be changed to 0.7 mg/L regardless of climatic conditions.[20] The reasons for the recommended change were (1) an increase in access to multiple sources of fluoride today, (2) a trend of increasing prevalence of fluorosis in the population attributed to the multiple sources of fluoride, and (3) the controlled climatic environment with air conditioning, resulting in similar water intake across the nation regardless of climatic conditions.[20]

As a safe drinking water standard, the Environmental Protection Agency (EPA) *requires* **defluoridation** when the natural fluoride level of the community water is greater than 4.0 mg/L. Furthermore, to reduce the risk of fluorosis, the EPA *recommends* defluoridation when the natural fluoride level of the community water is between 2.0 and 4.0 mg/L.[20] Ingestion of higher than recommended levels of fluoride by children has been associated with an increase in dental fluorosis in developing, unerupted teeth.

Fluoridation Campaigns

Antifluoridationists oppose community water fluoridation. Their reasons are based on their basic beliefs that fluoride is toxic, causing multiple harmful health effects, it does not prevent tooth decay, it is costly, and it interferes with freedom of choice and infringes on individual rights.[20] Antifluoridationists attempt to appeal to people's emotions by providing inaccurate, false information to the public and elected officials and attempting to link fluoridation with adverse health effects. However, their arguments against fluoridation do not have any merit based on scientific knowledge.[20]

Some states and cities have taken administrative action to implement fluoridation; this means that state legislatures or city government entities have voted to implement fluoridation. However, people usually prefer to have a voice in the decision-making process. More recently, communities have had to defend existing fluoridation that has been challenged by antifluoridationists. Between 2011 and 2014, 46 states in the U.S. faced fluoridation challenges at the state or local level,[23] and this trend

TABLE 6.4 Estimated Annual Per Capita Cost of Community Water Fluoridation, 1992[a] and 2019[b]

Community Population Size	COST/PERSON	
	1992	2019
<10,000 (small systems)	$2.12	$3.86
10,000–50,000 (medium-size systems)	$0.68	$1.24
>50,000 (large systems)	$0.45	$0.82

[a]Ringelberg ML, Allen SJ, Brown LJ. Cost of fluoridation: 44 Florida communities. J Public Health Dent 1992;52(2):75-80. Available at: https://www.ncbi.nlm.nih.gov/pubmed/1564695; [Accessed August 2019].
[b]2019 cost computed by adjusting for inflation on CPI Inflation Calculator. Bureau of Labor Statistics Databases, Tables & Calculators by Subject. Available at: <http://www.bls.gov/data/inflation_calculator.htm>; [Accessed August 2019].

has continued.[24] A referenced report of key lessons learned from these campaigns and individual reports of experiences in specific states and communities can serve to guide communities facing similar challenges.[25]

A number of factors are involved in fluoridation failing when put to a public vote. Among those factors are "a lack of funding, public and professional apathy, the failure of many legislators and community leaders to take a stand because of perceived controversy, low voter turnout, and the difficulty faced by an electorate in evaluating scientific information in the midst of emotional charges by opponents."[20] For antifluoridationists to be defeated, a community water fluoridation campaign must be executed in a well-planned, unified manner.[20,23] The steps necessary to win a fluoridation campaign are presented in Box 6.11. If a fluoridation *referendum* (a public vote) is planned in a community, it is critical to educate the public and encourage and even facilitate fluoridation proponents' going to the polls to vote[20,25] (Figure 6.6).

Dental hygienists have a professional responsibility to take an active role in assuring the passage and continuation of community water fluoridation in their own communities. The following duties specified in the ADHA Code of Ethics relate to this responsibility:[19]

- Promote access to dental hygiene services for all, supporting justice and fairness in the distribution of healthcare resources.
- Serve as an advocate for the welfare of clients.
- Provide clients with the information necessary to make informed decisions about their oral health.

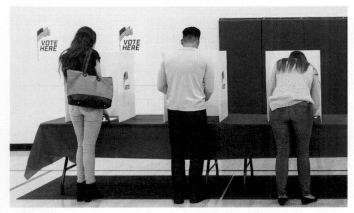

Fig 6.6 Proponents of water fluoridation need encouragement to go to the polls to vote for fluoridation. (@ iStock.com/SDI Productions.)

Whether for the purpose of the passage or continuation of fluoridation and whether by referendum or administrative action, education is crucial to the success of a fluoridation campaign. Knowledge is required for wise decision-making. Using evidence-based methods of health communication (see Chapter 8), dental hygienists in the roles of educators, resource persons, and advocates can be an effective force in the community by influencing public knowledge about the benefits of fluoridation in their community, providing accurate scientific information to community officials, and influencing future fluoridation decisions. In addition to providing community education, this can be accomplished by being a spokesperson for fluoridation with patients, family, and friends.

Multiple water fluoridation resources are available to help oral health professionals fulfill this responsibility. Some sources of these resources are SOHPs, ADA, ASTDD, American Academy of Pediatrics, CDC, state dental societies, and foundations such as the California Dental Foundation.

Other Fluoride Programs

Water fluoridation and fluoridated toothpaste have historically been the most common sources of fluoride in the U.S. and are the cornerstone of caries prevention.[21] Because of the ready availability of fluoride toothpaste to the public and its intense marketing by manufacturers in the U.S. and Canada, distribution of fluoride toothpaste is not considered a cost-effective public health program. Other fluoride modalities can be added for additional benefit in at-risk populations or individuals.[26] The public health application of these other means of delivering fluoride is discussed in this section.

The effectiveness of these various fluoride modalities in the reduction of dental caries is shown in Box 6.12. The addition of multiple sources of topical fluoride to water fluoridation has an additive effect on caries inhibition and can be beneficial when the caries risk is high. Addition of fluorides and other caries preventive treatments should be based on the presence of caries risk factors (Box 6.13). The ASTDD *Use of Fluoride in Schools* best-practice-approach report describes how community programs should be targeted to populations with multiple risk factors, especially fluoride deficiency and a high proportion of children from low-income families.[2]

Fluoride Varnish

Developed in Europe during the 1960s, the use of fluoride varnish was introduced to the U.S. in 1994 and remains in wide use in Europe and Canada. The varnish is applied by an operator, with a recommended application of two to four times a year for optimal benefit, depending on the risk level. The varnish is not intended to be permanent, like a sealant, but to hold the fluoride in contact with the tooth for a period of time.

Studies in Europe have demonstrated the efficacy of fluoride varnish historically, which has been confirmed by recent studies in the U.S.[27] (see Box 6.12). Compared with tray application of fluoride gel, fluoride varnish offers ease of application with less time, less patient discomfort, greater acceptability, and lower potential for harm in terms of nausea and vomiting, especially for infants, toddlers, and young children, disabled individuals,

BOX 6.12 Effectiveness of Various Fluoride Modalities

- **Community water fluoridation:** 50% to 70% caries reduction in early studies; 25% current caries reduction because of additional availability of other fluoride sources.
- **Fluoride varnish:** 37% reduction in primary teeth; 43% caries reduction in permanent teeth, including prevention of root surface caries in adults with gingival recession.
- **Fluoride mouthrinses:** 27% caries reduction in a structured program; cost-effective.
- **Dietary fluoride supplements:** Equivalent to water fluoridation with strict compliance of daily intake of recommended dosage over a long period.
- **Silver diamine fluoride:** 40%–80% caries reduction in the primary dentition; 25%–93% prevention factor in arresting and reducing the incidence of root caries, when used in combination with oral hygiene instruction and oral health education to reduce sugar consumption.

(From Quock RL. The evidence supporting fluoride varnish. J Decisions Dent 2017;3(1):50-53. Available at: <https://decisionsindentistry.com/article/evidence-supporting-fluoride-varnish/>; [Accessed September 2019]; Marinho VCC, Chong LL, Worthington HV, Walsh T. Highlighted review: Fluoride mouthrinses for preventing dental caries in children and adolescents. Cochrane Syst Rev 2016;7:CD002284. Available at: <https://doi.org/10.1002/14651858.CD002284.pub2>; [Accessed September 2019]; Fluoride: Topical and Systemic Supplements. American Dental Association; May 1, 2019. Available at: <https://www.ada.org/en/member-center/oral-health-topics/fluoride-topical-and-systemic-supplements>; [Accessed September 2019]; Contreras V, Toro MJ, Elias-Boneta AR, Encarnacion-Burgos A. Effectiveness of silver diamine fluoride in caries prevention and arrest: a systematic literature review. Gen Dent 2017;65(3):22-29. Available at: <https://www.ncbi.nlm.nih.gov/pmc/articles/PMC5535266/> [Accessed September 2019]; Subbiah GK, Gopinathan NM. Is silver diamine fluoride effective in preventing and arresting caries in elderly adults? A Systematic Review. J Int Soc Prev Community Dent 2018;8(3):101-199. Available at: <https://www.ncbi.nlm.nih.gov/pmc/articles/PMC5985673/>; [Accessed September 2019].)

BOX 6.13 Risk Factors for Dental Caries

- Lack of access to fluoridated water
- High intake of sugary foods or drinks
- Deep pit-and-fissure anatomy
- Eligibility for government assistance program; low socioeconomic status
- Active carious lesion; recent tooth extraction because of caries; recently restored lesion, especially if interproximal
- Recent caries experience of mother, caregiver, or sibling (if a child)
- Homeless or in otherwise unstable living conditions
- Low oral health literacy
- Special healthcare needs, chemo-radiation therapy, eating disorders, drug/alcohol abuse
- Lack of a dental home; poor dental utilization
- Inadequate salivary flow; use of medication that compromises salivary flow
- Visible plaque (poor oral hygiene)
- Presence of orthodontic appliances
- Exposed root surfaces

(From Caries Risk Assessment and Management. American Dental Association; December 14, 2018. Available at: <https://www.ada.org/en/member-center/oral-health-topics/caries-risk-assessment-and-management>; [Accessed September 2019]; Faller RV. Caries process and prevention strategies: Risk assessment (CE Course). Dentalcare.com; September 15, 2017. Available at: https://www.dentalcare.com/en-us/professional-education/ce-courses/ce377; [Accessed September 2019].)

hospitalized patients, and people with severe gag reflexes that cannot tolerate tray application of gels and foams.[21] Fluoride varnish is recommended over other fluoride regimens for application to primary and permanent teeth of children.[26] In addition, only a unit-dose fluoride varnish should be used in a program that targets children younger than age 6 years.[26]

Public health **fluoride varnish programs** are common today for at-risk children in clinical sites, schools, HS centers, and WIC sites and are implemented easily in community settings such as schools and HS programs.[28] These programs can be operated by various entities such as state and municipal health departments, local school districts, dental hygiene programs, and oral health professional organizations. Targeting programs to high-risk populations and repeating applications at least twice-annually for at least 2 years will increase the cost effectiveness.

An example is a school-based fluoride varnish program conducted by dental hygiene students at a local nonprofit preschool for 3- and 4-year-old children from low-income families with multiple other population caries risk factors (Figure 6.7). The program, which has been in operation since 2009,[29] is set up in an extra classroom of the facility with a minimum of resources. Children are screened and receive fluoride varnish application twice a year. The program includes classroom education and orientation to the varnish application in all 3- and 4-year-old classes and a parent education program. In addition, children brush daily at school, supervised by their teachers, and oral hygiene supplies are sent home to assure that children have the necessary tools to brush at home. A school staff member personally contacts the parents of children who are identified during the screening as needing urgent dental care. The program was started as a student project with financial assistance from a local dental hygiene society[29] and continues today with the support of the collaborating partners and in-kind corporate donations of supplies.

Because of the established effectiveness of fluoride varnish, program administrators should concentrate evaluation efforts on the ability to apply varnish multiple times, acceptability, and cost-effectiveness of the program.[28] Children enroll at this

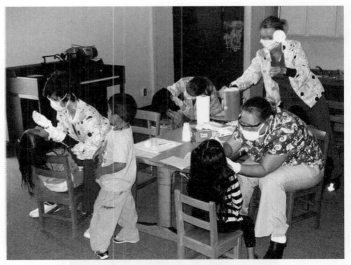

Fig 6.7 Dental hygiene students apply fluoride varnish in a preschool program for at-risk children, set up in an extra classroom of the facility.

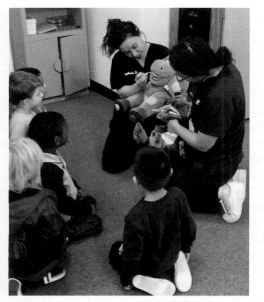

Fig 6.8 Dental hygiene students demonstrate fluoride varnish placement on a puppet; providing education in conjunction with a preschool-based fluoride varnish program increases student compliance during the varnish-application phase.

preschool as 3-year-olds and typically continue in the program for 2 years, receiving oral health education, screening, and fluoride varnish application twice a year for those 2 years. The program experienced 95% to 100% participation of children in varnish application from 2008 to 2015 as a result of the orientation and education phase (Figure 6.8) and teacher involvement in the program (Figure 6.9). Resources to assist with the development of a fluoride varnish program are included in the References and Additional Resources at the end of this chapter.

The U.S. Preventive Services Task Force recommends that primary care medical providers apply fluoride varnish to children two to four times a year, depending on risk, from the time of primary tooth eruption through age 5 years; this practice is reimbursable by Medicaid and many private insurance

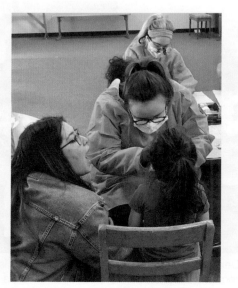

Fig 6.9 Teacher involvement in a preschool fluoride varnish program enhances the program and improves compliance.

carriers.[30] Nondental primary care clinicians are targeted to provide this treatment because they are more likely than oral health professionals to have contact with children younger than 6 years.[30] This is a means of reaching these high-risk children at the age of primary tooth eruption for maximum benefit.

Fluoride Mouthrinse Programs

In communities in which a public water source is not available or community water fluoridation is undesired for various reasons, school-based **fluoride mouthrinse programs** have been implemented. The efficacy and cost-effectiveness of fluoride mouthrinsing in a structured environment such as this has been demonstrated (see Box 6.12). According to the ASTDD, these programs are less common in the U.S. today because of the increased adoption of water fluoridation.[2] A school-based program requires involvement and cooperation of school personnel, oversight by a licensed oral health professional according to the individual state laws, and parental permission for participation of children.[31]

Mouthrinse programs are administered by school personnel or volunteers on a weekly basis to participating children who rinse for 60 seconds with 10 mL of 0.2% sodium fluoride.[31] The child then expectorates the fluoride rinse into a paper cup, places a napkin inside the cup to absorb the solution, and discards the cup. The procedure takes less than 5 minutes.[31] State and local health departments conducting these programs have manuals to guide their planning and implementation (see References and Additional Resources at the end of this chapter).

Dietary Fluoride Supplements

The use of **dietary fluoride supplements** is another recommended way to provide fluoride to children at high risk for caries.[32] The use of supplements is the only systemic alternative to fluoridation. These supplements are available only by prescription, and to reduce the risk of dental fluorosis in permanent teeth, they are recommended only for children living in nonfluoridated areas[32]

Supplements are available in two forms: (1) drops for infants aged 6 months and older and (2) chewable tablets for children and adolescents. The correct dosage is based on the child's age and the existing fluoride level in all available drinking water sources, including water in the home, bottled water, and water at the school or day care center and after-school care program[32] (Table 6.5). All sources of fluoride should be evaluated with a thorough fluoride history before dietary supplementation.[32] Patient exposure to multiple water sources can make proper prescribing complex. The need for continuation of fluoride supplements should be reevaluated in the event of a child's change of residence or increasing access to other sources of systemic fluoride.

See Box 6.12 for the effectiveness of fluoride supplements. The need for daily compliance over an extended period of time is a major procedural and economic disadvantage of community-based fluoride supplement programs.[32] This liability makes them impractical for dispensing by a community-based clinic for use at home.

School-based fluoride supplement programs are a way to overcome the problem of daily compliance. These programs were common several decades ago before water fluoridation became more prevalent. The ASTDD describes their use today in some nonfluoridated areas, especially with children younger

TABLE 6.5   Dietary Fluoride Supplement Schedule

Age	FLUORIDE ION LEVEL IN DRINKING WATER (PPM[a])		
	<0.3 ppm	0.3–0.6 ppm	>0.6 ppm
Birth–6 months	None	None	None
6 months–3 years	0.25 mg/day[b]	None	None
3–6 years	0.50 mg/day	0.25 mg/day	None
6–16 years	1.0 mg/day	0.50 mg/day	None

[a]1.0 part per million (ppm) = 1 milligram/liter (mg/L).
[b]2.2 mg of sodium fluoride contains 1 mg of fluoride ions.
(From American Academy of Pediatric Dentistry (AAPD). Fluoride therapy, 2018, Chicago, IL: AAPD Reference Manual 2018-19;40(6):250-253. Available at: <https://www.aapd.org/globalassets/media/policies_guidelines/bp_fluoridetherapy.pdf>; [Accessed September 2019].)

BOX 6.14   Recommendations to Prevent Fluorosis

- Counsel parents and caregivers about the use of fluoride (F) toothpaste by young children (<3 years old, smear of F toothpaste; 3–6 years old, no more than a pea-sized amount of F toothpaste).
- Counsel parents about the risk of fluorosis related to mixing concentrated infant formula with fluoridated water.
- Encourage parents, caregivers, and school/Head Start personnel to supervise children's toothbrushing to decrease their swallowing excess F toothpaste.
- Target F mouthrinses only to children at high risk for developing tooth decay.
- Base the prescribing and recommending of high F concentration toothpastes on comprehensive caries risk assessment.
- Advocate for the labeling of the F concentration of bottled water.
- Know the F concentration of a child's primary source of drinking water and all other possible sources of F in the child's diet at home and away from home to be able to make appropriate decisions about using other F products, especially dietary F supplements.
- Use an alternative source of water for children ≤8 years old whose primary drinking water has a F level >2 mg/L.
- Collaborate with professional healthcare organizations, public health agencies, and suppliers of oral care products in the education of healthcare professionals and the public.

(From Fluorosis. Centers for Disease Control and Prevention; March 8, 2019. Available at: <https://www.cdc.gov/fluoridation/faqs/dental_fluorosis/>; [Accessed September 2019]; American Academy of Pediatric Dentistry (AAPD). Fluoride Therapy, 2018. AAPD Reference Manual 2018-19;40(6):250-253. Available at: <https://www.aapd.org/research/oral-health-policies--recommendations/fluoride-therapy/>; [Accessed September 2019]; Wiener RC, Shen C, Findley P, Tan X, Sambamoorthi U. Dental fluorosis over time: A comparison of national health and nutrition examination survey data from 2001-2002 and 2011-2012. J Dent Hyg 2018;92(1):23-29. Available at: <https://www.ncbi.nlm.nih.gov/pmc/articles/PMC5929463/>; [Accessed March 2020].)

than 6 years who are unable to hold a fluoride rinse in the mouth for 60 seconds.[2] Program operation is similar to a school fluoride rinse program. Children are given a fluoride tablet daily at school, which they chew for 1 minute and then swallow.

Although the total costs of such a program are small, the overall cost is much greater than the per capita cost of community water fluoridation. Furthermore, unlike supplements, fluoridation provides caries prevention for the entire population regardless of age, socioeconomic factors, educational attainment, or other social variables, thus reducing disparities.[20] This is particularly important for families and individuals with limited access to oral healthcare services.

Silver Diamine Fluoride

Approved by the Federal Drug Administration in 2014 to treat sensitivity, 38% **silver diamine fluoride** (SDF) has been endorsed by the ADA and the American Academy of Pediatric Dentistry (AAPD) for off-label use to prevent caries and arrest cavitated carious lesions.[33,34] See Box 6.12 for the effectiveness of SDF.

It is thought that the use of SDF can greatly impact the cost of dental care in the U.S., with savings for Medicaid, CHIP, commercial insurance companies, community programs, families, and individuals.[33] As with most new procedures, it will take time for the profession to adopt its use; however, the ASTDD *Use of Fluoride in Schools* best-practice-approach report describes the initiation of school-based SDF programs by some SOHPs.[2]

Prevention of Fluorosis

With all the additional sources of fluoride available today, the prevalence of caries has decreased. However, the prevalence of dental fluorosis seems to have increased dramatically during the period from 1986 to 2012,[35] although the dramatic increase may be a result of research methodology (see Chapter 5). Fluoridated water, infant formula, and swallowed toothpaste are the main contributors to an increase in fluorosis.[35] Healthcare professionals, such as dentists, dental hygienists, and primary care medical providers, are important sources of information for patients regarding the use of fluoride-containing products and should provide education and recommendations on the appropriate use of these products to help reduce the prevalence of fluorosis (Box 6.14). Dental hygienists can be a valuable resource

to the community by providing public education on fluorides and consultation with primary care medical providers on water fluoridation and other sources of fluoride.

Dental Sealants

Used in combination with water fluoridation and other fluorides, dental sealants are a cornerstone of individual and community practice[36] (Figure 6.10). While fluorides primarily prevent smooth surface caries,[22] sealants are designed to prevent pit-and-fissure caries and are more effective than fluorides for this purpose.[37] Studies have shown that sealant placement in permanent molars prevents 80% of dental caries after 2 years, compared with molars not receiving sealants.[38]

School-based sealant programs (SBSP) are strongly recommended by the CDC and the ASTDD in their *School-Based Dental Sealant Programs* best-practice-approach report, as a way of reaching children at high risk for caries.[2,39] In some programs mobile dental vans are sent to schools, and sealants are applied in the van. In other programs, portable equipment is transported from school to school and set up in available spaces such as a gym, lunchroom, or extra classroom. Students are then brought to the designated room for the procedure.

Two recent reviews of SBSP revealed that these programs save society money and are cost-effective, especially when they

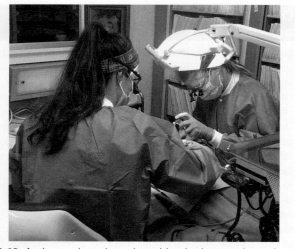

Fig 6.10 Active and student dental hygienists apply sealants at a faith-based community health center. (Courtesy Amy Teague.)

TABLE 6.6 Centers for Disease Control and Prevention Recommendations for School-Based Sealant Programs

Topic	Recommendations
Indications for sealant placement	Seal sound and noncavitated pit-and-fissure surfaces of posterior teeth, with first and second permanent molars receiving highest priority.
Tooth surface assessment	Differentiate cavitated and noncavitated lesions: • Unaided visual assessment is appropriate. • Dry teeth before assessment with cotton rolls, gauze, or compressed air when available. • An explorer may be used to gently confirm cavitation; do not use a sharp explorer under force. • Radiographs are unnecessary solely for sealant placement. • Other diagnostic technologies are not required.
Sealant placement and evaluation	Clean the tooth surface: • Toothbrush prophylaxis is acceptable. • Additional surface preparation, such as air or enameloplasty, is not recommended. • Use a four-handed technique when resources allow. • Evaluate sealant retention within 1 year. • Seal the teeth of children, even if follow-up cannot be assured.

(From Gooch BF, Griffin SO, Gray SK, et al. Preventing dental caries through school-based sealant programs. J Am Dent Assoc 2009;140(11):1356-1365. Available at: <http://jada.ada.org/article/S0002-8177%2814%2964584-0/fulltext> [Accessed September 2019]; Best Practice Approach: School-based Dental Sealant Programs. Association of State and Territorial Dental Directors; November 2017. Available at: <https://www.astdd.org/docs/sealant-bpar-update-11-2017-final.pdf>; [Accessed September 2019].)

target schools attended by a large number of children who are at high risk for caries.[38,40] It was projected that providing sealants in a school program to 1,000 children in 1 year would prevent 485 restorations and increase quality of life by adding 1.59 disability-adjusted life-years.[40] According to one of these reviews, labor accounts for two-thirds of the total cost, and even minimal improvements in efficiency or decreases in labor costs could greatly improve the cost-effectiveness. One way this has been accomplished is to maximize the use of dental auxiliaries and reduce supervision requirements for dental hygienists.[38]

The ASTDD also describes the use of *school-linked sealant programs* that are connected with a school, but the sealants are delivered at a different site such as a clinic or private dental office.[2] The program may present information, distribute consent forms, and conduct dental screenings at schools. Preschool-age children at high risk for caries can be reached with similar programs in HS settings (see the Head Start section later in this chapter).

A typical SBSP is described by the CDC.[39] SBSPs generally are focused on providing sealants to children aged 6 to 11 years or in grades 3 through 5. The program will visit a school over the course of 1 to 3 days. A licensed oral health professional will screen children for oral disease, existing sealants, and sealant retention; place sealants as needed, typically at no cost; and refer to a local dentist any child who requires follow-up dental care. For ethical reasons, referral is a critical step in any program that includes screening. A signed permission slip from a parent or guardian is required for a child to participate.

According to the ASTDD, targeting these ages allows the placement of sealants shortly after tooth eruption, which is considered a best practice to maximize the time of greatest susceptibility to caries.[2] The ASTDD also recommends targeting molars because about 90% of decay occurs in the pits and fissures of permanent posterior teeth with the molars being at highest risk.[2] To target schools that have a high percentage of children at high risk for caries, schools are selected that have a high rate of children participating in a free or reduced-price meal program.[38] Exemplary SBSPs highlighted on the ASTDD website at https://www.astdd.org/school-based-dental-sealant-programs

can serve as models for an oral health professional that is planning a SBSP.

Table 6.6 provides the 2009 CDC recommendations for SBSPs, which were prepared by an appointed CDC-expert workgroup.[41] According to the ASTDD *School-Based Dental Sealant Programs* best-practice-approach report, these recommendations and the referenced report by Gooch and colleagues continue to serve as an evidence-based guide for SBSPs.[2] Further resources to assist with developing a SBSP are included in the References and Additional Resources at the end of this chapter.

Although the percentage of preschool- and school-age children with sealants has risen in recent years, the increase has not been as great as needed, especially in the population that is at greatest risk for caries, namely children from low-income families.[38] The rate of sealed primary teeth is especially low.[36] A major national emphasis continues to be the increased use of sealants, which requires ongoing oral health promotion to increase the acceptance and use of sealants by the public and oral health practitioners.[36,38] Because research has demonstrated that most people acquire knowledge of the need for sealants from their oral health practitioners, it is important that oral healthcare providers be knowledgeable and have positive attitudes about the use of sealants.[42] Box 6.15 presents CDC-suggested ways that oral health professionals and others can assist with this goal.[40]

BOX 6.15 Actions to Promote an Increase in Dental Sealant Prevalence

The federal government is:
- Classifying pediatric dental services as an essential health benefit to be covered by dental insurance as part of the Affordable Care Act.
- Matching state costs of applying sealants to all children enrolled in Medicaid/Children's Health Insurance Program (CHIP) and tracking program performance.
- Encouraging community health centers with dental programs to start or expand school-based sealant programs (SBSPs) to reach more children from low-income families.
- Helping fund states to increase the number of sealant programs.
- Providing incentives for dentists to practice in underserved areas to increase access to dental services.

State officials can:
- Target SBSPs to the areas of greatest need.
- Track the number of schools and children participating in sealant programs.
- Implement policies that deliver SBSPs in the most cost-effective manner.
- Help schools connect to Medicaid and CHIP, local health department clinics, community health centers, and private community dental providers to encourage more use of sealants and reimbursement of services.

Oral healthcare providers can:
- Apply sealants to children at highest risk for dental caries, including those covered by Medicaid/CHIP.
- Learn about SBSPs and their effectiveness.

- Donate time and resources to a SBSP.
- Accept children into their practice who are identified as needing additional services when they receive sealants in schools.
- Educate parents about the benefits of and access to sealants and encourage them to have their children's teeth sealed.
- Partner with other health providers, especially school nurses and pediatricians, to devise a strategy for increasing knowledge about sealants among parents.

School administrators can:
- Work with local and state public health programs and local oral healthcare providers to start SBSPs
- Support having SBSPs; promote their benefits to teachers, staff, and parents.
- Help children enroll in SBSPs by putting information for parents in school registration packets.
- Encourage schools to develop relationships with local dental offices and community dental clinics to help children find a dental home.
- Facilitate and support programs to educate parents and children about sealants.

Parents can:
- Ask their child's dentist to apply sealants when appropriate.
- Register their child to participate in a SBSP; if a SBSP is not available, ask the school to start one.
- Find a dental home for their child.

(Modified from School Sealant Programs. Centers for Disease Control and Prevention; March 1, 2018. Available at: https://www.cdc.gov/oralhealth/dental_sealant_program/school-sealant-programs.htm; [Accessed September 2019]; Junger ML, Griffin SO, Lesaja S, Espinoza L. Awareness among US adults of dental sealants for caries prevention. Prev Chronic Dis 2019;16:180398. Available at: <http://dx.doi.org/10.5888/pcd16.180398>; [Accessed December 2019].)

Oral Health Education

Oral health education (OHE) is the process of teaching people about oral health to help them prevent oral disease. OHE should be included in all community oral health programs to supplement and support the provision of preventive services that avert and control oral diseases (Figure 6.11). Equally important is to include an interprofessional focus in OHE to connect oral health with overall health (Figure 6.12). The intent is to assist people in making decisions, choosing behaviors, and learning skills that support their oral health.

OHE should focus on interventions such as promoting the use of fluorides and sealants and stress skill acquisition and adoption of evidence-based risk-reducing behaviors such as regular oral hygiene and reduction of cariogenic food choices. Various factors, including social factors, attitudes, and the environment, influence these decisions and affect the outcomes of OHE. Thus, for OHE to be effective, it must be based on sound health education and promotion theory (see Chapter 8).

The school setting is ideal to reach children and, through them, their families and the community.[43] In this way, school-based OHE is important to the goal of optimal oral health for all citizens. OHE should be integrated into all aspects of a school program such as health education, health services, physical education and activity, nutritional environment and services, and physical environment.[43] (See School-Based Oral Health Programs section later in this chapter.)

Other community-based opportunities for OHE are available through various faith-based, community-based, social service, healthcare, and policymaking organizations and groups

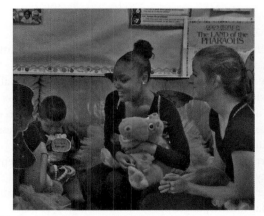

Fig 6.11 Oral health education is a critical component of fluoride varnish and other programs that provide a service in a community program.

such as the WIC Program, HS, service clubs, scouting and similar organizations, other youth organizations, sports clubs, hospitals, clinics, long-term care facilities, city councils, and other governmental groups. Information about diverse oral health topics can be presented in these settings. OHE can be directed to the general public, various priority populations, other health professionals who provide care for the public, and policymakers. Some examples follow:

- Prenatal and postnatal oral care for parents, infants, and toddlers
- Oral health concerns of special care patients with conditions such as diabetes and stroke

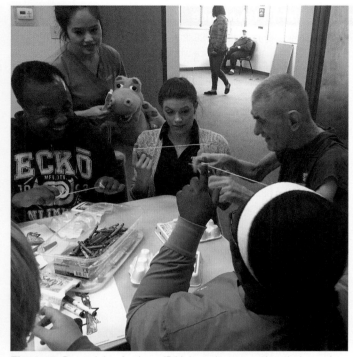

Fig 6.12 Dental hygienists (DHs) and occupational therapists (OTs) present an oral health education program with an interprofessional focus to physically and mentally challenged clients in an adult daycare center. OTs help clients with manual dexterity while DHs teach oral hygiene skills.

- Oral and denture care for older adults
- Oral health effects of tobacco products, oral cancer information, and tobacco cessation
- Daily oral care needs of physically and mentally challenged individuals (see Figure 6.12)
- Diet and nutrition related to oral health for all stages of life
- Oral-systemic link for other healthcare professionals (Figure 6.13)
- Information on access to oral health care presented to policymakers
- Water fluoridation information presented to a city council or similar municipal group

The dental hygienist in the role of health educator uses the knowledge of oral diseases and primary preventive measures to inform people about how to improve their oral health in connection with overall health. Critical to fulfilling this responsibility is the need to become an effective teacher (Box 6.16) and remain updated on health promotion and educational theory (see Chapter 8).

Developing an Oral Health Presentation

Careful planning is required to develop effective, evidence-based OHE presentations for the community. Structured oral health curricula and other resources for OHE are available through SOHPs, oral health professional organizations, oral health coalitions and nonprofits, universities, CDC and other federal agencies, and oral health industry (see Additional Resources at

---

BOX 6.16 Characteristics of an Effective Teacher

1. Has a thorough command of the topic being taught.
2. Is prepared and organized.
3. Begins class promptly and in a well-organized way.
4. Practices effective classroom management.
5. Provides the significance or importance of information to be learned.
6. Uses active, hands-on student learning.
7. Uses varied instructional techniques.
8. Uses examples, models, analogies, metaphors, and variety in modes of instruction to make materials understandable and memorable.
9. Provides clear explanations.
10. Provides many concrete, real-life, practical examples.
11. Provides frequent and immediate feedback to students on their performance.
12. Praises student answers and uses probing questions to clarify or elaborate answers.
13. Teaches at an appropriate pace, stopping to check student understanding and engagement.
14. Communicates at the level of all students in class.
15. Considers learning styles of the students.
16. Uses nonverbal behavior such as gestures, walking around, and eye contact to reinforce comments.
17. Stimulates student interaction.
18. Keeps the class focused on the objectives.
19. Provides clear, specific expectations for assignments.
20. Is sensitive to student motivation and understanding.
21. Uses effective public speaking skills.
22. Presents oneself as "real people."
23. Is dynamic and energetic.
24. Demonstrates self-confidence.
25. Has a sense of humor.
26. Treats students with respect and caring.
27. Creates a class environment that is comfortable for students.
28. Uses feedback and reflection to assess and improve teaching.

(Modified from 20 Observable Characteristics of Effective Teaching. TeachThought; December 12, 2018. Available at: <https://www.teachthought.com/pedagogy/20-observable-characteristics-of-effective-teaching/>; [Accessed October 2019]; Characteristics of Effective Teachers. Stanford Teaching Commons, Stanford University. Available at:<https://teachingcommons.stanford.edu/resources/teaching/planning-your-approach/characteristics-effective-teachers>; [Accessed October 2019].)

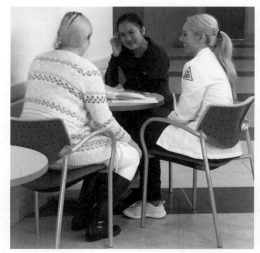

Fig 6.13 Dental hygiene students educate speech-language pathology students on the risk of poststroke oral complications as they collaborate to treat patients in a poststroke center.

BOX 6.17 Oral Health Education Lesson Plan Template

Title: Identify a title that reflects the topic of your lesson.

Concept/Topic to Teach: Clearly identify the topic of the lesson.

Goal: What is the purpose of the lesson? Record the general goal of your lesson.

Objectives: Begin with the end in mind. What do you want the students to learn from this lesson? Write no more than three specific objectives for the lesson.

Vocabulary: Create a key vocabulary list that you will add to as you develop your lesson plan. You will make sure the students understand these terms as they work through the lesson.

Materials: Create a materials list and add to this as you develop your lesson. This will help you prepare what you need for your lesson, such as audio/visual (A/V) equipment, number of copies, and teaching supplies.

Introduction: Plan your introduction, such as a simple oral explanation for the lesson, an introductory worksheet, or an interactive activity.

Teaching Method: Select the teaching strategy you will use, such as lecture, group discussion, an activity, or a combination.

Content Outline: Write out supporting content information as notes.

Instructions: Write out step-by-step instructions for the practice skills for the lesson.

Review: Create an end-of-lesson review of the most salient points of the lesson.

Evaluation Plan: Complete detailed assessments to determine the learning outcomes; tie the evaluation plan to the objectives.

Accommodations: Plan any necessary accommodations for English as a second language (ESL) or special education audience participants.

(Modified from Teaching Guide: Writing Lesson Plans Fort Collins, CO: Colorado State University. Available at: <http://writing.colostate.edu/guides/teaching/lesson_plans/>;[Accessed August 2019].)

the end of this chapter and Appendix A). Many of these materials can be adapted for use in presentations on various topics for diverse vulnerable populations.

These resources can be used to develop a **lesson plan**, which is a necessary step in planning an oral health presentation.[44] An outline of a lesson plan is provided in Box 6.17 as a guide. The components of the lesson plan should be based on the assessment of the audience to assure relevancy to their needs.[44] In addition, selection of teaching strategies and materials should be based on the advantages and disadvantages of the different methods (Table 6.7). Various teaching techniques are more suitable for different topics and for different audiences based on age, educational background, oral health literacy, and other factors. In general, more effective methods are those that involve active audience participation, use multiple senses, and combine teaching techniques to meet the needs of various learning styles and to maintain audience interest.[44] Health education theory (see Chapter 8) and the steps of the community program planning process (see earlier in this chapter) should be incorporated into all OHE efforts.

TABLE 6.7 Teaching Methods for Oral Health Presentations

Advantages	Disadvantages
Lecture—informative talk, prepared beforehand and given to a group; useful to introduce new topics, arouse interest in a subject, or review concepts	
<ul><li>Many various facts/ideas/concepts can be presented in an orderly fashion and in a short period</li><li>Information can be conveyed to a large audience</li><li>Allows for preparation before presentation</li><li>Instructor determines aims, content, organization, pace, and direction</li><li>Diverse materials can be integrated</li><li>Media can be incorporated</li><li>Builds on foundation knowledge</li><li>Difficult concepts can be developed</li></ul>	<ul><li>No active participation by the learner</li><li>Encourages one-way communication</li><li>Stifles creativity</li><li>Requires effective writing, speaking, and modeling skills; poor presentation technique is a barrier to learning</li><li>Difficult to monitor student learning</li></ul>
Lecture-Demonstration—informative talk; presents information supplemented by a demonstration to reinforce learning; can be used to introduce information and to demonstrate skills or techniques to supplement information; field trips can be used for the demonstration portion	
<ul><li>Illustrates information visually</li><li>Presents information in a complete format</li><li>Allows for concentration of attention and economical use of time</li><li>Useful for reinforcing material</li><li>Can use models, computer-generated slides, videotapes and other tools</li><li>Technology (e.g., computer monitors) allows viewing by more participants</li></ul>	<ul><li>Without appropriate technology, difficult for large groups to see demonstration</li><li>Requires careful preparation for success</li><li>Requires adequate equipment and facilities</li><li>Can be a passive approach</li></ul>

(Continued)

TABLE 6.7 Teaching Methods for Oral Health Presentations (*Cont.*)

Advantages	Disadvantages
Discussion—group activity in which the student and teacher define a problem and seek a solution; interaction between teacher and students to promote divergent thinking where closure is not expected; promotes understanding and clarification of concepts, ideas, and feelings; includes use of questions by the leader to stimulate interaction	
• Allows interaction among participants • Provides two-way communication between presenter and audience • Encourages individuals to participate/contribute • Engages participants in problem solving (higher order learning) • Encourages teamwork, tolerance of divergent opinion, and development of interpersonal skills • Can be focused on both cognitive and affective learning	• Strong personalities can influence a group • Poor discussion leader may contribute to failure of the discussion • Nothing may be achieved; discussion may go in many directions without closure • May not be profitable if group members do not have appropriate background • Difficult to manage among young children
Discovery Learning—uses a less direct questioning format to prod the learner into using logic or common sense to discover ideas or concepts; useful to build on foundational knowledge and to introduce new concepts	
• Promotes learner involvement • Requires application of knowledge (higher level learning) • Promotes critical thinking • Motivates student to discover the "right answer" • Promotes divergent thinking; useful when multiple answers are plausible	• May be interpreted as guessing • Learner needs to be guided so that correct information is concluded • Requires foundational knowledge
Brainstorming—free sharing of ideas generated by unstructured group interaction; may have a well-defined, clearly stated problem to address; ideas recorded for future discussion but never analyzed for merit during session; useful for group identification of an issue or problem	
• Useful for youth and adult groups • Encourages creativity • Encourages application of knowledge • Encourages contribution by all participants with no fear of a "wrong answer" • Encourages people to build on others' ideas	• Group dynamic may be influenced by stronger personalities • Requires careful management to maintain the purpose of the exercise • Not useful to share information, only for problem identification or issue clarification • Difficult to manage with children
Web-Based Learning—use of computer to present information in a way that can be interactive; includes use of the monitor to present photos, animation, video, print, and sound for lecture-demonstration, cases, discussion groups, simulation, testing, and other online teaching methods	
• Provides an alternative medium to present information • Accessible at all times if learner has access to a computer • Can be updated • Provides enhanced printed material • Provides ready access to wealth of resources on the web • Can be used for virtual field trips	• Useful for youth and adult groups • Some individuals may not have computer skills or access to appropriate technology • Cost of equipment and linkages
Cooperative and Collaborative Learning Activities—occur both inside and outside the classroom or learning environment; for example, group activities, projects, debates, and experiments	
• Encourages critical thinking • Promotes social environment for learning • Students can learn from each other	• Can be difficult to manage • Requires maturity of the students

SCHOOL-BASED ORAL HEALTH PROGRAMS

The following statistics demonstrate the continuing need for oral health programs for children in the U.S.[45]

• 20% of children ages 6 to 11 years have at least one untreated carious lesion.
• An average of 34 million school hours are lost each year because of emergency dental care.
• Approximately 100 million Americans do not have access to fluoridated tap water.
• 60% of children do not have dental sealants.

This information points to the necessity to have **school-based oral health programs** (SBOHP) to meet the needs of children who are not receiving the oral health care they need.

The Whole School, Whole Community, Whole Child (WSCC) model (https://www.cdc.gov/healthyschools/wscc/index.htm) is promoted by the CDC to address health in schools.[46] The model is student-centered and emphasizes the role of the community in supporting the school, the connections between health and academic achievement, and the importance of evidence-based school policies and practices. One of the 10 interacting essential elements of the WSCC model is health.

The success of a SBOHP depends on its integration with other school health programs. To this end, ASTDD policy "fully supports and endorses a strategic effort within school health programs to integrate oral health into the WSCC school health model."[43] Table 6.8 provides examples of incorporating oral health into other essential elements of the model.

A comprehensive SBOHP includes screening, multiple primary prevention programs, and dental treatment for the children as well as OHE of children (Figure 6.14) and their families. An example of a SBOHP is Miles of Smiles—Laredo

TABLE 6.8   Integration of Oral Health into the Essentials Elements of the Whole School, Whole Community, Whole Child School Health Model

Essential Element	Examples of Activities
Physical education/physical activity	• Requiring use of oral protective equipment during sports • Providing safe playground equipment and surface area
Nutrition environment and services	• Providing dentally healthy meals, snacks, and vending machine options • Controlling sugary snacks brought from home
Physical environment	• Requiring use of seat belts on school buses • Enforcing safety rules such as at the water fountain to avoid accidents that will injure the teeth or mouth
Health education	• Annual oral health curriculum that builds • Teaching preparation of dentally healthy meals in appropriate classes • Inclusion of the oral-medical connection in the curriculum
Other health services	• Interprofessional approach to school-based screenings • Inclusion of the oral-medical connection in relation to services offered
Community engagement	• Parent and student presentations by oral health professionals in the community • Community support of field trips to oral health facilities and oral health student assignments and projects
Family engagement	• One-on-one assistance to parents in establishing dental homes • Using parents as volunteers in school-based preventive programs

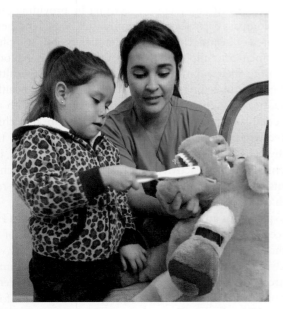

Fig 6.14 A dental hygienist helps a first-grade child practice toothbrushing. (Courtesy Nichole Salazar.)

(MOS-L), targeting children who attend economically disadvantaged elementary schools in the Mexico border area of a southwest state.[47] In existence since 2007 and funded by the **Health Resources and Services Administration** (HRSA) and DentaQuest Foundation, MOS-L is part of a larger program, Miles of Smiles, serving a metropolitan area. Housed at the local branch of the state university, MOS-L collaborates with multiple partners, including an associated dental school, government entities involved, the school districts, and a local community center.

The objectives of Miles of Smiles are the following:[47]
- Reduce barriers to receiving dental services.
- Provide preventive dental services to children.
- Refer children with urgent oral health problems to providers in the community.
- Keep children dentally healthy throughout their early school years.
- Disseminate this model to other communities.

The program is designed to maximize participation by targeting high-risk children unlikely to receive routine dental care in clinical settings that are not school based. Taking preventive dental services to the schools by using portable dental equipment that is transported and assembled on site is more cost-effective and eliminates barriers associated with lack of transportation, limited service hours, and lack of access to dental providers.[57] In 2014–2015, MOS-L provided the following dental services valued at over $450,000 to over 8500 children in 42 elementary schools at no cost to the families or schools:[47]
- Dental screening with the Basic Screening Survey (BSS; see Chapter 4)
- Referral for restorative or emergent care
- Primary preventive services such as fluoride varnish to children in kindergarten, first, second, and third grades, and dental sealants to children in second grade with follow-up and replacement in third grade
- OHE for children and their families

Children with urgent and routine oral healthcare needs identified during the BSS screening and who do not have a dental home are triaged into a case management system. Dental case managers and staff contact the parents and identify a source of dental care using public-private partnerships. School nurses are incorporated into the case management process.[47]

SmilesMaker, an innovative electronic data entry tool, was created for use by the Miles of Smiles program to record longitudinal BSS data.[47] The MOS-L dental team uses iPads to access SmilesMaker and enter screening data through a secure and encrypted connection to the dental school server. SmilesMaker is available free to other community oral health programs by contacting Miles of Smiles on the web at https://milesofsmiles.uthscsa.edu/.[47]

HEAD START

The **Head Start** (HS) program provides a unique opportunity to reach preschool-age children (Figures 6.15 and 6.16). Dental hygienists can be involved at multiple levels.

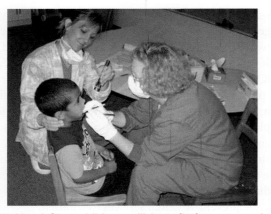

Fig 6.15 Head Start children will benefit from screening and fluoride varnish programs conducted by dental hygienists.

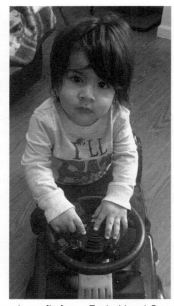

Fig 6.16 Toddlers benefit from Early Head Start oral health programs that put them on the road to healthy teeth and gingiva starting with "the first tooth." (Courtesy Anabel Ruiz.)

Head Start Program Description

HS was founded in 1965 as part of President Johnson's War on Poverty[48] and has been reauthorized consistently by subsequent presidents. The most recent HS reauthorization was funded when President Trump signed the Consolidated Appropriations Act in 2017, which included over $9.2 billion for HS programs, representing a 1% increase compared with 2016.[49]

The HS program was designed to break the cycle of poverty by providing a comprehensive early learning program for children from birth to age 5 years from low-income families. HS programs promote school readiness by enhancing the social and cognitive development of children through the provision of educational, health, nutritional, social, and other services to enrolled children and families. HS began as a summer program before kindergarten and progressed to a full-time year-round school program for children 3- to 4-years old at the time of enrollment. Recognizing the mounting

evidence of the importance of the earliest years to a child's growth and development, **Early Head Start** (EHS) was established in 1995 to serve children from age 6 weeks after birth until the child turns 3 years old at the time of enrollment into HS or another pre-kindergarten program. Parents are an integral part of these programs, engaging in their children's learning, learning about effective parenting skills, and making progress toward their own educational, literacy, and employment goals.[50]

HS and EHS programs are administered by the DHHS **Administration for Children & Families** (ACF) Office of Head Start (OHS). Based on specific criteria, HS grants are awarded directly to public agencies, private nonprofit or for-profit organizations, tribal governments, and school systems for the purpose of operating HS programs in local communities.[48] HS agencies receive grant funding directly from ACF (rather than from the state) and may directly operate the HS program, delegate operations to another agency, or use a combination of these means. The HS programs are located in schools, community centers, or family child-care homes in urban, suburban, and rural communities.[50]

Head Start annually reports general information about the program, including demographics for the children and families enrolled and program statistics. Children from families with incomes below the FPL are eligible for HS and EHS services.[50] For example, in 2019, a family of four was required to have an income at or below $25,750 to qualify to enroll their children.[51] Children from homeless families and families receiving public assistance are also eligible, and foster children are eligible regardless of their foster family's income.[51] The ages, racial/ethnic group representation, and primary language of children in HS programs are presented in Table 6.9.

Health Services

The HS staff partners with parents to support children's growth and development and facilitate learning by providing services that encompass early learning, family well-being, and health.[52] In the area of health, children's perceptual, motor, and physical development are supported to permit them to fully explore and function in their environment. All children receive health and development screenings, nutritious meals, and oral health and mental health support. Programs connect families with medical, dental, and mental health services to ensure that children are receiving the services they need.[50] Children are taught healthy behaviors, such as handwashing, toothbrushing, injury prevention, physical activity, and making healthy food choices. Parents participate in health education workshops or receive health education services in the home.[52]

HS programs are required to establish and maintain a Health Services Advisory Committee (HSAC) comprised of local healthcare professionals, parents, and other community volunteers.[52] The HSAC can be instrumental in identifying community resources, assisting programs in developing and implementing policies and procedures, keeping the program informed of emerging research and practice guidelines, and providing education to program staff and parents.[52] Participation on the

TABLE 6.9   Head Start Child and Family Demographics, 2017–2018

Total number of children and pregnant women served in the 50 states, District of Columbia, and six territories	1,050,000
Ages[a]	
5 years old and older	1%
4 years old	38%
3 years old	35%
2 years old	11%
1 year old	7%
Younger than 1 year old	6%
Pregnant women	1%
Racial/Ethnic Composition[a]	
White	44%
Black/African American	30%
Unspecified/Other	10%
Biracial/Multiracial	10%
American Indian/Alaska Native	2%
Hawaiian/Pacific Islander	1%
Ethnicity	
Hispanic or Latino Origin	37%
Non-Hispanic/Non-Latino Origin	63%
Language	
Families primarily speaking a language other than English at home	28%
Families primarily speaking Spanish at home	22%

[a]Percentage does not total 100% because of rounding.
(From Head Start Program Facts Fiscal Year 2018. U.S. Department of Health and Human Services, Office of the Assistant Secretary for Planning and Evaluation; 2018. Available at: <https://eclkc.ohs.acf.hhs.gov/sites/default/files/pdf/no-search/hs-program-fact-sheet-2018.pdf>; [Accessed November 2019].)

BOX 6.18   Requirements for Local Head Start Programs Related to Oral Health

- Within the first 90 days of enrollment, determine if each child is up-to-date on age-appropriate primary and secondary preventive oral health care, based on the Early and Periodic Screening, Diagnostic, and Treatment (EPSDT) dental periodicity schedules; if not up-to-date, assist parents with arranging to bring the child up-to-date as quickly as possible.
- Assist parents in understanding how to enroll and participate in ongoing family dental care (dental home).
- Help parents continue to follow recommended oral healthcare schedules.
- Implement periodic observations (screening) or other appropriate strategies to identify new or recurring oral health concerns.
- Respond to each child's individual needs based on dental evaluations and treatments
- Facilitate and monitor necessary oral health preventive care, treatment, and follow-up, including topical fluoride treatments, as recommended by an oral health professional.
- In communities where there is inadequate fluoride in the water supply and for every child with moderate to severe tooth decay, also facilitate fluoride supplements and other necessary preventive measures and further oral health treatment as recommended by the oral health professional.
- Provide assistance to parents related to obtaining prescribed medications and supplies related to an oral health condition.
- Establish and implement policies and procedures for rapid response to dental emergencies with which all staff are familiar and trained.
- Assist children who have teeth with once-daily toothbrushing with fluoride toothpaste at school.
- Provide oral health education for staff, parents, and families; include information on the principles of preventive oral health, incorporating the need for early dental treatment during pregnancy.
- Encourage parents to become active partners in their children's oral healthcare process and to accompany their children to dental examinations and appointments.
- Facilitate enrolled pregnant women in accessing comprehensive services through oral healthcare referrals.
- Develop a system for staff to track referrals and services provided and monitor the implementation of a follow-up plan to meet any oral health treatment needs.

From Head Start Program Performance Standards. U.S. Department of Health and Human Services Administration for Children and Families, Office of Head Start, 2016. Available at: <https://eclkc.ohs.acf.hhs.gov/sites/default/files/pdf/hspps-appendix.pdf>; [Accessed November 2019].)

HSAC is an opportunity for dental hygienists to get involved in local HS programs.

Oral Health Services

In recognition of the critical importance of oral health for young children, oral health requirements are incorporated into the *Head Start Program Performance Standards*[52] (Box 6.18). HS programs must provide high-quality oral health services that are developmentally, culturally, and linguistically appropriate and that will support each child's growth and school readiness.[53] Children learn about oral health through classroom education (Figures 6.17 and 6.18) and required daily tooth brushing at school (Figure 6.19), and parents receive OHE and encouragement to support preventive oral health practices at home.[53]

Also, local HS programs are required to work with every enrolled family to establish a dental home (see later section The Dental Home for Children and Adults) and assure that children receive dental examinations, necessary treatment, monitoring, and preventive measures such as fluoride. Because of the increased emphasis on dental homes by the medical community, the number of children who enter HS programs without a dental home has decreased in the past decade. The report *Head Start Program Facts: Fiscal Year 2018* indicates that the number of HS children with a dental home increased significantly during the 2017–2018 program year,[50] as it has during the previous years since 2011.[50] Nevertheless, the number of children without a dental home is still significant.[50]

Resources are available to assist HS programs in establishing dental homes and locating oral health professionals to provide services to meet the oral health performance standards. It is recommended that a HS program establish mutually beneficial collaborations with individuals and organizations

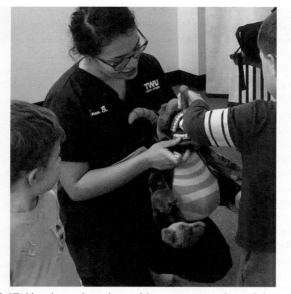

Fig 6.17 Hands-on learning with puppets and models makes learning about toothbrushing fun for preschool children.

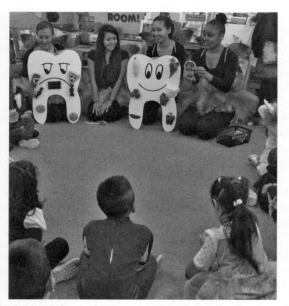

Fig 6.18 Head Start children need to learn the basics of oral health, including healthy food choices. (Courtesy Schelli Stedke.)

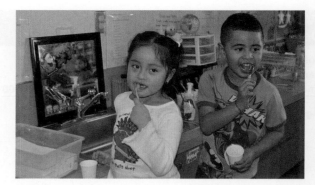

Fig 6.19 Head Start requirements include daily brushing at school to reinforce this important healthy lifestyle behavior.

Dental Hygienists Working with Head Start

Whether employed in an HS program or providing volunteer service, dental hygienists are a valuable resource to HS programs, potentially providing the following services:

- Offer, coordinate, and provide screenings, preventive services, education, and referral for treatment (Figures 6.7–6.11 and 6.15–6.19); many states have adopted less restrictive supervision regulations that allow dental hygienists **direct access** (see Chapter 2) to provide services in public health settings, including HS programs.[57]
- Assist in the coordination of follow-up care.[58]
- Provide leadership for the HSAC.[52]
- Advocate for HS children and families.[59]
- Facilitate establishing dental homes for HS children.[59] (Figure 6.20)

Dental hygienists also function as *dental hygienist liaisons.* The National Center on Early Childhood Health and Wellness (NCECHW), administered by the American Academy of Pediatrics, works in partnership with ADHA to coordinate the Dental Hygienist Liaison program.[59] In this program, one dental hygienist from each state volunteers to promote oral health for pregnant women and children enrolled in HS in the following ways:[59]

- Provide a communication link between NCECHW and HS programs.
- Work with state and local organizations, such as coalitions and SOHPs, to solve oral healthcare access problems for HS children.
- Meet with health professionals to share information about HS's commitment to oral health and to assist participants in acquiring oral healthcare services.
- Provide or work with oral health and health professionals to deliver fluoride varnish application for children and OHE and training to program staff.
- Share information and materials about the importance of oral health, oral health visits, good nutrition, oral hygiene practices, and oral-injury-prevention strategies with program staff and families.

Resources for dental hygienist liaisons are available from the ASTDD at https://www.astdd.org/head-start-state-dental-hygienist-liaisons-information. In these ways, dental hygienists working with HS are enabling the HS grantee to meet the oral health–related performance standards and to bring improved oral health to every HS child.[58]

that represent various parts of the community, such as public health and dental professionals, insurance providers, and universities.[54,55] Because they serve the same general population, reaching out to local community health centers is especially recommended.[54] By building partnerships and communicating a common interest to all, a HS program can work with the whole community to promote children's oral health.[54] The OHS also has resources on their website to help HS programs provide oral health services (https://eclkc.ohs.acf.hhs.gov/oral-health). In addition, case management systems developed by the states help caregivers navigate the complex dental care delivery and payment systems to help assure that children needing dental care can obtain it.[56]

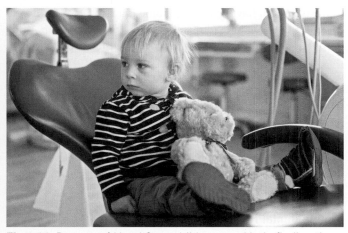

Fig 6.20 Parents of Head Start children need help finding them a dental home. (@ iStock.com/tatyana_tomsickova.)

The National Maternal and Child Oral Health Resource Center (OHRC) has the goal of enhancing the quality of oral health services for pregnant women, infants, and children. OHRC has developed a wealth of educational materials, such as brochures for pregnant women and parents of infants and young children, tip sheets for HS staff and parents, and fact sheets. These resources can assist dental hygienists who wish to become involved in HS and other pre-school programs (see Additional Resources at the end of this chapter).

SECONDARY AND TERTIARY ORAL HEALTH PREVENTION PROGRAMS

Dental Treatment

Primary preventive procedures can successfully reduce the prevalence and incidence of the major oral diseases. However, failure to receive primary preventive care results in the need for more costly secondary and tertiary preventive treatment of oral diseases.[1] Elimination of oral diseases in the U.S. population has not been achieved. In 2017, only approximately 84.9% of children (ages 2–17 years), 64% of adults (ages 18–64 years), and 65.6% of older adults (ages ≥65 years) in the U.S received dental treatment,[60] not all of which was part of comprehensive care. Various barriers are responsible for people failing to seek dental care or seeking it only in emergencies[1] (see Box 5.5 in Chapter 5). Nevertheless, dental treatment is an essential element of dental public health to promote optimal oral health of the population.[8]

The cost of secondary and tertiary treatment programs can be reduced by fully using alternative workforce models such as dental hygiene-based dental therapists (see Chapter 2) and **denturists** who have direct access to provide dentures.[61] In addition, in 2019, dental hygienists were permitted to administer local anesthesia in 45 states and nitrous oxide in 33 states,[62] facilitating and reducing the cost of secondary and tertiary dental treatment in public health.[63,64]

Delivery of dental and dental hygiene services in public health can be accomplished through stationary community-based dental clinics, which may be run by federal, state, county, city, or private nonprofit organizations.[61] This delivery of care can also be accomplished with the use of vans, portable dental equipment, or a combination (see Figures 2.3, 2.4, 2.7, and 2.11 in Chapter 2 and Figure 11.14 in Chapter 11).[66] Several resources in the Additional Resources at the end of this chapter can be helpful in designing and implementing a mobile clinical oral health program.

Dental hygienists are allowed to initiate treatment in community settings without the presence of a dentist (direct access) in 42 states.[57] This allows easier and less costly delivery of preventive services and provides patient entry into the delivery system to receive further dental care. In this way, direct access can result in the capacity to deliver increased secondary and tertiary dental treatment. Because of the low rates of dental utilization by the most vulnerable population groups, it is important to include screening and referral in OHE programs to assist people in identifying resources for necessary dental care[8] (Figures 6.15 and 6.21).

The Dental Home for Children and Adults

The dental home concept is important to the improvement of oral health for all (Figure 6.22). The dental home can be provided by a traditional dental office or by a dental public health clinic. In the public health setting, this can be a stationary clinical facility or a mobile clinic.[65,66] As long as a dental public health facility can provide comprehensive care on a consistent basis, it can be a dental home for any age group. Because of problems with inconsistent access to certain mobile facilities, some states have introduced legislation requiring mobile dentists and mobile clinical facilities to register with the state to assure that patients have access to dental records.[67]

The dental home has been emphasized in dental public health programs especially for children (Figure 6.20). According to the AAPD, the **dental home** is "the ongoing relationship between the dentist and the patient, inclusive of all aspects of oral health care delivered in a comprehensive, continuously accessible, coordinated, and family-centered way. The dental home should be established no later than 12 months of age to

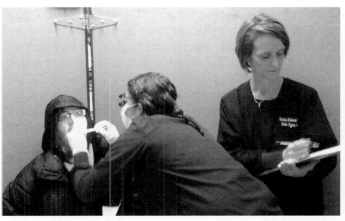

Fig 6.21 Dental hygiene students screen homeless and indigent individuals at a faith-based soup kitchen as part of a community program designed to provide oral health education and referral to local community clinics for treatment. (Courtesy Our Daily Bread, Denton, Texas.)

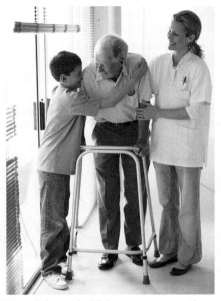

Fig 6.22 Older adults and children are among the underserved, vulnerable populations that need a coordinated dental home program. (@ iStock.com.)

help children and their families institute a lifetime of good oral health. A dental home addresses anticipatory guidance and preventive, acute, and comprehensive oral health care and includes referral to dental specialists when appropriate."[68] The AAPD *Policy on the Dental Home* outlines specific services that should be provided by the pediatric dental home.[69]

The passage of the **Patient Protection and Affordable Care Act** (ACA) of 2010 included the addition of the dental home concept to the medical home using an **interprofessional collaborative practice** (ICP) approach through the **Early and Periodic Screening, Diagnostic and Treatment** (EPSDT) benefit for children and adolescents under age 21 who are enrolled in Medicaid.[70] Growing evidence supports the need for this team-based delivery approach to achieve better primary and oral healthcare outcomes.[8,69]

Initiatives are in place to assist with the establishment of dental homes for children. As explained throughout this chapter, families are encouraged and assisted in establishing a dental home for children through HS and various school-based oral health programs. In addition, the American Academy of Pediatrics has published *Bright Futures*[71] and the *Oral Health Toolkit*[72] to support medical practitioners in using an ICP approach to encourage the establishment of dental homes for their pediatric patients. These resources provide healthcare providers with oral health guidelines and other necessary oral health information, including an oral care periodicity schedule, for use in their treatment, education, and referral of patients from pregnancy to adolescence. These resources are useful also to inform policymakers about children's oral health issues. (See the ICP section in Chapter 2 for more information on these resources and the ICP approach.)

A dental home is equally important for adults. Having a dental home provides the potential for greater utilization of oral health services and reduction of risk of oral diseases. According

to the ADA, not having a dental home is a risk factor for dental caries for children and adults of all ages.[73] The American Academy of Periodontology recommends routine dental hygiene care and early identification to prevent and control the progression of periodontal disease in adults.[74] Individuals with a dental home are more likely to receive this care. The dental home is critical also in relation to the potentially life-saving practice of routine oral cancer screening to identify oral and pharyngeal cancer in the early stages, which reduces mortality rates. According to the American Cancer Society, early identification often allows for more treatment options and can result in better treatment outcomes.[75]

I-Smile Dental Home Program

Greater coordination and case management of Medicaid and other government-funded healthcare coverage through state Medicaid offices will enhance the success of establishing dental homes. An exemplary program is *I-Smile*, a statewide dental home program operated by the Iowa Department of Public Health (IDPH) that connects people of all ages living in Iowa with dental, medical and community resources.[76]

Funded by the Iowa Department of Human Services, the I-Smile program is administered through contracts with local public health organizations that are part of the statewide Title V Child Health Program, which assures health services for low-income children, adolescents, and pregnant women. Each Child Health Program contractor has an I-Smile Coordinator working within their communities to help children and pregnant women access oral health services, prevent oral diseases, better understand the importance of good oral health, and establish a dental home.[76] I-Smile Coordinators are the point of contact within the dental network, assessing community needs, coordinating dental care, and addressing barriers that prevent access to dental care.[76] Responsibilities of I-Smile Coordinators are presented in Box 6.19.

Two specialized arms of the I-Smile program also operate. The first consists of 19 *I-Smile @ School* programs that provide

---

BOX 6.19 Responsibilities of the I-Smile Coordinator

- Develop relationships with dental offices to encourage acceptance of referrals of underserved families needing dental care.
- Develop partnerships within the community to promote and increase awareness of oral health.
- Link with local boards of health to address oral health issues affecting county residents.
- Train medical providers how to apply fluoride varnish and screen the mouth for disease.
- Coordinate dental care for families, including assisting them with finding a dental provider, scheduling dental appointments, finding transportation, and payment for dental care.
- Establish access to oral screening, fluoride, and sealant applications in public health settings (e.g., schools; Women, Infants, and Children (WIC) programs; Head Start programs).
- Educate community members about the importance of community water fluoridation.

dental screenings, dental sealants, fluoride varnish, and OHE for elementary- and middle-school-aged children and also help them establish a dental home.[76] To assure reaching children of low-income families, I-Smile @ School targets schools with no less than 40% of children receiving free and reduced-price lunches.[76] Second, recognizing the importance of the dental home for adults, the IDPH is piloting *I-Smile Silver* to help adults and older adults access oral health care.[76] I-Smile Silver is modeled after the I-Smile program for children. It is supported by a statewide oral health coalition for older adults and has additional funding from the Delta Dental of Iowa Foundation and HRSA.[76]

Oral Health Services for Older Adults

An expanding population in need of primary, secondary, and tertiary preventive services is the older adult population. The number of Americans aged 65 and older is projected to nearly double from 52 million in 2018 to 95 million by 2060, with an increase from 16% to 23% of the total population.[77] It is predicted that by 2034, older adults will outnumber children younger than age 5 years for the first time in American history.[77] The growth of this population is expected to affect every facet of American society.

Older adults are at high risk for developing chronic health conditions that can negatively affect their oral health. Approximately 80% of older adults have at least one chronic condition, and 70% of Medicare beneficiaries have two or more.[78] In recognition of the need to address the overall and oral health of older adults, an Older Adults topic area was added to the *Healthy People 2020* objectives, and the Oral Health topic area objectives included older adults.[79] This emphasis continues with *Healthy People 2030*.[79] Many opportunities exist to serve the oral health needs of older adults in the community (Figures 6.23 and 6.24).

Older adults are living longer and are more health conscious than their counterparts of past generations. As a result, they are

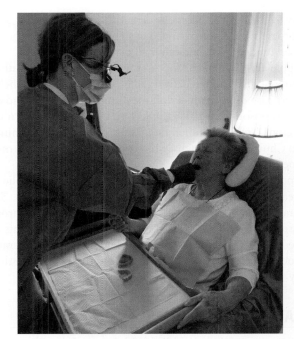

Fig 6.24 Oral cancer screening along with teaching self-examination for oral cancer is a priority oral health program for older adults in community settings.

retaining more of their natural dentition. Complete tooth loss has declined in the U.S., which has increased the need to provide preventive and restorative services to older adults.[80]

Many older adults experience a financial barrier to access to oral health care because of having to live on a fixed or reduced income and losing their dental insurance when they retire. This lack of access to affordable dental care can lead to higher expenditures for medical and emergent care associated with oral diseases.[81] It has been suggested that oral health care benefits need to be provided through Medicare (see Chapter 5) to ensure that seniors have access to good oral health throughout their lifetime.[81] A bill to provide this dental benefit was introduced in Congress in January 2019.[82] Although it did not pass, its introduction indicates a growing appreciation of the importance of oral health care for older adults and the recognition of the need to close the current gap in oral health equity for this vulnerable population.[81] When this proposal becomes reality, this benefit will improve access to oral health services by providing the necessary resources to be able to develop more and broader community-based programs for older adults. In addition, it will expand the prospects for dental hygienists who are interested in serving older adults. To this end, in the role of advocate, dental hygienists can support legislation and programs that will improve access to dental care for older adults.[19]

Apple Tree Dental

An example of a program to increase access to dental care for older adults is Apple Tree Dental, a nonprofit organization that brings dental care to older adults in long-term care facilities via mobile equipment at a reduced fee.[83] Primary, secondary, and tertiary preventive services are provided, including dentures. This program began in Minnesota in 1985, when a few dental professionals

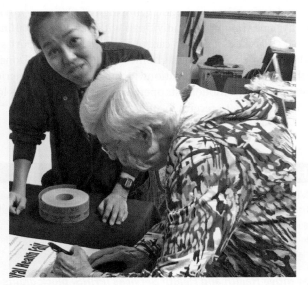

Fig 6.23 Older adults living in a retirement community participate in an oral health fair to gain information and resources that can empower them to maintain their oral health.

organized to provide access to dental care for frail older adults. The program has since expanded to eight locations across the state that serve older adults and other vulnerable populations.[83]

Apple Tree Dental collaborates with state and local authorities to establish mobile delivery sites. Funding sources include a broad base of individual donors, foundation grants, and corporate sponsors.[83] In 2019, Apple Tree Dental received a multiyear grant pledge to launch the newest dental center within the Mayo Clinic Health System, which opened in 2020 in Fairmont, Minnesota.[83]

Apple Tree Dental provides a model that can be replicated to treat older adult populations in other communities. Such programs should be based on an established need through assessment using standardized data collection instruments and procedures (see Chapters 4 and 7) and taking into consideration the social, demographic, health, and economic characteristics of today's older adult population.

FINANCING PROGRAMS

The financing of dental public health is complex, with a combination of public and private monies supporting programs, the availability of which varies according to the national economy. Federal publicly financed initiatives cut across multiple agencies, have multiple federal and state funding streams, and are only as strong as the government policies that support them. These factors can make financing of oral health programs challenging and sometimes risky in terms of depending on future financing.[8]

Public funding is insufficient to address all the oral health needs in the nation, making it important that oral health programs seek diversified funding from other sources such as foundations and philanthropic organizations.[8] At present the majority of public health funding addresses the health and well-being of pregnant women and children and is accomplished through numerous federal initiatives. Several of these and others are described in Box 6.20. Funding for oral health care for other population groups is limited.[1] ACA healthcare reform increased access to oral health services for children and other limited population groups; however, it has been suggested that a more comprehensive health financing system is needed to also improve oral health for other vulnerable groups.[1]

Successful financing of programs results when government leaders collaborate with private entities to establish networks of community, county, city, and state systems to strengthen the core foundation of oral healthcare financing.[8] To this end, the private sector and the business community work with state governors on initiatives that strive to improve the health status of citizens. (See Chapter 5 for additional information regarding financing of oral health care.)

Volunteer Dental Services Programs

Oral health professionals have responded to the need for greater access to dental care for underserved populations by donating their time and finances to provide oral health services free of charge through **volunteerism**. They volunteer in various community programs, some of which have been described in this and other chapters. They also frequently do this through organized **volunteer dental services programs**. For example, volunteer members of various dental hygiene societies operate and staff sealant and fluoride programs in their communities.[84] Another example is the ADA Give Kids a Smile program. Since 2003, over 5.5 million children without access to dental care have been treated free of charge by more than half a million volunteers, including dentists and dental hygienists.[85]

As a nonprofit organization, Dental Lifeline Network (DLN) operates several programs through which volunteer dental personnel provide dental care in their own private practices for people who cannot afford it and have a permanent disability, are aged 65 or older, or are medically fragile.[86] Donated Dental Services (DDS) is their flagship program that provides free, comprehensive dental treatment to this vulnerable population. With programs in every state, DDS is a volunteer network of more than 15,000 dentists and 3500 dental labs and has surpassed $378 million in donated dental services to more than 120,550 people since its inception in 1985. Another DLN program, Dental HouseCalls, uses mobile dental equipment to take dental care to people in Colorado who cannot easily travel, including residents of nursing homes and people who are homebound. Local dentists staff the mobile clinic and, because of financial limitations and lack of insurance, frequently provide donated or reduced-fee services. Colorado Campaign of Concern provides oral hygiene training for individuals with developmental/intellectual disabilities or their caregivers, family, or support staff and helps to establish dental homes for these clients. Donated Orthodontic Services is a nationwide program of the American Association of Orthodontists operated by DLN that enables low-income children to receive in-office orthodontic treatment.[86]

BOX 6.20   Federal Initiatives Used to Finance Oral Health Programs

Block Grants Programs
- Examples of state and local initiatives with significant **block grant** funding include state oral health programs (SOHPs), community water fluoridation, comprehensive school-based programs, safety net programs, and development of state oral health plans based on the *Healthy People* objectives.[1–3]

Maternal and Child Health Services (MCHS) block grants (Title V)
- MCHS is the oldest and one of the largest federal block grant programs.[2]

- MCHS is a key source of funding to promote and improve the health and well-being of the nation's mothers, children, including children with special needs, and their families.[2]
- In 2017, 86% of all pregnant women, 99% of infants, and 55% of children nationwide benefited from a Title V–supported service.[2]

Preventive Health and Health Services (PHHS) block grants
- PHHS block grants allow states to address their own unique public health needs and challenges with community-driven methods.[3]

BOX 6.20 Federal Initiatives Used to Finance Oral Health Programs (*Cont.*)

Women, Infants, and Children (WIC) Program

- WIC provides grants for supplemental foods, nutritional education, immunizations, and healthcare referrals to local communities for low-income pregnant women, mothers of young children and infants, and children aged 5 years and younger who are found to be at nutritional risk.[4]
- A total of $5.7 billion in WIC grants were awarded in 2019 to local WIC programs.[5]
- Oral health is incorporated into the educational component and as assistance in establishing a dental home.[6]
- Local programs collaborate with other agencies and organizations such as SOHPs for oral health information, screening, primary preventive services, and referrals for dental treatment; clinical services such as fluoride varnish application are financed through Medicaid.[7]

Medicaid/Children's Health Insurance Program (CHIP)

- Medicaid and CHIP are federally financed insurance programs that provide dental insurance coverage for dental services in community oral health programs (see Chapter 5).[8]

Administration for Children and Families (ACF)

- ACF is a Department of Health and Human Services agency that promotes the economic and social well-being of families, children, individuals, and communities of vulnerable populations.[9]
- A budget of $52 billion is used to administer more than 60 programs that are operated by 16 different government offices.[9]
- Head Start (HS) is one of the programs administered by ACF (see earlier in this chapter); HS program funds can be used for professional oral health services for HS children when no other source of funding is available.[13]

Community Health Centers

- These centers provide comprehensive health care, including dental (see Community Health Center section in Chapter 5).
- In 2018, almost $9.1 billion in federal and nonfederal grants and contracts supported health centers; the Health Resources and Service Administration (HRSA) Health Center Program is the greatest source of funding.[11]
- They are also funded by Medicare and Medicaid benefits of patients served.[11]
- They generate approximately $54 billion in healthcare services each year; this included almost $3.5 billion in dental services in 2018.[11]
- The program saves the U.S. healthcare system an estimated $24 billion dollars annually by avoiding more costly healthcare services.[12]
- A community health center that serves an underserved area or population as defined by HRSA and receives grants under Section 330 of the Public Health Service Act (PHS) is referred to as a **Federally Qualified Health Center** (FQHC).[13]
- FQHCs must adhere to government regulations pertaining to the scope and quality of health services provided to anyone, regardless of ability to pay.[14]
- A community health center that meets the PHS eligibility requirements but does not receive PHS funding is referred to as a *FQHC Look-alike*; these centers receive other sources of federal and state funding, including Medicare and Medicaid reimbursement.[13]

1. Summary Report: 2019 Synopses of State Dental Public Health Programs: Data for FY 2017-2018. Association of State and Territorial Dental Directors; 2019. Available at: <https://www.astdd.org/docs/synopses-summary-report-2019.pdf>; [Accessed October 2019].
2. Title V Maternal and Child Health Services Block Grant Program. Maternal and Child Health Bureau; 2019. Available at: <https://mchb.hrsa.gov/maternal-child-health-initiatives/title-v-maternal-and-child-health-services-block-grant-program>; [Accessed October 2019].
3. About the PHHS Block Grant. Centers for Disease Control and Prevention; November 15, 2018. Available at: <https://www.cdc.gov/phhsblock-grant/about.htm>; [Accessed October 2019].
4. Special Supplemental Nutrition Program for Women, Infants, and Children (WIC). Food and Nutrition Service. Available at: <https://www.fns.usda.gov/wic>; [Accessed November 2019].
5. WIC Program Grant Levels by State Agency. U.S. Department of Agriculture; 2019. Available at: <https://www.fns.usda.gov/wic/wic-funding-and-program-data>; [Accessed October 2019].
6. Carlson S, Neuberger Z. WIC Works: Addressing the Nutrition and Health Needs of Low-Income Families for 40 Years. Center on Budget and Policy Priorities; March 29, 2017. Available at: <https://www.cbpp.org/research/food-assistance/wic-works-addressing-the-nutrition-and-health-needs-of-low-income-families>; [Accessed November 2019].
7. Lipper J. Advancing Oral Health through the Women, Infants, and Children Program. Center for Health Care Strategies; April 2016. Available at: <https://www.chcs.org/media/NH-State-WIC-Profile_041316.pdf>; [Accessed November 2019].
8. Medicaid/CHIP. Centers for Medicare & Medicaid Services. Available at: <https://www.cms.gov/>; [Accessed November 2019].
9. Budget Information. Administration for Children & Families; 2019. Available at: <https://www.acf.hhs.gov/olab/olab/budget>; [Accessed November 2019].
10. Head Start Program Performance Standards. ACF Office of Head Start; 2016. Available at: <https://eclkc.ohs.acf.hhs.gov/sites/default/files/pdf/hspps-appendix.pdf>; [Accessed November 2019].
11. 2018 National Health Center Data. Bethesda MD: Health Resources and Services Administration; 2018. Available at: <https://bphc.hrsa.gov/uds/datacenter.aspx>; [Accessed November 2019].
12. Letter from Congress to House Appropriations Subcommittee on Labor, HHS, Education, and Related Agencies About FY 2020 Community Health Center Funding. U.S. Congress; March 28, 2019. Available at: <http://www.nachc.org/wp-content/uploads/2019/04/FY20-CHC-Letter_DeGette-Bilirakis_March-2019-1.pdf>; [Accessed November 2019].
13. What is an FQHC? FQHC.org. Available at: https://www.fqhc.org/what-is-an-fqhc>; [Accessed November 2019].
14. Federally Qualified Health Center (FQHC). HealthCare.gov. Available at: <https://www.healthcare.gov/glossary/federally-qualified-health-center-fqhc/>; [Accessed November 2019].

SUMMARY

The various community oral health programs introduced in this chapter offer practicing dental hygienists an extension of their private practice experience. Becoming acquainted with the oral healthcare needs of the community at large—in conjunction with an understanding of the best practices for available oral health programs; funding resources from the local, state, and national levels; and effective program planning processes—provides an opportunity for dental hygienists to become part of the solution to oral healthcare access problems in their communities.

APPLYING YOUR KNOWLEDGE

1. Research and prepare a report on fluoride concentration levels in existing water supply sources in the communities served by your dental hygiene program clinic.
2. Have a classroom debate on fluoridation. Appoint people to take pro and con positions, and research your position before the debate. Research the changes made related to the CDC recommendation for the optimum level of fluoride in the community water supply, and what brought about the changes. Have a mock city council decide the outcome.
3. Develop a community oral health program. Describe the use of all five steps of the community program planning process in your program, including a goal and specific, measurable objectives, and identify potential resources to fund the program.
4. Discuss how you, as a private practice dental hygienist, might help implement the core essential public health functions and oral health services in your community.
5. Research the possibility of forming an oral health coalition in your community using the web to find a toolkit or other source that provides information about how to form a coalition. Whom would you invite to join the coalition? Decide on the goals and objectives of the organization.

LEARNING OBJECTIVES AND COMPETENCIES

This chapter addresses the following community oral health learning objectives and competencies for dental hygienists that are presented in the revised May 2015–2016 *ADEA Compendium of Curriculum Guidelines for Allied Dental Education Programs:*

Learning Objectives

- Identify and use the current practiced public health preventive modalities.
- Defend the need for preventive modalities in dental public health practice.
- Identify appropriate levels of supplemental fluoride for a community.
- Describe the history, efficacy, efficiency, and implementation of community water fluoridation.
- Identify and use community dental health activities related to prevention and control of oral conditions and promotion of health.
- Explain the role of dental providers, with emphasis on the dental hygienist, in activities related to the practice of public health.
- Compare the federal, state/provincial and local presence of government in dental care delivery.
- Evaluate the role of the government in financing dental care.
- Describe how a dental hygienist could best educate a target population.
- Describe the process of lesson plan development.
- List and describe teaching strategies.
- List the characteristics of an effective teacher.
- Develop and present a lesson plan on oral health education.
- Identify target populations to whom dental hygienists may provide services.
- Describe the various program planning paradigms.
- Describe various dental public health programs.
- Develop a dental public health program plan.
- Plan a community program based on the needs assessment.
- Identify possible constraints, alternatives and evaluation tools for the program.
- Describe the mechanisms of program evaluation.
- Compare qualitative and quantitative evaluation.
- Describe various government-related opportunities for dental public health programs.

Competencies

- Providing health education and preventive counseling to a variety of population groups.
- Identifying services that promote oral health and prevent oral disease and related conditions.
- Assessing, planning, implementing and evaluating community-based oral health programs.
- Using screening, referral and education to bring consumers into the healthcare delivery system.
- Providing dental hygiene services in a variety of settings, including offices, hospitals, clinics, extended care facilities, community programs and schools.

COMMUNITY CASE

The dental hygiene school in your nonfluoridated community has received a 3-year federal grant from the U.S. Public Health Service to establish a pilot school-based interprofessional collaborative health center in a Title 1 elementary school that also has a Head Start program. The community is classified as a medical and dental health professional shortage area by HRSA, which provided the basis for the funding. The program will include oral health education, primary oral disease prevention services, and dental treatment. As the newly employed dental hygienist at the school, you will supervise dental hygiene students on-site at the elementary school and in the clinic.

1. All of the following are components of establishing this oral health initiative EXCEPT one. Which is the EXCEPTION?
   a. Assessment
   b. Evaluation
   c. Assurance
   d. Implementation
   e. Planning

2. The program goal is to improve the oral health of the school-age children. Which of the following instructional objectives for the educational component in the second-grade class is specific and measurable?
   a. The students will completely understand the connection of oral health to general health.
   b. The students will label six parts of the tooth accurately on a diagram.
   c. The students will know how to brush and floss.
   d. The students will remember the cause of tooth decay.

3. Which preventive program would have the most benefit for all the school-age children in this community?
   a. School-based fluoride mouthrinse program
   b. School-based fluoride varnish program
   c. School-based sealant program
   d. Water fluoridation

4. Which program is the most likely source of funding for dental treatment in the school clinic?
   a. Medicaid
   b. Medicare
   c. Head Start
   d. Women, Infants, and Children (WIC) program

5. Which dental hygiene service provided by the dental hygiene students is considered the most effective, best practice for the prevention of dental caries?
   a. Parent educational session at a parent-teacher association (PTA) meeting
   b. Development of brochures on good oral health practices
   c. Application of fluoride varnish on children's teeth
   d. Referral of children to the dental clinic for treatment

6. You could use all of the following EXCEPT one as resources to help establish dental homes for individuals in this population. Which is the EXCEPTION?
   a. Association of State and Territorial Dental Directors (ASTDD)
   b. Federally Qualified Health Center (FQHC)
   c. State oral health program (SOHP)
   d. Administration for Children and Families (ACF)

REFERENCES

1. Bersell CH. Access to oral health care: A national crisis and call for reform. J Dent Hyg 2017;91(1):6–14. Available at: <https://jdh.adha.org/content/jdenthyg/91/1/6.full.pdf>; [Accessed October 2019].

2. Best Practice Approaches. Reno, NV: Association of State and Territorial Dental Directors. Available at: <https://www.astdd.org/best-practices/>; [Accessed November 2019].

3. Community Tool Box. Work Group for Community Health and Development, University of Kansas; 2019. Available at: <https://ctb.ku.edu/en>; [Accessed October 2019].

4. U.S. Department of Health & Human Services. Available at: <www.hhs.gov>; [Accessed October 2019].

5. Location-Based Oral Health Programs. Atlanta, GA: Centers for Disease Control and Prevention; October 1, 2019. Available at: <https://www.cdc.gov/oralhealth/funded_programs/index.htm>; [Accessed October 2019].

6. Guidelines for State and Territorial Oral Health Programs: PART II State Roles, Activities and Resources. Reno, NV: Association of State and Territorial Dental Directors; 2018. Available at: <https://www.astdd.org/docs/astdd-guidelines-section-II-matrix-for-state-roles-examples-and-resources-1-2018-revisions.pdf>; [Accessed October 2019].

7. Wisconsin Oral Health Coalition. West Allis, WI: Children's Health Alliance of Wisconsin; 2019. Available at: <https://www.chawisconsin.org/initiatives/oral-health/wisconsin-oral-health-coalition/>; [Accessed October 2019].

8. Guidelines for State and Territorial Oral Health Programs Part I. Association of State and Territorial Dental Directors; December 2015. Available at: <https://www.astdd.org/docs/astdd-guidelines-part-I-2015-update-january-2016.pdf>; [Accessed October 2019].

9. Healthy Smiles in Rural Nevada. Chicago, IL: ADHA Institute of Oral Health. Available at: <https://www.adha.org/healthy-smiles-in-rural-nevada>; [Accessed October 2019].

10. Child Nutrition Programs: Income Eligibility Guidelines (July 1, 2019–June 30, 2020). U.S. Department of Agriculture Food and Nutrition Service; 2019 Mar 20. Available at: <https://www.fns.usda.gov/cnp/fr-032019>; [Accessed March 2020].

11. Dental Health Arlington. Available at: <https://www.dentalhealtharlington.org/>; [Accessed October 2019].

12. Children's Oral Health Coalition. Fort Worth, TX: Cook Children's Health Care System; 2019. Available at: <https://www.centerforchildrenshealth.org/en-us/Counties/tarrantcounty/ChildrensOralHealthCoalition/Pages/default.aspx>; [Accessed October 2019].

13. Local Oral Health Coalitions. Wilsonville, OR: Oregon Oral Health Coalition; 2018. Available at: <https://www.orohc.org/coalitions>; [Accessed October 2019].

14. Local Coalition Grantees. West Allis, WI: Midwest Collaborative Initiative, 2019-2020. Children's Health Alliance of Wisconsin; 2019. Available at: <https://www.chawisconsin.org/download/mci-map/>; [Accessed October 2019].

15. Northern Nevada Dental Coalition for Underserved Populations. Nevada Dental Hygienists' Association; 2019. Available at: <https://nvcha.com/coalitions/>; [Accessed October 2019].

16. McKenzie JF, Neiger BL, Thackeray R. Planning, Implementing & Evaluating: Health Promotion Programs: A Primer. 7th ed. Glenview, IL: Pearson Education; 2017.

17. About the Community Guide. The Community Guide. Washington, DC: U.S. Department of Health and Human Services. Available at: <https://www.thecommunityguide.org/about/about-community-guide>; [Accessed March 2020].

18. Bowen DM, Pieren JA. The dental hygiene profession. In: Bowen DM, Pieren JA, editors. Darby and Walsh Dental Hygiene Theory and Practice. 5th ed. Maryland Heights, MO: Elsevier; 2020.

19. Code of Ethics for Dental Hygienists. In: ADHA Bylaws & Code of Ethics, pp. 32-38. Chicago, IL: American Dental Hygienists' Association; 2018. Available at: <https://www.adha.org/resources-docs/7611_Bylaws_and_Code_of_Ethics.pdf>; [Accessed August 2019].

20. Fluoridation Facts. Chicago, IL: American Dental Association, Council on Advocacy for Access and Prevention, National Fluoridation Advisory Committee; 2018. Available at: <file:///C:/Users/Admin/AppData/Local/Temp/Fluoridation_Facts-3.pdf>; [Accessed February 2020].

21. Featherstone JDB, Rechmann P, Zellmer IH. Dental caries management by risk assessment. In: Bowen DM, Pieren JA, editors.

Darby and Walsh Dental Hygiene Theory and Practice. 5th ed. Maryland Heights, MO: Elsevier; 2020.

22. Community Water Fluoridation. Atlanta, GA: Centers for Disease Control and Prevention. October 23, 2019. Available at: <https://www.cdc.gov/fluoridation/index.html>; [Accessed November 2019].

23. Crozier S. Resolution OKs social media campaign for fluoridation. ADA News; 2014 Dec 8. Available at: <http://www.ada.org/en/publications/ada-news/2014-archive/december/resolution-oks-social-media-campaign-for-fluoridation>; [Accessed August 2019].

24. Manchir M. Water fluoridation on the ballot. ADA News; 2018 Mar 14. Available at: <https://www.ada.org/en/publications/ada-news/2018-archive/november/water-fluoridation-on-the-ballot>; [Accessed August 2019].

25. Community Water Fluoridation Brief: Highlights and Lessons Learned from 2014. Boston, MA: DentaQuest Foundation; 2015. Available at: <http://www.astdd.org/docs/community-water-fluoridation-lessons-learned-2015.pdf>; [Accessed August 2019].

26. Fluoride therapy. Chicago, IL: American Academy of Pediatric Dentistry (AAPD); 2018. AAPD Reference Manual 2018-19;40(6),250-253. Available at: <https://www.aapd.org/globalassets/media/policies_guidelines/bp_fluoridetherapy.pdf>; [Accessed September 2019].

27. Quock RL. The evidence supporting fluoride varnish. J Decisions Dent 2017;3(1):50–3. Available at: <https://decisionsindentistry.com/article/evidence-supporting-fluoride-varnish/>; [Accessed September 2019].

28. School-based Fluoride Varnish Program Report, August 2015-2016. Reno, NV: Association of State and Territorial Dental Directors; 2017. Available at: <https://www.astdd.org/docs/fluoride-varnish-program-report.pdf>; [Accessed September 2019].

29. Beatty CE, Beatty CF, Marshall D. Small steps for big smiles: A community fluoride varnish pilot program (poster). Portland, OR: National Oral Health Conference; 2009.

30. Silk H, McCallum W. Fluoride: The family physician's role. Am Fam Physician 2015;92(3):174–9. Available at: <https://www.aafp.org/afp/2015/0801/p174.html#afp20150801p174-b15>; [Accessed September 2019].

31. Oral Health Program: School-Based Fluoride Mouthrinsing Program. Madison, WI: Wisconsin Department of Health Services; April 17, 2019. Available at: <https://www.dhs.wisconsin.gov>; [Accessed September 2019].

32. Fluoride: Topical and Systemic Supplements. Chicago, IL: American Dental Association; 2019 May 1. Available at: <https://www.ada.org/en/member-center/oral-health-topics/fluoride-topical-and-systemic-supplements>; [Accessed September 2019].

33. Use of Silver Diamine Fluoride for Dental Caries Management in Children and Adolescents, Including Those with Special Health Care Needs. Chicago, IL: American Academy of Pediatric Dentistry (AAPD); 2017. AAPD Reference Manual: Recommendations: Clinical Practice Guidelines, 2018-19;40(6),152-161; 2018-19. Available at: <https://www.aapd.org/media/Policies_Guidelines/G_SDF.pdf>; [Accessed September 2019].

34. Slayton RL, Urquhart O, Araujo MWB, Fontana M, Guzmán-Armstrong S, Nascimento MM, … Carrasco-Labra A. Evidence-based clinical practice guideline on nonrestorative treatments for carious lesions. J Am Dent Assoc 2018;149(10):837–849e19. Available at: <https://doi.org/10.1016/j.adaj.2018.07.002>; [Accessed September 2019].

35. Neurath C, Limeback H, Osmunson B, Connett M, Kanter V, Wells CR. Dental fluorosis trends in US oral health surveys: 1986 to 2012. Tranl Res 2019;4(4):298–308. Available at: <http://dx.doi.org/10.1177/2380084419830957>; [Accessed November 2019].

36. Healthy People 2020 Midcourse Review. Hyattsville MD: National Center for Health Statistics; 2018 Jun 5. Available at: <https://www.cdc.gov/nchs/healthy_people/hp2020/hp2020_midcourse_review.htm>; [Accessed September 2019].

37. Fannon ME, Yamamoto J. Pit and fissure sealants. In: Bowen DM, Pieren JA, editors. Darby and Walsh Dental Hygiene Theory and Practice. 5th ed. Maryland Heights, MO: Elsevier; 2020.

38. Griffin SO, Naavaal S, Scherrer C, Patel M, Chattopadhyay S. Evaluation of school-based dental sealant programs: An updated community guide systematic economic review. Am J Prev Med 2017;52(3):407–15. Available at: <https://doi.org/10.1016/j.amepre.2016.10.004>; [Accessed September 2019].

39. School Sealant Programs. Atlanta, GA: Centers for Disease Control and Prevention; October 15, 2018. Available at: <https://www.cdc.gov/oralhealth/dental_sealant_program/school-sealant-programs.htm>; [Accessed November 2019].

40. Griffin S, Naavaal S, Scherrer C, Griffin PM, Harris K, Chattopadhyay S. School-based dental sealant programs prevent cavities and are cost-effective. Health Aff (Millwood) 2016;35(12):2233–40. Available at: <https://www.ncbi.nlm.nih.gov/pmc/articles/PMC5870880/>; [Accessed September 2019].

41. Gooch BF, Griffin SO, Gray SK, et al. Preventing dental caries through school-based sealant programs. J Am Dent Assoc 2009;140(11):1356–65. Available at: <http://jada.ada.org/article/S0002-8177%2814%2964584-0/fulltext>; [Accessed August 2019].

42. Junger ML, Griffin SO, Lesaja S, Espinoza L. Awareness Among US Adults of Dental Sealants for Caries Prevention. Prev Chronic Dis 2019;16:180398. Available at: <http://dx.doi.org/10.5888/pcd16.180398>; [Accessed December 2019].

43. Integrating Oral Health into the Whole School, Whole Community, Whole Child School Health Model. Reno, NV: Association of State and Territorial Dental Directors; 2015. Available at: <https://www.astdd.org/www/docs/integrating-oral-health-into-the-whole-school-whole-community-whole-child-school-health-model.pdf>; [Accessed September 2019].

44. Benes S, Alperin H. Lesson Planning for Skills-Based Health Education. Champaign, IL: Human Kinetics; 2019.

45. Division of Oral Health at a Glance. Atlanta GA: Center for Disease Control and Prevention, 2019. Available at: <https://www.cdc.gov/chronicdisease/resources/publications/aag/oral-health.htm>; [Accessed October 2019].

46. Whole School, Whole Community, Whole Child. Atlanta, GA: Centers for Disease Control and Prevention; May 29, 2019. Available at: <https://www.cdc.gov/healthyschools/wscc/index.htm>; [Accessed November 2019].

47. Miles of Smiles—Laredo. San Antonio TX: University of Texas Health Science Center San Antonio Dental School; Available at: <https://milesofsmiles.uthscsa.edu/about/>; [Accessed October 2019].

48. History of Head Start. Washington DC: Administration for Children and Families, Office of Head Start; 2019. Available at: <https://www.acf.hhs.gov/ohs/about/history-of-head-start>; [Accessed October 2019].

49. Linehan, L. FY 2017 Head Start Funding Increase ACF-PI-HS-17-02. Washington DC: Administration for Children and Families, Office of Head Start, Head Start Policy & Regulations; May 12, 2017. Available at <https://eclkc.ohs.acf.hhs.gov/policy/pi/acf-pi-hs-17-02>; [Accessed November 2019].

50. Head Start Programs. Washington DC: Administration for Children and Families, Office of Head Start; February 11, 2019. Available at: <https://www.acf.hhs.gov/ohs/about/head-start>; [Accessed November 2019].

51. Poverty Guidelines and Determining Eligibility for Participation in Head Start Programs, 2019. Washington DC: Administration for Children and Families, Office of Head Start; October 29, 2019. Available at: <https://eclkc.ohs.acf.hhs.gov/eligibility-ersea/article/poverty-guidelines-determining-eligibility-participation-head-start>; [Accessed October, 2019].

52. Head Start Program Performance Standards. Washington DC: Administration for Children and Families, Office of Head Start; September 2016. Available at: <https://eclkc.ohs.acf.hhs.gov/sites/default/files/pdf/hspps-appendix.pdf>; [Accessed November, 2019].

53. Head Start Program Performance Standards Related to Oral Health. Washington DC: Administration for Children and Families, Office of Head Start; 2018. Available at: <https://eclkc.ohs.acf.hhs.gov/oral-health/article/head-start-program-performance-standards-related-oral-health>; [Accessed October, 2019].

54. Spiegel M. Improving Access to Oral Health Services for Head Start and Early Head Start Children. San Francisco CA: University of California, San Francisco Public Health Department, San Francisco Children's Oral Health Initiative, San Francisco Health Improvement Partnership; December 2016. Available at: <https://www.sfdph.org/dph/files/dentalSvcsdocs/HS-FQHC_Dental-Handbook.pdf>; [Accessed November 2019].

55. Effective Partnership Guides: Improving Head Start for Migrant and Seasonal Head Start Children and Their Families. Bethesda MD: Health Resources and Services Administration; 2018. Available at: <https://eclkc.ohs.acf.hhs.gov/sites/default/files/pdf/effective-partnerships-guide-oral-health-mshs-v3.pdf>; [Accessed November 2019].

56. Phipps K. MI Head Start Smiles 2017-2018. Lansing MI: Michigan Department of Health and Human Services; July 2018. Available at: <https://www.michigan.gov/documents/mdhhs/Head_Start_Smiles_Report_2017_633306_7.pdf>; [Accessed November 2019].

57. Direct Access. Chicago, IL: American Dental Hygienists' Association. Available at: <http://www.adha.org/direct-access>; [Accessed November 2019].

58. Oral Health Assessment, Follow-Up, and Treatment. Washington DC: Administration for Children and Families, Office of Head Start, Early Childhood Learning & Knowledge Center; 2019 Jan 2. Available at: <https://eclkc.ohs.acf.hhs.gov/oral-health/article/oral-health-assessment-follow-treatment>; [Accessed November 2019].

59. Holt K. National Center on Early Childhood Health and Wellness Dental Hygienists' Liaison Program. Pediatrics 2018;141(1):601. Available at: <https://pediatrics.aappublications.org/content/141/1_MeetingAbstract/601>; [Accessed November 2019].

60. Oral and Dental Health: Dental Visits. Hyattsville, MD: National Center for Health Statistics; 2017 May 3. Available at: <https://www.cdc.gov/nchs/fastats/dental.htm>; [Accessed November 2019].

61. Denturist: License Requirements. Olympia WA: Washington State Health Department; Available at: <https://www.doh.wa.gov/LicensesPermitsandCertificates/ProfessionsNewReneworUpdate/Denturist/LicenseRequirements>; [Accessed November 2019].

62. Scope of Practice. Chicago IL: American Dental Hygienists' Association; 2019. Available at: <https://www.adha.org/scope-of-practice>; [Accessed November 2019].

63. Smith AM, Gurenlian JR, Freudenthal J, Appleby KM. Patients' perspective regarding the administration of local anesthesia by dental hygienists. J Dent Hyg 2019;93(5):40–7. Available at: <https://jdh.adha.org/content/93/5/40>; [Accessed November 2019].

64. Richardson AM. Dental hygiene and anesthesia: Even government is perplexed by doublespeak. DentistryIQ; March 9, 2015. Available at: <https://www.dentistryiq.com/dental-hygiene/career-development/article/16349502/dental-hygiene-and-anesthesia-even-government-is-perplexed-by-doublespeak>; [Accessed November 2019].

65. Health Center Program. Bethesda MD: Health Resources and Services Administration, Bureau of Primary Health Care. Available at: <https://bphc.hrsa.gov/>; [Accessed November 2019].

66. Langelier M, Moore J, Carter R, Boyd L, Rodat C. An Assessment of Mobile and Portable Dentistry Programs to Improve Population Oral Health. Albany NY: Oral Health Workforce Research Center, Center for Health Workforce Studies, School of Public Health, SUNY at Albany; August 2017. Available at: <http://www.oralhealthworkforce.org/wp-content/uploads/2017/11/OHWRC_Mobile_and_Portable_Dentistry_Programs_2017.pdf>; [Accessed November 2019].

67. Ingles J. Ohio bill prescribes rules for mobile dental units. Cincinnati OH: Cincinnati Public Radio; December 4, 2019. Available at: <https://www.wvxu.org/post/ohio-bill-prescribes-rules-mobile-dental-units#stream/0>; [Accessed December 2019].

68. American Academy of Pediatric Dentistry. Definition of Dental Home. The Reference Manual of Pediatric Dentistry 2019-2020, p. 15; 2018. Available at: <https://www.aapd.org/media/Policies_Guidelines/D_DentalHome.pdf>; [Accessed February 2020].

69. American Academy of Pediatric Dentistry. Policy on the Dental Home. The Reference Manual of Pediatric Dentistry 2019-2020, pp. 34-35; 2018. Available at: <https://www.aapd.org/globalassets/media/policies_guidelines/p_dentalhome.pdf>; [Accessed February 2020].

70. Early and Periodic Screening, Diagnostic, and Treatment. Medicaid.gov. Available at: <https://www.medicaid.gov/medicaid/benefits/epsdt/index.html>; [Accessed November 2019].

71. Bright Futures. Washington DC: American Academy of Pediatrics; 2019. Available at: <https://brightfutures.aap.org/Pages/default.aspx>; [Accessed October 2019].

72. Oral Health Toolkit. Washington DC: American Academy of Pediatrics; 2019. Available at: <https://www.aap.org/en-us/about-the-aap/aap-press-room/campaigns/tiny-teeth/Pages/default.aspx>; [Accessed September 2019].

73. Caries Risk Assessment and Management: ADA Caries Risk Assessment Forms. Chicago, IL: American Dental Association; 2018 Dec 14. Available at: <https://www.ada.org/en/member-center/oral-health-topics/caries-risk-assessment-and-management>; [Accessed November 2019].

74. Preventing Periodontal Disease. Chicago, IL: American Academy of Periodontology; 2019. Available at <https://www.perio.org/consumer/prevent-gum-disease>; [Accessed November 2019].

75. Oral Cavity and Oropharyngeal Cancer: Early Detection, Diagnosis, and Staging. Atlanta, GA: American Cancer Society; 2019. Available at: <http://www.cancer.org/cancer/oral-cavity-and-oropharyngeal-cancer/detection-diagnosis-staging.html>; [Accessed November 2019].

76. I-Smile. De Moines, IA: Iowa Department of Public Health; 2019. Available at: <https://idph.iowa.gov/ohds/ismile>; [Accessed November 2019].

77. Vespa J, Medina L, Armstrong DM. Demographic Turning Points for the United States: Population Projections for 2020 to 2060: Population Estimates and Projections: Current Population Reports. Washington, DC: U.S. Census Bureau; 2020. Available at: <https://www.census.gov/content/dam/Census/library/publications/2020/demo/p25-1144.pdf>; [Accessed March 2020].

78. Healthy Aging: Fact Sheet. Arlington, VA: National Council on Aging; 2018. Available at: <https://d2mkcg26uvg1cz.cloudfront.net/wp-content/uploads/2018-Healthy-Aging-Fact-Sheet-7.10.18-1.pdf>; [Accessed March 2020].

79. Healthy People 2020. Washington, D.C.: Department of Health & Human Services, Office of Disease Prevention and Health Promotion; 2019. Available at: <https://www.healthypeople.gov/2020>; [Accessed October 2019].

80. Dye BA, Weatherspoon DJ, Mitnik GL. Tooth loss among older adults according to poverty status in the United States from 1999 through 2004 and 2009 through 2014. J Am Dent Assoc 2019;150(1):9–23e3. Available at: <https://jada.ada.org/article/S0002-8177(18)30644-5/fulltext>; [Accessed November 2019].

81. Aravamudhan K, Burroughs M, Chaffin J, Chávez EM, Goldberg J, Jones J…Yarbrough C. An Oral Health Benefit in Medicare Part B: It's Time to Include Oral Health in Health Care. Oral Health America; 2019. Available at: <https://www.justiceinaging.org/wp-content/uploads/2018/07/Medicare-Dental-White-Paper.pdf>; [Accessed October 2019].

82. S.22 - Medicare Dental Benefit Act of 2019. Congress.gov; 2019 Jan 3. Available at: <https://www.congress.gov/bill/116th-congress/senate-bill/22>; [Accessed November 2019].

83. Apple Tree Dental; 2020. Available at: <https://www.appletree-dental.org/>; [Accessed October 2020].

84. Sealants Across Texas. Available at: <https://www.facebook.com/events/tstc-in-harlingen/sealants-across-texas/1492320974409914/>; [Accessed November 2019].

85. Give Kids a Smile 15th Anniversary. Chicago IL: ADA Foundation. Available at: <https://www.adafoundation.org/~/media/ADA_Foundation/GKAS/Files/GKAS-15th-Anniv-Gratitude-Report.pdf?la=en>; [Accessed November 2019].

86. About Us: About Our Programs. Denver CO: Dental Lifeline Network; 2019. Available at: <https://dentallifeline.org/about-us/our-programs/#dds>; [Accessed November 2019].

ADDITIONAL RESOURCES

ASTDD Competencies for State Oral Health Programs
https://www.astdd.org/docs/CompetenciesandLevelsforState
OralHealthProgramsfinal.pdf

Campaign for Dental Health (fluoridation), American Academy of Pediatrics
http://ilikemyteeth.org/
Cavity Free Kids
http://cavityfreekids.org/
CDC Division of Oral Health
http://www.cdc.gov/oralhealth/index.htm
Colgate Bright Smiles, Bright Futures
http://www.colgate.com/app/BrightSmilesBrightFutures/US/EN/HomePage.cvsp
Crest + Oral B
http://www.dentalcare.com/en-US/home.aspx
Delta Dental Community Care Foundation
https://www.deltadentalins.com/about/community/philanthropy/
Fluoridation Facts, 2018, American Dental Association
https://www.ada.org/en/public-programs/advocating-for-the-public/fluoride-and-fluoridation/fluoridation-facts
Fluoride Varnish Guide, State of Tennessee
https://www.tn.gov/content/dam/tn/health/program-areas/Dental%20Fluoride%20Varnish%20Guide%202017.pdf
Head Start Health Services Competencies: A Tool to Support Health Managers and Staff
https://eclkc.ohs.acf.hhs.gov/sites/default/files/pdf/health-competencies.pdf
Mobile-Portable Dental Manual
http://www.mobile-portabledentalmanual.com
Mouth Healthy Oral Health Curriculum, American Dental Association
http://www.mouthhealthy.org/en/
National Maternal and Child Oral Health Resource Center
https://www.mchoralhealth.org/
National Spit Tobacco Education Program (NSTEP)
https://www.rwjf.org/en/library/research/1999/01/to-improve-health-and-health-care-1998-1999/the-national-spit-tobacco-education-program.html
Oral Health Foundation
https://www.dentalhealth.org/
Oral Health Resources for Head Start
https://eclkc.ohs.acf.hhs.gov/oral-health
School-based Dental Sealant Program Manual, Ohio Department of Health
https://www.astdd.org/docs/ohio-dental-sealant-manual-february-2018.pdf
School Based Fluoride Mouthrinse Manual, Wisconsin Department of Health Services, Division of Public Health, Oral Health Program
https://www.dhs.wisconsin.gov/publications/p0/p00309.pdf
Seal America: The Prevention Invention. 3rd ed., 2016
https://www.mchoralhealth.org/seal/

7

Research

Risa Handman-Nettles and Christine French Beatty

OBJECTIVES

1. Explain the importance of research in relation to dental hygiene practice.
2. Describe evidence-based decision-making (EBDM) and explain the levels of evidence used for EBDM in relation to the process of EBDM.
3. Explain the significance and use of the scientific method in researching questions related to dental hygiene practice.
4. Differentiate between the null hypothesis and the alternate hypothesis of a research study.
5. Contrast qualitative and quantitative research and describe the use of each in relation to dental hygiene.
6. Recognize various research designs and explain the characteristics and uses of each.
7. Explain sampling, describe sampling techniques and their uses, and explain the importance of sample size.
8. Describe the groups used in experimental, quasi-experimental, and observational studies, and describe the use of randomization and matching to form groups.
9. Contrast independent and dependent variables; explain the significance and relationship of relevant and extraneous variables to research study results.
10. Explain procedures that control errors and bias in research, including blinding, length of study, sampling, collection of data, treatment of data, and other important considerations.
11. Explain validity, reliability, and associated terms relative to data collection and generalization; describe how to minimize threats to validity.
12. Explain the standards of ethical conduct of research.
13. Explain the types of data and measurement scales and the significance of each.
14. In relation to the presentation of data and data analysis:
    a. Compute and use the mean, median, and mode to summarize data; compute and use measures of dispersion to define distribution curves; and interpret percentiles.
    b. Discuss the uses of and interpret the results of descriptive, correlation, and inferential statistics.
    c. Develop and use different types of chart displays to present data; determine which type of graph to use with different types of data.
    d. Determine when it is appropriate to use parametric versus nonparametric statistics.
    e. Explain the significance of 68%, 95%, and 99% of the scores in relation to the normal distribution.
    f. Contrast the use of the following inferential statistical tests: t-test, analysis of variance (ANOVA), confidence intervals, chi-square, Wilcoxon signed-rank test, and Mann-Whitney U test.
    g. Explain probability, statistical significance, power, and the role of sample size in relation to power and statistical significance.
    h. Explain the p value required for statistical significance and its relationship to inferential statistical tests.
    i. Explain the statistical conclusion.
    j. Explain the difference between and how to prevent type I and type II errors.
15. Express the importance of and the criteria for evaluating dental literature; review a research report related to dentistry or dental hygiene; and explain the differences between clinical significance and statistical significance.

OPENING STATEMENT: Questions in Research

- How does a public health team decide that community water fluoridation is needed in a specific community and plan ways to promote it?
- What does a dental hygienist say to a patient who asks if a particular mouthrinse really reduces dental plaque biofilm buildup as claimed in advertising?
- How does a dental hygienist advocate with public officials for a change in regulations that would allow older adults direct access to dental hygienists in extended-care facilities?
- How do communities decide what diseases/conditions or target groups on which to focus when allocating public health funds for dental public health programs?
- How does a dental hygienist answer a question about the best brand of toothpaste posed by a member of the audience of a community oral health presentation?
- What health communication channels, formats, and materials are most effective for patients served by a specific community health clinic?
- What is the most effective school-based caries prevention program?
- How does a dental hygienist answer patients' questions about the results of nonsurgical periodontal therapy compared with surgical treatment of periodontitis?
- What are the benefits to the public's oral health of implementing a dental hygiene-based dental therapist workforce model?
- How does a dental hygienist explain the relative advantages of dental floss, a water flosser, and other interproximal oral hygiene aids?

USING RESEARCH TO ANSWER QUESTIONS

Dental hygienists must seek answers to the questions in the Opening Statements and others that relate to the various dental hygiene career paths (see Careers of Public Health section of Chapter 2). Even though students may commonly learn answers to such questions from instructors or colleagues, they must learn where and how to find reliable answers independently, which requires an understanding of the research process. Research via the **scientific method** is the basis by which answers are produced, and **evidence-based decision-making** (EBDM) is critical to the process of applying these answers to different practice situations.

The dental hygiene profession has a research agenda adopted by the American Dental Hygienists' Association (ADHA)[1] and the Canadian Dental Hygienists' Association (CDHA)[2] for their respective countries. The areas of research of each one are summarized in Box 7.1. Their breadth demonstrates the importance of research to dental hygiene practice in all areas of practice a

dental hygienist may select. All the questions presented in this chapter relate to these research agendas.

Research reports published in reputable scientific journals and on the web disseminate the results of independent research. To determine whether the information contained therein is indeed reliable, valid, and useful, certain knowledge and skills must be a part of the repertoire of every competent dental hygienist. This chapter provides a basic overview of what research entails and a means of evaluating the results of that research.

Evidence-Based Decision-Making

Evidence-based practice (EBP) in dental hygiene is the conscientious, explicit, and judicious use of current best evidence in answering questions about the care of individual patients.[3] This means that dental hygienists practicing according to EBP are meticulous in carefully and wisely using clear scientific evidence from research results to make practice-based decisions. EBP applies to all dental hygiene career paths and professional roles. Most applications of EBDM are made to clinical practice; however, EBDM

BOX 7.1   Dental Hygiene Research Agendas

American Dental Hygienists' Association

Professional Development

- Education—Assessment of curricula, delivery and adaptation of educational programming for addressing evolving models of health care and practice, assessment of educational institutional investment in alternative delivery methods, alternative educational programming, community return on investment, articulation, transferability and academic educational laddering for ongoing growth of the profession, implementation of and evaluation of new or redesigned educational delivery models, assessment of learners' and educators' performance, examining research associated with the Scholarship of Teaching and Learning (SoTL) and alternative career pathways, interprofessional education
- Regulation—Discovery of emerging workforce models, evaluation of changes to professional regulations, use of interprofessional collaborations
- Occupational Health—Determination and assessment of risks for occupational injury; methods to reduce occupational stressors; testing and evaluation of techniques to reduce or eliminate hazards to occupational health; dissemination and translation into practice of methods that reduce harmful effects of occupational stressors on practitioners

Client Level

- Basic Science—Discovery of new tools for diagnosis of conditions and diseases, evaluation of the use of knowledge of emerging science to determine client conditions or needs as related to dental hygiene care, research validating the dental hygiene diagnosis and the translation of outcomes into tools used in clinical practice
- Oral health care—Testing new therapies and prevention modalities for oral health care; evaluating clinical care products, services, behavioral interventions, and new and alternative treatments; developing and evaluating clinical guidelines resulting from successful treatment and prevention modalities which are translated into routine clinical practice

Population Level

- Health Services—Surveys of oral health status and related needs of specific populations and other health services data related to oral health and dental hygiene, community interventions, ongoing strategies to improve translation of population health and community interventions
- Access to Care—Discovery of vulnerable populations, research on access to care, use of outcomes assessment to translate research into population-level health

Canadian Dental Hygienists Association

Risk Assessment and Management

- Caries, oral/mucosal cancer, periodontal, quality of life assessments, treatment planning
- Inflammation
- Impact of aging
- Adjunctive therapies
- Behavior change—Tobacco cessation, nutritional counseling, motivational interviewing
- At risk populations

Access to Care and Unmet Needs

- Healthy public policies to address complex issues
- Seniors and aging
- First Nations, Métis, Inuit
- Low income families
- Other unmet oral health population group needs

Capacity Building of the Profession

- Dental hygiene degree versus diploma
- National standards
- Interprofessional collaboration
- Optimizing/advancing scope of practice
- Higher education
- Integration of new knowledge and emerging research

(From Canadian Dental Hygienists' Association. 2015–2020 Dental Hygiene Research Agenda; 2013. Available at: <https://files.cdha.ca/profession/research/DHResearchAgenda_EN_updated_2020.pdf>; [Accessed July 2019].)

(Modified from American Dental Hygienists' Association. National Dental Hygiene Research Agenda; 2016. Available at: <https://www.adha.org/resources-docs/7111_National_Dental_Hygiene_Research_Agenda.pdf>; [Accessed July 2019]; Canadian Dental Hygienists Association. 2015-2020 Dental Hygiene Research Agenda; 2013. Available at: <https://files.cdha.ca/profession/research/DHResearchAgenda_EN_updated_2020.pdf>; [Accessed July 2019].)

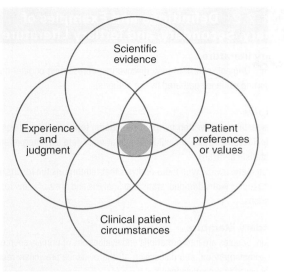

Fig 7.1 Evidence-based decision-making. (From Forrest JL, Miller SA. Evidence-based decision-making. In Bowen DM, Pieren JA. Darby & Walsh Dental Hygiene: Theory and Practice, 5th ed. Maryland Heights, MO: Elsevier; 2020.)

also forms the foundation of decisions about the delivery of oral health education, community oral health program planning and evaluation, advocating for the oral health of the public and the profession, and even appropriate ways to conduct research.

EBDM involves a combination of relevant components: (1) scientific evidence, (2) professional expertise and judgment of the practicing dental hygienist, (3) patient or community preferences or values, and (4) circumstances of the situation[4] (Figure 7.1). These factors require critical evaluation to determine the best decision for the individual patient, community group, or other practice circumstance. All of these components are important.[4] Decisions based on only one or a few of these elements can result in ineffective treatment and programs. EBDM improves a dental hygienist's ability to integrate scientific evidence into dental hygiene practice. This will ensure that dental hygiene practice is informed and strengthened by current research findings.[4]

An example will illustrate these components of EBDM. If an early childhood caries (ECC) prevention program is being planned for a group of teenage mothers, it is important to consider research results relative to specific preventive strategies for ECC; the values and preferences of the young mothers, such as the importance they place on oral health and their preferred learning environments and methods; circumstances of these young teenage mothers such as their specific concerns, age, living situation, family support, financial resources, and children's current health status and oral health needs; and the oral health professional's expertise and judgment relative to working with this population. All these elements are important in planning the most effective ECC prevention program for this priority population.

Ranking of Evidence for Evidence-Based Decision-Making

Scientific research evidence for EBDM is ranked according to its value, founded on the relative authority of various types of research (Figure 7.2). The highest level of evidence available based

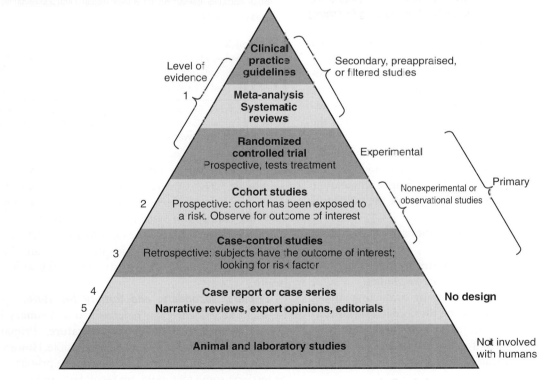

Based on ability to control for bias and to demonstrate cause and effect in humans

Fig 7.2 Ranking of evidence for evidence-based decision-making. The gold standard of evidence (best clinical evidence available) is at least one published systematic review of multiple, well-designed studies of the type that is best to answer the research question. (From Forrest JL, Miller SA. Evidence-based decision-making. In Bowen DM, Pieren JA Darby & Walsh Dental Hygiene: Theory and Practice, 5th ed., pp. 25-33. Maryland Heights, MO: Elsevier; 2020.)

on the type of question and study methodology should be used for EBDM.[3] A dental hygienist must be able to efficiently retrieve scientific information and correctly identify the type of study to ensure the literature is appropriate for EBP.[4]

The traditional **narrative review** that is commonly found in some dental hygiene journals is actually at the lower end of the hierarchy of evidence, so students must learn to find, recognize, and read other types of research reports. The systematic review, especially with a meta-analysis, is the highest ranked evidence for EBDM. Between are various types of individual original research studies, which will be explained throughout the chapter. The systematic review and meta-analysis are described here.

In a **systematic review**, the scientific method is applied to comprehensively review all previously published research studies on a topic that fit prespecified eligibility criteria. The results are critically appraised and synthesized to answer a precise research question. Explicit, systematic methods are used to minimize bias and are communicated to the reader to provide transparency. Applying the following key methods to the systematic review results in an unbiased, comprehensive answer to the research question:

- Use of clearly stated objectives with predefined eligibility criteria for studies included in the review to focus on a single question
- An unequivocal, reproducible methodology
- A systematic search for all studies that would meet the eligibility criteria
- Assessment of the quality and validity of the findings of the included studies by evaluating the research methodology and risk of bias
- A systematic presentation and synthesis of the features and findings of the included studies[5]

The addition of **meta-analysis** to a systematic review provides a higher level of evidence because statistical methods are applied to combine the results of all relevant, independent studies, resulting in new information. Use of meta-analysis has the following advantages:[6]

- Greater power is derived when more data are available for the statistical analysis by combining the data from individual studies; this can result in statistical significance where none was found with the smaller study samples of the individual studies.
- Research results are more valid when they are based on more data.
- New research questions can be answered by identifying consistency of evidence and differences across studies.
- Controversies resulting from apparently conflicting studies can be settled by formally assessing the conflict, statistically analyzing the combined data, and exploring and quantifying reasons for different results of individual studies.
- Knowledge gaps that indicate the need for more research are identified.

A major source of reputable systematic reviews with meta-analysis related to oral health and other healthcare topics is the Cochrane Collaboration. This is an international, not-for-profit, independent organization dedicated to making up-to-date,

---

> **BOX 7.2   Definitions and Examples of Primary, Secondary, and Tertiary Literature**
>
> **Primary literature**
> Definition: Original reports of new discoveries representing original thinking and reporting evidence gathered by the author(s).
>
> *Examples*
> - A research report written by the researcher(s) to relate the findings of an original research study, including presentation of data and interpretation of the statistical results.
> - A systematic review with meta-analysis that reinterprets the results of previous studies with additional statistical analysis and answers new research questions.
>
> **Secondary literature**
> Definition: Sources are interpretations and evaluations of primary sources that offer a commentary on, and discussion of, the evidence previously reported; does not contribute new evidence.
>
> *Examples*
> - Critical literature reviews and many dental sciences textbooks that refer to primary sources.
> - A systematic review without meta-analysis. Although a secondary source, it is still a higher level of evidence than individual primary research reports. This is because it is a critical, comprehensive review of all available studies on the topic, and its transparency avoids the limitations of other secondary sources.
>
> **Tertiary literature**
> Definition: Sources that compile and summarize primary and secondary sources; do not provide evidence for EBDM but can sometimes be suitable in a literature review for certain purposes (e.g., use of a medical or dental dictionary to define terminology).
>
> *Examples*
> - Dictionaries, encyclopedias, fact books, manuals, almanacs, atlases, some textbooks, and compilations of abstracts.
> - Indexes used to locate primary and secondary sources.

(From Richard G. Trefry Library of the American Public Library System. What are Primary, Secondary, and Tertiary Sources? 2019. Available at: <https://apus.libanswers.com/faq/2299>; [Accessed July 2019].)

---

accurate information related to health care readily available worldwide.[6] The Cochrane Collaboration produces and disseminates systematic reviews with meta-analysis through their *Cochrane Database of Systematic Reviews*, available at the online Cochrane Library. At this site hundreds of reviews are available on various relevant health topics, including many that are cataloged under the topics of dentistry and oral health, and public health.

Primary, secondary, and tertiary literature. The sources of scientific evidence can be classified as **primary literature**, **secondary literature**, or **tertiary literature**.[7] Primary sources should be used for EBDM whenever possible. However, this can be confusing in that journal articles can be primary, secondary, or tertiary; some textbooks are secondary, and some are tertiary; and some books are even primary. See Box 7.2 for definitions and examples of primary, secondary, and tertiary literature. A research librarian can help one determine the type of literature and level of evidence of a specific work.

THE SCIENTIFIC METHOD AND DEVELOPMENT OF A RESEARCH QUESTION

Understanding the basics of research entails gaining an appreciation for the components of a good research study, that is, understanding how a research idea is formulated, how a study is designed and executed, and how the resulting data are critically evaluated so that one can infer appropriate conclusions from the results. Research can be thought of as a search for truth and the knowledge gained from this search. A true definition of research is the process of systematically and carefully investigating a subject to discover new insights about the world.[8]

Dental hygiene research involves an organized search for knowledge about issues that relate to the professional practice of dental hygiene. To increase the chance that research will be valid, reliable, and relevant, the scientific method—a series of logical steps starting with the formulation of a problem—is employed. These steps are listed and illustrated in relation to ECC

in Figure 7.3. The discoveries provided by research may lead to new knowledge or to the revision of existing knowledge. Box 7.3 describes the evolution of a research problem, research question, and ensuing clinical trials that led to revising existing knowledge, a process that occurred over more than a decade. This methodical search for knowledge impacted the profession's current standard of practice in relation to the use of fluoride varnish for prevention of dental caries, having a significant effect on the oral health of young children in the United States (U.S.).

Formulating a Research Question

The first step in beginning a research study is the formulation of a research problem, which is the topic to be investigated, or the focus of the research. As this idea is narrowed or clarified it leads to a research question to be answered (see Figure 7.3). Studies can have several research questions. They should be clear, specific, relate to the research problem, and be relevant to the population of interest. Also, research questions should

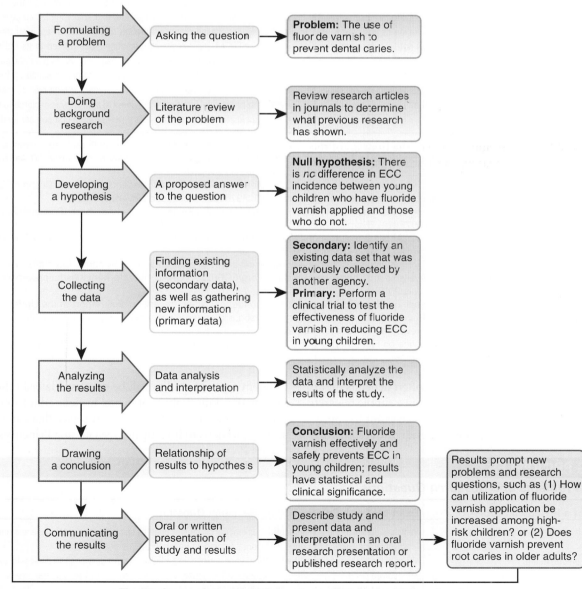

Fig 7.3 Steps of the scientific method. *ECC,* Early childhood caries.

BOX 7.3 **Application of the Research Process to a Current Topic of Interest: Fluoride Varnish**

Research is a continual process that starts with a research problem and ends with answers to research questions, frequently along with identifying the need for additional research. The application of fluoride varnish for dental caries prevention can be used to illustrate this process in relation to a current topic of interest. The review and evaluation of this preventive procedure and its acceptance as a standard of care to prevent caries is an ideal example of applying the scientific method to the research process and using the results for evidence-based decision-making (EBDM).

In the 1990s, the Centers for Disease Control and Prevention (CDC) established a group to develop recommendations for using fluorides to prevent dental caries. The recommendations of this group were based on critical analysis of all available evidence regarding the efficacy and effectiveness of various fluoride modalities. The group critically reviewed studies from Canada and Europe related to the use of fluorides and the effectiveness of fluoride varnish in preventing dental caries. At that time, the use of fluoride varnish in the U.S. was limited to the treatment of dentin hypersensitivity. In 2001, the CDC released guidelines on the use of fluorides to prevent caries based on this review of the evidence available at that time. These guidelines included the statement that "a prescribing practitioner can use fluoride varnish for caries prevention as an *off-label* use, based on professional judgment."[1]

In 2002, the Cochrane Collaboration published a systematic review with meta-analysis of fluoride varnish studies. The conclusion of this review was that fluoride varnish substantially inhibited caries in both the permanent and deciduous dentitions. However, the authors noted that most studies were of poor quality and included little information concerning acceptability of treatment or possible side effects. Furthermore, the authors recommended that further clinical trials be conducted and that they be of high quality and include assessment of potential adverse effects.[2]

After this review, clinical trials were conducted in this country to test the effectiveness of fluoride varnish in preventing dental caries for the purpose of building a stronger body of research on the topic. Based on the results of this research, in 2007 the Association of State and Territorial Dental Directors published a research brief supporting the use of fluoride varnish and promoting its greater effectiveness compared with other professionally applied topical fluorides.[3] The next year, the American Association of Public Health Dentistry passed a resolution recommending the use of fluoride varnish for caries prevention.[4]

In 2013, Cochrane Collaboration published a second systematic review with meta-analysis, updating their first systematic review of 2002. Conclusions of the 2013 review "suggested substantial caries-inhibiting effect of fluoride varnish in both permanent and primary teeth using fluoride varnish."[5] Also, in 2013 the American Dental Association (ADA) adopted evidence-based clinical guidelines on the use of fluoride varnish in dental and dental hygiene practice, supported by a systematic review conducted by the ADA Center for Evidence-Based Dentistry.[6] The American Academy of Pediatric Dentistry reiterated their support of the use of fluoride varnish to prevent dental caries in their updated guidelines in 2014 and 2018.[7] Currently, the clinical procedure is used regularly in private and community-based practice to prevent caries and treat dentin hypersensitivity.[7]

In summary, the use of fluoride varnish to prevent dental caries was questioned, evaluated, researched, supported, and finally implemented into private and community-based practice. Through this process of applying the scientific method to EBDM, more research questions arose related to its utilization. For example, questions about acceptance of the procedure by patients, parents, and oral health professionals were important to address to speed up its diffusion as a dental caries preventive measure, especially in high-risk children. In addition, utilizing medical healthcare providers to apply it was explored to expand its timely application to young children's newly erupted first primary teeth.

---

[1] Centers for Disease Control and Prevention, Fluoride Recommendations Work Group. Recommendations for using fluoride to prevent and control dental caries in the United States. MMWR 2001;50(RR14):1-42. Available at: <http://www.cdc.gov/mmwr/preview/mmwrhtml/rr5014a1.htm>; [Accessed July 2019].

[2] Marinho VC, Higgins JP, Logan S, et al. Fluoride varnishes for preventing dental caries in children and adolescents (Abstract). Cochrane Database Syst Rev 2002;(3):CD002279. Available at: <http://www.ncbi.nlm.nih.gov/pubmed/12137653>; [Accessed November 2019].

[3] Association of State and Territorial Dental Directors, Fluorides Committee. Fluoride Varnish: An Evidence-Based Approach: Research Brief; 2007. Available at: <http://www.astdd.org/docs/Sept2007FINALFlvarnishpaper.pdf>; [Accessed November 2019].

[4] American Association of Public Health Dentistry. AAPHD Resolution on Fluoride Varnish for Caries Prevention; Adopted January 2008. Available at: <https://www.aaphd.org/resolution-statements>; [Accessed November 2019].

[5] Marinho VCC, Worthington HV, Walsh T, et al. Fluoride varnishes for preventing dental caries in children and adolescents. Cochrane Libraries (Web) 2013; doi:10.1002/14651858. CD002279.pub2. Available at: <http://www.cochrane.org/CD002279/ORAL_fluoride-varnishes-for-preventing-dental-caries-in-children-and-adolescents>; [Accessed July 2019].

[6] ADA Center for Evidence-Based Dentistry, Council on Scientific Affairs. Topical Fluoride for Caries Prevention: Full Report of the Updated Clinical Recommendations and Supporting Systematic Review; 2013. Available at: <https://ebd.ada.org/en/evidence/evidence-by-topic/8735/ada-clinical-recommendations-on-topical-fluoride-for-caries-prevention>[Accessed July 2019].

[7] American Academy of Pediatric Dentistry. Guideline on Fluoride Therapy. Clinical Guidelines; 2018. Available at: <https://www.aapd.org/globalassets/media/policies_guidelines/bp_fluoridetherapy.pdf> [Accessed July 2019].

---

be simple and concise; a successful study often depends on an uncomplicated research design resulting from a simple research question. A well-written research question can point to appropriate research methods. Variations of research questions for different types of studies will be discussed later in the chapter. During the clinical phase of dental hygiene education, students might debate about simple, relevant topics that can lead to research questions to investigate (see Guiding Principles).

GUIDING PRINCIPLES

Research Problems and Research Questions

Examples of a Research Problem	Examples of a Corresponding Research Question
Greater difficulty probing various areas of the mouth	Which quadrant in the human dentition is least accurately probed by second-year dental hygiene students at University X when using the Periodontal Screening Record (PSR) method of probing?
Effects of diet on oral health	What is the carbohydrate content of the diet of patients in an Indian Health Service (IHS) clinic who exhibit moderate periodontitis compared with the diet of those who exhibit no signs of periodontal disease?
Level of difficulty maintaining oral health for different people	What is the effect of modifying the brushing techniques of disabled patients in long-term care facilities on their gingival health?

The germane available literature is reviewed in the process of refining a research problem and developing important research questions. Thorough examination of a general topic in the literature will help to bring it into sharper focus and enable the researcher to create pertinent research questions that will address unknown or unexplained areas of the problem. Analysis of the literature is described later in this chapter. An abstract and other information related to a research study conducted by the primary author of this chapter is presented in Box 7.4. This sample study will be used to illustrate various concepts throughout this chapter, starting with the research question for the study. Referring to the study in Box 7.4 in relation to the concepts presented will aid the reader's understanding of how the concepts connect in creating, designing, carrying out, and reporting a study.

Development of a Hypothesis

After a research question is formulated, a **hypothesis** is developed. This is a statement that provides a proposed answer to the research question. The **alternate hypothesis** is stated in positive terms that represent the researcher's prediction or opinion. An example of an alternate hypothesis for the first research question in the Guiding Principles (*Which quadrant in the human dentition is least accurately probed by second-year dental hygiene students at University X when using the PSR method of probing?*) is "*Second-year dental hygiene students at University X using the PSR method are most inaccurate when probing the distal lingual surface of teeth in the upper right quadrant of the human mouth.*"

The hypothesis is often expressed as a **null hypothesis**, which assumes that there is no statistically significant difference between the groups being studied. The null hypothesis is a negative statement of the researcher's prediction or opinion. It is actually the null hypothesis that is tested statistically. An example of a null hypothesis for the preceding question is "*Second-year dental hygiene students at University X show no difference in the accuracy of probing any quadrant in the human mouth when using the PSR method.*" In Box 7.4 the alternative and null hypotheses are illustrated in relation to the research question for the sample study.

GENERAL METHODS OF RESEARCH

Three major categories of research are qualitative, quantitative, and mixed methods. Qualitative research methods require the use of language to answer the research question, whereas with quantitative research, numbers are used to answer the research question. The type of research question determines which method of research is required.[8] Sometimes a research project calls for a combination of qualitative and quantitative methods, called mixed methods. The words provide a clue to help you remember the difference between qualitative and quantitative.

Qualitative = Language
Quantitative = Numbers

BOX 7.4   Sample Quantitative Research Study

Research Question

How do competence and comfort in treating the transgender patient change after dental hygiene students participate in an educational workshop about transgender patient care?

Hypotheses

Alternate Hypothesis: There is a difference between the pre- and posteducational workshop measurements of competence and comfort in treating the transgender population among dental hygiene students.

Null Hypothesis: There is no difference between the pre- and posteducational workshop measurements of competence and comfort in treating the transgender population among dental hygiene students.

Abstract

Introduction: Transgender individuals face barriers to health care such as harassment, violence, and the refusal of care. Findings in the current scientific literature indicate a lack of instruction about caring for sexual minority patients in dental and allied dental education programs, which contributes to the barriers to care faced by this population. The purpose of this quasi-experimental study was to determine the effect of an educational workshop on dental hygiene student competence and comfort levels in treating transgender patients.

Methodology: The study was granted exempt status by the institutional review boards at Texas Woman's University and A. T. Still University. Dental hygiene student competence and comfort in treating transgender individuals were evaluated using an adapted version of the *Assessing Medical Attitudes Toward Transgender Care* survey before and after students attended an educational workshop. A convenience sample of dental hygiene students (n = 45), 55.6% first-year students and 44.4% second-year students ranging in age from 19–37 years, attended an educational workshop about caring for

transgender individuals after completing the pretest survey. Participants completed the posttest survey 2 weeks after attending the educational workshop.

Results: The nonparametric Wilcoxon signed-rank test (n = 45) was used to determine if there was a statistically significant difference between pre- and postintervention competence and comfort median scores. The results showed an overall statistically significant ($p < .001$) increase in dental hygiene student competence and comfort in providing care to transgender patients after attending the educational workshop. The results were considered significant at the preset level of $p < .05$.

Conclusion: Findings support that education about transgender health care can increase competence and comfort among dental hygiene students and should be included in dental and allied dental education curricula.

Additional Methodology

Descriptive Statistics

- Mean age of participants: 23.49 (standard deviation [SD] 3.59)
- Gender of participants: 93.3% female; 6.7% male
- Knew a transgender individual: 24.4%
- Had provided care to a transgender patient: 13.3%
- Mean competence scores: before intervention = 1.89 (SD = 0.65); after intervention 2.99 (SD = 0.56)
- Mean comfort scores: before intervention = 2.97 (SD = 0.81); after intervention 3.7 (SD = 0.44)

Inferential Statistics

- Competence: pretest median = 1.67; posttest median = 3.00, $z = 922.50$, ($p < .001$)
- Comfort: pretest median = 3.00; posttest median = 3.80, $z = 577.70$, ($p < .001$)

(From © Risa Handman-Nettles, RDH, MDH. Used with permission.)

Qualitative Research

Qualitative research methods rely on language to answer the research question. If a researcher cannot explain a particular concept with numbers, a qualitative research design is used. For example, a researcher may be looking for the perceived barriers of parents who fail to acquire dental sealants for their children. To gather data, the researcher could interview parents within that population and analyze the interview manuscripts to discover a common theme. **Qualitative data** can be collected via documented narratives, interviews, documented observations, focus groups, or manuscripts. The analysis phase of a qualitative research study is lengthier than that of a quantitative study because the researcher is required to review responses individually. Analysis of qualitative data provides a context-specific understanding and interpretation of experiences. Qualitative data are coded to summarize the findings, and the codes are organized into categories. The categories give rise to themes that reveal concepts and theories supported by the observations.[8] Qualitative research reports are written narratives that include descriptions of these summaries, categories, concepts, and theories, as well as multiple quotes.[9] Qualitative research methods are used for community needs assessment and preliminary research done for the purpose of identifying research questions and hypotheses.[9]

Quantitative Research

Quantitative research methods rely on numbers to answer the research question. For example, a researcher may want to determine whether a relationship exists between the number of sports drinks consumed by athletes and their caries experience. The researcher could measure the number of sports drinks consumed by athletes in a particular population and the number of DMF teeth or surfaces in the same participants. Such **quantitative data** can be collected using a clinical examination, survey, observation, or patients' charts. Quantitative data are analyzed by applying statistics and communicated with numerical values, charts, and graphs.[11] Box 7.4 includes an explanation about how quantitative data were collected and analyzed for the sample research study presented.

This chapter focuses on the methods used to conduct and analyze quantitative research. Aids for conducing qualitative research are provided in the references and resources at the end of this chapter. Table 7.1 contrasts qualitative and quantitative research methods for greater understanding.

Mixed-Methods Research

Mixed-methods research combines quantitative and qualitative research methods to answer the research question. Data collection and reports of outcomes consist of a combination of techniques used for quantitative and qualitative studies.[8] For example, a researcher may want to investigate the effectiveness of an oral cancer presentation to an older adult community group. The researcher could evaluate their knowledge increase with a posttest for comparison to a pretest (quantitative) and their perception of the personal relevance of the program on a scale of 1 to 5 (qualitative data that is coded quantitatively) along with a brief narrative about how the information related to their own situation and individual changes they plan to make (qualitative).

RESEARCH DESIGNS

There are three main types of research designs used for oral health research: observational, quasi-experimental, and experimental.[10] See Table 7.2 for a summary of these designs and examples of research questions for the different designs. Selection

TABLE 7.1   Qualitative Versus Quantitative Research Methods

Criteria	Qualitative	Quantitative
Purpose	Understand, describe, discover, give meaning, generate hypotheses	Test hypotheses, determine cause and effect, and make predictions
Sample	Generally smaller purposive samples	Larger random samples preferred whenever possible
Data collection approach	Unstructured or semistructured interviews, focus groups, and participant observations	Structured surveys and interviews with closed-ended questions; measurement of specific variables
Types of data collected	Words, interactions, behaviors using rich description rather than numbers	Based on precise measurements using validated data collection instruments; can be reduced to numbers
Type of data analysis	Identify patterns and themes; inductive	Identify statistical relationships; deductive
Results	Specialized findings that are less generalizable; cite participants' responses	Generalizable findings that can be applied to other populations
Scientific method	Exploratory or bottom-up; generation by the researcher of a new hypothesis and theory from the data	Confirmatory or top-down; use of data by the researcher to test a hypothesis and theory
Focus	Wide-angle lens; examines the extensiveness of phenomena	Narrow-angle lens; tests a specific hypothesis
Final report	Narrative report with contextual description and direct quotes	Statistical report with correlations, comparisons of means, and statistical significance findings

(From Merriam S, Tisdell E. Qualitative Research: A Guide to Design and Implementation, 4th ed. San Francisco, CA: John Wiley & Sons, Inc.; 2017; Patten M, Newhart M. Understanding Research Methods: An Overview of the Essentials, 10th ed. New York, NY: Routledge; 2018; Jacobsen K. Introduction to Health Research Methods: A Practical Guide, 2nd ed. Burlington, MA: Jones & Bartlett Learning; 2017.)

TABLE 7.2   Various Research Designs

OBSERVATIONAL RESEARCH APPROACH

Type of Study Design	Observational Characteristics	Use/Purpose	Relative Advantage(s)	Example of Research Question[a]
Cohort study: One group is observed over time; can be compared with a comparison group	Longitudinal; prospective or retrospective	Determine incidence; determine risk; estimate causality	Highest level of evidence of all observational studies; multiple outcomes can be measured for one exposure; demonstrates direction of causality	Will the knowledge of early childhood caries (ECC) of young mothers change over the time period that their children are enrolled in Head Start?
Case-control study: Two groups, one with disease (cases) and one without (controls) are compared to identify factors in their history that can be associated with the disease or condition (exposures)	Retrospective	Determine risk; estimate causality; examine relationships among variables that cannot be studied prospectively because of ethical or practical concerns	Less costly, shorter in duration, and easier to conduct compared with cohort studies	Will a relationship be evident between ECC knowledge of mothers and their own oral health when a group with high oral health status is compared with a group that has low oral health status?
Cross-sectional study: Representative cross-section of the population is observed at one point in time; disease attributes and potential risk attributes are measured to test association	Snapshot of the health status of a population at one point in time	Determine prevalence; can indicate associations between risk attributes and outcome of interest; cannot be used to confirm risk factors or estimate causality; useful to generate hypotheses	Easy to conduct; weaker design than others to show associations between exposure to risk factors and outcome of interest; bias of response and level of nonresponse are concerns of design	Is there a relationship between the ECC knowledge level of a group of teenage mothers and their own oral health?
Ecological study: Existing group-level data (rather than data collected from individuals) are used to relate risk attributes to health or other outcomes Two types: 1. Ecological comparison: assessment of correlation between exposure rates and disease rates among different populations over same time period 2. Ecological trend: correlation of changes in exposure with changes in disease over time within the same community or other group to establish trends	Longitudinal or cross-sectional; retrospective	Identify prevalence and incidence should be used to generate hypotheses rather than to establish definite relationships	Inexpensive, less time consuming, and easy to carry out; less reliable than other designs; prone to bias, confounding of variables and ecological fallacy (observed association for groups may not represent the association that exists for individuals within the groups)	Is the prevalence of ECC in a country associated with per-capita consumption of sugar in the country?

EXPERIMENTAL RESEARCH APPROACH

Type of Study Design	Observational Characteristics	Use/Purpose	Relative Advantage(s)	Example of Research Question[a]
Experimental study: Experimental treatment is manipulated, and dependent variable is measured in two or more randomized groups; characterized by controlled methods; also called a randomized controlled trial; variations include pretest/posttest, repeated measures, crossover, split-mouth, factorial	N/A	Test hypotheses; establish causality	Greatest control of all study designs; highest level of evidence of all studies	Will the ECC knowledge level of a group of teenage mothers increase as a result of an educational program, compared with an equivalent group that does not receive the educational program, when the groups are randomly formed?

(Continued)

TABLE 7.2	Various Research Designs (*Cont.*)				
EXPERIMENTAL RESEARCH APPROACH					
Type of Study Design	**Observational Characteristics**	**Use/Purpose**	**Relative Advantage(s)**	**Example of Research Question[a]**	
Quasi-experimental study: Shares similarities with the traditional experimental design but lacks randomization and control; also referred to as nonrandomized	N/A	Test hypotheses; establish causality	Used when randomization is not practical or is impossible	Will the ECC knowledge level of a group of teenage mothers in one high school increase as a result of an educational program, compared with another high school that does not receive the educational program?	

[a]All research question examples relate to the same research problem of ECC.
(From Kumar KS. Epidemiology for Practitioners; 2017. Available at: <https://www.healthknowledge.org.uk/e-learning/epidemiology/practitioners>; [Accessed September 2019]; Jacobsen K. Introduction to Health Research Methods: A Practical Guide, 2nd ed. Burlington, MA: Jones & Bartlett Learning; 2017; Kviz F. Conducting Health Research Principles, Process, and Methods. Thousand Oaks, CA: Sage Publications; 2020; Himmelfarb Health Sciences Library. Study design 101; 2019. Available at: <https://himmelfarb.gwu.edu/tutorials/studydesign101/casecontrols.cfm>; [Accessed September 2019]; Beatty CF, Dickinson C. Oral Epidemiology. In: Nathe CN, Dental Public Health & Research: Contemporary Practice for the Dental Hygienists, 4th ed. Upper Saddle River, NJ: Pearson; 2017.)

of a design is based on the purpose and hypothesis of the study. Reviewing the literature for previous studies on a topic can guide the choice of a research design for a new study. The selected design can emulate accepted research designs that have been validated previously by others and reported in the literature.

Observational Research

In an **observational research** design, the researcher strictly observes participants' behaviors, actions, or other exposures to disease-related factors in relation to the presence of disease.[9] There is no treatment applied or manipulated and no randomization of participants; rather, individuals are observed in the natural progression of events. For this reason, observational research is below the experimental approach on the ranking of evidence for EBDM (Figure 7.2). Observational studies establish prevalence and incidence. **Prevalence** is the proportion of the population with a given trait, disease, or health condition measured at some designated time.[8] **Incidence** is the rate of *new* disease or other condition in a population during a designated period (number of new cases divided by the total population at risk over a time period multiplied by a multiplier, e.g., 100,000).[8]

Observational research is sometimes referred to as developmental and can be descriptive or analytic. **Descriptive studies** define characteristics of a population, for example, case reports, case series, and simple cross-sectional surveys. **Analytic studies** provide information about association of risk attributes with an outcome such as disease and are aimed at helping to establish risk for developing the outcome and estimate causality. Examples are **case-control studies**, **cohort studies**, and **ecological studies**. **Cross-sectional studies** are also analytic if factors are measured to associate with the variable of interest. Cohort, case-control, and some ecological studies are **longitudinal** in nature, meaning that multiple observations occur over time.[8] This is in contrast to cross-sectional, which indicates that data describing exposures to suspected risk or protective factors and disease outcomes data are collected at the same time.[8] Case-control studies are **retrospective**, indicating that the study looks backward to

identify prior exposures in relation to an outcome that is established at the start of the study.[12] On the other hand, cohort and longitudinal ecological studies are **prospective** in that outcomes, such as development of a disease, are observed forward in time and related to other factors.[8] Table 7.2 provides more information and examples of these various types of observational studies.

Experimental Research

A true **experimental study** design has the greatest control; thus, it provides the highest level of evidence of all the study designs[11] (Figure 7.2). The aim of experimental research is to discover the effects of a treatment in a controlled setting. An experimental design is used to discover if there is a benefit to receiving treatment compared with not receiving treatment.[11] A critical element of control in experimental studies is the randomization of participants to assure equivalency of groups.

A specific example of experimental research is a **clinical trial**, a type of study that tests the safety, efficacy, and effectiveness of new procedures, therapies, drugs, or other interventions to prevent, screen for, diagnose, or treat disease in humans.[8] Clinical trials are conducted on volunteer participants and include a control group to compare the new treatment with a control. These studies are particularly valuable in EBDM.

Various experimental design variations can be applied to clinical trials. Several that are common to oral health research are described here.

Pretest-Posttest Design

In this design, the dependent variable is measured before (called the **baseline** measure) and after the treatment intervention is introduced. The aim is to compare two groups to determine whether the treatment produces a change in the dependent variable in the group that received the treatment or intervention.[12] For example, a study could be carried out to test the effectiveness of a water flosser compared with dental floss in reducing gingivitis. A baseline measure of the dependent variable gingivitis is recorded as a pretest before introducing the intervention (the two types of interdental cleaning procedures). After the study participants use the water flosser or floss for the designated period, gingivitis is measured again, called the posttest, for comparison with the pretest. The **pretest-posttest study** design is classic and can be combined with other experimental designs described here. Sometimes a study is conducted with a **posttest only**. This design has inherent threats to validity in that group similarities prior to introducing the intervention cannot be verified. It also has the weakness of being unable to determine a change in the treatment group resulting from the treatment or intervention.

Repeated Measures Design

Sometimes the dependent variable is measured several times, usually at posttest, to ascertain if the effect of the independent variable on the dependent variable will hold over time. For example, in the study comparing the water flosser to floss, gingivitis could be measured several times as posttest measures (3 months, 6 months, 9 months, 12 months) to be certain that any improvement in gingivitis is not temporary. The **repeated measures** design is sometimes referred to as a *time series* design.[11]

Crossover Design

Study participants can be given a sequence of different treatments with a period of time between, during which no treatment is applied. All groups in a **crossover study** design receive the same treatments, just in a different order. After using the first treatment for the designated period, participants are switched (crossed over) to the opposite treatment after an appropriate **washout period** intended to prevent any carryover effects from the first treatment to the next.[8] This design helps to control any differences between experimental and control group members in that both groups are made up of the same people, namely all the study participants.

An example of this design is to have one group use the water flosser and have the other group use the dental floss for 3 months. At the end of the 3 months, the two groups cease using their interdental cleaning for a month (the washout period). Then the groups switch to use the other interdental cleaning product for 3 months. In this way, both groups will have used both products with a washout period between.

Split-Plot (Split-Mouth) Design

This design is convenient to apply to oral health research because of the ability to assign equivalent pairs (teeth, pockets, arches, sides of mouth, quadrants) to experimental and control groups. In the **split-mouth study** design, all study participants receive two or more treatments to a separate unit of the mouth. This design also has the advantage of exactly matching the control and experimental groups.[12]

An example of this design is to have all study participants use the water flosser on one side of the mouth and the floss on the other side of the mouth. Combining different experimental designs can be illustrated via adding a crossover component by switching sides after a period of time.

Factorial Design

When the researcher is interested in studying several different interventions in various combinations within the same study, a

TABLE 7.3 Combination of Factors for Six Groups of a 3 × 2 Factorial Design	
Group 1 ○ Varnish application 2 times a year ○ Use of xylitol chewing gum ○ Use of antimicrobial rinse	**Group 2** ○ Varnish application 4 times a year ○ Use of xylitol chewing gum ○ Use of antimicrobial rinse
Group 3 ○ Varnish application 2 times a year ○ No xylitol chewing gum ○ Use of antimicrobial rinse	**Group 4** ○ Varnish application 4 times a year ○ No xylitol chewing gum ○ Use of antimicrobial rinse
Group 5 ○ Varnish application 2 times a year ○ Use of xylitol chewing gum ○ No antimicrobial rinse	**Group 6** ○ Varnish application 4 times a year ○ Use of xylitol chewing gum ○ No antimicrobial rinse

Design consists of two levels of three factors:
- Frequency of fluoride: 2 times a year and 4 times a year
- Use of xylitol gum: Yes or no
- Use of antimicrobial rinse: Yes or no

factorial study is used.[8] This design allows the simultaneous assessment of how multiple factors affect the dependent variable and interact with each other. The number of factors can be many. An example of this design is a study to investigate the effects of combining various dental caries prevention therapies on the incidence of caries in high-risk children. Multiple groups would be formed with various combinations of factors, such as fluoride varnish applied at different frequencies, use of xylitol gum, and rinsing with an antimicrobial agent. These designs are identified by the number of factors and the levels being examined. Table 7.3 provides an illustration of a 3 × 2 factorial study (three factors and two levels of each factor, resulting in six groups).

Quasi-Experimental Research

A **quasi-experimental research** design is similar to an experimental design. The purpose is the same, and the design is experimental in nature in that there is manipulation of a treatment in the study. The experimental design variations can be used in quasi-experimental studies as well. The difference is that the participants are not randomized; therefore, other strategies are used to address threats to internal validity and rule out alternative explanations of a possible treatment effect.[12] Also called nonrandomized research designs, quasi-experimental designs are used when randomization is not practical or is impossible.[12] The quantitative study in Box 7.4 is a quasi-experimental study with a pretest-posttest design. It is considered quasi-experimental because instead of using a control and an experimental group, there was only one group. All participants completed the pretest, received the intervention, and completed the posttest. The concepts of randomization and validity will be discussed in more detail later in the chapter.

Another type of quasi-experimental study is a **community trial**, in which a community, rather than a group of individuals, receives the intervention. Such trials can be used to evaluate policies, programs, or preventive treatments at the community level.[10] By their nature community trials cannot be randomized because intact community groups are used. Even though community trials have less control than clinical trials, they are useful to assess the effect of a community intervention on the incidence of disease within that community. Community water fluoridation trials are an example. Another example is to compare the benefits of smoke-free community policies on health outcomes at the community level. A final example of a community trial is an evaluation of a tobacco education program implemented in one high school, compared with a different program or no program in another high school.

RESEARCH METHODOLOGY

When a research question and hypothesis are identified, a plan is developed to conduct the study. This plan consists of selecting a research design (see previous section) and then identifying groups to be involved in the study, methods for data collection, procedures to manipulate the treatment being tested, and statistics and tests to summarize and analyze the data collected. Following a well-thought-out research plan with appropriate research methods is important to control errors and bias (any influence that produces a distortion in the study results).[8] This is critical to generate valid research results that provide legitimate evidence for EBDM. Ways to avoid sources of error and bias are summarized in Box 7.5.

Population and Sampling

It is important to clearly understand what is meant by the population and sample and how they relate to each other. Equally

---

BOX 7.5   Ways to Avoid Sources of Error and Bias in Clinical Trials

- Have a researchable hypothesis
- Base the study on valid assumptions
- Operationally define variables clearly
- Use the appropriate population for the type of study
- Use a representative sample
- Have an adequate sample size to accommodate for loss of participants
- Control extraneous variables
- Use an appropriate type of control or comparison group
- Control group differences by using randomization and stratification
- Use participants as their own control when appropriate
- Use blind and double-blind procedures (masking)
- Use a pretest for comparison
- Control for pretest sensitization
- Use valid and reliable instruments
- Control examiner error with standardization and calibration
- Carefully control and supervise procedures
- Control errors in measuring the dependent variable
- Standardize study conditions in all groups
- Use repeated measures when appropriate
- Use several measures of the dependent variable when called for
- Have a long enough trial to detect new disease or change
- Use statistical procedures that are appropriate for the data

(Adapted from Beatty CF, Dickinson C. Oral epidemiology. In Nathe CN, Dental Public Health & Research: Contemporary Practice for the Dental Hygienist, 4th ed. Upper Saddle River, NJ: Pearson; 2017.)

---

important is comprehension of the various ways that samples can be formed and the value of randomization.

Population

In research the **population** is the entire group of individuals having similar characteristics targeted for study.[12] The term **parameter** refers to numeric characteristics of the population.

Populations can be large or small, depending on the topic to be studied. For example, in the second research question in the Guiding Principles (*What is the carbohydrate content of the diet of patients in an IHS community clinic who exhibit moderate periodontitis compared with the diet of those who exhibit no signs of periodontal disease?*), the population consists of all patients who have been treated in the IHS clinic and have a diagnosis of moderate periodontitis. This population might be difficult to access if it is a large clinic that treats patients from a large geographic area. However, the population of the first research question in the Guiding Principles (*Which quadrant in the human dentition is least accurately probed by second-year dental hygiene students at University X when using the Periodontal Screening Record (PSR) method of probing?*) is likely small and easily accessed, making data collection from the entire population realistic. The population of interest in the quantitative study in Box 7.4 is all dental hygiene students. This is a large population that would be difficult to access; therefore, a sample of the population was used to conduct the study.

A population must be selected that is suitable for the study. For example, a study to test the efficacy of a home care product to control gingivitis must be conducted on a population that exhibits an appropriate level of gingivitis and possesses other necessary characteristics (e.g., age, ability to use the product) to be able to participate.

Sampling

The process of obtaining a representative portion of the population is known as sampling. A **sample** is a part or subset of the population that, if properly selected, can represent the population and provide meaningful information about the entire population.[9] The term **statistic** is used to refer to numeric characteristics of samples.

Samples too can be large or small and are chosen to reflect the research design most appropriately. Large representative samples are especially important for descriptive surveys. Smaller samples are used frequently for clinical trials. A small sample is typically used in a **pilot study**, which is a trial implemented to assess the feasibility of a study.[12] A pilot study cannot be employed to test a hypothesis; therefore, it does not produce evidence for EBDM.[13]

The importance of using a sample can be illustrated in relation to the same research question (*What is the carbohydrate content of the diet of patients in an IHS community clinic who exhibit moderate periodontitis compared with the diet of those who exhibit no signs of periodontal disease?*). Although it might be optimal to collect data from all patients in the IHS clinic with moderate periodontitis to arrive at the answer, this may not be realistic. Because of time constraints, lack of resources, or financial issues, it may be decided that selecting a sample from within the population can make it possible to conduct the study.

TABLE 7.4 Types of Samples

Type of Sample	Definition	Result	Example
Random[a]	Study participants are chosen independently of each other, with known opportunity or probability for inclusion; each member of a population has an equal chance of being included; table of random numbers can be used for selection	Increases external validity by controlling differences in study participants; decreases possibility of selection bias; allows for valid generalization of results to the population; yields a representative sample only when drawn from a homogeneous population	Sample is randomly selected from a list of patient numbers in the computerized patient records who have the diagnosis of moderate periodontitis; if 50 clinic patients have the diagnosis of moderate periodontitis, and a 50% sample is desired, 25 patients can be randomly selected
Stratified random[a]	Study participants are randomly selected from two or more subdivided groups (strata) in the population that have similar characteristics; strata used to stratify are according to any relevant (confounding) variables that could affect the study outcome	Results in a sample that proportionately and accurately represents the subgroups (strata) in the population; yields the most representative sample for a heterogeneous population; controls for effects of confounding variables to prevent extraneous variables	Sample can be stratified for gender by randomly selecting in a manner that results in a sample that represents the percentage of males and females in the population; if 60% of the 50 patients with moderate periodontitis are male, and 40% are female, 60% of the sample will also be male and 40% female (30 males and 20 females)
Systematic[a]	Selection of every nth member of the population from a list or file of the total population; the n depends on the size of the sample desired in relation to the population, for example, 10% is every tenth member of the population	Considered to be random when the list or file of members of the population is in random order and the first member of the sample is selected randomly	From the computerized list of patient numbers with the diagnosis of moderate periodontitis, a 50% systematic sample of 25 patients can be generated by randomly selecting the first patient and then selecting every second patient
Judgmental or purposive[a]	Selection, through personal judgment, of study participants who would be most representative of the population and meet the specific required disease levels and/or characteristics for the purpose of the study; selected by the researcher or someone else with knowledge of the population	Nonprobability sample (not random) that introduces bias, which reduces validity of the sample and limits the generalizability of study results; appropriate to use when very specific criteria are required such as certain disease levels or exclusion criteria for drug or treatment trials	Sample selection by the dental hygienist who has treated the patients, is aware of their disease levels and potential for cooperation and compliance, and is aware of the purpose of the study and the participant qualifications needed
Snowball[b]	Selection by referral to potential subjects in studies where subjects are hard to locate; one or more member(s) of the desired population is (are) identified and asked to help find further members of the population and so on until the sample size is met	Nonprobability sample (not random) that introduces bias; appropriate to use when it is the only way to reach the population	Sample of the homeless population in the community to determine their oral health needs, generated by a dental hygienist who approaches a homeless man and woman who regularly attend her church's meal ministry and asking them to find others to participate in the survey
Convenience[a]	Study participants are chosen on the basis of ease and availability; used when access to the total population is not feasible for random sample selection	Nonprobability (nonrandom) sample; introduces bias, which reduces validity of the sample and limits the generalizability of study results; requires multiple studies with different samples	Sample consisting of the first 25 patients with a diagnosis of moderate periodontitis who volunteer to participate after a call for volunteers is posted in the clinic and on social media

[a]Example relates to the research question: What is the carbohydrate content of the diet of patients in an Indian Health Service community clinic who exhibit moderate periodontitis compared with the diet of those who exhibit no signs of periodontal disease?
[b]Example relates to the research question: What are the oral health needs of homeless individuals in the local community?

If it is decided that a sample of the population is to be used, different sampling techniques can be employed. Each type of sample has its uses, advantages, and disadvantages.[9] Several common types of sampling, namely **random sampling, stratified random sampling, systematic sampling, judgmental** or **purposive sampling, snowball sampling,** and **convenience sampling** are described in Table 7.4. In addition, an example of each type of sample is provided in relation to a research question. Box 7.4 includes a description of the sample and sampling technique used in the study example.

Study Groups

Experimental, some quasi-experimental, and some analytic research types use groups to conduct the study. These groups are compared to answer the research question.

Experimental and Control Groups in the Experimental Approach

The sample is divided into groups for an experimental and quasi-experimental study in which a treatment or intervention is imposed or manipulated to determine its effectiveness. The

experimental group is exposed to or receives the experimental treatment. The **control group** does not receive the intervention; it provides a comparison group against which the effects of the intervention on the experimental group can be contrasted.[12]

The control group can receive a *placebo*, a *traditional or standard treatment,* or *no treatment*. A placebo is an inert substance or an alternative intervention that is not expected to affect the dependent variable. It is used to control the effect produced when study participants behave or respond differently by virtue of knowing whether they are receiving the treatment or the control.[12] For example, they may be more compliant if they know they are using a new mouthrinse that is being tested to control gingivitis rather than no mouthrinse.

Use of the standard treatment is important in some cases when it would be unethical to withhold a standard level of treatment or therapy. To illustrate, if a new dentifrice formula is being tested, it would be unethical to withhold a current therapeutic dentifrice product from the control group because the benefits of the standard toothpaste have been established. Also, using the standard treatment as a control can demonstrate if the experimental treatment is more effective than the current treatment. Applying no treatment to the control would establish only the value of the new treatment compared with no treatment.

In experimental research, assuring that groups are equivalent for any relevant variables is important (see Variables section later in chapter). This will control bias, which will help ensure that any positive study results are not a function of group differences. Equivalent groups are achieved through **randomization**, which is the process of randomly assigning members of the sample to the study groups.[12] If randomization is not possible, **matching** the groups for relevant variables should be attempted to ensure group equivalency.[12] When groups are not equivalent, the study is quasi-experimental rather than experimental.

When conducting a study to test the effects of a new antimicrobial mouthrinse in controlling gingivitis in the IHS clinic patients with moderate periodontitis (the population previously used for various examples), random assignment ensures equivalency of the experimental and control groups. The sample is randomly assigned to two groups: the experimental group uses the new mouthrinse, and the control group uses a standard therapeutic mouthrinse. If randomization cannot be applied to group assignment, it would be important to match the groups for gender and age, both of which are risk factors for periodontitis. If a small sample size is used, randomization may not achieve group equivalency. In this case, matching could be combined with randomization to ensure group equivalency.

If the groups were formed without random procedures or matching, for example, using *intact groups,* the study would be quasi-experimental. An example of this would be using patients from two different clinics, with one clinic using one mouthrinse and the other clinic using the other mouthrinse. Although the experimental treatment could be assigned randomly to the intact groups, equivalency of groups is not controlled.[10,12]

The participants in a research study can demonstrate a change in their behavior simply in response to receiving attention or being observed.[9] This inherent confounding effect in research is referred to as the *observer effect or attention effect*.[9] It

is also called the **Hawthorne effect**, named after the industrial plant in which research was conducted that first identified this phenomenon.[9] Because it cannot be controlled and it can affect any participant in research, use of a control group and randomization of groups are critical.

Cases and Controls in Observational Studies

In observational research, the terms *cases* and *controls* are used.[8] Groups are formed according to their current disease or other outcome of interest. For example, in a case-control study the researcher identifies a group of individuals with a disease (cases) and a group of individuals without the disease (controls) to retrospectively investigate what factors in their history are associated with the disease (called *exposures*). Another example is an ecological study in which the different disease rates of two populations are studied to identify an associated factor. The group with the higher rate of disease is the cases group, and the group with the lower rate is the control.

Variables

A **variable** is a characteristic or concept that varies within the population under study. The different types of variables in an experimental study are the **independent variable**, the **dependent variable**, **relevant variables**, and **extraneous (confounding) variables** (see Box 7.6). Understanding these terms can

---

BOX 7.6 Types of Variables Associated with Experimental Research

Independent Variable
- The experimental treatment or intervention that is imposed on the experimental group of an experimental or quasi-experimental study.
- The variable that is manipulated by the researcher and is believed to cause or influence the dependent variable.

Dependent variable
- The variable that is thought to depend on or to be caused by the independent variable.
- The outcome variable of interest that is always measured during the course of an experimental study.
- Sometimes referred to as the outcome or measurement variable.

Relevant variable
- Any variable that should be controlled because it can influence how the independent variable affects the dependent variable; relevant variables vary for the condition being studied.

Extraneous variable (or confounding variable)
- A relevant variable that is not controlled in a study.
- Variables that can influence (confound) the relationship between the independent and dependent variables and potentially be sources of error in relation to any observed effects in the study outcomes.
- Reduce the internal validity of an experimental study.
- Must be controlled in experimental and nonexperimental studies through either the research design or statistical procedures to prevent their interference in establishing relationships among study variables and to increase internal validity.

(From Ravid R. Practical Statistics for Educators, 5th ed. Lanham, MD: Rowman & Littlefield; 2015; Kviz F. Conducting Health Research: Principles, Processes, and Methods. Thousand Oaks, CA: Sage; 2020.)

help you appreciate the importance of using appropriate research designs, data collection methods, data analysis, and interpretation of research results.

Variables can be illustrated by using the example presented in the previous section of an experimental study to test the effectiveness of a new antimicrobial mouthrinse in controlling gingivitis in moderate periodontitis patients. The independent variable is the mouthrinse, and the dependent variable is gingivitis. Age and gender are relevant variables because they are associated with periodontal disease. Both are controlled by using randomization for group assignment. Oral hygiene is also a relevant variable for gingivitis and can be further controlled by keeping it constant via training and monitoring of oral hygiene throughout the study. If it is not controlled, it becomes an extraneous or confounding variable that can be a source of error for interpretation of results, thus reducing the internal validity of the study. In other words, if the groups have different levels of daily self-care (oral hygiene), the observed effect of the mouthrinse on gingivitis could be a result of that difference in oral hygiene rather than the mouthrinse being tested. Some other potential relevant variables for gingivitis are diet, standard of living, homelessness, gender, age, and dental history. The independent and dependent variables are also illustrated in the study example in Box 7.4.

Blinding (Masking)

One way to control bias is to use a **blind study**, which uses a procedure called blinding or *masking*.[9] Typically in a *single-blind study*, the examiners are unaware of the group assignment; hence, they are not aware which group is receiving the treatment and which is the control. In a *double-blind study*, the study participants, as well as the researchers and examiners who interact with the study participants, are unaware of group assignment. Masking the study participants prevents participant reactivity, which is any possible difference in a participant's behavior that could result from their knowledge of group assignment. Masking the researchers can control for any bias in the way study participants are treated. Blinding the examiners prevents any influence of bias, even subconscious bias, in observations or measurement of the dependent variable.

Using blind study procedures, especially masking the examiners, is critical and should be done whenever possible. In some cases, it is not possible to mask study participants even though examiners can be masked. For instance, in the previous example of a study to compare the water flosser to dental flossing, it would be impossible for study participants not to know which device they are using.

Length of Study

The appropriate length of a study depends on the variables being studied and the type of study. For example, survey research that requires measurement of the variables only one time will take less time to complete than an experimental study that requires multiple measures of the dependent variable. Also, the nature of the dependent variable will affect the ideal length of a clinical trial. The study must be long enough to allow detection of new disease and extension of current disease. General recommendations are 2 to 3 years for caries studies, 8 to 21 days for plaque-inhibiting studies, 90 days for supragingival calculus-inhibition studies, longer for subgingival calculus-prevention studies, and 6 months for gingivitis-reduction studies.[14]

Collecting Data

Many different techniques can be used to collect data (see Chapters 3 and 4). The research design determines the appropriate method of data collection. During data collection, it is important to use calibrated instruments (e.g., indexes, surveys, tests, actual dental examination instruments such as a probe or explorer) and equipment (e.g., x-ray machine). Reliability of an instrument or of equipment refers to its dependability and consistency.[11] When examiners are involved in data collection, it is imperative that they too be reliable. This is achieved through **calibration** (see Figure 7.4), which will be discussed further later in this section.[15]

Two important concepts relate to data collection: validity and reliability. **Validity** is accuracy, and the term is used to refer to the accuracy of data and to the accuracy of the methods and instruments used to collect the data. In essence, it means that the outcomes of data collection accurately represent the presence or absence of the variable being measured.[11] Examiner calibration affects the validity of the data. Also, because self-report by study participants to measure a variable can be unreliable, it too can be a source of measurement error and threaten the validity of the data.

The term validity is used also to refer to the validity of a study, meaning that the study correctly answers the question that it asks.[9] Two types of validity exist in relation to research results. The first, *internal validity*, refers to how well a study is conducted and depends on the controls placed during the conduct of the research study. For example, if a study concludes that one therapeutic technique is superior to another, how confident we can be that it actually is superior is a function of how well the study design controlled for any sources of error. In other words, internal validity refers to the fact that the therapeutic technique being

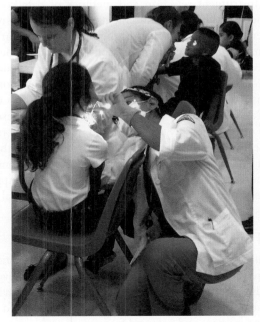

Fig 7.4 Calibration of examiners is critical during data collection to assure reliability of data. (Courtesy Schelli Stedke.)

tested is responsible for the observed effects and that these effects are not caused by some other uncontrolled factor. All sources of error related to data collection must be controlled to ensure internal validity, such as using valid and calibrated instruments, calibrating examiners, controlling variables (see earlier discussion), carefully planning and supervising study procedures, and using appropriate statistical procedures[8] (see Box 7.5).

For example, if dental caries is measured with the DMF index (see Appendix F), the resulting data must accurately identify the presence or absence of caries on those teeth. The examiners must evaluate the correct surfaces and accurately apply the criteria for measurement of caries; and the instruments and procedures used must be capable of accurately identifying the presence and absence of caries.

To assure validity of data and thus contribute to the internal validity of the study, standard instruments and dental indexes with documented validity should be used (see Appendix F). If new surveys, instruments, or indexes are developed for a study, they must be validated to ensure validity of measures.

The second form of study validity is *external validity*, which refers to the extent to which study results can be generalized accurately to other situations and people. External validity is affected by the population and how well the sample represents the population.[9] When a population is well suited for the research question and the sample is strongly representative of the population, external validity is said to be high, and the results can be generalized to other members of the population. External validity also refers to the extent to which the study results can be generalized to other situations and settings in the "real world". Thus, there is an inherent trade-off between external and internal validity. The more applicable a study is to a broader context, the less control there is of confounding or extraneous factors that can reduce internal validity, and vice versa.

The term **reliability** refers to the consistency and stability of the data.[12] Reliability of data is critical to assure valid research results. Instrument selection and methods of data collection affect the reliability of measurements. For data to be reliable, examiners, also called raters, must be calibrated (see earlier) to assure that their measurements are consistent and can be reproduced. For example, if two dental hygienists screen children in a school-based program, both should be trained and monitored on the use of the various dental indexes so their results will accurately and consistently reflect the criteria of the indexes. The findings of the dental hygienists should match. This is referred to as **interrater reliability**.[12] Also, a rater who inspects the same child on multiple occasions should detect the same conditions each time. This is called **intrarater reliability**. Review Appendix F for the common dental indexes used to measure oral health variables.

Ethical Conduct of Research

The dental hygiene profession addresses ethical expectations related to research in the ADHA *Code of Ethics for Dental Hygienists*. Standards concerning the ethical conduct of research with human participants have also been established[9] and are required by the federal government and enforced by research review committees of organizations involved in research[16,17] (see Guiding Principles).

For details of these ethical standards, refer to the Collaborative Institutional Training Initiative (CITI) tutorial *Human Subjects Research* in the Additional Resources at the end of this chapter.

GUIDING PRINCIPLES

Standards of Ethical Conduct of Human Subjects Research

- *Respect and Dignity.* Human participants should be treated with respect and dignity.
- *Informed Consent.* Informed consent is required, including full disclosure of the research plan and a description of the risks and benefits of participation.
- *Voluntary Participation.* Participation must be completely voluntary, and participants may withdraw from a study for any reason at any time without penalty or loss of benefits.
- *Confidentiality/Anonymity.* Confidentiality and anonymity must be protected during and after the study, including in relation to reporting results of the study.
- *Protection of Human Research Participants.* Participants must be protected to assure beneficence, nonmaleficence, and a risk-benefit ratio that favors the benefits side.
- *Social Justice.* Individuals and groups participating in a study must be treated fairly and equitably in terms of bearing the burdens and receiving the benefits of research. Also, when placebos are used, participants must be treated fairly.
- *Research Misconduct.* Research misconduct must be avoided, including plagiarism, copyright or patent infringement, falsifying or fabricating data, misrepresenting data, and conducting frivolous research.

Communication of Research Results

In addition to these standards, a responsibility discussed in the *Code of Ethics for Dental Hygienists* is to share the results of research.[16] Failure to communicate results means they are not available to the community of practitioners; conversely, sharing results of research adds to the profession's body of knowledge. Dental hygienists in a research role, regardless of the primary professional role, have an ethical responsibility to communicate research results in a meaningful way, either in writing or through a professional presentation (see Chapter 8). This will allow other practitioners access to the information for the benefit of the public. For example, unusual clinical cases, innovative procedures, and successful community programs can benefit other professionals and the patients and communities they serve.

PRESENTATION OF THE DATA AND DATA ANALYSIS

After variables have been defined and measured, and the data have been collected from the study participants, the next steps of the scientific method are to analyze the data and present the results. Understanding data and statistics is important to be able to use appropriate statistics correctly and according to the types of data, to avoid data analysis as a source of error in the research results.

Data

A discussion of data analysis must begin with an understanding of data itself. Pieces of information, such as numbers collected

TABLE 7.5 Types of Data

Type of Data	Characteristics	Examples	Scales of Measurement	Appropriate Data Display
Categorical	• Descriptive • Have no numerical value • Each individual data point is assigned to a group or category • There is no rank order to the categories • Considered to be qualitative in nature (descriptive)	• Socioeconomic status • Ethnicity • Political preference • Religion • Stages of cancer • Periodontal classification	• Nominal • Ordinal	• Frequency distribution table • Bar graph
Dichotomous	• Categorical data with exactly two categories • Considered to be qualitative in nature (descriptive)	• Male/Female • Yes/No • Dentulous/Edentulous • Pass/Fail	• Nominal • Ordinal	• Frequency distribution table • Bar graph
Discrete	• Numeric data with a set of fixed or finite values • Can be counted only in whole numbers; fractions have no real meaning • Considered quantitative in nature	• How many times a person brushes their teeth • Number of decayed, missing, or filled (DMF) teeth or surfaces • Number of dental visits in a year	• Interval • Ratio	• Frequency distribution table • Bar graph
Continuous	• Numeric data • Can be expressed by a large or infinite number of measures along a continuum • Have real value when expressed as fractions • Considered to be quantitative in nature	• Test scores • Millimeter probe depths • Height • Weight • Time	• Interval • Ratio • Ordinal data with many categories can be treated as continuous	• Frequency distribution table • Histogram • Frequency polygon

from measurements, counts obtained during the course of a research study, and responses to surveys and interviews, are known as **data.** Although the concept of data itself may seem fairly straightforward, there are different types of data, and the type of data determines how they are handled during statistical analysis and graphic representation.[12] **Categorical data, dichotomous data, discrete data,** and **continuous data** are explained and illustrated in Table 7.5.

The various types of data are represented by different *scales of measurement* (Table 7.5). The scale of measurement that data possess also determines the appropriate statistical procedures for summary and analysis of the data. The scales of measurement, in order of complexity, are as follows:[11]

- **Nominal scale**—Consists of named, mutually exclusive categories that have no order. For example, females are in one category of gender, and males are in another. Other examples of nominal scale data are ethnic group membership and religious preference. The nominal scale is the simplest or least complex of the four scales of data.
- **Ordinal scale**—Consists of categories of variables that have rank order, but there is no equal or defined value between the ranks. For example, cancer staging for tumors is grouped into five stages: 0, I, II, III, IV, and IV. In general, the different stages represent advancing levels of increased tumor size and/or spread of the cancer to adjacent tissues or organs, nearby lymph nodes, or both. Although the higher stages represent more extensive disease, differences from one stage to another are inexact, and each type of cancer is staged a little differently, making it difficult to define differences between stages precisely.[18] Other examples of ordinal scale data are stages of periodontal disease, socioeconomic status, and rating or ranking scales such as satisfaction and preferences.

Many dental indexes are ordinal scale (see Appendix F). The competence and comfort data collected and reported in the sample study described in Box 7.4 are ordinal scale data.

- **Interval scale**—Has an equal distance between measures along the continuum, but there is no true zero point, meaning there is no absence of the variable. Examples are temperature, IQ scale, and time on a clock. Oral health variables are not typically interval scale
- **Ratio scale**—Has equal intervals between the measures along a continuum, and there is a meaningful absolute zero point determined by nature, meaning there can be absence of the variable being measured. Examples are height and weight, number of teeth or sealants, and blood pressure.

Each scale of measurement takes on the characteristics of the previous one, building up to the ratio scale, which is the most complex. Because of their greater complexity, ratio scale data are considered most powerful and are preferred whenever possible to provide stronger research results.

Statistics

Statistics is a science used to describe, summarize, and mathematically analyze quantitative data for the purpose of making an inference about a population based on the sample data.[9] Two broad categories of relevant statistics are as follows:[11]

- **Descriptive statistics** are used to classify, organize, and summarize data. Their objective is to communicate results without generalizing beyond the sample to any population. Some ways in which data are described or summarized are with measures of central tendency, measures of dispersion, frequency counts and percentages, charts, percentiles, and correlation statistics. In Box 7.4 the use of descriptive statistics is described for the variables measured in the sample study.

TABLE 7.6   Selected Descriptive and Inferential Statistics

Types of Statistics	Uses/Characteristics	Measurements/Statistical Techniques
Descriptive	• Describe and summarize data in sample • Not generalized to another group • Show relationships among variables (correlation)	• Measures of central tendency (mean, median, mode) • Measures of dispersion (range, variance, standard deviation) • Frequency counts and percentages • Tables and graphs • Percentiles • Correlation
Inferential	• Generalize or apply information from the sample to the population • Includes categories of parametric and nonparametric	• Parametric: t-test, analysis of variance (ANOVA) • Nonparametric: chi-square, Wilcoxon signed-rank test, Mann-Whitney U test • Confidence intervals

• **Inferential statistics** are used to analyze sample data to make inferences about the larger population from the sample data. In other words, descriptive statistics tell us something about the sample, whereas inferential statistics tell us something about the population that the sample comes from. In Box 7.4 the use of inferential statistics is described to test the hypothesis of the sample study.

Descriptive and inferential statistics are contrasted in Table 7.6. Different types of questions are answered by descriptive and inferential statistics. Descriptive statistics answer questions about the status and relationship of variables in a group (e.g., rates of caries, number of sealants placed, oral hygiene status). Inferential statistics answer questions about differences and probability (e.g., effectiveness of methods to prevent or control disease, differences in rates of disease, improvement in dental utilization over time; see Guiding Principles).

GUIDING PRINCIPLES

Different Research Results Derived by Using Descriptive Versus Inferential Statistics

• *Only 26% of the patients treated in a specific community-based health center report using dental floss regularly.*
  This is an example of a research result derived with *descriptive statistics*. The data from the sample exactly describes the status of the variable (regular use of dental floss), relates only to that group, and provides no inference or generalization to a larger population.
• *The regular use of dental floss can help prevent periodontal disease.*
  This statement exemplifies a research result determined with *inferential statistics*. It is a result of generalizing to a larger population based on the analysis and interpretation of sample data. Also, a judgment is required, for example, contrasting periodontal disease rates of those who floss regularly to rates of those who do not.

Descriptive Statistics

Measures of central tendency. Measures of central tendency include the mean, median, and mode (Table 7.7). As the first step in describing a distribution of data, they communicate the middle or centrality of a distribution of scores.[11]

The **mean** is the arithmetic average of the data distribution. It is statistically noted as $\bar{x}$ and is calculated by adding all the values and dividing by the number (n) of items according to the following formula:

$$\text{mean} = \frac{\sum \bar{x}}{n}$$

The positive aspect of the mean is that it includes the value of each score; the negative aspect is that it can be distorted by extreme scores in the distribution and thus may not give a true picture of the central tendency. For example, if a test is administered in a class of 12 people and 10 people in the class score an 85 and 2 people score a 30, the class average is 75.83. This is not a true representation of the distribution of class scores because the vast majority scored 85. The use of the mean requires ratio data,[12] although it is common practice to use it with rating scales that have a large number of values, including dental indexes. An advantage to the mean is that it is amenable to further mathematical calculation and can be used in many statistical tests. Therefore, it is the measure used most often.

The **median** represents the exact middle score or value in an ordered distribution of scores; it is the point above and below which 50% of the scores lie. When the total number of scores is even, the median is computed by adding the two middle scores and dividing by 2. The median can be used with ratio, interval,

TABLE 7.7   Measures of Central Tendency

Measure	Characteristics	Type of Data
Mean	• Arithmetic average • Affected by extreme scores • Used in further statistical procedures to test hypotheses	• Ratio (continuous, discrete), interval • Common practice to use with dental indexes and rating scales that have numerous values
Median	• Middle score • Not distorted by outliers	• Ratio, interval, ordinal
Mode	• Most frequently occurring score • Distribution may be unimodal, bimodal, multimodal, or have no mode	• Ratio, interval, ordinal, nominal (categorical, dichotomous)

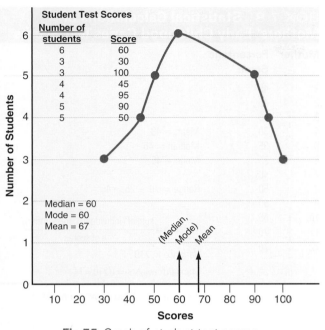

Fig 7.5 Graph of student test scores.

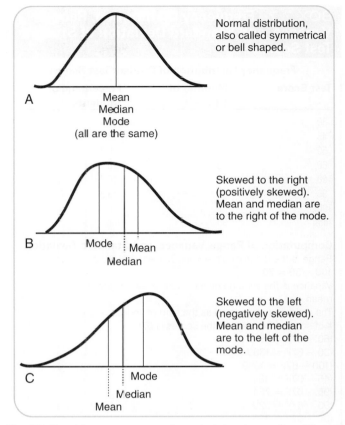

Fig 7.6 Graphing measures of central tendency for different types of curves.

and ordinal data. However, because it is not used in many statistical tests, it is sometimes not useful.

Unlike the mean, the median has the advantage that it is not distorted by outliers (extremely high or low scores) or skewed data. In the previous example described in the Mean section, the median score would be 85. However, it is not difficult to imagine what would happen if scores were not evenly distributed and the median were used to communicate the central tendency with no further information. In this case the information provided also may not demonstrate a true midpoint for the test scores. Communicating both the mean and the median might provide a clearer representation of the central tendency of the data distribution.

The **mode** is the score or value that occurs most frequently in a distribution of scores. Once again, the mode for the preceding example would be 85. The distribution of scores may be unimodal, bimodal, or multimodal, or there may even be no mode. The greatest usefulness of the mode is to communicate the central tendency of categorical or nominal data.

Figure 7.5 presents the mean, median, and mode of a group of test scores. The curve of the distribution represented by the line graph varies slightly from a symmetric bell-shaped curve, so the mean is a slightly higher value than the median and mode. Figure 7.6 illustrates the relationship of the mean, median, and mode in different types of distributions. In the symmetric distribution of a bell-shaped curve (A), the mean, median, and mode are the same value. In a positively skewed curve (B), the mean is to the right (higher score in the distribution) of the median and mode. In a negatively skewed curve (C), the mean is to the left (lower score in the distribution) of the median and mode. Note that in a skewed distribution, the median is always between the mode and the mean because it is the midpoint of the distribution, and the mean is toward the tail of the curve. This illustrates that if one knows the mean and median of a

distribution of scores, one can tell if the distribution is normal or skewed and, if skewed, the direction of the skew.

Measures of dispersion. In addition to the measures of central tendency (mean, median, and mode), measures of dispersion (also known as measures of variation) are used to describe data. Measures of dispersion (Table 7.8) communicate how much individual scores differ or vary from the mean.[11] For example, to provide a clearer picture of the distribution of scores, a measure of dispersion would help to communicate the effect of the extreme scores in the previous sample application of the mean to provide a clearer picture of the distribution.

The simplest measure of dispersion is the **range**, which communicates the difference between the highest and lowest values in a distribution of scores (Box 7.7). A more sophisticated measure of dispersion, called **variance**, is a method of ascertaining the way individual scores are located on a distribution in

TABLE 7.8	**Measures of Dispersion**
Measure	**Characteristics**
Range	• Simplest • Computation includes only the highest and lowest scores in the distribution
Variance	• Most sophisticated • Computation includes all scores in the distribution
Standard deviation	• Square root of the variance • Has same characteristics as the variance • Commonly reported in oral health research reports

BOX 7.7   Frequency Distribution, Range, Variance, and Standard Deviation of Student Test Scores

Frequency Distribution of Student Test Scores

Test Score	Number of Students	Percentage of Students
30	3	10
45	4	13.3
50	5	16.7
60	6	20
90	5	16.7
95	4	13.3
100	3	10
Total	30	100

Computation of Range, Variance, and Standard Deviation

Range is the difference between highest and lowest score: $100 - 30 = 70$.

Variance is the average deviation or spread of scores around the mean.

The variance is calculated as the sum of (individual score – mean)^2 / # of scores (the mean of the scores is 67).

$(60 - 67)^2 = 49$

$(30 - 67)^2 = 1369$

$(100 - 67)^2 = 1089$

$(45 - 67)^2 = 484$

$(95 - 67)^2 = 784$

$(90 - 67)^2 = 529$

$(50 - 67)^2 = 289$

49×6 (# of scores of 60) $= 294$

1369×3 (# of scores of 30) $= 4107$

1089×3 (# of scores of 100) $= 3267$

484×4 (# of scores of 45) $= 1936$

784×4 (# of scores of 95) $= 3136$

529×5 (# of scores of 90) $= 2645$

289×5 (# of scores of 50) $= 1445$

Sum of above (individual score – mean)$^2 = 16,830$

$16,830 \div 30$ (total number of scores) $= 561$

561 is the variance

Standard deviation is the positive square root of the variance: $\sqrt{561}$

The square root of 561 = 23.7

23.7 is the standard deviation

BOX 7.8   Statistical Calculations of Mothers' Early Childhood Caries Test Scores

Mother	Percentage Score
1	45
2	45
3	45
4	30
5	35
6	25
7	40
8	50
9	60
10	65
11	70
12	70

Mean = 48

Median = 45

Mode = 45

Range = $70 - 25 = 45$

$$Variance = \frac{sum\ of\ (individual\ scores - mean)^2}{\#\ of\ scores}$$

Variance = 210

Standard deviation = $\sqrt{210} = 14$

Note: All scores and calculations are rounded to whole numbers.

It makes sense, then, that the farther away the data points on the distribution are from the mean, the greater the variance and SD. A large SD value in relation to the value of the mean indicates a wide spread of scores. For the data in Box 7.7, the SD of 23.7 in relation to the mean of 67 represents the large spread of scores presented in the frequency distribution. Also, the SD of two distributions can be compared to determine whether the variance of scores around the mean is similar or different, and if different, which distribution has the larger spread of scores.

As another example, Box 7.8 demonstrates the data calculations for pretest scores that were collected in a community research project involving 12 unwed teenaged mothers and their knowledge of ECC. In the case of this distribution, although the mean, median, and mode are close in value, the mean is slightly higher than the median and mode (the distribution is slightly positively skewed) because of several higher scores. In addition, the large SD of 14 in relation to the mean of 48 communicates the wide spread of scores (range of 25 to 70) in this distribution.

Correlation. The relationship or association of one variable to another is demonstrated with a **correlation statistic**.[11] For example, height and weight often show a strong correlation because taller people usually have a higher weight than shorter people. As another example, age and periodontal disease are correlated because periodontal disease is associated with age (older adults have a higher incidence of periodontal disease than young adults).

Various correlation statistics are available for use with different types of data (categorical, discrete, and continuous) and measurement scales (nominal, ordinal, interval, and ratio). Regardless of the type and scale of data, the correlation coefficient is interpreted the same way.

The results of the calculation for correlation always have a range between +1 and −1. The sign (+ or −) indicates either a positive or negative (inverse) relationship. The relationship is *positive* (+ value of the coefficient) when the value of one variable increases as the value of the other also increases. An example is the relationship between heart disease and periodontal disease; the values increase and decrease together.

relation to the mean. The **standard deviation** (SD), which is the square root of the variance, is frequently reported rather than the variance. The advantage of the variance and SD compared with the range is that every data point in relation to the mean is used in calculating the statistic, which provides a truer picture of how the individual scores relate to the mean.

The steps to calculate the variance and SD are as follows (see Box 7.7):

1. Subtract each data point from the mean.
2. Square these differences.
3. Add the squared differences.
4. Divide by the total number of data points.
5. Figure out the square root of the result.

The formula for the SD is as follows:

$$SD = \sqrt{\frac{sum\ of\ (data\ point - mean)^2}{\#\ of\ values}}$$

TABLE 7.9 Interpretation of Correlation Coefficient: Direction and Strength

Sign of Coefficient Value (+ or −)	Direction of Relationship/ Interpretation
+	Positive As one variable increases, the other also increases; and vice versa
−	Negative As one variable increases, the other decreases; and vice versa

Value of Coefficient	Strength of Association/ Interpretation
0.00–0.25	Little if any
0.26–0.49	Weak
0.50–0.69	Moderate
0.70–0.89	High
0.90–1.00	Very high

(Modified from Munro BH. Statistical Methods for Health Care Research, 6th ed. Philadelphia, PA: Lippincott; 2013.)

TABLE 7.10 Summary of Mothers' Pretest and Posttest Knowledge Scores and Hours of Education

Group Number	Group Type and Pretest Scores	Hours of Education	Average % Increase from Pretest to Posttest
1	Four mothers with an average pretest score of 50	2	60
2	Four mothers with an average pretest score of 50	4	70
3	Four mothers with an average pretest score of 50	6	80
4	Four mothers with an average pretest score of 50	8	90

In contrast, a *negative* correlation shows a negative or inverse relationship between variables (Table 7.9). For example, oral hygiene practices are negatively associated with gingivitis; as oral hygiene practices increase, gingivitis decreases, and vice versa: as oral hygiene practices decrease, gingivitis increases.

Continuing with the sample study described earlier, using the sample pretest data in Box 7.8, additional data presented in Table 7.10 shows that as the amount of time educating the mothers increased, the difference between their pretest and posttest scores also increased. The scattergram in Figure 7.7 graphically displays this same positive relationship between the two variables (the diagonal of the line shows that as one variable increases in value, the other also increases). The greater the incline of the diagonal line in a scattergram, the stronger the relationship. However, without a correlation coefficient, it is impossible to know the strength of the relationship. Suppose the correlation coefficient for the data for these two variables was +0.85. This would provide a numeric value that can be interpreted to determine the strength of the association.

Table 7.9 also provides a guide to interpreting the value of the correlation coefficient in representing the strength of the relationship. Using this guide, +0.85 would be considered a high correlation. However, the purpose of each study and the potential use of the results must also be considered along with the correlation coefficient to determine what a noteworthy relationship is.[11] In all cases, the closer the relationship is to +1 or −1, the stronger the relationship.[11]

As an example of a negative correlation, Figure 7.8 is a scattergram showing a negative relationship between a diet that includes fruits and vegetables each day and the occurrence of certain cancers. In this case, as the intake of fruits and vegetables increases, the incidence of cancer decreases, and vice versa: as the intake of fruits and vegetables decreases, the incidence of cancer increases. The diagonal line of a negative relationship on a scattergram is in the opposite direction, compared with its position in a positive relationship (compare with Figure 7.7). The

value of the correlation coefficient for an inverse relationship is interpreted the same way as the value of a positive correlation. For example, a correlation coefficient of −0.91 in this case would indicate a very high inverse correlation.

A perfect positive (+1) or negative (−1) correlation coefficient is possible in theory. However, it would be rare to find a perfect relationship because other variables can be associated also with the variables that are being evaluated with the correlation analysis. For example, although dental caries and use of fluorides are strongly associated, the relationship is not perfect because other variables such as diet, oral hygiene, and genetics are also associated with dental caries.

It is important to remember that correlation communicates only association of variables, which indicates risk, not causation.[11] It cannot be used to indicate cause and effect without follow-up longitudinal studies. For example, correlation between Alzheimer's disease and periodontal disease only indicates they are associated. The nature of the relationship is not clear until longitudinal studies are conducted to test if one causes the other or if a third factor is causally associated with both, such as in the case of dental caries and fluorosis.

Percentiles. A percentile is a statistical measure that represents the value below which a specific percentage of observations fall in a distribution of values. **Percentiles** are often used to report scores on a norm-referenced test. For example, if a score is in the 90th percentile, it is higher than 90% of the other scores. Another common use is the assessment of infants' and children's weight and height compared with national averages and percentiles found in growth charts. Similarly, body mass charts used to identify obesity are based on percentiles. Quartiles and deciles, which split data into 25% and 10% groups, respectively, are specific percentiles used in some cases. Percentiles are important to us because they are used by many dental insurers to determine their highest reimbursable fees (e.g., usual, customary, and reasonable [UCR] fees; see Table 5.6 in Chapter 5).[19]

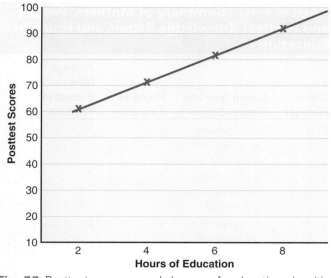

Fig 7.7 Posttest scores and hours of education (positive correlation).

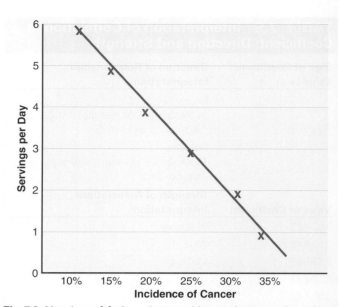

Fig 7.8 Number of fruit and vegetable servings per day related to percent incidence of cancer (negative correlation).

Displaying the Data

Data can be presented in *tables* and *graphs,* also called charts, for easier understanding and interpretation. Tables and graphs should be used to organize and present statistical results that cannot be discussed easily in a sentence or two of text. In some cases, tables are preferred, and in some cases, graphs are preferred; however, any image used should be meaningful and should not repeat information in the text. Tables interact with the reader's verbal system and work best when the data presentation is used to look up or compare individual values, requires precise values, or has values that involve multiple units of measure. Graphs are perceived by the reader's visual system and work best when communicating the shape of a distribution of values or a relationship among values.[8,20]

Frequency distribution tables. Frequency distribution tables can be produced for all types of data. They show the frequency or number of times that values or categories occur in a data distribution.[11] To create a **frequency distribution table**, the raw data are put in order and then the frequency for each value or category is calculated. Frequencies can be expressed as an actual frequency or counts, or as a relative frequency or percentages. By examining a frequency distribution table, one can easily determine the mode and get a sense of the shape of the distribution. As an example, the data in Box 7.7 are presented in a frequency distribution table with the test scores in order and with frequency counts and percentages. The data can be grouped into intervals in a frequency distribution table, which will be discussed later.

Graphs. Various types of graphs, also called charts, can be used to present data pictorially.[11] Several are described in this section. The appropriate graphs to use for various types of data are presented in Table 7.5. Creating a frequency distribution table (see Box 7.7) is the first step of constructing a graph of frequency data.

Bar graph. A visual representation of categorical (nominal or ordinal scale) data can be provided with **bar graphs**. The data

are plotted with rectangular bars or columns that represent the values for the various categories. The bars are of equal width and separated to show the discrete nature of the categories. Bar graphs can be displayed with vertical columns (see Figure 7.9), horizontal bars (see Figure 5.19 in Chapter 5), comparative bars (multiple bars to show a comparison between values; see Figures 5.2, 5.3, 5.4, and 5.9 in Chapter 5), or stacked bars (bars that contain multiple types of information; see Figure 5.21 in Chapter 5). In a column bar graph, the categories of data appear along the horizontal (x) axis, and the height of each bar corresponds to the frequency or value of the category it represents, which is indicated on the vertical (y) axis. Figure 7.9 visually depicts the frequency of "yes" and "no" responses to a survey question used in the sample research study presented in Box 7.4.

Histogram. While a bar graph compares the values of various categories, a **histogram** shows the distribution of continuous data for a variable. A histogram is similar in appearance to a

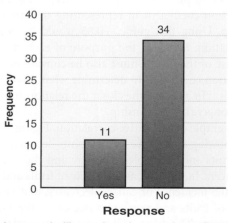

Fig 7.9 A bar graph illustrating the number of study participants (frequency of "yes" and "no" responses) who knew a transgender individual.

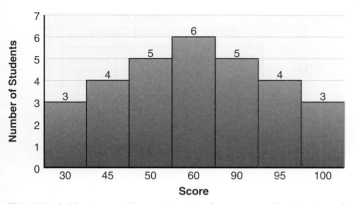

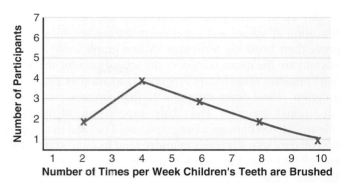

Fig 7.10 A histogram illustrating the frequency distribution of student test scores.

Fig 7.11 Number of times per week participants brush their children's teeth as shown in a frequency polygon.

bar graph except the bars of a histogram are joined (touching). This is because each column represents a group defined by the continuous, quantitative variable, and the values of the variable are on a continuum. Therefore, a histogram is used to depict frequency data for a continuous (interval or ratio scale) variable. Figure 7.10 visually illustrates the frequency distribution of the test scores presented in Box 7.7.

Frequency polygon. A **frequency polygon** is a line graph also used to portray the frequencies of continuous data. A histogram is converted into a frequency polygon by connecting the top center point of each bar to create a line that pictorially presents the frequency distribution with a line instead of with bars. Figure 7.11 is a frequency polygon that displays how many times per week the mothers in a study brush their children's teeth. This data could be presented easily as a histogram instead. An advantage of using a frequency polygon rather than a histogram is that several data distributions can be presented in the same graph for a clear comparison. For example, a study could be conducted to test the effect of using social media to educate young mothers on their frequency of brushing their children's teeth. A frequency polygon with two lines could be used to compare the brushing frequency of the group that used social media and the group that did not.

Time series graph. Graphs can be used also to show change in the measure of a variable over time. For example, monthly

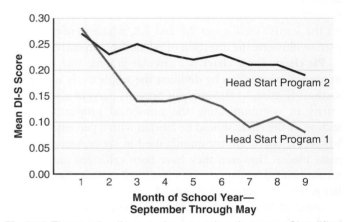

Fig 7.13 Time series line graph comparing the mean Simplified Debris Index (DI-S) of children in two Head Start programs over the school year.

mean Simplified Debris Index (DI-S) scores (see Appendix F) of children who brush daily at school in a Head Start program could be communicated with a bar graph to show progress of brushing ability over the school year (Figure 7.12). **Time series graphs** are more frequently presented as line graphs (Figure 7.13). An advantage of the line graph is the ability to compare two groups. For example, let's suppose the children

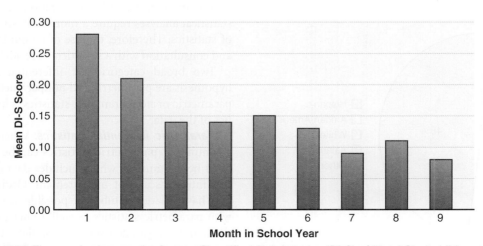

Fig 7.12 Time series bar graph of mean Simplified Debris Index (DI-S) of Head Start children over the school year.

in this Head Start program routinely received oral health education at school and supervision during brushing to improve their brushing technique. A line graph could be used to compare the mean DI-S over the school year for this Head Start program (Head Start Program 1) to another Head Start program (Head Start Program 2) that did not provide an educational program and daily supervision of brushing (Figure 7.13). Although a bar graph could be used to compare the two data sets, it is easier to understand in a line graph. Both are referred to as time series graphs because they plot a variable over time.

Scattergram. The relationship between variables that is communicated statistically with the correlation coefficient (see previous section) can be visually depicted with a **scattergram** or scatter plot. For each study participant, the value of one variable is plotted on the *x* axis against the value of the second variable on the *y* axis (see Figures 7.7 and 7.8, which were previously used to illustrate the direction of relationship in correlation).

Pie chart. A **pie chart** is a circular graphic that illustrates numerical proportion by dividing the whole circle or pie into sections (Figure 7.14). Simply, it presents parts of a whole. For clarity in communicating the numerical proportions, each section of the circle should be labeled with a percentage of the whole. Pie charts are commonly used in lay presentations and mass media. However, they have been criticized and are not recommended by experts for scientific literature. Employing a bar graph is recommended instead.

Some of the graphs described in the previous section are used for frequency data, and some are not. When a table or graph presents frequencies, the data can be presented as individual data points or in groups. These groupings are referred to as *intervals* and must be of equal sizes for accurate presentation and interpretation. A grouped frequency distribution can be converted to a histogram or frequency polygon in the same way that an ungrouped frequency distribution is changed over. For example, the individual test scores in Box 7.8 are presented in Figure 7.15 as a grouped frequency distribution table and a frequency polygon showing frequencies and percentages for specified intervals or ranges of test scores.

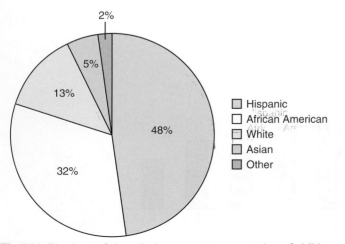

Fig 7.14 Pie chart of the ethnic group representation of children in a Head Start program.

**Test Scores on
Early Childhood Caries**

Test Scores	Frequency	Percent
20–40	4	33.3
41–60	5	41.7
61–80	3	25.0
Total	12	100

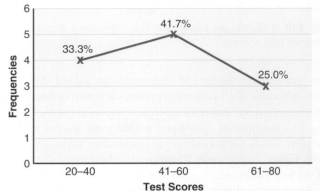

Fig 7.15 Frequency distribution table and histogram of grouped frequency data.

Although tables and graphs may be incorporated into a written report with text, the data in these charts should be understandable even without complementary text. To communicate data accurately, it is important that proper technique be used to construct effective tables and graphs (see Box 7.9). Statistics texts and websites can be referenced for more details about constructing charts or graphs.

Inferential Statistics

Inferential statistics are used to test hypotheses and generalize results from the sample studied to the actual population that the sample was drawn from and represents.[11] Computing inferential statistics is a more complex process than other statistical procedures that have been discussed in the chapter up to this point. Such computations and interpretation of results of inferential statistical analyses require a more sophisticated understanding of statistics. Therefore, the use of computers for computation and consultation with a statistician are advised.

Two broad categories of inferential statistics to test a hypothesis are parametric and nonparametric. The selection of parametric or nonparametric statistics is based on characteristics of the data.

Parametric inferential statistics. When data meet certain assumptions, **parametric statistics** can be used. First the data must be continuous, which includes data that represents ratio and interval scales of measurement. Ordinal or discrete data that have a large number of possible scores can be analyzed with parametric statistics as well. Other assumptions are that the sample size is adequate, the population distribution is normal, and the group variances are similar.[11] Examination of the mean, median, and mode, as well as the variance or SD, will help indicate if the assumptions have been met. Data are more likely to meet these assumptions when the sample is drawn randomly from the population, hence the greater value placed on experimental studies versus quasi-experimental studies.

An understanding of the normal distribution will help with grasping these required assumptions for using parametric statistics. A **normal distribution** is a theoretical symmetric bell-shaped curve that is characteristic of data representing most natural occurrences in this world. The distribution of the data

in this curve is such that approximately 68% of the scores fall within one SD above or below the mean, approximately 95% lie within two SDs of the mean, and 99% are within three SDs of the mean[11] (Figure 7.16). We saw earlier in the chapter that the symmetry of the normal distribution results in the mean, median, and mode being equal, in contrast to skewed curves (see Figure 7.6). Thus, to decide whether parametric statistics are warranted, one can examine the similarity of the mean, median, and mode of the population data to determine whether the distribution is normal. To decide whether the group variances are equal, the variances or SDs of both study groups (experimental and control) are examined to determine their similarity.

There are numerous parametric statistical tests. This chapter will present only a few that are commonly used in oral health research. Others can be found in statistics reference books, some of which are included in the references listed for this chapter.

t-test. One of the most common parametric statistics is the *t*-test, which is applied to analyze the difference between the means of two data sets.[11] It provides the researcher with a statistical analysis of the difference between two groups, each receiving a different treatment or control, a change in one group resulting from a treatment, or a comparison of a group to an established norm for the population. Each of these two situations requires the use of a different version of the *t*-test.

The *independent samples t-test*, also known as the *Student t-test* and sometimes referred to as the *two-sample t-test*, is employed to determine the significance of differences between the means of two independent groups such as an experimental group compared with a control group. For example, a study might investigate the effect of a new toothbrushing method on gingivitis. Patients with gingivitis are randomized into two groups: (1) an experimental group asked to practice a new method of toothbrushing and (2) a control group receiving no instruction and asked to brush with their usual method. Gingivitis is measured with appropriate indexes at the beginning of the study and again 3 and 6 months later. The hypothesis is that the new method of toothbrushing will decrease gingivitis. The hypothesis is tested by applying the Student *t*-test to compare the mean gingivitis improvement of the two groups.

When the *t*-test is applied to a single group to compare pretreatment and posttreatment scores, the *t*-test for dependent samples (also called *paired samples*, *matched samples*, or *repeated measures t-test*) is used. This analysis is required when only one

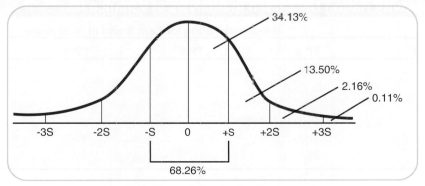

Fig 7.16 Normal distribution (bell curve).

group is studied, such as in a cohort study. To illustrate, a researcher may want to examine the difference in blood glucose levels of diabetic patients before and after treatment with a new diet. Assuming that all patients in the study have similar characteristics, such as age and degree of disease present, the *t*-test for dependent samples can be used to test the difference between pretreatment and posttreatment glucose levels.

The *one-sample t-test* can be applied to compare the mean of a group on a variable to a specified constant such as a known or hypothesized value in the population. For example, the average daily production of a new staff member could be compared with the average daily production of all similar staff over the last 5 years.

Analysis of variance. Another commonly used parametric test is **analysis of variance (ANOVA)**. A more powerful test than the *t*-test, ANOVA allows for comparison of two or more sample means by analyzing interactions between and among the variances of the multiple groups.[11] When used to compare two group means, ANOVA yields the same results as the *t*-test. When three or more group means are compared, ANOVA must be used instead of the *t*-test.

An example of the application of ANOVA is the comparison of five brands of toothpaste that claim relief of tooth sensitivity. Volunteers are recruited, and each one is randomly given a different brand disguised in a plain white tube. Each study participant is asked to use this tube until it is finished. When the tube is empty, after a washout period, each patient is given a different brand in an unmarked tube to use until it too is emptied. This is repeated until all five patients exhaust all five brands of sensitivity-relief toothpaste. Patients are asked to rate their tooth sensitivity on a numeric scale of 1 to 10 each day for each tube of toothpaste. The mean sensitivity ratings for each of the five toothpaste brands for each patient would look something like the data in Table 7.11.

ANOVA allows the dental hygienist to compare the mean sensitivity scores of the various brands of toothpaste used in the study. ANOVA will yield information about which actually reduce sensitivity and how each brand compares with the others. In essence, ANOVA compares differences within groups (within each brand of toothpaste) and between groups (between the different brands). If a difference is found to be significant, a follow-up statistic is applied to determine where the significant difference lies, in other words, which brand produced a statistically significant lower mean sensitivity rating.

Nonparametric inferential statistics. When the data do not meet the assumptions for parametric statistics (see earlier), it is necessary to apply **nonparametric statistics**.[11] Nonparametric techniques are most useful for data that is measured on the nominal or ordinal scale because of their qualitative nature. Although these data are represented by numbers, such as a rating scale, the numbers are derived subjectively. Nonparametric tests involve fewer assumptions about the population so they can be used also with all types of data when sample and group sizes are small. Variations of nonparametric tests exist for different sample sizes (five or less and greater than five).

Several nonparametric statistical tests are used regularly in oral health research.[21] One of the most common is the **chi-square test** (χ^2), two versions of which are used in different ways. The χ^2 *test of independence* is used to compare counts of categorical variables between two or more independent groups, similar to using the *t*-test or ANOVA to compare group means. This version of χ^2 is also used to test the statistical significance of the relationship between variables that has been established with a correlation coefficient. The *goodness of fit χ^2* is used to test the differences between observed and expected frequencies of categorical variables within distributions.

The **Wilcoxon signed-rank test** and the **Mann-Whitney U test** are nonparametric equivalents to the *t*-test for use with ordinal data. See Box 7.4 for reporting of results derived from the Wilcoxon signed-rank test. Other nonparametric tests can be reviewed in various statistics books listed in the references of this chapter.

Confidence intervals. Another inferential statistic is a **confidence interval** by which researchers estimate the accuracy of a sample statistic such as the sample mean.[11] It consists of two parts: an interval and a percentage level of confidence. For example, with the mean of 48 for the test scores in Box 7.8, the confidence interval is 48 ± 7.94 (interval of 40.06 to 55.94) at a 95% level of confidence. The interpretation is that if the test were repeated on multiple different samples from the same population, the calculated confidence interval of 48 ± 7.94 would encompass the true population mean 95% of the time. Researchers usually use a 95% or 99% level of confidence. Increasing the confidence level to 99% would necessitate increasing the interval of values as well. Therefore, increasing the confidence interval also decreases the specificity of the data, and vice versa. Parametric and nonparametric approaches can be applied to

TABLE 7.11	Sensitivity Rating Data Used in Analysis of Variance Test				
	Sensitivity Rating for Each Brand of Toothpaste				
Patient Number	**TP 1**	**TP 2**	**TP 3**	**TP 4**	**TP 5**
1	6	5	4	5	2
2	5	5	3	4	3
3	7	5	4	5	3
4	5	4	4	3	4
5	6	5	5	4	4
Mean sensitivity rating	5.8	4.8	4.0	4.2	3.2

TP, Toothpaste brands 1 to 5.
Key: 1–10 = Sensitivity rating scale (10 is maximum).

the computation of confidence intervals, depending on whether parametric assumptions are met for the data.

Determining Statistical Significance

The final outcome of a statistical analysis with inferential statistics is to determine whether the results are statistically significant. **Statistical significance** is a way of indicating that the results found in an analysis of data are unlikely to have been caused by chance; in other words, statistical significance communicates the chance that the results have been caused by the independent variable.[9]

Power analysis. A **power analysis** is used to determine how many study participants are needed to provide significance.[22] This analysis is calculated according to a specific statistical formula. The power of a study, or its ability to detect differences among groups and relationships among variables, is directly and positively related to sample size and the precision with which the study is planned and conducted.[22]

Sample size is important because using too small or too large a sample can influence the statistical significance. Generally, when applying parametric statistics, the use of less than 30 in a sample or 25 in a study group will provide too little information to make generalizations about the populations and demonstrate statistical significance of results. With too large a sample, statistical significance can occur more easily, possibly indicating statistical significance when there is none.[11] When a sample is too small to apply parametric statistics, the appropriate nonparametric test must be selected for the sample size to assure accurate interpretation of statistical significance.

The true importance of determining statistical significance is that the greater the statistical significance, the more chance that any differences between or among groups are real and not caused by chance. When study results are statistically significant there is added assurance that they can be generalized to the population from whom the sample was taken.

p values. Researchers use a **p value** to determine statistical significance.[11] Regardless of the inferential statistic used to test the hypothesis, a p value is found for the statistical result. The p value is the probability that the statistical result could be a false scientific conclusion. The p value is affected by the sample size, the differences between or among the distributions of scores, and the variance of the scores in the distributions.

Normally, an acceptable p value is 0.05 or less.[11] This means that results with a p value of 0.05 or less ($p \leq .05$) are generally considered statistically significant and provide the basis for rejection of the null hypothesis. A p of 0.05 means that the results can be caused by chance 5 times in 100. Another way to say this is that there is a 5% chance that the observed results or differences are due purely to chance and not a true difference caused by the independent variable. Lower p values (e.g., 0.01, 0.001, or less) are more statistically significant. The smaller the p value, the more significant the findings of the study are considered. The results of the study described in Box 7.4 were found to be significant at $p < .001$. This means there is less than a 0.1% chance that the results were because of chance.

The statistical conclusion. The researcher comes to the conclusion to either accept or reject the null hypothesis of the study

TABLE 7.12 Errors Related to the Statistical Decision About the Null Hypothesis

Null Hypothesis Is Actually:	Null Hypothesis Is	
	Accepted	Not Accepted
True	No error	Type I α (alpha) error
False	Type II β (beta) error	No error

based on the statistical results of the data analysis.[11] For example, let us suppose that a study compares the effectiveness of two teaching methods in a community setting in relation to increasing oral health knowledge and improving routine oral health behaviors. At the end of the study the increase in knowledge of the two groups is compared, resulting in a p value of 0.05. In this case the **statistical conclusion** is to reject the null hypothesis, meaning that one teaching method resulted in a greater increase in knowledge. Based on the statistical significance of $p = .05$, there is a 95% chance that the greater increase in knowledge in that group was a result of the teaching method. Stated another way, there is a 5% chance that the greater increase in knowledge is because of chance occurrence rather than a result of the superiority of the teaching method. The conclusion of the study in Box 7.4 is presented there: "education about transgender health care can increase competence and comfort among dental hygiene students and should be included in dental and allied dental education curricula."

Because the statistical analysis is based on probability rather than certainty, there is the possibility of error in the statistical conclusion.[11] Errors can be minimized by using appropriate research designs, carefully following suitable research procedures, controlling confounding variables and other sources of error or bias, and having an adequate sample size.[11] Two types of errors exist, and they tend to cancel each other out (Table 7.12). Efforts to reduce one type of error generally result in increasing the other type.

When the researcher rejects the null hypothesis based on the statistical results, but the null is actually true, this is referred to as a **type I alpha (α) error**. In this case the statistical conclusion states that a difference exists when in actuality it does not. With a significance level of 0.05 ($p = .05$), there is a 1 in 20 chance that a conclusion will state that a difference exists when there is no difference. The type I error rate can be reduced by lowering the p value, for example, to 0.01 or 0.001.

However, when the opposite occurs, in other words, when the null hypothesis is accepted although it is actually false, this is called a **type II beta (β) error**. In this case the statistical conclusion states that no relationship exists when one actually does exist.

ANALYSIS OF THE LITERATURE

A thorough review of the literature is the first step of the research process and is critical to every stage of the research process: synthesizing the research problem, developing the research question, selecting the research design, formulating the research plan including data collection, and interpreting the results. Additionally, regularly reviewing and critically analyzing the literature is a professional responsibility that is necessary regardless of the professional role of the dental hygienist.[23]

Familiarity with the literature is important in relation to being informed and up to date on dental hygiene foci that affect one's practice, such as theories, methods, therapies, and products. This assimilation of information requires more than listening to colleagues with clinical expertise or attending continuing education programs and professional conferences, which are at the lower end of the hierarchy of evidence for EBDM (see Figure 7.2). Regular review of published literature, whether in print or on the web, is an important step in remaining current in the discipline. Meeting this professional responsibility[16,23] helps to enable the dental hygienist to answer questions posed by patients, intradisciplinary and interdisciplinary colleagues, and community partners; maintain competency; and be identified as an exceptional oral health professional.[3]

Every dental hygienist should have access to regular subscriptions of scientific journals and Internet services to be able to conduct their own research on various topics related to dental hygiene practice (Figure 7.17). Sometimes this can be achieved via access to a library with a scientific collection associated with a nearby university or college health sciences program, dental school, or medical school. Also, these may have research librarians who can help a dental hygienist find literature on a scientific topic.

Becoming skillful in obtaining scientific information is not as easy as one may expect. However, it is a skill that must be cultivated by every professional dental hygienist because it is necessary to be able to access current information for EBDM. This section describes an overview of what is available in the form of written resources, how to choose the best sources of this information, and how to critically review this literature. Remaining focused on the research related to specific topics to be reviewed should help to provide simple yet intelligent answers to the questions at hand.

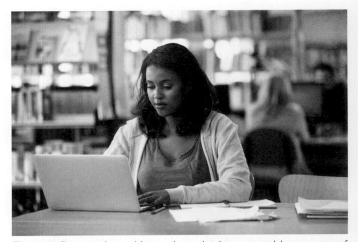

Fig 7.18 Peer reviewed journals and other reputable sources of scientific literature are accessible through university and college libraries as well as online. (@ iStock.com/monkeybusinessimages)

Selection of Literature

Various factors must be considered when selecting journal articles and other sources of information for a literature review (see Figure 7.18).[24] This section will discuss the selection of an appropriate journal, the author, and the date of publication of research articles. In addition, use of web sources of information is discussed. Working with a research librarian, either in person or or online, will help to assure that valid resources are selected.

Selecting a Journal

To begin a literature review, the dental hygienist or researcher must select appropriate journals. The scientific writing in a journal should be comprehensible to the average dental hygienist who is knowledgeable about the topic area. Selecting literature that is pertinent to the field of dental hygiene will allow the researcher to obtain a complete understanding of the research topic while focusing the research on issues of importance to dental hygiene. For example, because of the technical and intricate scientific detail of its topics, the *Journal of Biochemical Research* may not be the ideal place to start looking for information on periodontal host factors; the *Journal of Periodontology* may be preferable. Although both journals publish in-depth scientific literature, the material in the second is tailored to dentistry and dental hygiene, thus making it relevant and understandable to the average oral health researcher.

Equally important is the selection of a reputable journal. Several aspects lend credibility to a journal, including an editorial review board that evaluates each contributed article for accuracy and reflection of current knowledge, relevancy of content, and issues involving appropriate scientific style and method of writing. This process is known as **peer review**, and the journal that uses peer review is referred to as a **refereed journal** or a peer-reviewed journal. Individuals who are considered experts on the content of a manuscript review it to make recommendations concerning its publication. A reputable journal is commonly affiliated with a professional group or society, a specialty group, or a reputable scientific publisher. Sometimes professional groups will have a political stance or agenda, which should be considered in selecting literature on some topics.

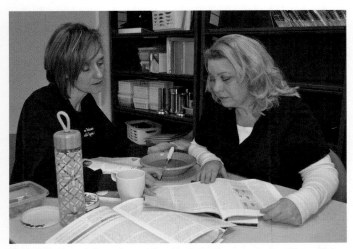

Fig 7.17 Practicing dental hygienists discuss scientific articles for evidence-based decision-making during a lunch break. (Courtesy Charlene Dickinson & Christine French Beatty.)

Popular magazines and periodicals published by commercial firms are not considered reliable sources of scientific information. Examples of poor choices for scientific literature are any of the typical newsstand health and recreation journals and glamour and beauty magazines. Also, although many attractively presented dental and dental hygiene publications exist, some are simply glorified advertising brochures and do not represent an acceptable source of scientific material.

Authors

When selecting a journal article, the reader should be careful to note that the author has the appropriate qualifications. Authors should possess credentials and have experience in or a current relationship with the field about which they are writing. If the written work is a research study, there should also be information about the research facilities where the research was conducted and information about financial support for the project.

Date of Publication

Most often readers need to depend on the most current information although older information may be considered classic or have historical significance and therefore may be useful occasionally in conducting a review. One classic study often mentioned in scientific writing is the Vipeholm study, conducted by Gustafsson and colleagues in Sweden in the 1950s to investigate dental caries in relation to sugar intake.[25] Another example is Dr. Harold Löe's classic study of the role of plaque bacteria on gingivitis, published in 1965.[26]

Although these are foundational studies, it is important to review current studies that provide the newest information because newer research can change one's understanding of a disease and its prevention or control. Additionally, the most recent literature on a topic is necessary to identify the current prevalence of oral diseases in the population and up-to-date national oral health priorities and strategies to address the problems. Information usually is considered current if it has been published within the last 3 to 5 years. However, it is important to be persistent in research efforts to find the most current information, which may be even more recent.

Also, when reading a research article, references cited in the journal article should be carefully screened to validate their relevancy and age. Sometimes only a limited amount of information is available on a given topic, which is reflected in the article. For example, there is still a scarcity of true research involving herbal or alternative dental therapies.

Other Sources of Literature

In today's age of electronics, journals are not the only source of valid literature.[27] Reliable electronic resources are available through websites of various organizations and government agencies (see Appendices A and D). When using literature from websites, it is important to critically evaluate web sources based on specific criteria (Box 7.10). Generally, reliable websites for scientific information have an extension of .edu or .gov, and other valuable information can be found at .org and .net sites (Box 7.11). Websites with a .com extension are less reliable

---

BOX 7.10 Criteria to Evaluate Web Sources of Literature

Authority
- Who is the author?
- What are the author's qualifications?
- Has the author published articles or books other than web pages?
- Is the source peer-reviewed or edited?
- Does the author belong to an organization?
- If the page is authored by an organization, what additional information about that organization is available?

Accuracy
- Are there clues to tell you that the information on the page is true?
- Does the author list sources? Is there a bibliography of citations on the page to show where the data are coming from?
- Can the information be verified elsewhere, perhaps in a print source?
- Are there obvious errors (e.g., spelling, grammar)?

Currency
- Are the copyright dates and time period of the page current?
- When was the page last updated?
- Is the information on the page current or outdated?
- Are the links current or are there any dead links on the page?
- Do links lead to current or foundational material or outdated, useless information?

Coverage
- Is the page a complete document or an abstract/summary?
- Does the author adequately cover the topic? Is important information left out?
- Does the page contain information that is pertinent to the research topic? Does it contain enough information to be useful? How can you use this information?

- Are there good links to additional coverage? Are the links appropriate to the topic?
- Is the information free or is there a fee to access more detailed data?

Purpose or Type of Page
- What does the Statement of Purpose, Mission Statement, or About Us link tell you?
- What kind of web page is this: advocacy business, informational, news, advertising/sponsorship, or personal?
- Does the page have the required level of scholarship for scientific information?
- Does the page include enough information to be useful?

Intended Audience
- For whom was the page written, readers of scientific or professional information or the general public?
- Is the purpose to inform or entertain?

Biased Opinion
- Does the page or author reflect a particular bias or viewpoint? Does research done on the author indicate a bias?
- Is inflammatory or provocative language included that reflects a particular agenda? If so, it is biased.
- Why was this page written? Is the page trying to sell readers a product or service or persuade them to a particular position (biased), or is it reporting on information (unbiased)?
- Is there advertising on the page? Can it be differentiated from the informational content?

(Modified from Web Page Evaluation. Binghamton University Libraries, State University of New York; 2017. Available at: <http://www.binghamton.edu/libraries/research/guides/web-page-checklist.html>; [Accessed July 2019].)

BOX 7.11 Reliable Web Sources of Literature

- Professional organizations (e.g., American Dental Hygienists' Association [ADHA], American Academy of Periodontology [AAP], American Dental Association [ADA]) = .org
- Government agencies (e.g., National Institutes of Health [NIH], Centers for Disease Control and Prevention [CDC], military) = .gov, .mil
- Universities and colleges = .edu
- Foundations and other nonprofits = .org, .net
- Community agencies = .org, .net
- Scientific sites (e.g., American Council of Science and Health, Mayo Clinic) = .org, .net

Note: .org and .net have been used recently by less reliable sites; care should be taken to evaluate sites with these extensions.
(Modified from Web Page Evaluation. Binghamton University Libraries, State University of New York; 2017. Available at: <http://www.binghamton.edu/libraries/research/guides/web-page-checklist.html>; [Accessed July 2019].)

sources of scientific information because they reflect individual web pages and web pages of commercial establishments. Sometimes use of these sites is appropriate, depending on the information sought, but they should be used with care when conducting a literature review. Articles found on a website should be evaluated using the same criteria used to evaluate journal articles.

Evaluation of the Selected Literature

Regardless of the source of research articles for the literature review, print or web-based, different types of research articles can be used as indicated in the ranking of evidence for EBDM (Figure 7.2). It is important to seek study designs in the literature

that provide the highest level of evidence available.[4] Because they are foundational to EBDM, systematic reviews, preferably with meta-analysis, should be searched out whenever possible.[4] However, many times you will not find a strong systematic review and will have to depend on other levels of evidence; therefore, it is also important to be able to evaluate a primary research report.

Validation of a research report, whether it is a systematic review or a primary research report, should include evaluation of the criteria already discussed, including author's expertise; comprehensive, accurate, and current references; and the reputation, scientific credibility, potential political stance, and peer review of a journal. Also, regardless of the type of literature reviewed, a dental hygienist should consult full-text materials rather than abstracts. Because an abstract is a brief summary and does not include the detail of information, it can be misinterpreted and is at the lower end of the levels of evidence for EBDM.

When reviewing a systematic review, the following questions should be asked:[28] (1) Did the review explicitly address a sensible question? (2) Was the search for relevant studies detailed and exhaustive? (3) Were the primary studies of high methodological quality? (4) Were selection and assessments of the included studies reproducible? Additional information to guide evaluation of systematic reviews is available from the references included in this chapter.

When reviewing a primary research report, it is important also to evaluate all components of the content of the research report to assure its value in contributing sound evidence on the topic[29] (Box 7.12). The following section discusses what to look for in each section of the primary research report.

BOX 7.12 Evaluation of a Primary Research Report

Journal
- Use of peer review (refereed)
- Nature of the journal; political stance
- Reputation of the journal
- Respectable scientific or professional publisher or sponsor
- Not commercially published; limited advertising; not a magazine

Author(s)
- Credentials and qualifications
- Scholarly experience; previously published
- Professional affiliation
- No affiliation of author or research facility with funding agency

Date of Publication
- Within 3 to 5 years, except for classic studies or historical perspective
- More recent if rapidly changing topic of study

Abstract
- Approximately 200 words
- Clear statement of purpose of study in the first few sentences
- Clear profile of article with brief description of the type of research, population and sample, methods, overview of statistics, results, and conclusions

Introduction
- Review of the background, supporting literature
- Description of research problem or purpose/reason for the study
- Statement of research question or hypothesis (alternate or null)

Materials and Methods
- Appropriate type, design, and methods of research to answer the research question
- Clear description of research procedures
- Appropriate materials and methods used (see Box 7.13)

Results
- Appropriate treatment of data
- Clear and understandable presentation of data
- Appropriate statistical tests
- Correct statistical conclusion

Discussion/Conclusions
- Interpretation of results
- Discussion of results in relation to previous research results presented in introduction
- Inferences and opinions stated as such
- Discussion of clinical significance
- Description of limitations of study
- Discussion of plans or recommendations for further research
- Valid conclusions, based on facts

References
- Valid sources
- Current references

BOX 7.13 Questions to Answer in Evaluating the Materials and Methods Section of a Primary Research Report

- Was the type and design of the research (descriptive, observational, correlational, experimental, retrospective, prospective, randomized, nonrandomized appropriate for the research question?
- Were the research procedures clearly described, both for understanding and to allow replication?
- Were the population and sample described and appropriate for the research question?
- Was the type of sample appropriate, and does the sample consist of individuals who represent the population?
- Were there enough participants in the study and in the groups of the study to allow for valid data analysis and generalization of findings to the population of interest?
- Was the use or non-use of a control group appropriate? If used, was the type of control group appropriate for the study design?
- Were all relevant variables controlled in the study to prevent extraneous variables?
- Were appropriate, valid, and reliable data collection methods used? If instruments (e.g., questionnaire, survey, index, actual dental instrument, or dental equipment) were used to collect data, were they previously established as valid and reliable? If a dental index was used to measure an oral disease or condition (see Appendix F), was it applied appropriately? If an instrument was

- developed for this study, was it tested for validity and reliability as part of this study? Was self-report used unnecessarily?
- Were the examiners calibrated and their reliability established?
- Were blind (masking) procedures followed to assure that examiners were unaware of which participants were assigned to the treatment and control groups?
- Were the research conditions consistent for all groups and completely described? Were the treatment and control groups treated in the same manner except for the independent variable?
- Was the length of the study appropriate for the dependent variable being studied?
- Were all groups monitored for an adequate period of time to assess long-term results of the treatment?
- Were all other sources of error and bias controlled?
- Were appropriate statistical methods correctly applied for data analysis?
- Were ethical procedures followed such as approval of research by a research review committee, informed consent, voluntary participation, protection of confidentiality and anonymity, and protection of human research participants?
- Were any potential sources of bias (e.g., study participants also being patients of the researcher who developed the technique being studied, relationship of research facility and researcher[s] to the funding agency) present?

Components of a Primary Research Report

It is essential to include primary research when conducting a literature review. A primary research report describes original research and includes the methods, materials, results, discussion and interpretation of results, and conclusions of the study. The contents of a published research report go by the following outline; each component of the report should be evaluated.

Abstract. An **abstract** is a brief description of the published work and appears at the beginning of a research report to provide the reader with an overview of the study. This helps the reader determine whether the research report is relevant to the topic under review. An abstract of a research report usually is confined to approximately 100 to 300 words[9] and concisely defines the study's purpose, methods, materials, results, and conclusions. The abstract does not present a complete picture of the study nor the results; therefore, it should not be relied on exclusively. The only way to evaluate a scientific article and assess its usefulness as a source of reliable information is to read the details within the full-text article. An abstract of the study of dental hygiene student competence and comfort in treating transgender patients is provided in Box 7.4.

Introduction. A primary research article begins with a review of the relevant current literature to introduce the study. An accurate and complete description of the research problem is provided, and the purpose or objective of the study is clearly explained. The research question or hypothesis should be clear.

Materials and Methods. This section of the primary research report describes the population, sample, and data collection methods, as well as the other methods and materials used to manipulate the independent variable and control confounding or extraneous variables and other sources of error and bias. Enough detail should be provided in this section that other researchers can replicate the study. The purpose of **replication** is

to reproduce the results to add to the body of research on the topic. Another reason to provide details of materials and methods is to allow researchers to modify the study design as needed to refine the conclusions or answer new related questions.

The reviewer will need to determine the appropriateness of the various methods used to conduct the study.[29] The overall question to answer is whether the methods controlled extraneous variables and other sources of error, and avoided bias (see Box 7.5). Questions to answer in evaluating the materials and methods used in the study are presented in Box 7.13.

Results. This section includes a summary of the data, a description of the statistical analysis, justification of the statistical tests used, results of the statistical analysis, and a statement of the statistical decision. Data should be described and visually presented in tables and graphs, which should be clear and understandable to the reader. How the hypothesis of the study was tested should be described. Statistical tests should be designated and should be appropriate for the data collected in the study.

Discussion. In this section the author interprets the statistical results and links them to the relevant literature discussed in the introduction. Frequently, additional literature is introduced in this section in relation to interpreting and applying the results. This section should also include an account of any complications observed during the research and a description of the study's strengths and weaknesses. The author should especially focus the reader on any limitations of the study that could affect interpretation and generalization of results.

A discussion of the conclusions and the inferences drawn from the results of the research are presented in this section as well. These conclusions should communicate clearly the statistical decisions to reject or accept the null hypotheses and define outcomes of the research study. Conclusions are based on the facts derived from the research, directly reflecting the findings of the study. It is never appropriate to make statements that are not based on fact or that are not derived from study results. However, the author can speculate on the meaning of the results. Although speculation may be appropriate, it should be stated as such. When applicable, the researcher also should discuss the clinical significance of the research results. Based on the conclusions, the researcher may mention further research necessary to obtain additional information or clarify questions identified by the results of the study.

Clinical significance versus statistical significance. When statistical results of a study indicate statistical significance, it is important also to consider the practical or **clinical significance** of the results. Clinical or substantive significance has to do with clinical judgment, not with statistics.[28] Results can be statistically significant without having clinical importance or practical implications.[12]

Several circumstances can lead to results that are statistically significant without being clinically significant. When study groups are very large, even slight differences can result in statistical significance, which may not be clinically important.[23] Even with appropriate sample size, sometimes the actual reduction in disease in a study group or difference in disease levels between groups may be statistically significant but not important.[28] For example, an experimental group using a new mouthrinse may experience a statistically significant greater reduction of gingivitis than the control group using the standard mouth rinse. Yet, close scrutiny of the data might reveal that the experimental group still has a clinically significant level of gingivitis, potentially meaning that neither mouthrinse is the best treatment to recommend to patients. Another possibility is that the new mouthrinse is not as acceptable to patients so they may not be willing to use it. In both cases it is important to consider the lack of clinical significance of the results of the study.

However, study results may not be statistically significant, yet have clinical application.[28] For example, very small study groups can lead to a lack of statistical significance, and yet the differences in disease can have clinical importance. Another example is if a new treatment procedure is tested and found to be no more effective than the current standard treatment, but the new treatment has other benefits (e.g., easier to use, more comfortable for the patient, or less costly). In this case the new treatment could be considered clinically significant without being statistically significant. Thus, it is essential that the professional dental hygienist critically interpret results of investigations when making evidence-based decisions to apply these research outcomes to their dental hygiene practice. It is also critical that the whole body of literature on a topic be considered, not just the results of one study, in determining clinical significance of research results and application to EBDM.

SUMMARY

This chapter provides an overview of the basics of research, including the steps in the scientific method, the methods of research and data analysis, how to interpret research results, keys in analyzing the literature, and the components of a primary research report. In addition, the role of research and critical analysis of the literature are discussed in relation to EBDM. Although all research should be conducted according to the scientific method to provide results with a measure of validity and reliability, scientific research remains an inexact science. However, when studies are properly designed, results are accurately analyzed with the use of the appropriate statistical procedures, and results are thoughtfully and critically interpreted, valid and up-to-date information can be obtained that can improve current dental hygiene practice and serve as a springboard for further studies. The inventive and inquisitive practitioner will seek to discover information that enhances the practice of dental hygiene in all its contemporary roles and keeps the profession moving in a forward direction.

APPLYING YOUR KNOWLEDGE

1. Design a mock experimental research study based on a question you have that is related to the field of dental hygiene. Formulate a research problem and develop an alternate hypothesis and a null hypothesis for the research problem. Then define or describe the following for the mock study:
   a. Population
   b. Sample
   c. Experimental group
   d. Control group
   e. Independent variable
   f. Dependent variable
   g. Data—classify it as categorical, continuous, or discrete, and identify the scale(s) of measurement of the data as nominal, ordinal, interval, or ratio
2. Complete a literature review for the research problem formulated in No. 1.
3. Using data that you have reviewed or collected, determine the mean, median, and mode, and develop a table and graphs to present the data.
4. Give five examples of positive and negative correlations using variables related to dental hygiene or to data from articles you have read.
5. Using one of the research studies from your literature review, describe the statistical analysis. Evaluate appropriateness of the statistical techniques used and the charts to display the data.
6. Evaluate a primary research report that you read as part of your literature review.
7. Design and complete a research study or community project following the steps of the scientific method; present a poster on the results of the study or project.
8. Complete the CITI tutorial *Human Subjects Research* at https://about.citiprogram.org/en/series/human-subjects-research-hsr/; report to the class what you learned from the course.

LEARNING OBJECTIVES AND COMPETENCIES

This chapter addresses the following community dental health learning objectives and competencies for dental hygienists that are presented in the *ADEA Compendium of Curriculum Guidelines for Allied Dental Education Programs*:

Learning Objectives

- Describe the reasons for conducting research in dental hygiene.
- Define the purpose of dental hygiene research.
- List, explain, and describe the various research approaches appropriate in community dental health.
- Define and describe data analysis and interpretation techniques used in community dental health literature.
- Identify data by their type and scale of measurement.
- Define and describe descriptive and inferential statistics.
- Select and compute appropriate measures of central tendency and measures of dispersion.
- Describe and construct frequency distributions and graphs.

- Effectively critique oral health research reported in dental publications.

Competencies

- Recognize and use written and electronic sources of information.
- Evaluate the credibility and potential hazards of dental products and techniques.
- Evaluate published clinical and basic science research and integrate this information to improve the oral health of the patient.
- Recognize the responsibility and demonstrate the ability to communicate professional knowledge verbally and in writing.
- Accept responsibility for solving problems and making decisions based on accepted scientific principles.
- Expand and contribute to the knowledge base of dental hygiene.

COMMUNITY CASE

Marco is a registered dental hygienist practicing in a community health center dental clinic. Most of the adult clients treated in this clinic present with moderate to severe periodontal disease with cementum exposure and accompanying dentin hypersensitivity. Marco currently treats his patients who have dentin hypersensitivity with a fluoride gel. Based on his reading of journal articles about the treatment of dentin hypersensitivity with fluoride and the superior performance of fluoride varnish compared with other fluoride products, Marco decides to evaluate whether fluoride varnish would work better for his own patients than the fluoride gel he has been using. He plans to pursue a change in the clinic's treatment protocol for dentin hypersensitivity if the varnish is more effective. After clearing the idea with his employer and gaining regulatory approval for his project, Marco recruits 100 of his own patients to participate in his study, all of whom are diagnosed with moderate to severe dentin hypersensitivity as recorded in their patient records. He randomly assigns half of them to a group to be treated with fluoride gel and the other half to a group to be treated with fluoride varnish. Before starting each patient on the assigned treatment, Marco records the patient's self-assessment of the severity of their hypersensitivity the day before the appointment. The self-assessment is based on a scale of 0 for little to no dentin hypersensitivity experienced during the day to 10 for severe dentin hypersensitivity experienced during the day. He also assesses the level of sensitivity by spraying air on the exposed root surfaces with an air water syringe and by dragging an explorer across the exposed root surfaces. Marco hypothesizes that the group treated with fluoride varnish will experience less severe dentin sensitivity than those treated with fluoride gel. After treatment, the patients will be assessed monthly for 3 months using the same measures. At the

end of the 3-month period, he will compare the patients' pretrial dentin hypersensitivity scores with the 1-month, 2-month, and 3-month scores.

1. The experimental group in this study is which of the following?
   a. All the volunteers that Marco enrolls in the study
   b. The patients who receive the fluoride gel treatment
   c. The patients who receive the fluoride varnish treatment
   d. The patients who do not complete the study
   e. All the patients treated in the clinic who have moderate to severe periodontitis and dentin hypersensitivity
2. The data that Marco collects for this study are which of the following types of data?
   a. Discrete data
   b. Ordinal scale data
   c. Categorical data
   d. Ratio scale data
   e. Continuous data
3. Which two of the following statistics can be used to summarize the data?
   a. Parametric
   b. Chi-square
   c. Correlation coefficient
   d. Counts and percentages
   e. Means and standard deviations
4. All of the following EXCEPT one can negatively affect the internal validity of this study. Which is the EXCEPTION?
   a. Self-report measure of the dependent variable
   b. Use of a convenience sample
   c. Potential examiner bias
   d. Potential lack of intrarater reliability

5. Which of the following graphs is the best method for Marco to present the final study outcome data to his employer to recommend a new protocol for the clinic?
   a. Bar graph
   b. Frequency polygon
   c. Histogram
   d. Time series graph
   e. Scattergram

6. Which two of the following describe the type of study used by Marco?
   a. Quasi-experimental
   b. Repeated measures
   c. Pretest-posttest
   d. Observational
   e. Blind (masked)

REFERENCES

1. American Dental Hygienists' Association. National Dental Hygiene Research Agenda; 2016. Available at: <https://www.adha.org/resources-docs/7111_National_Dental_Hygiene_Research_Agenda.pdf>; [Accessed July 2019].

2. Canadian Dental Hygienists' Association. 2015-2020 Dental Hygiene Research Agenda; 2013. Available at: <https://files.cdha.ca/profession/research/DHResearchAgenda_EN_updated_2020.pdf>; [Accessed July 2019].

3. UNC Health Science Library. Evidence Based Dentistry; 2019. Available at: <http://guides.lib.unc.edu/c.php?g=8433&p=43431>; [Accessed July 2019].

4. Forrest JL, McGovern Kupiec L. Evidence-based decision making: Introduction and formulating good clinical questions. Dentalcare.com Continuing Education Courses, Course Number 311; 2018. Available at: <www.dentalcare.com/en-us/professional-education/ce-courses/ce311>; [Accessed July 2019].

5. Curtin University. Systematic Reviews: What is a Systematic Review?; 2017. Available at: <https://libguides.library.curtin.edu.au/c.php?g=202420&p=1332858>; [Accessed July 2019].

6. Deeks JJ, Higgins JPT, Altman DG. Why perform a meta-analysis in a review? Part 2, Chapter 9, Section 9.1.3. In: Higgins JPT, Green S. Cochrane Handbook for Systematic Reviews of Interventions; 2011. Available at: <http://handbook.cochrane.org/>; [Accessed March 2015].

7. Richard G. Trefry Library of the American Public Library System. What are Primary, Secondary, and Tertiary Sources?; 2019. Available at: <https://apus.libanswers.com/faq/2299>; [Accessed July 2019].

8. Jacobsen K. Introduction to Health Research Methods: A Practical Guide. 2nd ed. Burlington, MA: Jones and Bartlett Learning; 2017.

9. Patten M, Newhart M. Understanding Research Methods: An Overview of the Essentials. 10th ed. New York, NY: Routledge; 2019.

10. Friis RH. Epidemiology 101 (Essential Public Health). 2nd ed. Burlington, MA: Jones and Bartlett Learning; 2018.

11. Ravid R. Practical Statistics for Educators. 5th ed. Lanham, MD: Rowman & Littlefield; 2015.

12. Kviz F. Conducting Health Research: Principles, Processes, and Methods. Thousand Oaks, CA: Sage; 2020.

13. Bogel S, Draper-Rodi J. The importance of pilot studies, how to write them and what they mean. Internat J Osteopath Med 2017;23(2):2–3.

14. Beatty CF, Beatty CE. Biostatistics. In: Nathe CN, editor. Dental Public Health & Research: Contemporary Practice for the Dental Hygienis. 4th ed. Upper Saddle River, NJ: Pearson; 2017.

15. Gunnerll KL, Fowler D, Colaizzi K. Inter-rater reliability calibration program: Critical components for competency-cased education. Competency-based Educ 2016;1(1):36–41.

16. American Dental Hygienists' Association. Code of Ethics for Dental Hygienists; 2020. Available at: <http://www.adha.org/resources-docs/7611_Bylaws_and_Code_of_Ethics.pdf>; [Accessed November 2020].

17. Collaborative Institutional Training Initiatives. Human Subjects Training (tutorial); 2018. Available at: <https://about.citiprogram.org/en/series/human-subjects-research-hsr/>; [Accessed July 2019].

18. National Institutes of Health, National Cancer Institute. Cancer Staging; 2015. Available at: <http://www.cancer.gov/cancertopics/factsheet/detection/staging>; [Accessed July 2019].

19. American Dental Association Center for Professional Success. Typical Dental Plan Benefits and Limitations; 2019. Available at: <https://success.ada.org/en/dental-benefits/typical-dental-plan-benefits-and-limitations>; [Accessed August 2019].

20. Lozovsky V. Table vs. Graph; 2019. Available on Information Builders website at: <https://techsupport.informationbuilders.com/public/wfn/9-2/05_lozovsky.html>; [Accessed July 2019].

21. Jain S, Gupta A, Jain D. Common statistical tests in dental research. JAMSDR 2015;3(3):38–45.

22. Statistics Solutions, Statistical Power Analysis. 2019. Available at: <https://www.statisticssolutions.com/statistical-power-analysis/>; [Accessed July 2019].

23. Forrest JL, Miller SA. Evidence-based decision making. In: Bowen DM, Pieren JA, editors. Darby and Walsh Dental Hygiene: Theory and Practice. 5th ed. Maryland Heights, MO: Elsevier Saunders; 2020. p. 25–33.

24. Pyrczak F, Tcherni-Buzzero M. Evaluating Research in Academic Journals: A Practical Guide to Realistic Evaluation. 7th ed. New York, NY: Routledge; 2019.

25. Ng A. Vipeholm study. Cariology (Web); 2009. Available at: <http://cariology.wikifoundry.com/page/Vipeholm+Study>; [Accessed March 2019].

26. Löe H, Theilade E, Jensen SB. Experimental gingivitis in man (abstract). J Periodontol 1965;36:177–87. Available at: <https://onlinelibrary.wiley.com/doi/abs/10.1111/j.1600-0765.1967.tb01901.x>; [Accessed July 2019].

27. Binghamton University Libraries, State University of New York. Web Page Evaluation; 2017. Available at: <http://www.binghamton.edu/libraries/research/guides/web-page-checklist.html>; [Accessed July 2019].

28. Duke University Medical Center Library, University of North Carolina at Chapel Hill Health Sciences Library. Introduction to Evidence-Based Practice (tutorial); 2019. Available at: <http://guides.mclibrary.duke.edu/c.php?g=158201&p=1036002>; [Accessed July 2019].

29. Gall MD, Gall JP, Borg WR. Applying Education Research: How to Read, Do, and Use Research to Solve Problems of Practice. 7th ed. Hoboken, NJ: Pearson; 2015.

ADDITIONAL RESOURCES

American Dental Association Research Agenda
http://www.ada.org/en/about-the-ada/ada-positions-policies-and-statements/research-agenda
American University literature review tutorial
http://subjectguides.library.american.edu/litreview
Centre for Evidence Based Dentistry
http://www.cebd.org/
Cochrane Library
http://www.cochranelibrary.com/
Collaborative Institutional Training Initiative (CITI)
https://about.citiprogram.org/en/series/human-subjects-research-hsr/
Critically Reading Journal Articles
Subramanyam RV. Art of reading a journal article: Methodically and effectively. J Oral Maxillofac Pathol 2013;17(1) 65–70. https://www.ncbi.nlm.nih.gov/pmc/articles/PMC3687192/

DHNet National Center for Dental Hygiene Research & Practice
https://dent-web10.usc.edu/dhnet/
Journal of Dental Hygiene online articles
https://jdh.adha.org/
National Dental Hygiene Research Agenda
https://www.adha.org/resources-docs/7111_National_Dental_Hygiene_Research_Agenda.pdf
Qualitative Research Methods: A Data Collector's Field Guide
https://course.ccs.neu.edu/is4800sp12/resources/qualmethods.pdf
Research Center, American Dental Hygienists' Association
http://www.adha.org/research-center

8

Health Promotion and Health Communication

Beverly Ann Isman

OBJECTIVES

1. Discuss the scope of health promotion and the wide range of activities involved.
2. Apply various health promotion strategies, theories, and models to situations for promotion of oral health.
3. Follow a sequence of steps in the health communication process when developing, implementing, or evaluating a health communication plan or project.
4. Discuss ways to assess needs of diverse populations before designing health promotion and health communication strategies.
5. Describe health communication in relation to health information technology, as well as strategies to appropriately frame health messages for different audiences and different mobile and social media applications.
6. Identify uses and limitations of strategies for delivering health information to consumer groups in terms of the materials, activities, communication pathways, and evaluation methods.
7. Outline the basic considerations, advantages, and limitations of various formats for communicating scientific information to health professionals.
8. Identify and take advantage of opportunities for personal growth and development in health promotion, health communication, and health information technology.

OPENING STATEMENTS: Challenges to Promoting Oral Health

- Despite years of research on prevention of oral diseases, very little is known about how best to promote oral health.
- Assuring oral health for all people will be difficult until the World Health Organization's (WHO) eight prerequisites for health are achieved: peace, shelter, education, food, income, stable ecosystem, sustainable resources, social justice, and equity.[1]
- More community-based participatory research, in which community members are involved at all stages, and more interdisciplinary research, with nondental behavioral scientists, might shed more light on effective health promotion and communication strategies.
- More evidence is needed to document that changes in attitudes and beliefs about oral health lead to improved oral health outcomes.
- Improved knowledge levels alone rarely translate into healthy behaviors, so approaches need to be designed around proven behavioral and communication theories.

- Most behavioral change that occurs after oral health education or promotion is short term and not sustained without periodic reinforcement; it is important to continue to seek an answer to what it takes to create sustainable changes.
- Today dental hygienists have unique and unlimited opportunities to become involved in community health promotion activities and health communication strategies; more advocacy is needed to create community-focused career opportunities for using these skills.
- Exponential use of social media and online resources can increase knowledge but also can inundate users with information, as well as misinformation that is not evidence-based.
- The main goal of this chapter is to help dental hygienists incorporate a thought process for assessing needs, forming evaluation questions, and planning health promotion and communication strategies before jumping to implement what seems like a *good idea*.

HEALTH PROMOTION

Defined in Chapter 1, **health** is a personal resource that permits people to lead productive lives.[1] **Health promotion** is a broad concept defined by the WHO as "the process of enabling people to increase control over, and to improve their health,"[2] thus involving **empowerment**. Health promotion introduces the role of behaviors, not just attitudes and knowledge, into the health equation and goes beyond a focus on individual behavior toward a wide range of social and environmental interventions.

Oral health promotion is more than oral health education (see Chapter 6) and links oral health to other health issues. Thus, this chapter focuses on the concepts of oral health promotion, strategies to affect behavioral and community changes, and the dental hygienist's role in selecting communication pathways and communicating health messages to other health professionals and to the public.

The Ottawa Charter, a global health promotion imperative created in 1986, identified the WHO prerequisites for health and three basic health promotion strategies to address these prerequisites: (1) advocating for health, (2) enabling people to achieve their full health potential, and (3) mediating different societal interests in pursuit of health.[1] At the ninth global conference held in Shanghai, China in 2016, pathways were offered to advance health promotion and address the determinants of health through sound governance, healthy cities, health literacy, health-promoting schools, and social mobilization.[2] These strategies have direct relevance to oral health, the health promotion theories enumerated in this chapter, and healthcare reform efforts in the United States and other countries.

Oral health promotion efforts can increase the use of oral health and wellness services and preventive self-care measures. The anticipated outcome of these efforts is a reduced incidence and severity of oral diseases, reduced oral health disparities among population subgroups, and improved oral and overall health. Yet, as highlighted by the challenges in the Opening Statements, applied oral health promotion research is still not well integrated or coordinated with research and theories developed by other health disciplines. An important goal of health promotion is to achieve oral **health equity**[3] (see Chapters 4 and 9)."

Watt and Sheiham promoted the use of the "**common risk factor approach**" to identify and address multiple diseases, including oral diseases, and to implement preventive strategies and health promotion messages that can have an enhanced impact.[4] In this approach they posed a "theoretical basis for a social determinants framework for oral health inequalities"[4] that has influenced the integration of oral health into general health improvement strategies.[5] This perspective focuses on socio-political-economic factors that are common to many chronic conditions as the key determinants of health, providing the basis for a collaborative approach to address oral health within the context of overall health promotion and policy development.[4]

Health Promotion Theories

When promoting health and preventing disease, a **theory** helps us analyze and interpret health problems and then develop and evaluate interventions based on the analysis. According to Glanz, a theory is "a set of interrelated concepts, definitions, and propositions that present a systematic view of events or situations by specifying relations among variables to explain and predict the events or situations."[6] This abstract notion comes to life only when it is applied to specific topics and problems. Sometimes theories are called *conceptual frameworks* or *models*.

How can theories be applied to dental hygiene and public health practice? Every day, dental hygienists face challenging oral health problems. Some examples are members of underserved, vulnerable groups who have have trouble accessing dental care, babies who develop early childhood caries from sweetened liquids in baby bottles, athletes who sustain oral injuries because they refuse to wear a mouth guard or other facial protection, teens who develop oral lesions from using tobacco products, or patients who present with poor oral hygiene and related oral health issues (Figure 8.1). Theories can help us analyze these situations and apply effective solutions.

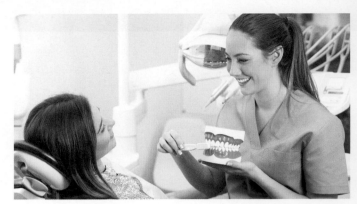

Fig 8.1 Health promotion theories apply to all health education encounters. (© iStock.com/AntonioGuillem.)

Dental hygienists often assume oral health problems are because of a person's laziness or unwillingness to follow simple oral care recommendations. Lecturing the person about facts to improve oral health is a doomed approach because it is a generic intervention, does not assess or validate the person's point of view or health beliefs, and does not consider the environmental, literacy, or cultural circumstances that have influenced the person's attitudes, beliefs, or health practices. Analyzing oral health problems from more than one perspective is important for understanding how each perspective affects the others.

Health behaviors and health status are influenced by health determinants at various levels, as described in Table 8.1 and illustrated in Figure 8.2.[7] These levels provide an **ecological approach** to health promotion that focuses on both population-level and individual-level health determinants and interventions.[7] The ecological approach is based on the idea that health behaviors and health both shape and are shaped by the social environment[7] (see Chapter 3). Thus, to effectively initiate and sustain changes in health behaviors and health status, multiple interventions are often needed to address all levels of influence.

The following sections describe selected health promotion and **health education** theories that relate to the intrapersonal, interpersonal, community, and organization levels of influence

TABLE 8.1 Levels of Influence of Health Promotion Models

Level of Influence	Definition
Intrapersonal factors	Individual characteristics that influence behavior, such as knowledge, attitudes, beliefs, and personality traits
Interpersonal factors	Interpersonal processes and primary groups, including family, friends, and peers, that provide social identity, support, and role definition
Institutional factors	Rules, regulations, policies, and informal structures that may constrain or promote recommended behaviors
Community factors	Social networks and norms or standards that exist formally or informally among individuals, groups, and organizations
Public policy	Local, state, and federal policies and laws that regulate or support healthy actions and practices for disease prevention, early detection, control, and management

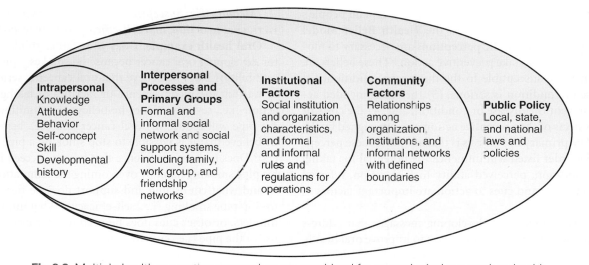

Fig 8.2 Multiple health promotion approaches are combined for an ecological approach to health promotion. (Modified from Ecological Model. Healthy Campus; 2018. Available at: <https://www.acha.org/HealthyCampus/HealthyCampus/Ecological_Model.aspx>; [Accessed February 2020].)

in the ecological approach and that have the most relevance to oral health issues. A narrative of each theory, including an oral health example and tips for remembering the theory, is accompanied by a table that contains key concepts, definitions, and general applications. For further elaboration or additional theories, see the References at the end of the chapter.

The use of public policy to influence oral health behavior is not addressed in this chapter; rather, it is threaded throughout the textbook. Some specific examples are the national initiatives and policy development in Chapter 1, advocacy in Chapter 2, assessment best practices in Chapter 3, surveillance policies in Chapter 4, water fluoridation and other policies related to specific community programs in Chapter 6, legislative advocacy in Chapter 9, public policy related to cultural competence and health literacy in Chapter 10, and interprofessional education policies in Chapter 11.

Intrapersonal Level

Stages of Change Theory (Transtheoretical Model). Years of research have shown that a *one-time* educational intervention without follow-up is totally ineffective for long-term retention of knowledge or behavior change. The **Stages of Change Theory** views change as a process or cycle that occurs over time rather than as a single event.[8] This theory allows the dental hygienist to assess a person's readiness to change a behavior toward a more healthful lifestyle such as daily brushing to prevent gingivitis. The theory assumes that at any point in time everyone is at a different stage of readiness to make lifestyle changes and that people cycle through the various stages over time, depending on the behavior to be changed and whether the environment is supportive. Relapse can occur as temptation to revert to old behaviors overcomes one's ability to maintain the desired behavior change. For changes in behavior to occur, counseling must address the individual in relation to their current stage of readiness to change.[8] This theory is focused on strategies rather than information. The major stages of this model with definitions and applications are outlined in Table 8.2.

TABLE 8.2 Stages of Change (Transtheoretical Model)

Concept	Definition	Application
Precontemplation	Being unaware of problem; not having thought about change	Increase awareness of need for change; personalize information on risks and benefits
Contemplation	Thinking about change in the near future	Motivate and encourage the making of specific plans
Decision/ determination	Making a plan to change	Assist in developing concrete action plans or setting gradual goals
Action	Implementing specific action or plans	Assist with feedback, problem solving, social support, and reinforcement
Maintenance	Continuing desirable actions or repeating periodic recommended steps	Assist in coping, using reminders, finding alternatives, and avoiding slips or relapses

(Modified from McKenzie JF, Neiger BL, Thackeray R. Planning, Implementing & Evaluating Health Promotion Programs: A Primer, 7th ed. Glenview, IL: Pearson Education, Inc; 2017.)

[Memory Tip: Readiness to change cycles through stages]

Oral health example. The cycle starts by assessing and increasing one's awareness of a problem (e.g., a person has gingivitis) to determine the level of readiness to change and then initiate behavior change (e.g., brushing and flossing effectively and using antimicrobial rinses), and then progresses to maintaining motivation to continue preventive actions (e.g., exchanging text messages with motivational reminders and status checks). To be effective in changing behavior, health messages and programs should be matched to an individual's current stage of change-readiness. The dental hygienist's goal is to help the individual move to the next stage on the cycle of adopting effective preventive behaviors.

Health Belief Model. Described as a way to explain people's use of preventive health services, the **Health Belief Model** (HBM) suggests that specific perceptions are necessary to motivate an individual to take preventive action.[8] These beliefs are that (1) they are susceptible to the disease or condition, (2) the disease or condition is serious, (3) the recommended action will prevent the disease or condition, and (4) the costs or negative aspects of the preventive action are outweighed by the benefits. The primary hypothesis is that adopting these perceptions in the order listed will influence the potential for taking action. In addition, perceived ability to take action, referred to as **self-efficacy**, and cues to action are important factors in this model.

The HBM is applied by developing messages that address these perceptions to influence decisions to improve oral health. In contrast to the Stages of Change Theory, the HBM is focused on information. Although it has been used successfully in many situations, the model has been criticized because it is strictly information-based and does not factor in attitudes, beliefs, motivation, habitual behaviors, individual determinants of health decisions, and environmental or economic influences on health behaviors. The components of the model and some applications are presented in Table 8.3.

TABLE 8.3   Health Belief Model

Concept	Definition	Application
Perceived susceptibility	One's opinion of chances of getting a condition	Define population at risk and risk levels; personalize risk based on a person's features or behavior; heighten perceived susceptibility if too low
Perceived severity	One's opinion of how serious a condition and its sequelae are	Specify consequences of the risk and the condition
Perceived benefits	One's opinion of the efficacy of the advised action to reduce risk or the seriousness of the effect	Define action to take: How, where, when; clarify the positive effects to be expected
Perceived barriers	One's opinion of the tangible and psychological costs of the advised action, and that any actual costs are outweighed by the benefits	Identify and reduce barriers through reassurance, incentives, and assistance; assist the individual in doing a cost/benefit analysis of the recommended preventive action
Cues to action	Strategies to activate readiness	Provide how-to information; promote awareness; identify and reduce barriers through reassurance, incentives, and assistance; send reminders
Self-efficacy	Confidence in one's ability to take action	Provide training, guidance, and encouragment

(Modified from McKenzie JF, Neiger BL, Thackeray R. Planning, Implementing & Evaluating Health Promotion Programs: A Primer, 7th ed. Glenview, IL: Pearson Education, Inc; 2017.)

[Memory Tip: Susceptibility, risk, seriousness, benefits, barriers, cues to action, and self-efficacy are key terms]

Oral health example. Does your father think he is at risk for developing oral cancer because he smokes a pipe (i.e., susceptibility)? Does he believe that oral cancer is serious enough to warrant the inconvenience or sacrifice of taking preventive action (i.e., severity)? Does he believe that limiting his use of the pipe will reduce his oral cancer risk (i.e., benefits)? Does he believe that it is possible to stop smoking a pipe (i.e., barriers)? Does he have confidence that he can succeed in changing his pipe smoking habit by overcoming the temptation to smoke it, and what counseling and support does he need to be able to stop pipe smoking (i.e., self-efficacy)? What information, reminders, or other cues does he need to appropriately limit his use of the pipe (i.e., cues to action)?

Interpersonal Level

Social Learning Theory. The **Social Learning Theory** (also known as the Social Cognitive Theory) posits that people learn primarily in the following four ways:[8]

1. Vicarious learning, also called observational learning, as a result of observing others' behavior.
2. Remembering and imitating the observed behaviors of others (modeling).
3. Inferences made from the *evidence* of observed outcomes of behavior.
4. Motivation from judgments voiced by others such as testimonies or promotions by experts.

The basic premise of this theory is that people learn by observing the actions of others and the results of these actions, as well as their own cognitive processing of that information and environmental influences on behavior. Behavioral change is accomplished through the interaction of behaviors, environmental influences, and personal cognitive processes. According to this theory, the world's environment and one's behavior influence each other—a concept known as *reciprocal determinism*. Self-efficacy is also an important concept in this theory. Table 8.4 lists the relevant definitions and applications of the major concepts.

[Memory Tip: Learning by observing, copying, processing consequences, and listening to others]

Oral health example. While visiting a day care center, you are asked to help a single mother increase her confidence about brushing her toddler's teeth. First you assess what she is currently doing, how she has determined to do things this way, and what questions or concerns she has. Then you help her refine her current skills or learn a new skill. You use techniques such as having her observe others who do it well, asking her to research what "experts" recommend, giving her the opportunity for guided practice of what she has learned, having her process what she is learning through reflection and discussion, providing ongoing encouragement, and giving periodic feedback. When she gains some confidence in her skills, you ask her to help you assist the day care workers and other day care parents to improve their skills so they can support each other and so oral hygiene care becomes a daily activity for all the children.

TABLE 8.4 Social Learning Theory (Social Cognitive Theory)

Concept	Definition	Application
Reciprocal determinism	Behavioral changes result from interaction between the person and the environment; change is bidirectional	Involve the individual and relevant others; work to change the environment, if warranted
Behavioral capability	Knowledge and skills to influence behavior	Provide information and training related to action
Expectations	Beliefs about likely results of action	Incorporate information about likely results of action in advance
Self-efficacy	Confidence in ability to take action and to persist in action	Point out strengths; use persuasion and encouragement; approach behavioral change in small steps
Observational learning	Beliefs based on observing others like oneself and/or visible physical results	Point out others' experience and physical changes; identify role models to emulate
Reinforcement	Responses to a person's behavior that increase or decrease the chances of recurrence	Provide incentives, rewards, praise; encourage self-reward; decrease possibility of negative responses that deter positive changes

(Modified from McKenzie JF, Neiger BL, Thackeray R. Planning, Implementing & Evaluating Health Promotion Programs: A Primer, 7th ed. Glenview, IL: Pearson Education, Inc; 2017.)

Community Level

Community Organization Theory. **Community Organization Theory** is the process of involving and activating members of a community or subgroup to (1) identify a common problem or goal of importance to them, (2) identify and mobilize resources to address the problem, (3) implement the chosen strategies, and (4) evaluate their efforts.[8] The community can be large or small and can represent a diverse definition of community, based on geographic location, an organization, a workplace setting, or even a group with a common cause. Community organization involves social planning, social action, group consensus about common concerns, collaboration in problem solving, and formation of community partnerships or coalitions. It is based on the community's emotional and social commitment to action. People usually refer to this process as *community empowerment* because it is a grassroots approach to health promotion, rather than an effort that is initiated and conducted solely by health professionals. The goal is to guide and facilitate the community organization process as the community learns the skills to solve their own problems. Table 8.5 outlines the key components.

[Memory Tip: Grassroots organization and empowerment]

Oral health example. What might the role of a church pastor and a congregation be in relation to oral health promotion? The pastor notices that many of the older adult members have stopped coming to church suppers because they have lost their teeth or dentures and are embarrassed to eat in public. The pastor forms a committee of the congregation that includes older adult members to discuss potential solutions to the problem. They contact a local dental school to help develop a program to assist the older adults, and they involve the congregation to raise funds to help defray the cost of examinations and new dentures. Dental and dental hygiene student teams work together to assess the participants' needs, attitudes, and interests; to fabricate and fit dentures; and to develop programs for the older adults based on their input. Group discussions focus on oral health in relation to overall health, getting used to dentures, denture care, and the challenges of eating various foods with dentures. Gradually, the older adult members become comfortable eating and speaking with their new dentures, and they resume their attendance at church suppers. In addition, the selection of food at these suppers is changed to accommodate the varied dietary practices and chewing abilities. Recognizing the multiple benefits from this collaboration, the following year the congregation continues to work with the student teams to strategize ways to promote oral health to people of all ages within their parish.

Diffusion of Innovations Theory. The **Diffusion of Innovations Theory** helps assess and plan for the spread of new ideas, products, or services within a society or other groups.[8] Attention is directed to (1) characteristics of the innovation, (2) communication channels, and (3) social systems. A key aspect of this theory is *relative advantage*, which is how much the innovation

TABLE 8.5 Community Organization Theory

Concept	Definition	Application
Empowerment	Process of gaining mastery and power over oneself or one's community to produce change	Give tools and responsibility to individuals and communities for making decisions that affect them
Community competence	Community's ability to engage in effective problem solving	Work with community to identify problems, create consensus, and reach goals
Participation relevance	Learner (community) should be active participant; work should start "where the people are"	Help community set goals within the context of preexisting goals, and encourage active participation
Issue selection	Identifying winnable, simple, and specific concerns as the focus of action	Assist community members in examining how they can communicate the concerns and whether success is likely
Critical consciousness	Developing understanding of root causes of problems	Guide consideration of health concerns in broad perspective of social problems

(Modified from McKenzie JF, Neiger BL, Thackeray R. Planning, Implementing & Evaluating Health Promotion Programs: A Primer, 7th ed. Glenview, IL: Pearson Education, Inc; 2017.)

TABLE 8.6 Diffusion of Innovations Theory

Concept	Definition	Application
Relative advantage	The degree to which an innovation is seen as better than the idea, practice, program, or product it replaces	Point out unique benefits such as monetary value, convenience, time saving, prestige, and others
Compatibility	How consistent the innovation is with values, habits, experience, and needs of potential adopters	Tailor innovation to the intended audience's values, norms, or situation
Complexity	How difficult the innovation is to understand or use	Create a program, idea, or product that is easy to use and understand
Trialability	Extent to which one can experiment with the innovation before a commitment to adopt is required	Provide opportunities to implement the innovation on a limited basis (e.g., free samples, introductory sessions, money-back guarantee)
Observability	Extent to which the innovation provides tangible or visible results	Ensure visibility of results through feedback or publicity

(Modified from McKenzie JF, Neiger BL, Thackeray R. Planning, Implementing & Evaluating Health Promotion Programs: A Primer, 7th ed. Glenview, IL: Pearson Education, Inc; 2017.)

TABLE 8.7 Characteristics of Adopter Categories and Suggested Strategies to Encourage Adoption

Adopter Category	Characteristics	Suggested Strategies
Innovators	Want to be the first to try the innovation; are venturesome and interested in new ideas; very willing to take risks; often the first to develop new ideas	Very little, if anything, needs to be done to appeal to this group
Early adopters	Represent opinion leaders; enjoy leadership roles; embrace change opportunities; already aware of the need to change and so very comfortable adopting new ideas	How-to manuals; information sheets on implementation; do not need information to convince them to change
Early majority	Rarely leaders but do adopt new ideas before the average person; typically need to see evidence that the innovation works before they are willing to adopt it	Success stories; evidence of the innovation's effectiveness
Late majority	Skeptical of change; will only adopt an innovation after it has been tried by the majority	Information on how many others have tried the new idea and adopted it successfully
Laggards	Bound by tradition; very conservative; very skeptical of change; the hardest group to bring on board	Statistics; fear appeals; pressure from people in the other adopter groups

(Modified from McKenzie JF, Neiger BL, Thackeray R. Planning, Implementing & Evaluating Health Promotion Programs: A Primer, 7th ed. Glenview, IL: Pearson Education, Inc; 2017.)

is perceived to be better than an approach or product that it replaces. As this perception affects the adoption of innovations, it is important to attempt to change perceptions when necessary. Another important concept is the different categories of adopters that embrace a new idea quickly, in moderation, or slowly. Diffusion of an innovation can be extremely slow or very rapid, depending on the characteristics of the population. Understanding these characteristics is necessary to determine how to introduce a new idea. Different strategies are useful to appeal to the various adopter categories. Table 8.6 displays the components of this theory, and Table 8.7 presents the adopter categories, their characteristics, and suggested strategies to appeal to them.

[Memory Tip: How innovations are adopted]

Oral health example. Let's use a historical example. Researchers in the 1990s found that despite numerous clinical trials showing the effectiveness and safety of dental sealants in caries prevention, their adoption by practitioners proceeded slowly. Adoption occurred much sooner in public health clinics, where higher caries rates resulted in a more critical need for low-cost, effective, caries-preventive measures and strong advocacy for the procedure. By contrast, in private dental offices many children had lower caries rates, some insurance companies did not reimburse for sealants, and practitioners were wedded to the use of amalgam restorations to manage rather than prevent dental caries. Over time caries rates in occlusal surfaces declined dramatically in children who received regular care and sealants at the clinics, whereas caries rates remained stable in the children treated in private or public dental practices that did not apply sealants.

In addition, the clinical procedure for sealant placement was technique-sensitive and required additional training for oral healthcare providers. Eventually, sealant materials improved, more oral health professionals received the required training, and the public became aware of the benefits of sealants. Major educational and advocacy efforts finally changed attitudes, patterns of practice, and reimbursement policies, thus resulting in increased use of sealants and reduced rates of occlusal caries in children treated in both the public and private sectors. Depending on their adopter category, some dentists needed to see for themselves the value and effectiveness of dental sealants before they were willing to accept their use.

Organizational Change Theory. Organizations pass through a series of stages as they initiate change. **Organizational Change Theory** describes the process of this change based on various theories that explain change in relation to the following:[9]

- The organizational structures and processes that influence workers' behavior and motivation for change.
- Specific strategies that are required at each stage of change, depending on where the organization is in the process of adopting, implementing, and sustaining new approaches.

Table 8.8 presents a summary of the stages as adapted from the various theories. For organizational change to be successful, all stages must be implemented, including integration of new policies within the organization.

TABLE 8.8 Organizational Change Theory

Concept	Definition	Application Strategies
Definition of problem	Problems recognized and analyzed; solutions sought and evaluated	Involve management and other personnel in awareness-raising activities
Initiation of action	Policy or directive formulated; resources for beginning change allocated	Provide process consultation to inform decision makers and implementers of what adopt on involves
Implementation of change	Innovation is implemented; reactions and role changes occur	Provide training, technical assistance, and aid in problem solving
Institutionalization of change	Policy or program becomes entrenched in the organization; new goals and values internalized	Identify high-level champion, work to overcome obstacles to institutionalization, and create structures for integration

(Modified from Baras D, Duff C, Smith BJ. Organizational change theory: implications for health promotion practice. Health Promot Int 2016;31(1):231-241. Available at: <https://academic.oup.com/heapro/article/31/1/231/2355918>; [Accessed October 2019].)

[Memory Tip: Organizations change in stages]

Oral health example. For months dental hygiene students had asked the cafeteria staff in their college to offer healthier foods as they had noticed too many high fat, high carbohydrate foods and sweetened beverages and not enough fresh produce. Many stages were involved in promoting a change (e.g., pricing different food items and calculating costs of buying from local farmers, interviewing students and faculty about food preferences, reviewing sample menus, incorporating new food items on a trial basis, and re-interviewing students and faculty about the changes). Over time more people began to select the healthy food options and suggest new recipes, thus creating healthier lunches. The dental hygiene students and the cafeteria staff then collaborated to host a weekly onsite farmers' market and to distribute health-promoting recipes so that everyone was encouraged to also prepare healthy meals at home. This process not only resulted in institutional change but also created healthier lifestyles.

Combining Health Promotion Theories

Health promotion theories often are combined within an intervention. Components of different theories can be brought together to address a specific health issue. In this way the strengths and limitations of the diverse theories can be balanced when they are used in combination.[8] For example, the HBM can be used to design educational materials, and the strategies used to implement the educational materials can be formulated around the Stages of Change Theory to assess readiness to change and to motivate movement through the stages. Furthermore, the Social Learning Theory can be used to add activities and encounters that will provide experiential learning and motivation to move from one stage to the next.

Multiple theories are combined to enhance the ecological dimension.[7] For example, a community-wide intervention can include policy development, community organization, organizational change, and individual behavior change to include all levels of influence (see Figure 8.2). Having an understanding of various health promotion theories enables the development of a successful, comprehensive oral health promotion program.

Expanding Dental Hygiene Knowledge and Strategies

To use these theories effectively, dental hygienists need to acquire the knowledge and approaches necessary to assess and change oral health behaviors, integrate them into healthcare and dental care systems, and evaluate outcomes (see Guiding Principles). They also need to stay abreast of innovative programs occurring in other professions and ways that other healthcare systems and countries address oral health problems.

GUIDING PRINCIPLES

Knowledge and Skills Needed to Assess, Change, and Evaluate Oral Health Behaviors and Systems of Oral Health Care

- Factors that are considered a risk for development of oral diseases and those factors that can be modified through preventive efforts at the primary, secondary, and tertiary levels
- Common risk factors for oral and other health problems and their interaction in relation to oral health problems
- How to assess a person's risk for development of oral diseases, and how to counsel the individual about risk reduction
- The level of scientific evidence for and the extent of certainty of the effectiveness of various preventive measures
- Which categories of interventions (e.g., personal behaviors, programs, societal and environmental modifications, policies) yield the desired impact
- How to deliver effective services and education to individuals and groups
- Selection and delivery of appropriate and effective oral, written, and electronic communication methods and channels
- Ways to motivate people to access services and return for continuing care
- Ways in which innovations are diffused and ways of bringing about organizational change
- The structure and function of various healthcare systems and community-based organizations
- How to evaluate efforts (e.g., effectiveness, costs, access, quality, outcomes) using both qualitative and quantitative methods

Adapted from: ADEA Compendium of Curriculum Guidelines (Revised Edition) Allied Dental Education Programs: Dental Hygiene May 2015–2016. American Dental Education Association. Available at: <https://www.adea.org/cadpd/allied-dental-education-resources.aspx>; [Accessed February 2020].

Some information and skills may be learned during the dental hygiene educational process, with additional strategies acquired through professional development, advanced degrees, work experience, and personal research. Resources for professional development are discussed later in this chapter.

HEALTH COMMUNICATION AND HEALTH INFORMATION TECHNOLOGY

Beliefs and behaviors about health are shaped by communication formats and technology that people interact with daily. These formats and uses of technology influence the way people search for, understand, and use health information to make decisions and act on these decisions.

The Community Guide defines **health communication** as "the study and use of communication strategies to inform and influence individual and community decisions that enhance health."[10] One of the channels of health communication is **health information technology**, which "includes digital tools and services that can be used to enhance patients' self-care, facilitate patient-provider communication, inform health behaviors and decisions, prevent health complications, and promote health equity."[10] The importance of using technology in health communication continues to grow to be able to meet consumer expectations in today's age of technology.[11]

Box 8.1 demonstrates the CDC's framework of the important steps in the health communication process that center around the community health program planning process consisting of assessment, planning, implementation, and evaluation (see Chapters 3 and 6). Embedded in this framework is the critical identification of the most effective content, channels, and context to capture people's attention and motivate them to use health information. This process has application to oral health education and promotion.

The importance of health communication and health information technology is reinforced by their inclusion in *Healthy People (HP)*.[11] Health communication emerged as a separate focus area in *HP 2010* objectives, and health communication and health information technology became a combined topic area (HC/HIT) in *HP 2020*.[11] A mid-course review of the *HP 2020* objectives revealed that almost half of the 25 measurable HC/HIT objectives reached their targets or improved, including the following: [12]

- Increased use of the Internet by patients to track personal health information and access health websites.
- Improved patient/provider communication.

BOX 8.1   Essential Strategic Planning Steps for Effective Health Communication

1. Review background information to describe the public health problem.
2. Define the specific desired behavior-change goal and set communication objectives.
3. Segment target audiences and perform market research to analyze their characteristics, attitudes, beliefs, values, behaviors, determinants, and benefits and barriers to behavior change.
4. Identify and pretest message concepts that need to be communicated.
5. Select methods and channels to communicate the message.
6. Select, create, and pretest messages and products.
7. Develop a production and promotion plan to launch the communication program.
8. Implement communication strategies and evaluate the process.
9. Conduct outcome and impact evaluation to determine if change took place.

(From Health Communication Basics: How Do I Do It? Atlanta, GA: Centers for Disease Control and Prevention; August 12, 2019. Available at: <https://www.cdc.gov/healthcommunication/healthbasics/HowToDo.html>; [Accessed October 2020].)

- Continuing disparities in use of the Internet and patient/provider communication, by race/ethnicity, country of birth, and educational attainment.
- Increased health-related conversations by adults with friends and family.
- Increased use of technology by medical practices.

In *HP 2030*, HC/HIT objectives are included in the topic area Health Communication.[11] Also included are other topic area objectives related to specific populations and health conditions that involve health communication.[11] Some of the Health Communication topic area objectives have specific application to oral health (see Guiding Principles).

GUIDING PRINCIPLES

Selected Healthy People 2030 Health Communication Objectives that Apply to Oral Health

- Increase in adults who talk to friends or family about their health.
- Increase in state health department use of social marketing in health promotion programs.
- Increase in health literacy of the population.
- Increase in persons who are counseled or engage in shared decision-making relative to cancer prevention.
- Increase in adults whose healthcare provider checked their understanding.
- Reduction in persons reporting poor communication with their healthcare provider.
- Increase in persons whose healthcare provider maximized their involvement in shared decision-making.
- Increase in persons with limited English proficiency who report adequate explanations by their healthcare provider.
- Increase the use of information technology in relation to accessing, viewing, exchanging, and sharing medical records.

(Adapted from Health Communication Objectives. Healthy People 2030. Available at: <https://health.gov/healthypeople/objectives-and-data/browse-objectives/health-communication>; [Accessed October 2020].)

Creating and Delivering Health Communication Messages

Several techniques can be used to increase the potential effectiveness of health communication messages. Some are discussed here. In all cases, use of needs assessment and risk assessment will enhance outcomes of health communication.

Health Marketing

According to the CDC, **health marketing** "involves creating, communicating, and delivering health information and interventions using customer-centered and science-based strategies to protect and promote the health of diverse populations."[13] Basically, it is the application of **social marketing** to health communication. This can be accomplished by integrating four fundmental marketing elements, sometimes called the four Ps of marketing, into health communication: Product, Price, Place and Promotion.[13] Table 8.9 defines these four Ps and provides examples in relation to an oral health education message.

Framing Health Messages

New forms of health information technology and perspectives on integrating oral health with other health messages are changing our options for framing, delivering, and evaluating

TABLE 8.9	**The Four Ps of Marketing in Relation to Health Messages**	
Oral Health Message: The Importance of Giving Up the Use of Tobacco		
P	**Explanation of the P**	**Oral Health Example**
Product	Represents the desired behavior you are asking your audience to perform and the associated benefits, tangible objects, and/or services that support behavior change	*Behavior:* Stop smoking *Benefits:* Improved general health and prevention of future health problems *Tangible objects:* Immediate health benefits such as improved cough or asthma, savings of cost of cigarettes, improved breathing *Services that support the change:* Available counseling or family support
Price	The cost (financial, emotional, psychological, or time-related) of overcoming the barriers the audience faces in making the desired behavior change	*Financial:* Cost of counseling or medical support *Emotional:* Necessity of staying away from family and friends who smoke and changing places to "hang out"; giving up other triggers such as coffee and alcohol *Psychological:* Withdrawal symptoms, learning to deal with temporary failures in the process of quitting *Time-related:* Appointments for counseling or medical support; self-analysis, journaling, and planning for change
Place	Where the audience will perform the desired behavior, where they will access the program, products, and services, or where they are thinking about your issue	*Performance of desired behavior:* Changes needed in the home, work, or leisure environments to support the change *Access to program:* Computer-based and social media support *Thinking about the issue:* Effect of environment on desire to continue smoking
Promotion	Communication messages, materials, channels, and activities that will effectively reach your audience	*Messages:* Information that needs to be conveyed *Materials:* Actual health education materials such as a brochure or a blog *Channels:* Media used to communicate messages (e.g., visual, written, or oral) *Activities:* Something the client participates in to receive the health message (e.g., reading a blog, viewing a video, developing an action plan, or attending counseling sessions)

(Modified from Centers for Disease Control and Prevention. Health Marketing Basics. Gateway to Health Communication. Available at: <https://www.cdc.gov/healthcommunication/toolstemplates/Basics.html>; [Accessed October 2020].)

health messages for the public. The concept of **framing health messages** relates to how messages are crafted rather than the content of the messages. Certain cues in a message (e.g., sounds, symbols, words, and pictures) can signal how and what to think about an issue. In the process of framing messages, an attempt is made to connect to people's values, beliefs, knowledge levels, and emotions, and to exclude information they consider irrelevant. In this way, framing brings meaning to a message.

Gain-framing a message is focusing on what is to be gained by adopting the recommended health behavior. *Loss-framing* is the opposite, focusing on the negative effect of an unhealthy behavior.[14] An oral health example of gain-framing is to focus on the benefits of seeking dental treatment (e.g., comfort and appearance), while loss-framing would focus on the pain and loss of teeth that can result from not seeking treatment. Recent research has suggested that the effectiveness of gain- and loss-framed messages differ, depending on the health behavior and anticipated outcome to which they are directed. Gain-framed health messages are more effective when targeting prevention behaviors and when behaviors have a relatively certain outcome.[16] Conversely, loss-framed messages are more effective for screening and treatment messages and when individuals perceive the health issue as highly relevant, the consequences as negative, and the intervention or health behavior as efficacious.[14–16]

Recent research by the FrameWorks Institute shows that the public has limited understanding of oral health issues and does not see a connection to overall health.[17,18] The researchers note the need to better understand more effective ways to elevate and explain oral health as a public concern so that appropriate messages about oral health will "stick" and create more public

awareness and discussion. For example, most people still equate oral health only with teeth, "no cavities," and visiting the dentist rather than as a general health issue that affects the whole mouth and body with identifiable risk factors for multiple preventable conditions and diseases. The Institute's publications listed in the References and Additional Resources at the end of this chapter propose a framing matrix that shows communication strategies and messages to avoid and those to advance when getting the public's or lawmakers' attention.

Targeting the Audience

With a more focused approach, health professionals can *target* materials to reach a specific subgroup or population, usually based on demographic characteristics (e.g., older adults, pregnant women, Latino teens). The assumption that underlies this approach is that enough homogeneity exists in the group to justify the messages and formats used. Subgroups such as frail elders and healthy active seniors, however, often are very heterogeneous, thus reducing the effectiveness of this approach in some situations.[13]

Personalizing Communication

Oral health messages often are packaged as *generic* messages such as, "See your dentist/dental hygienist twice a year" or "Brush twice a day." Such messages are not based on current behavior or individual risk assessment and, therefore, may not be completely relevant or effective. The most effective way to *personalize* information is to highlight only the information and key messages that apply to the person who receives it, based on assessment and risk assessment results.[19] **Tailored health messages** reach a specific person based on features unique to that person, which are discovered through assessment and an understanding of characteristics such as level of health literacy.[20]

Tailoring is the basis of many risk assessment/risk reduction and self-care programs in medicine (e.g., heart disease, diabetes, and osteoporosis) and dentistry (e.g., caries management by risk assessment). The use of personal trainers for health improvement through exercise is an example. Tailored messages provide a more meaningful and motivating strategy built on a person's specific input and needs. Tailoring a message without going through the essential assessment process, however, will result in an ineffective message because it won't be based on the individual's characteristics, gains, or lapses.

Limiting Content of Messages

A common error in health promotion is to use health messages that cover *several concepts* to appeal to the greatest number of people. For example, one brochure might cover brushing, flossing, and the use of fluorides, sealants, antimicrobials, and other preventive measures. It might also describe diagnostic procedures such as radiographs, periodontal probing, and microbial tests. This type of brochure assumes that dental hygienists should provide as much information as possible at one time, and that people will sort through the information to select the pieces that apply to them. Numerous studies have shown that this assumption is invalid.[21] Overwhelming people with information is not an effective strategy for changing behaviors. This is particularly true when people are busy, the information is above their reading level, or only some information is immediately relevant to their needs. Information needs to conform to the three A's: "Accurate, Accessible and Actionable."[21]

Health communication specialists recommend creating "elevator speeches" to practice limiting messages.[22] The goal of this strategy is to convey a concept or topic in a simple, genuine, short, direct, concise, interesting manner. Often used to promote policies or programs, the content should answer the who, what, why and how questions in 30 seconds to 2 minutes (the time it takes some elevators to go between a few floors). The first two sentences are the most important for grabbing attention.

Using Technology

The use of **social media** is increasing. In 2018, 70% of the U.S. population used social media to connect with each other or with the Internet, to share information, or for entertainment, compared with 5% in 2005 and 50% in 2011.[23] Young adults and teens are the most frequent users and early adopters of new programs, but use by older adults has increased in recent years. Users also vary by race/ethnicity, education level, and geographic location. Favored platforms change over time, especially among young adults, so it can be important to verify use by the targeted audience.

Mobile technologies using specific apps or text messaging and social media create unique opportunities for delivering personalized messages.[12] For example, individuals can receive messages that allow them to find where vaccinations or flu shots are being given by entering their zip code. CDC tweets provide updates on which states are most affected during flu season. New parents can sign up to receive messages that include oral health tips for their babies. Emergency management systems can alert us to wildfires or floods and ways to mitigate our risks.

The Internet allows for current information through frequent updates. It also promotes individualization by allowing people to search for and discuss information that applies to their situations, answers their specific questions, or assists them in communicating with their dental team and other healthcare providers. For example, Facebook Groups is a place for health professionals and patients to interact for education, support, or motivational sessions. Short videos on YouTube address many oral health topics.

Selecting and Evaluating Communication Formats for Different Audiences

Consumer-Oriented Communication

Before providing oral health information to an individual or group, an assessment and planning process is crucial (see Chapter 3). Depending on the audience and topic, a needs assessment can be accomplished through a literature review, informal observations or conversations, health literacy assessments, in-depth interviews, or focus groups. A needs assessment reveals important cultural beliefs, health practices, health literacy, and knowledge levels that can result in misconceptions and can serve as barriers, stumbling blocks, or enablers to care, communication, and behavior change.

Health literacy, oral health literacy, and the use of **plain language** are discussed at length in Chapter 10. Communication should also be culturally sensitive and linguistically competent. In other words, language and graphics should be inclusive and not promote stereotypes (see Chapter 10). Special considerations are needed when designing or translating materials for non-English speakers.[24] Box 8.2 lists some problems associated with translating materials and suggestions for

---

BOX 8.2   Language Translation Barriers and Suggestions for Overcoming Them

Problems with Translating Materials

- Medical and dental terms may not be understood, may have different meanings, or may not be directly translatable to another language. Even within languages such as Spanish, people from different nations or regions may use different words for dental terms such as *x-ray* or *baby teeth*.
- Translating word for word (literally) often is confusing because there may be no direct translation or a variety of phrases may be used, depending on the person's age, gender, social standing, or other characteristics. Literal translations without considering local language patterns and word usage may be annoying to the intended audience, causing them to ignore the information or reducing its credibility.
- Some people may speak a language that does not have a written equivalent, or they may speak a language but not be able to read it.

Suggestions for Overcoming Translation Barriers

- Use materials originally developed in that language or have new materials developed in the target languages rather than using a literal translation from English.
- Field test translated materials with a variety of members from the intended audience. Some researchers recommend two-way translation—one person translates the text from English to the other language, and a second person translates it back to English to identify any inconsistencies or mistranslations.
- It is best to use translators who are both bilingual and bicultural.
- Use only trained translators who are familiar with language used by readers who are at different literacy levels.

preventing or overcoming these problems.[24] These should also be considered during any needs assessment and when field-testing materials. Some educational materials are produced in a dual language format so that both English and the other language are included. This can be useful for both print and video productions.

Studies have shown that some types of health education and health promotion programs are more likely to change health outcomes. Intensive disease-management programs appear to reduce disease prevalence and severity, and self-management interventions increase self-management behavior. Effective interventions were those that were of high intensity, had a theory basis, were pilot tested before full implementation, emphasized skill building, and were delivered by a health professional. Interventions that change outcomes such as the use of healthcare services and health outcomes appear to work by increasing knowledge and/or self-efficacy, or by changing behavior.[25]

The planning process. Using findings from a needs assessment (see Chapters 3 and 6), a health promotion/health **communication plan** should be developed before any interventions are started (see Box 8.1). This plan should include objectives; activities; key messages; target audiences; timelines; resources needed and available; responsible parties; and evaluation methods, measures, and anticipated outcomes.[26] Selecting the communication formats, channels, and materials to be used in a program or campaign is part of the planning process. Evaluation measures should be planned with consideration given to the kinds of information needed (see Evaluation Considerations later in this section). Resources to assist with this process are included at the end of the chapter.

A variety of resources are available for dental hygienists to use when selecting communication formats and channels and designing and evaluating health messages. Examples of formats for presenting information to the public are included in

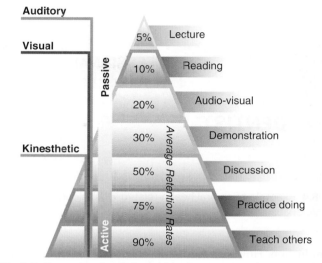

Fig 8.3 Example of an infographic that communicates retention rates of various learning formats and recommended formats based on learnings styles. (From Education Corner. The Learning Pyramid; 2019. Available at: <https://www.educationcorner.com/the-learning-pyramid.html>; [Accessed December 2019].)

Table 8.10, along with some of their uses and limitations. Using *infographics* is a way to pair words with graphics (Figure 8.3), with the intention of making health communication more understandable. However, their overuse and overcrowding or use of vague or complex graphics, especially when using small size font, can be confusing or misleading.

Word clouds (Figure 8.4) are becoming trendy and can be quickly generated by breaking text into component words and counting how frequently they appear in the text or as responses to a question.[27] Then different font sizes, styles, and colors are used to create a visual "cloud" based on the frequency of specific words, with more frequent words displayed larger. Colorful and drawing one's attention, word clouds are useful as an

TABLE 8.10	Uses and Limitations of Various Health Communication Formats for the Public	
Category and Examples	**Uses**	**Limitations**
Visual displays: posters, bulletin boards, information kiosks, billboards	Combines graphics and written information; best in public places to highlight key messages; most useful to bring issues to audience's attention	Requires legwork to post; has to be eye-catching; may not reach target population; not as effective as other formats to change behavior
Written media: newsletters, newspaper articles, fact sheets, booklets, fotonovelas, blogs, storybooks, pamphlets	Can include multiple messages in multiple languages; covers topic in more depth; tells a story; can be tailored to different ages/groups	Increases knowledge but may not change behaviors; graphics needed for low literacy readers; may not reach target audience
Audiovisual materials: CDs and DVDs, public service announcements, websites, TV, streaming video	Taps into audio and visual learning paths; can use champions or celebrities; can be tailored to specific audiences and ages; may help with adoption of new behaviors	Some expensive to produce; need to market for purchase or viewing; may not reach target audience; technology may not be available or have glitches; discussion or some other interaction is needed to improve potential for behavior change
Interactive formats: songs, role-playing, storytelling, gaming, theater or puppet shows, demonstrations, interactive computer programs, science experiments or science fairs, debates, simulations, text messages, other social media	Uses multiple learning pathways to increase understanding, retention, and behavior change; allows interaction/participation; can share different perspectives; can adapt for different audiences	Some can be expensive to produce and require human resources for interaction; need to match format to target audience and be culturally and linguistically appropriate

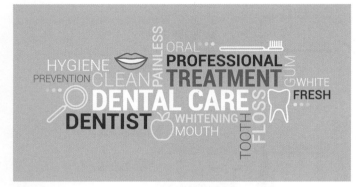

Fig 8.4 Example of an oral health-related word cloud. (@ iStock.com/elenabs.)

introduction. However, they tend to be overused, convey little useful information, and can be confusing, disorienting, and meaningless.[27]

Retention rates vary according to the format or method of communicating information as depicted in the Learning Pyramid or Cone of Learning in Figure 8.3.[28] Although studies have debunked the percentages, educators promote the application of this progression to the selection of formats, depending on the population group, setting, and other factors, and

suggest that using a variety of learning methods will lead to deeper learning and longer-term retention.[28,29] Each person has a preferred learning style (see Figure 8.3) and type of intelligence (see Box 8.3).[28,29] **Learning styles** describe how we learn or approach learning tasks, whereas **multiple intelligences** represent different intellectual abilities. Both are important in that they affect learning. The most effective format for learning depends on the individual's learning style and type of intelligence.[28,29] Assessing these characteristics before designing messages makes it easier to plan messages to reach a group of people with diverse learning styles and multiple intelligences.

Using a variety of formats can accommodate for an audience's differences in learning styles and multiple intelligences.[28,29] In addition, hands-on and interactive multimedia formats can account for these differences in a group and are usually more effective for retaining knowledge than simply reading or listening to a message.[29] This is true for other health professionals as well as the general public. Finally, research indicates that the use of multiple strategies has a greater effect on improved health literacy and increased use of healthcare services.[25]

Using **focus groups** is one effective way to determine, before launching a program, whether messages are at the appropriate language and literacy level, are culturally acceptable, have a pleasing appearance, and appeal to the people in

---

BOX 8.3   Multiple Intelligences and Instructional Techniques Related to Learning

Multiple Intelligences

All individuals have multiple intelligences that affect how they learn. Each person possesses each intelligence to an extent, but there is always a primary, or more dominant, intelligence.

Verbal-Linguistic Intelligence: Well-developed verbal skills and sensitivity to the sounds, meanings and rhythms of words.

Mathematical-Logical Intelligence: The ability to think conceptually and abstractly, and the capacity to discern logical or numerical patterns.

Musical Intelligence: The ability to produce and appreciate rhythm, pitch and timbre.

Visual-Spatial Intelligence: The capacity to think in images and pictures, to visualize accurately and abstractly.

Bodily-Kinesthetic Intelligence: The ability to control one's body movements and to handle objects skillfully.

Interpersonal Intelligence: The capacity to detect and respond appropriately to the moods, motivations and desires of others.

Intrapersonal Intelligence: The capacity to be self-aware and in tune with inner feelings, values, beliefs and thinking processes.

Naturalist Intelligence: The ability to recognize and categorize plants, animals and other objects in nature.

Existential Intelligence: The sensitivity and capacity to tackle deep questions about human existence, such as the meaning of life, why we die and how we got here.

Modes of Multimedia and Instructional Techniques

To engage the varied intelligences, use of a variety of modes of multimedia and instruction techniques is more effective for all learners.

Visuals: Use visuals to help learner acquire concrete concepts, such as object identification, spatial relationship, or motor skills.

Printed words: Although the printed word is the most common method used to dispense information, use audio as some argue that it is superior.

Sound: Use sound media as a stimulus for sound recognition or recall. Audio narration is useful for learners who struggle with reading.

Motion: Use motion to depict human performance so learners can copy the movement.

Color: Provide color choices that match what is being learned (e.g., the sky is blue).

Realia: Teach cognitive and motor skills by using objects and material form everyday life as teaching aids.

Instructional Setting: Design the instructional setting based on teaching materials being used, the environment, and use of individualized printed materials to allow the learner to set the pace.

Learner Characteristics: Select teaching models that consider learner characteristics.

Reading ability: Use pictures to aid learning with poor readers who understand spoken words rather than printed words.

Categories of Learning Outcomes: Develop learning outcome that align with learning categories: intellectual skills, motor skills, verbal information, overall attitudes, and use of cognitive strategies.

Events of Instruction: During planning and before selecting appropriate media, select external events that support internal learning and instructional event.

Performance: Provide opportunity for learner to perform tasks that demonstrate learning and retention and select media that corresponds with the desired performance of task.

(Modified from Herndon E. What Are Multiple Intelligences and How Do They Affect Learning? Cornerstone University; February 6, 2018. Available at: <https://www.cornerstone.edu/blogs/lifelong-learning-matters/post/what-are-multiple-intelligences-and-how-do-they-affect-learning>; [Accessed February 16, 2020]; Gardner H. Frames of Mind. New York, NY: Basic Books; 2011.]

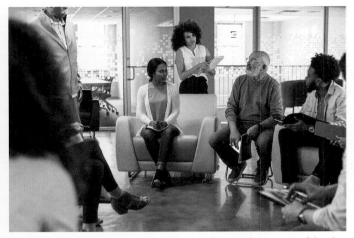

Fig 8.5 A moderator uses structured questions to guide the discussion in a focus group. (© iStock.com/SDI Productions.)

the group.[30] Group interviews, 30–60 minutes in length, are conducted with 5–10 members of the intended target audience in each group. A moderator guides the group discussion with structured questions (see Figure 8.5). When developing or testing health messages or materials, the moderator can use one or more versions of the materials to ask questions. For example, in field-testing a media campaign about dental sealants, you might ask the following:

- What is one message you remember from the campaign?
- Were there any messages that were confusing?
- Which materials were most informative? Motivational? Attractive? Appealing?
- Did you relate to the people in the photographs? How were they like you? Different from you?
- Were the campaign messages too short, just right, or too long?
- Should the campaign include more resources for those who want more information on dental sealants?
- Would this campaign motivate you to ask about dental sealants for your child's teeth?

The focus group participants' responses are summarized and analyzed to help make decisions on final content and format of the campaign materials before release to the public.

Evaluation considerations. Evaluation of communication formats, channels, and materials is critical to document that they are working (see Box 8.1).[31] This is not only a best practice but also necessary to assure program sustainability. Evaluation can occur both during and after educational interventions (formative and summative evaluation, respectively). The evaluation methods should be linked directly to the objectives, and both short-term and long-term outcomes should be considered. See Guiding Principles for some sample questions to be answered by the evaluation. Measures can be quantitative (e.g., how many people increased their knowledge of the causes of early childhood caries and how much increase in knowledge occurred) or qualitative (e.g., why people participated in the activity and how they intend to change their parenting behaviors). See Chapter 6 for a detailed discussion of program evaluation.

Evaluation plans do not always have to be complicated or use sophisticated statistical analysis. The key is to plan how to evaluate your efforts before executing a health promotion or health communication intervention and then document the outcomes of the evaluation. It is important to document intended outcomes and impact, as well as barriers to success, lessons learned, and unintended outcomes.[31] See Box 8.4 for examples of simple evaluation strategies.

Presentations to Health Professionals

The purpose of most professional presentations is to deliver thought-provoking information to a group of health professionals in a short period of time in a clear, concise, and appealing format that will be educational and promote discussion. Presentations often focus on new research or programs, emerging issues, clinical techniques, products or materials, career opportunities, educational techniques, policies or legislation, healthcare systems, or methods for disease prevention or detection. Information should cover a specific topic with key messages highlighted and sources documented. Presentations can be made to small groups, to large groups at conferences, or via webinars, podcasts, or other online learning formats.

The same principles and processes that apply to communicating with the general public also apply to communicating with health professionals. While direct needs assessment of the audience may not be possible before a presentation, acquiring some background information from the organizers or at the beginning of the presentation can help with tailoring information to the audience.

This section provides general information about four common types of professional presentations, although specific guidelines for presentations may vary by the sponsoring organization. Additional information on professional presentations is available in the online resources at the end of this chapter. Specific questions should be considered when selecting a topic and a format for a presentation (see Guiding Principles).

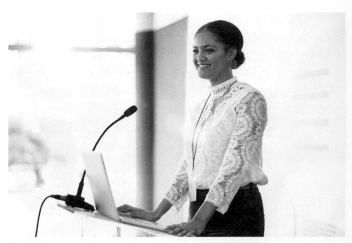

Fig 8.7 Presentation of an oral paper at a conference. (© iStock.com/Mikolette.)

GUIDING PRINCIPLES

Questions to Answer When Selecting a Topic and Format for a Professional Presentation

- Who will be the audience? How large will the group be?
- What is the audience's level of knowledge or interest in my topic?
- What level of interaction will I have or do I want with the audience?
- What questions might they ask? What questions can I ask to learn new information related to my topic from some members of the audience?
- How much time will I need to cover my key points?
- What audiovisual materials will most enhance my key points?

Professional presentations typically are organized around a similar flow or order. Regardless of the type of presentation, most are based on the following basic outline:

1. Introduction and background of the topic/project/presentation
2. Methods and materials, research or intervention strategies, and evaluation questions
3. Findings/results and key points
4. Discussion and significance
5. Summary and conclusions

Presentation of a poster display. The **poster** presentation display format (Figure 8.6) is popular because several presentations can be accommodated in a short time frame and no audiovisual equipment is needed.

Time: Session lasting 1 to 2 hours; each poster presentation lasting 5 to 10 minutes, depending on criteria of organization hosting the event

Format: Presenter discusses visual display with people who stop to look; posters lined up next to each other; poster usually attached by pushpins or a temporary adhesive to a display board

Size of audience: Varies greatly; some people "cruise by" quickly, some just pick up handouts, and others stop to read display and discuss topic

Appropriate audiovisuals: Text, data, artwork, or photographs usually printed as one large banner; audio or video applications not allowed; handouts encouraged

Benefits and limitations: Opportunity to discuss topic with individuals, share ideas, and acquire additional ideas; unpredictable attendance (sometimes crowded and noisy but at other times attendance is sparse); not appropriate for topics that require videos or other types of media

Tips: Use color and photographs to attract attention and highlight key points; use large, readable print and catchy title; intersperse categories of information with charts, graphics, and photographs, allowing enough white space to assure readability; consider setup logistics and transport; include copy of abstract, which is usually printed in the meeting program

Presentation of an oral paper or panel discussion. The **oral paper** format (Figure 8.7) usually is part of a session or a panel with a theme.

Time: Usually 10 to 15 minutes per paper, including time for questions; a panel may be one or more hours

Format: Oral presentation of information using notes and accompanied by audiovisuals

Size of audience: Usually more than 30 people but suitable for hundreds of people, especially if part of a satellite session broadcast to many sites

Appropriate audiovisuals: PowerPoint slides, short videos, other computerized applications; wireless Internet connectivity may be available

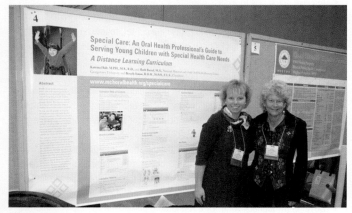

Fig 8.6 Format for a poster presentation. (Courtesy Beverly Isman.)

Benefits and limitations: Large group can be reached; presenter can speak from printed notes or directly from slide notes on computer usually standing behind a podium with a microphone; room lighting sometimes fairly dark so presenter cannot see notes or audience; no place to put notes on podium; interaction with audience often limited, except responding to questions; varying degrees of knowledge about topic in audience

Tips: Try to maintain some eye contact and do not simply read from your papers or slides; use uncomplicated and effective audiovisual materials that highlight important information rather than detract from or repeat information you give orally; practice delivery, timing, and use of audiovisuals before the presentation; decide what information to delete if you are running over the time allowance; include transitions between sentences and sections; upload your presentation per the sponsor's directions and check computer controls, placement for notes, room environment/lighting, and availability/reliability of Internet connectivity before your session

Presentation as a roundtable discussion. The **roundtable discussion** format (Figure 8.8) is gaining in popularity for a more informal presentation.

Time: 30 to 60 minutes; presentation sometimes repeated to a new group if session is longer and participants can select two topics

Format: Oral presentation and discussion supplemented by limited audiovisuals to people seated at a table or in a circle

Size of audience: Usually 8 to 10 people

Appropriate audiovisuals: Handouts, materials, or products; can use laptops with video application but not usually audio; Internet connectivity may be too expensive unless free wireless is available

Benefits and limitations: Format promotes interactive discussion with presenter serving more as a facilitator; participants can introduce themselves and share information with the whole table; good for controversial topics or new ideas and programs; limited number of people hear the topic; too many tables close together makes hearing the information difficult

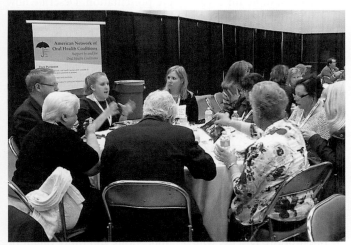

Fig 8.8 Roundtable discussion. (Courtesy Beverly Isman.)

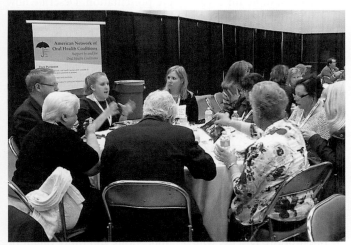

Fig 8.9 Web-based presentation. (Courtesy Charlene Dickinson.)

Tips: Speak from notes, handouts, or laptop; facilitation skills and ability to refocus discussion is important if discussion is off-track or is monopolized by an individual

Web-based presentation. A **web-based presentation**, also called a webinar or webcast (Figure 8.9), has become a preferred means of presenting material to selected groups of professionals because no travel costs or additional time are involved, and the presentation can be recorded for future viewing. Participants can connect to audio via computer or phone.

Time: Most last 30 to 60 minutes, depending on how many people are presenting the webinar

Format: Can do live video streaming or use prepared slides with live audio; many options for audience interaction via live chats, polling and evaluation questions, and unmuting audio lines; can also record and save to a website for later viewing

Size of audience: Depends on online package being used; some limited to 100 phone lines although others are unlimited

Appropriate audiovisuals: Videos, slides, and personal demonstrations if using video

Benefits and limitations: Can reach large audience with various levels of two-way interaction; if using live video, can see presenter and sometimes audience if they are gathered in a room with a video camera or have cameras on their computers; can download slides before or after presentation; can provide links to online resources; unintended noise or line interference has been a major problem especially if audience lines are not muted

Tips: Schedule a practice run before the presentation to assure you are familiar with navigating the web interface; reduce any sources of noise during your presentation

Audience evaluation of a professional presentation. The effectiveness of professional presentations can be assessed through the use of course and conference evaluation forms completed onsite or online by attendees or by asking the audience directly for some immediate feedback. Evaluation measures usually address the presenter's organization and clarity of information, effective use of audiovisuals, accuracy and relevancy of content, relation of theory to practice, knowledge of subject area, introduction of new information and ideas, and presentation style. In addition, questions can be asked about applicability to an individual's work, intent to use or share the information, and interest in future presentations or sharing resources on the topic.

RESOURCES FOR PROFESSIONAL DEVELOPMENT

Multiple avenues are available to dental hygiene students and practitioners to develop skills in health promotion and health communication. Chapter 7 outlines the importance of continual review of the scientific literature to keep abreast of new research and trends in dental hygiene and public health research and practice. Because public health covers such a broad array of topics, dental hygienists would benefit by reading literature from other subject areas such as injury prevention, cancer prevention and early detection, maternal and child health, geriatrics, and school health to gain different perspectives on health promotion and health communication. The many Internet sites and social media postings devoted to health topics facilitate quick perusal and acquisition of information on any topic. Self-study continuing education courses, podcasts or webinars are now more available and affordable or free. Useful online resources on health promotion and health communication are listed in the References and Additional Resources at the end of this chapter.

Another avenue for updating knowledge, practicing presentation skills, and **networking** with other professionals is attending professional association meetings. Many of these organizations promote student involvement through reduced membership rates, free or reduced registration fees, and special contests and awards. Dental hygienists' horizons also are broadened by attending general public health or health communication meetings. The CDC and other groups sponsor annual learning institutes and conferences on topics such as health literacy, health communication, and evaluation. The annual National Oral Health Conference, sponsored by the Association of State and Territorial Dental Directors and the American Association of Public Health Dentistry, offers the type of presentations and learning opportunities discussed in this chapter on a wide range of public health topics of current significance to all oral health practitioners.

SUMMARY

We live in a multicultural, global society in which some people are bombarded with health information and others are isolated from scientific advances, new communication technologies, and current health information. To create a more equitable distribution of resources and information, dental hygienists must broaden their perspectives on how to acquire and provide health information in a credible, appropriate, efficient, and effective manner. Ways to accomplish this include (1) applying well-researched health promotion and communication theories to oral health programs, (2) assessing people's learning styles, preferences, information needs, and other characteristics to be able to frame and tailor health communications, (3) delivering health communication using plain language in a culturally and linguistically appropriate manner based on needs assessment data, (4) selecting appropriate communication channels and strategies for the target audiences, and (5) evaluating the outcomes and impact of the interventions, activities, and teaching materials used.

Endless opportunities exist for using new communication modalities in a variety of settings outside a clinical private practice setting. Online courses, professional associations, and a variety of conferences can be valuable resources for preparing dental hygienists to meet today's health promotion and health communication challenges.

APPLYING YOUR KNOWLEDGE

1. Work in groups to design role-playing scenarios based on the types of behaviors described in the health promotion theories. You might use actual family or personal situations/behaviors and brainstorm how to change the behaviors using the theories.

2. Choose a topic, audience, and three key messages for designing a handout. Describe how you would vary the design and tailor the messages for three additional audiences based on different ethnicity, age, or other factors. Using the same audiences, describe how you would adapt the messages for four different communication channels, for example, tweets, YouTube videos, or blogs.

3. Choose an oral health topic for designing a health promotion activity for consumers. Each student should select a different audience (e.g., different age or ethnic group) for the materials. Then (a) describe how you would conduct a needs assessment, (b) select an appropriate educational format, and (c) evaluate the outcomes of your approach.

4. Choose a topic for a 10-minute presentation. Describe how you would present this topic as (a) a scientific poster, (b) an oral paper, (c) a roundtable discussion, and (d) a web-based presentation.

5. Review calls for abstracts/presentation proposals and agendas of annual meetings from various professional associations. Include at least one dental-related group, one public health group, and one health promotion or communication group. Compare the organizations for similarities and differences in topics and formats, including the potential for student presentations.

6. Select three online or print journals that focus on health promotion or health communications research or programs. Compare the journals in terms of target audience, array of topics, whether they are peer reviewed, and frequency of publication. Discuss which publications you think might be most useful to you in your career.

LEARNING OBJECTIVES AND COMPETENCIES

This chapter addresses the following community dental health learning objectives and competencies for dental hygienists that are presented in the *ADEA Compendium of Curriculum Guidelines for Allied Dental Education Programs*:

Learning Objectives
- Describe health education and promotion principles.
- Outline the different learning and motivation theories.
- Describe how a dental hygienist could best educate a target population.

Competencies
- Providing health education and preventive counseling to a variety of population groups.

- Promoting the values of good oral and general health and wellness to the public and organizations within and outside of the professions.
- Assessing, planning, implementing and evaluating community-based oral health programs.
- Recognizing and using written and electronic sources of information.
- Recognizing the responsibility and demonstrating the ability to communicate professional knowledge verbally and in writing

COMMUNITY CASE

You are a dental hygienist who has been working in clinical private practice for 3 years and now wants to work part-time in a public health setting. The local health department has hired you to work on a project to help mothers of children ages 0 to 5 years learn about: (1) the relationship between consumption of sugar, including sweetened beverages, and dental caries, (2) how to determine the amount and type of sugar from food labels, (3) how to select foods low in refined sugars, and (4) how to use these foods to create healthy snacks for their young children. Your target population is approximately 2000 low-income women whose children are eligible for Medicaid benefits and services from the Women, Infants, and Children (WIC) program, and whose children attend Early Head Start or Head Start programs. According to the most recent health department data, 50% of the women are Hispanic, 10% are Caucasian, 25% are African American, 10% are Asian, and 5% are of other ethnic backgrounds.

1. Your first task is to review the various health promotion theories and determine which would be useful for this project. You decide that you need to assess whether the women in the target population perceive that their children are consuming foods high in sugars and, if so, whether the mothers perceive that it puts them at risk for dental caries. Which one of the following theories is best to use for this purpose?
   a. Social Learning Theory
   b. Stages of Change Theory
   c. Health Belief Model
   d. Organizational Change Theory

2. Your next task is to select and tailor health messages you want to include in your health communication approaches. Which one of the following approaches is an example of tailoring a message?
   a. Use separate brochures for each ethnic group.
   b. Develop learning modules that focus on the women's roles as mothers.

   c. Design short learning modules geared to each level of caries risk identified during the assessment process.
   d. Use a short booklet that leaves a blank place in which to write the child's name.

3. All of the following EXCEPT one are useful strategies to help the target population learn the information. Which is the EXCEPTION?
   a. Ask them to demonstrate a skill to help reinforce the written instructions.
   b. Have them read rather than hear and see the information; they will learn more from reading it.
   c. Ask them to repeat instructions in their own words to help them remember the information.
   d. Use a hands-on, interactive, multimedia approach.

4. You decide that the project materials need to be available in at least English and Spanish. Which of the following approaches is LEAST likely to result in effective and culturally relevant materials?
   a. Use translators who are bilingual and bicultural.
   b. Test the materials in three focus groups: (1) English-only readers, (2) Spanish-only readers, and (3) partially bilingual readers.
   c. Do a literal translation from the English version to Spanish.
   d. Create the materials in dual language format.

5. During the project you have an opportunity to present information on the project at a statewide public health association meeting. You are most interested in discussing and getting feedback on ways to improve the materials and messages. Which presentation format would allow you the best opportunity to accomplish this?
   a. Roundtable discussion
   b. Poster presentation
   c. Oral presentation
   d. Informal networking with individuals

REFERENCES

1. World Health Organization. The Ottawa Charter for Health Promotion. Available at: <https://www.who.int/healthpromotion/conferences/previous/ottawa/en/>; [Accessed November 2019].
2. World Health Organization. What is Health Promotion. Available at: <https://www.who.int/healthpromotion/fact-sheet/en/>; [Accessed November 2019].
3. Centers for Disease Control and Prevention. Health Equity. August 28, 2019. Available at: <http://www.cdc.gov/chronicdisease/healthequity/index.htm>; [Accessed September 2019].
4. Watt RG, Sheiham A. Integrating the common risk factor approach into a social determinants framework. Community Dent Oral Epidemiol 2012;40(4):289–96. Abstract available at: <https://onlinelibrary.wiley.com/doi/abs/10.1111/j.1600-0528.2012.00680.x>; [Accessed September 2019].
5. Kumar CS, Somasundara SY. Common Risk Factor Approach: Finding Common Ground for Better Health Outcomes. Int J Contemp Med Res 2017;4(6):1367–70. Available at: <https://www.ijcmr.com/uploads/7/7/4/6/77464738/1524_jul_18.pdf>; [Accessed February 2020].
6. Glanz K, Rimer BK, Viswanath K. Health Behavior and Health Education. 5th ed. San Francisco, CA: Jossey-Bass; 2015.
7. American College Health Association. Healthy Campus. Ecological Model. Available at: <https://www.acha.org/HealthyCampus/HealthyCampus/Ecological_Model.aspx>; [Accessed November 2019].
8. McKenzie JF, Neiger BL, Thackeray R. Planning, Implementing & Evaluating Health Promotion Programs: A Primer. 7th ed. Glenview, IL: Pearson Education, Inc; 2017.
9. Baras D, Duff C, Smith BJ. Organizational change theory: implications for health promotion practice. Health Promot Int 2016, March;31(1):231–41. Available at: <https://academic.oup.com/heapro/article/31/1/231/2355918>; [Accessed October 2019].
10. The Community Guide. Available at: <https://www.thecommunityguide.org/topic/health-communication-and-health-information-technology>; [Accessed October 2020].
11. Healthy People 2020. Available at: <https://www.healthypeople.gov/2020>; [Accessed September 2019].
12. National Center for Health Statistics. Healthy People 2020 Midcourse Review; June 5, 2018. Available at: <https://www.cdc.gov/nchs/healthy_people/hp2020/hp2020_midcourse_review.htm>; [Accessed October 2020].
13. Centers for Disease Control and Prevention. Health Communication Basics. Available at: <https://www.cdc.gov/healthcommunication/healthbasics/index.html>; [Accessed October 2020].
14. Toll BA, O'Malley SS, Katulak NA, et al. Comparing Gain- and Loss-Framed Messages for Smoking Cessation with Sustained-Release Bupropion: A Randomized Controlled Trial. Psychol Addict Behav 2007;21(4):534–44. doi:10.1037/0893-164X.21.4.534. Available at: <https://www.ncbi.nlm.nih.gov/pmc/articles/PMC2527727/>; [Accessed February 2020].
15. Akl EA, Oxman AD, Herrin J, et al. Framing of Health Information Messages. Cochrane Database of Systematic Reviews; 2011, December 7. Abstract available at: <https://www.cochranelibrary.com/cdsr/doi/10.1002/14651858.CD006777.pub2/full>; [Accessed February 2020].
16. Bosone L, Martinez F. When, How, and Why is Loss-Framing More Effective than Gain- and Non-Gain-Framing in the Promotion of Detection Behaviors? Int Rev Soc Psychol 2017;30(1):184-192. Available at: <https://www.rips-irsp.com/articles/10.5334/irsp.15/>; [Accessed October 2020].
17. FrameWorks Institute. Unlocking the Door to New Thinking: Frames for Advancing Oral Health Reform; 2017. Available at: <https://frameworksinstitute.org/assets/files/PDF_oralhealth/oral_health_messagememo_may_2017.pdf>; [Accessed September 2019].
18. FrameWorks Institute. Getting Stories to Stick: The Shape of Public Discourse on Oral Health; 2017. Available at: <https://www.frameworksinstitute.org/assets/files/PDF_oralhealth/dentaquest_mcffa_final_2017.pdf>; [Accessed September 2019].
19. Hiligsmann M, Ronda G, van der Weijden T, Boonen A. The development of a personalized patient education tool for decision making for postmenopausal women with osteoporosis. Osteoporos Int 2016;27:2489–96. Available at: <https://www.ncbi.nlm.nih.gov/pmc/articles/PMC4947108/>; [Accessed February 2020].
20. Schapira MM, Swartz S, Ganschow PS, et al. Tailoring Educational and Behavioral Interventions to Level of Health Literacy: A Systematic Review. MDM P&P 2017, June 15;2(1). :2381468317714474(e). Available at: <https://journals.sagepub.com/doi/full/10.1177/2381468317714474>;[Accessed February 2020].
21. Centers for Disease Control and Prevention. Health Literacy: Develop & Test Materials; October 17, 2019. Available at: <https://www.cdc.gov/healthliteracy/developmaterials/index.html>; [Accessed December 2019].
22. Elevator Pitches for Scientists; 2013. Available at: <https://medschool.vanderbilt.edu/wp-content/uploads/sites/9/files/public_files/Elevator%20Pitches%20for%20Scientists_Uyen_0.pdf>; [Accessed September 2019].
23. Pew Research Center. Social Media Fact Sheet; 2019. Available at: <https://www.pewinternet.org/fact-sheet/social-media/>; [Accessed September 2019].
24. Nápoles AM, Santoyo-Olsson J, Stewart AL. Methods for Translating Evidence-Based Behavioral Interventions for Health-Disparity Communities. Prev Chronic Dis 2013, November 21;e. Available at: <http://dx.doi.org/10.5888/pcd10.130133>; [Accessed December 2019].
25. Berkman ND, Sheridan SL, Donahue KE, et al. Health Literacy Interventions and Outcomes: An Updated Systematic Review. Evidence Report/Technology Assessment No. 199. Prepared by RTI International–University of North Carolina Evidence-Based Practice Center under contract No. 290-2007-10056-I. AHRQ Publication Number 11-E006. Rockville, MD: Agency for Healthcare Research and Quality; 2011. Available at: <http://archive.ahrq.gov/research/findings/evidence-based-reports/literacyup-evidence-report.pdf>; [Accessed December 2019].
26. Community Tool Box. Chapter 6, Section 1. Developing a Plan for Communication; 2019. Available at: <http://ctb.ku.edu/en/table-of-contents/participation/promoting-interest/communication-plan/main>; [Accessed December 2019].
27. Temple S. Word clouds are lame; 2019. Available at: <https://towardsdatascience.com/word-clouds-are-lame-263d9cbc49b7>; [Accessed October 2020].
28. Education Corner. The Learning Pyramid; 2019. Available at: <https://www.educationcorner.com/the-learning-pyramid.html>; [Accessed December 2019].
29. Herndon E. What Are Multiple Intelligences and How Do They Affect Learning? Cornerstone University; February 6, 2018. Available at: <https://www.cornerstone.edu/blogs/lifelong-learning-matters/post/what-are-multiple-intelligences-and-how-do-they-affect-learning>; [Accessed February 2020].
30. Community Tool Box. Chapter 3, Section 6. Conducting Focus Groups; 2019. Available at: <http://ctb.ku.edu/en/table-of-contents/assessment/assessing-community-needs-and-resources/conduct-focus-groups/main>; [Accessed December 2019].
31. National Cancer Institute. Making Health Communication Programs Work. Available at: <https://www.cancer.gov/publications/health-communication/pink-book.pdf>; [Accessed December 2019].

ADDITIONAL RESOURCES

American Evaluation Association: Guidelines for Roundtable
Presentations
www.eval.org/p/cm/ld/fid=171

American Marketing Association and ReadyTalk: Best Practices for
Webinar Planning and Execution
https://www.readytalk.com/sites/default/files/docs/support-training/
ReadyTalk_and_AMA_Webinar_Best_Practices.pdf

Association of State and Territorial Dental Directors: Communication
Plan Template for a Goal-Specific Project or Document and Year at
a Glance Template
https://www.astdd.org/docs/communication-plan-template-for-
a-goal-specific-project-or-document-and-year-at-a-glance-
template-april-2018.docx

Centers for Disease Control and Prevention: CDC Clear
Communication Index
https://www.cdc.gov/ccindex/index.html

FrameWorks Institute: Reframing Oral Health: A Communications
Toolkit for Advancing Oral Health Reform
https://www.frameworksinstitute.org/toolkits/oralhealth/

National Maternal and Child Oral Health Resource Center.: A Way
with Words: Guidelines for Writing Oral Health Materials for
Audiences with Limited Literacy
http://www.mchoralhealth.org/PDFs/AWayWithWords.pdf

Public Health Ontario: Partners for Health: At a Glance: The Six Steps
for Planning a Health Promotion Program
http://www.publichealthontario.ca/en/eRepository/Six_steps_
planning_health_promotion_programs_2015.pdf

Public Health Ontario: Partners for Health: At a Glance: The Twelve
Steps to Developing a Health Communication Campaign
http://www.publichealthontario.ca/en/eRepository/Twelve_steps_
developing_health_communication_campaign_2012.pdf

Purrington C: Designing Conference Posters
www.swarthmore.edu/NatSci/cpurrin1/posteradvice.htm

Radel J: Oral Presentations
http://people.eku.edu/ritchisong/oralpers.html

World Helath Organization: WHO Strategic Communications
Framework for Effective Communications
https://www.who.int/mediacentre/communication-framework.pdf

BOOK

Gagliardi L. Dental Health Education: Lesson Planning and
Implementation. 3rd ed. Long Grove, IL: Waveland Press; 2021

9

Social Responsibility

Sharon C. Stull

OBJECTIVES

1. Discuss why healthcare systems are in crisis domestically and globally.
2. Relate social responsibility and professional ethics to each other and to community oral health practice.
3. Discuss the various opinions surrounding healthcare access as a right or a privilege.
4. Discuss the government's role in healthcare delivery in the United States (U.S.).
5. Discuss the dental hygienist's professional responsibility related to leadership, advocacy, policy development, access-to-care and workforce issues, patient responsibility for health actions oral health promotion, and risk communication.
6. Facilitate patient confidentiality and patient responsibility in accordance with applicable legislation, methods of communication, and ethical codes.
7. Identify the roles of governmental organizations, nongovernmental organizations, and healthcare professionals as they operate within a community in relation to policy development and advocacy to strengthen the oral healthcare delivery system.
8. Discuss the functionality of an interprofessional oral health workforce model; provide leadership in interprofessional collaboration.
9. Describe the responsible use of social media in the provision of oral health care.

OPENING STATEMENTS: Status and Future of Health Care

- The healthcare system in the U.S. is in crisis.
- The public health system in the U.S. is fragmented and insufficient.
- Oral health is a component of overall health, and access to all healthcare services should be considered to promote the general welfare of society.
- Human rights should be the foundation of public health practice, research, and policy.
- Leadership involves social and civic responsibility, professionalism, and communication.
- Comprehensive oral health benefits were excluded for most adults in the Patient Protection and Affordable Care Act of 2010, commonly referred to as the Affordable Care Act (ACA).

A SYSTEM IN CRISIS

The Preamble of *The Constitution of the United States of America* states that one of the reasons for creating the Constitution was to "promote the general Welfare."[1] Society faces a crisis of substantial inequality in the distribution of healthcare and oral healthcare services despite stated goals to reduce poverty and establish viable common-ground solutions. Also, it is apparent the healthcare crisis has been recognized, reported, discussed, and debated for more than 50 years.

The *2000 Surgeon General's Report on Oral Health* quantified the disparities in oral health status among underserved populations and the barriers many people face in obtaining care.[2] The limited capacity of the oral health professions at national and state levels, including private- and public-delivery systems, coupled with public apathy and a general lack of social responsibility of society as a whole, have contributed to the failure of making oral health care accessible to everyone. Health reforms have been recommended for several decades with little success, and, in most cases, oral healthcare services have been curiously excluded until the passage of the **Patient Protection and Affordable Care Act** (ACA) in 2010.

Poverty, at various levels, impacts access to those citizen's fundamental right to oral health care. Although there is no universal definition of **poverty**, the World Health Organization (WHO) recognizes the crisis of poverty and health: Poverty is associated with the undermining of a range of key human attributes including health. Morbidity and mortality rates are significantly higher in low-income countries compared with middle- and high-income countries.[3] The poor are exposed to more health risks and illness, which can reduce productivity, thus perpetuating or increasing poverty. In general, the lower an individual's socioeconomic status (SES) is, the worse is their health.

In 2017, 39.7 million (12.3%) Americans were living below the **federal poverty level** (FPL); this is a slight and insignificant decrease from the previous year and the third decrease since 2014.[4] Of greater significance is a study measuring "economic insecurity" which found that 79% of people in the U.S. live in danger of poverty or unemployment at some point in their lifetime. In this case, poverty is defined as a year or more of periodic joblessness, reliance on government aid such as food stamps, or income below 150% of the FPL.[4]

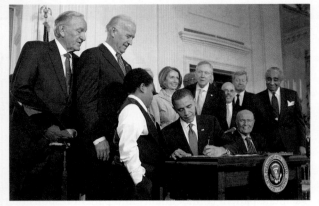

Fig 9.1 President Obama signing the Affordable Care Act on March 23, 2010. (Source: Pete Souza/Wikimedia Commons/Public Domain.)

Since the passage of the ACA in 2010 (Figure 9.1), more recent data (2019) indicates that 35 states and the District of Columbia have adopted the ACA, thereby expanding coverage of Medicaid to millions of previously uninsured individuals and decreasing the uninsured rate from 18% in 2013 to 10% in 2016.[5] The expansion of eligibility for Medicaid to people with incomes up to 138% of the FPL is the largest such expansion since the inception of the program in 1965.[5] However, in 2017 and 2018 the rate of uninsured increased slightly with 10.4% uninsured Americans in 2018.[6] The major contributing factor is reported to be the cost of coverage.[6]

Debate about providing universal health care to U.S. citizens has continued even after the passage of the ACA. In 2017, the 115th U.S. Congress considered several ACA repeal bills. Although all these bills were defeated by the Senate,[7] their introduction and passage by the House reflects a continuing problem with healthcare coverage in the U.S.

While the ACA remains law, certain aspects of it have been altered such as repealing the individual mandate by a presidential executive order in December 2017 through the Tax Cuts and Job Act of 2017.[8] As a consequence, only 9.2 million individuals signed up in the healthcare national exchange, which was a considerable decrease of 400,000 individuals of those seen in 2016.[8] A society that accepts the responsibility to care for the welfare of others should expect the government to establish strong **social justice** policies that answer the access-to-healthcare issues. Furthermore, a government that expects equality and fairness among citizens has a responsibility for the health of its citizens through adequate health and social initiatives.

SOCIAL RESPONSIBILITY AND PROFESSIONAL ETHICS

What should be our social responsibility as concerned citizens and ethical oral healthcare professionals? It is imperative to have licensed dental hygienists included in social justice initiatives and **advocacy** that address the general and oral health crisis in America.

Social Responsibility

Frequently, dental hygiene students ask questions about the social responsibilities of dental hygienists (see Guiding Principles). The responsibilities of the dental hygienist include all of these and more, as will be discussed in this chapter.

GUIDING PRINCIPLES

Questions in Relation to the Social Responsibilities of Licensed Dental Hygienists

- What are the hygienist's social responsibilities to the profession of dental hygiene, to all patients, and to society as a whole?
- Do these responsibilities entail taking a leadership role in a professional organization or in public health, and/or in advocating for evolving governmental policies?
- Do these responsibilities include maintaining competency in clinical skills and being current on evidence-based research in dental and dental hygiene sciences so as to provide the best possible care for the patient and to meet the needs of the community?
- Do these responsibilities look beyond the patients of record in a practice to individuals and communities that lack access to needed oral health care?
- Do these responsibilities embrace the art of health promotion communication to assure that the public is empowered to improve its own oral health?

Social responsibility is a broad term meaning the expectation that people and organizations behave ethically and with sensitivity toward social, cultural, economic, and environmental issues. Striving for social responsibility helps individuals, organizations, and governments positively impact development, business, and society. Social responsibilities include the concepts of a person's right to health care, the profession's obligation to raise the oral health literacy of the community, and government's responsibility to promote the health and well-being of the public.

Professional Ethics

Often equated with social responsibility, **ethics** is commonly defined as the general study of right and wrong conduct. Oral health professionals continue to make an ethical commitment to address the oral health needs of society. If individuals' oral health needs are not being met because the system stands in the way, then correcting that system is part of the ethical responsibility of society and of the oral health professions.[9]

Professional ethics is the code by which the profession regulates actions and sets standards for its members, with the recognition that professionals are accountable for their actions. This code serves as a guide to the profession to ensure a high standard of competency, to strengthen the relationships among its members, and to promote the welfare of the entire community. Dental hygienists are required daily to make choices in practice that necessitate ethical decision-making.

The *Code of Ethics for Dental Hygienists* adopted by the American Dental Hygienists' Association (ADHA) guides requisite ethical decision-making through seven basic values (Box 9.1).[9] Commitment to ethical conduct is the foundation of society's trust and confidence in the dental hygiene profession. Ethical conduct is not confined to a particular practice setting; it is knowing and applying the core values in all aspects of life while serving the common good. The ADHA ethical code describes ethical responsibilities related to the community and

BOX 9.1 Seven Basic Values of the Dental Hygiene Profession in the American Dental Hygienists' Association *Code of Ethics for Dental Hygienists*

Individual Autonomy and Respect for Human Beings—The right of people to be treated with respect, to informed consent before treatment, and to full disclosure of all relevant information so they can make informed choices about their care.

Confidentiality—Respect for the confidentiality of client information and relationships as a demonstration of the value placed on individual autonomy, and acknowledgement of the obligation to justify any violation of a confidence.

Societal Trust—Value of client trust and understanding that public trust in the profession is based on the actions and behavior of the members of the profession.

Nonmaleficence—Acceptance of the fundamental obligation to provide services in a manner that protects all clients and minimizes harm to them and to others involved in their treatment.

Beneficence—Acceptance of a primary role in promoting the well-being of individuals and the public by engaging in health promotion and disease prevention activities.

Justice and Fairness—Value of justice and support of the fair and equitable distribution of healthcare resources based on the belief that all people should have access to high-quality, affordable oral health care.

Veracity—Acceptance of the obligation to tell the truth and expect that others will do the same, based on the value of self-knowledge and seeking truth and honesty in all relationships.

society.[9] As members of both the society and the profession, dental hygienists are challenged to fairly and justly distribute oral healthcare services to all individuals in need.[9] Several thought-provoking questions will guide the discussion in this chapter about the professional application of ethics to access to care. (see Guiding Principles).

GUIDING PRINCIPLES

Questions about Dental Hygiene's Responsibility to Address Access to Oral Health Care

- What is the responsibility of the dental hygienist to the broader group of *public* or *society*, which includes the following: people without access to oral healthcare services, culturally diverse populations, and individuals with special healthcare needs?
- Do individuals have a right to receive quality oral health care at a cost they can afford?
- What is a fair or just distribution of limited oral healthcare resources?

HEALTH CARE: A PRIVILEGE OR A RIGHT?

It is important to understand the U.S. healthcare delivery system, how it operates, who participates in it, what legal and ethical issues arise as a result of it, what problems continue to plague it, and if health care, including oral health care, is a *right* or a *privilege* for each citizen. These questions will be discussed.

Health Care as a Privilege

For years research has linked health and the economy.[10] "Healthier populations contribute to a stronger local economy, and a stronger local economy contributes to a healthier population."[10] Thus, focusing on the health of our nation has multiple benefits, both to individuals and to society as a whole. Historically, the U.S. has not offered healthcare coverage as a right of citizenship. The U.S. healthcare system is one of individualism and self-determination, focusing on the individual rather than the collective needs of the population. It is a privileged system of healthcare access, not answering the needs of all the citizenry. The people who receive the benefits and privileges of health care are those who have employer-based insurance or can afford to pay for it in a fee-for-service healthcare system. Those who are without insurance or have limited resources tend to seek health care only when it becomes an emergency (Figure 9.2).

Our current healthcare delivery system is *fragmented* between an individually funded private system and a government-mandated and funded model of healthcare delivery, even since the passage of the ACA in 2010. This combination of private and public forces is referred to as **pluralistic**. For 70% of the U.S. population, health care is still provided through a complex system of various health insurance funding networks.[5]

Oral healthcare access has significantly increased in the last decade for low-income children through the ACA and the expansion of Medicaid. Yet, adults and older adults continue to experience more limited access to oral healthcare services through the current private dental care delivery system. According to the National Association of Dental Plans, approximately 74 million Americans had no dental coverage in 2016, and only 52.9% of adults over age 65 reported having dental coverage.[11] Additionally, as of January 1, 2016, there were nearly 49 million people living in over 5000 dental health professional shortage areas (dental HPSAs) across the country.[12] (See Chapters 2 and 5 for more information on dental HPSAs.)

The Senate Special Committee on Aging introduced the Medicare and Medicaid Dental, Vision and Hearing Benefit Act of 2019. Although it did not pass, this proposed bill represents another milestone in recent efforts to underscore the need for

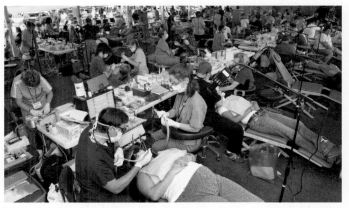

Fig 9.2 Mission of Mercy: A coordinated national dental access event for underserved adults who do not have a dental home or access to oral healthcare services. (Courtesy Virginia Dental Association.)

improved coverage of oral health benefits in government-funded programs, especially for older adults.[13]

Health Care as a Right

The country made an ethical decision that a sound basic education was the right of each child, and by 1918 all states required elementary education for all children.[14] Furthermore, during its development the U.S. decided it was a right of citizens to have security provided through government-funded police, fire, and defense forces and to have access to other government-provided public services such as fresh water, waste removal, libraries, roads, and bridges. All these assumed rights of a modern citizen are possible through taxation.

What about health care? In 1965, the passage of legislation establishing Medicare and Medicaid placed this country on the path of government funding of health care for seniors and the poor and disabled. Additionally, the country decided that anyone who presents at a hospital emergency room will be treated, regardless of insurance coverage or ability to pay. More recently, the ACA addressed the problem of uninsured individuals. Thus, the U.S. has made incremental decisions toward the position that health care is a right of all American citizens.

The Constitution of the United States does not specifically guarantee a "right to health" just as it does not guarantee a right to an education. Health is a dynamic and is unique to each individual.[14] One interpretation is that health and access to health care are not so much a legal right as they are a *moral* right. As such, society as a whole has an obligation to provide care in response to that right, with providers playing an important role. This is reflected in the professional responsibility to the community and society highlighted in the ADHA *Code of Ethics for Dental Hygienists*: "Recognize and uphold our obligation to provide pro bono service."[9]

The duty to ensure basic health and oral health for all Americans is shared by federal, state, community, public, and private entities. Entrusted by society, the oral health professions are obliged to lead the effort to ensure access to oral health care by all.[15] However, society has not universally accepted their share of responsibility despite several key events that have attempted to highlight the relationship among individual rights, human dignity, and the human condition.

In 1946, the *Constitution of the World Health Organization* defined health as "a state of complete physical, mental, and social well-being, and not merely the absence of disease or infirmity."[16] This view of health was reinforced in the *Universal Declaration of Human Rights* adopted by the United Nations General Assembly in 1948: "Everyone has the right to a standard of living adequate for the health and well-being of himself and of his family, including food, clothing, housing, and medical care."[17] This definition of health is still used by WHO today.[18]

In an amendment to the U.S. Public Health Service Act in 1966, Congress declared "that fulfillment of our national purpose depends on promoting and assuring the highest level of health attainable for every person."[19] The fundamental basis of human rights is the recognition of the equal worth and dignity of everyone and implies that individuals, institutions, and society as a whole should protect and promote health and ensure that it is neither impaired nor at risk.

GOVERNMENT ROLE IN HEALTHCARE DELIVERY

The U.S. government plays an important role in healthcare delivery. Three governmental levels participate in the U.S. healthcare system: federal, state, and local (see Chapter 1). The federal government provides a range of regulatory and funding mechanisms. It adopts a national healthcare budget, and it funds, sets reimbursement rates for, and establishes standards of care for providers in the Medicare and Medicaid program. It also provides ongoing surveillance and evaluation of the healthcare system. The individual states are responsible for regulatory and funding mechanisms and provide healthcare programs as dictated and funded by the federal government. The local level is responsible for implementing programs dictated and supported by the federal and state levels (see Chapter 6).

Many healthcare systems, including that of the U.S., have been evaluated using William Kissick's **iron triangle of health care**, a concept that consists of three essential aspects: quality, cost, and access[20] (Figure 9.3). According to health economists, the three legs of the triangle are in competition and thus balance each other through inherent trade-offs. The theory is that one, or possibly two, of the legs can be improved, but it is always at the expense of the other(s). In other words, an increase in access will result in a decrease of quality and/or an increase in cost, an increase in quality will result in an increase in cost and/or a decrease in access, and a decrease in cost will result in a decrease in access and/or a decrease in quality. Additionally, because the relationship among these three aspects of the healthcare system is reciprocal, it is difficult to have any significant overall structural change in the healthcare system.

However, as our current healthcare system has become more consumer driven, greater patient *choice* and promotion of

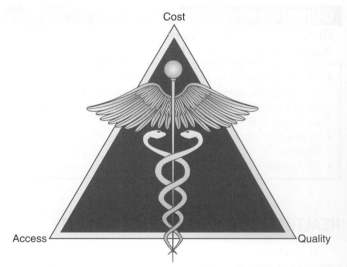

Fig 9.3 The iron triangle of health care. (Modified from Karadimos A. The Iron Triangle of Healthcare in the Blockchain era. Data Driven Investor; 2018 Sep 29. Available at: <https://medium.com/datadriveninvestor/the-iron-triangle-of-healthcare-in-the-blockchain-era-85cd66f5777e>; [Accessed October 2019].)

competition in health care have shown that increases in access to high-quality care can be found at affordable prices. When federal and state health policies give consumers more control over their healthcare dollars, they can use that power to demand greater value. A popular model that often shows improvement in patient healthcare outcomes is the lifting of unnecessary regulations.[21] It has been suggested also that some of today's changes can disrupt the balance of the iron triangle, for example, alternative modes of healthcare delivery such as the use of mid-level providers (e.g., dental therapists), retail clinics, telehealth services, and online access to consultation with health professionals, medication management, and medical supplies.[21] These disrupters have the potential to drive down costs while maintaining quality.[21] Other disrupters are the structural changes suggested for the healthcare system in the 2018 report *Reforming America's Healthcare System Through Choice and Competition*[22] (Box 9.2).

Dental Safety Net Providers

The dental **safety net** refers to the structures that support populations facing considerable barriers to accessing health and oral healthcare services (see Chapters 2 and 5). This typically involves individuals without private insurance and unable to pay for services out of pocket. The dental safety net is comprised of practitioners, payment programs, and facilities that provide clinical, nonclinical, and support services. Many of these are funded, regulated, and/or operated by the government. The safety net includes nonprofit free and charitable clinics, Medicaid, Children's Health Insurance Program (CHIP), Federally Qualified Health Centers (FQHCs), school-based health

---

BOX 9.2 Structural Changes Suggested for the Healthcare System in the United States

Healthcare Workforce and Labor Markets
Implementing policies that broaden providers' scope of practice while improving workforce mobility and reducing restrictions to encourage innovation and allow providers to meet patients' needs; includes direct access and direct reimbursement for dental hygienists and telehealth.

Healthcare Provider Markets
Encouraging the development of value-based payment models that offer flexibility and risk-based incentives for providers, especially without burdening small or rural practices.

Healthcare Insurance Markets
Scaling back government mandates, eliminating barriers to competition, and allowing consumers maximum opportunity to purchase health insurance that meets their needs.

Consumer-Driven Health Care
Developing price and quality transparency initiatives to ensure that newly empowered healthcare consumers can make well-informed decisions about their care.

(From Reforming America's Healthcare System Through Choice and Competition. Washington, D.C.: Department of Health and Human Services, Department of the Treasury, Department of Labor; 2018 Dec. Available at: <https://www.hhs.gov/sites/default/files/Reforming-Americas-Healthcare-System-Through-Choice-and-Competition.pdf>; [Accessed September 2019].)

---

centers, and academic dental institutions, among other entities. If not for the dental safety net, millions more Americans would be without access to healthcare and oral healthcare services.[23]

Policy Development

One of the professional roles of a dental hygienist is to advocate for health policy initiatives to improve the inequities of the current oral healthcare delivery model (see Chapter 2). According to our professional code of ethics, it is our ethical responsibility to the community and society to "promote access to dental hygiene services for all, supporting justice and fairness in the distribution of healthcare resources."[9] This requires the establishment of procedural standards.

As one of the core functions of public health, **policy development** is often intertwined with the social responsibility of promoting oral health initiatives. According to the WHO, leadership and governance involves ensuring that strategic health policy frameworks are in place.[24] The CDC describes health policy as "the advancement and implementation of public health law, regulations, or voluntary practices that influence systems development, organizational change, and individual behavior to promote improvements in health."[25] Such policies can be executed within the health sector as well as within other sectors such as education, agriculture, employment, and the tax code. Having an explicit health policy serves several purposes:
1. Defines a vision for the future, thus helping to establish targets and reference points for the short and medium term.
2. Outlines priorities and expected roles of different groups.
3. Builds consensus and informs people.

Understanding the policymaking process is crucial to serving public needs. Policy is used to connect the results of community *assessment* to *assuring* that the oral health needs of the public are addressed. Thus, the three core functions of public health (assessment, assurance, and policy development) function synergistically in public health practice (see Chapter 1).

To be successful, all oral health policy initiatives should involve collaborative efforts between partners and stakeholders, including professionals, community leaders, coalitions, and the public; consider cultural, generational, and economic barriers; and address the important oral health issues identified by the nation (see Chapter 1). According to the CDC, although policy development is rarely linear, the process involves identifying a problem; identifying, analyzing, and prioritizing potential policy solutions; and adopting and evaluating the best solution.[25]

The dental hygienist's social or civic responsibility includes knowing their individual congressional legislators and state delegates. Establishing these political advocacy relationships is beneficial for educating and influencing legislators who will vote on bills that may impact oral health initiatives and the practice of dental hygiene to improve oral healthcare access. In the role of political advocate, the dental hygienist thereby influences the oral health status of the public and society. Participating in advocacy at the state level in this manner frequently involves lobbying, which may be done through a professional organization or coalition. Understanding the legislative process by which an idea becomes a bill and ultimately a law is important when involved in lobbying for passage of a state statute (Figure 9.4).

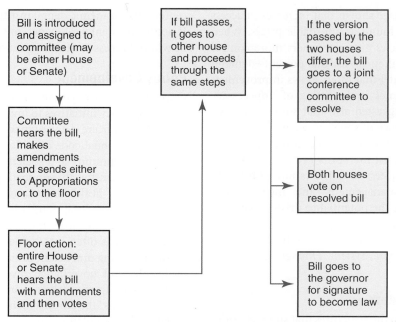

Fig 9.4 How a bill becomes a law at the state level.

A similar process occurs at the federal and local levels. The same legislative process at the federal level culminates in signing by the President. Also, dental hygienists are called on frequently to assist with local or state oral health issues such as establishing and protecting water fluoridation, seeking funding for school-based sealant programs, initiating changes in scope of practice and supervision regulations for dental hygienists, and other program and policy development that will impact the oral health of citizens (see Chapters 2 and 6). Regardless of the level of policy desired, the order of procedures to develop policy is nearly identical (Box 9.3).

Demand Versus Resources

Today differences exist between need and demand, and between supply and requirements of the citizenry.[12] It is imperative that healthcare providers educate the public and policymakers on how to bring public healthcare capacity to a level that will provide the resources necessary to optimally meet the demand for healthcare services.[9] Herein lies a major social responsibility of all healthcare providers. For dental hygienists, this translates

into the social responsibility to advocate for and promote oral health and wellness by: (1) communicating, educating, and advocating for the prevention of oral health risks and (2) advocating for changes in the oral health professions that can increase oral healthcare capacity (see Chapters 2, 5, and 6). Such advocacy efforts must be based on what is best for the public rather than on the individual needs of healthcare providers or that of the profession.[9]

PATIENT RESPONSIBILITY AND PATIENT CONFIDENTIALITY

"Although the U.S. continues to spend more on health care than any other country, it is unclear whether this higher expenditure is yielding better healthcare outcomes with system-wide outcomes measurement fraught with challenges, including confounding social and environmental factors, as well as inconsistent and unavailable data."[26] Based on this quote, it is important to seek effective ways to improve the health of our nation. In a society such as ours where a pluralistic healthcare system exists, greater emphasis is placed on individual responsibility for health. Thus, it has been suggested that "the single greatest opportunity to improve health and reduce premature death lies in personal behaviors. In fact, behavioral causes account for a significant number of deaths in the U.S."[27]

However, today, although emphasis is sometimes placed on behavioral change and improved technology to improve health,[26] heightened consideration is being given to the **social determinants of health** (SDOH), which are the underlying social status, wealth, ethnicity, education, geographic location, and other social factors that impact health outcomes.[28,29] SDOH are conditions in the places where people live, learn, work, and play that affect a wide range of health risks and outcomes.[28] Based on these SDOH, not all people have opportunities for the same health outcomes. Applying what is known about

---

BOX 9.3   Order of Procedures for Policy Development

- Develop personal and professional relationships with policymakers and decision makers
- Collaborate with partners to identify data needed
- Assess and quantify oral health needs and existing resources
- Share data with partners and identify possible strategies and solutions
- Share data and desired solutions with policymakers
- Be available to policymakers for questions at all stages of the process and to provide information and testimony
- Thank the policymakers, regardless of the outcome, and continue to maintain relationships for future efforts
- Consider supporting other health policy initiatives supported or sponsored by this policymaker that may not have an oral health focus

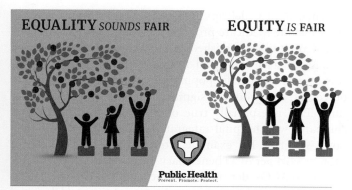

Fig 9.5 Achieving health equity makes it possible for everyone to reach an "apple". (From Health Equity. Healthy Communities; 2020. Available at: <https://www.mmshealthycommunities.org/collective-action/health-equity/>; [Accessed February 2020].)

SDOH can improve individual and population health and advance **health equity** by addressing 80% of the determinants of health.[30] (See Chapters 3 and 4 for further discussion of the social determinants of health and health inequities.)

The relationship of access to care and SES as one of the SDOH can be viewed as bidirectional. An individual's oral healthcare inequity can foster a decline in personal confidence and reduced employment opportunities. This in turn can further distance the individual from improved oral and overall health, thus perpetuating an inability to improve SES. This societal inequality is an example of disparities in health equity. According to the CDC, "health equity is achieved when every person has the opportunity to attain his or her full health potential and no one is disadvantaged from achieving this potential because of social position or other socially determined circumstances"[30] (see Figure 9.5).

Patient responsibility for health is more significant today because of the increase in chronic diseases that result in greater morbidity and mortality rates. Seven of the 10 leading causes of death in the U.S. are chronic diseases, accounting for more than 64% of deaths[27]; several relate to oral health. Prevention is a key to reducing the need for emergency and episodic health care, as well as reducing the incidence of related oral diseases. Such prevention requires patient responsibility to adopt protective health behaviors. Effective health communication and improvement of the public's health literacy are critical to this process (see Chapters 8 and 10).

In relation to oral health, patient responsibility depends partially on access. Various protective factors involve professional treatment, many of which can be accomplished by a dental hygienist. The direct access of the dental hygienist to the public is important to increase accessibility for this purpose (see Chapter 2). Lack of access to oral health care produces a downward cycle of poor oral health.

Health Insurance Portability and Accountability Act

When an individual is able to access oral healthcare services, confidentiality becomes a primary ethical responsibility to patients and clients.[9] Also, assurance of protection of privacy in the transfer of personal health information between providers is mandated by the **Health Insurance Portability and Accountability Act** (HIPAA).[31] Patient confidentiality must be adhered to in all practice settings in both private and public sectors such as public health sites, service-learning events, health fairs, with community stakeholders, and in the academic environment.[9] (See HIPPA Privacy Rule in Additional Resources.) The more recent emphasis placed by Congress on health information exchange and electronic health records is assisting providers in sharing crucial confidential information for the purpose of improving health outcomes.[31]

HEALTH CARE: A COMPREHENSIVE APPROACH

Strengthening the Current Dental Care Delivery System

It is essential to understand the term **access to care** and its relationship to social responsibility. According to the Access to Health Services topic area of *Healthy People 2020,* "access to comprehensive quality healthcare services is important for promoting and maintaining health, preventing and managing disease, reducing unnecessary disability and premature death, and achieving health equity for all Americans."[32] This understanding of the importance of equity in relation to access to care is even more significant in *Healthy People 2030.*[33] The WHO adds to the definition of access to care: "ease in reaching health services or health facilities in terms of location, time, and ease of approach."[18] Access involves ensuring that conditions are in place for people to obtain the care they need and want. Access to health care varies across countries, groups, and individuals, largely influenced by social and economic conditions. Access is affected also by the health policies that are in place, such as those that relate to available coverage, approved services, timeliness of care, and an available, well-qualified workforce.[34]

Oral health professions have a social responsibility to advocate for health equity policies that assure the necessary conditions to enhance access to oral health care.[9] Even with the current programs, access to care is unreliable.[12,29,34] Furthermore, the ACA has challenged the capacity of the delivery systems to accommodate the influx of people who have insurance coverage for the first time. Individuals with limited resources and isolated populations especially will continue to experience numerous barriers to overall healthcare and oral healthcare services.[12] The existing gap between the current dental workforce capacity and the increasing oral health demands of the community will provide a challenge. However, the ACA has significantly increased oral health provisions for children from low-income families in the following ways:[35]

- Mandated oral health benefits for children with no out-of-pocket costs for preventive services
- Improved oral health surveillance in all states
- Made available grants to school-based health centers, which include oral health services
- Promoted oral health, including a focus on early childhood caries, prevention, oral health of pregnant women, and oral health of at-risk populations
- Increased school-based sealant programs
- Established training, workforce development, and loan repayment provisions.

Several unifying messages emerged from the Sixth Leadership Colloquium titled *Strengthening the Dental Care Delivery System* sponsored by the U.S. National Oral Health Alliance in 2013.[36] These themes point to the social responsibility of oral health professions to strengthen the oral care delivery system so that access to oral health care can be realized by all, not just a select few (see Guiding Principles).

GUIDING PRINCIPLES

What it Will Take to Strengthen the Oral Healthcare Delivery System

- Focus oral health care on prevention and wellness for individuals, families, and communities.
- Move toward interprofessional healthcare teams, cost-effective workforce models, and care delivery systems.
- Transform education for a future strengthened by team-based oral health care and medical care.
- Empower communities to support highly effective oral healthcare systems.
- Align payment and systems approaches to promote and support prevention and wellness.

Previous chapters highlight many recent strides made by the oral health professions to strengthen the current oral health delivery systems, some of which address these recommendations. The dental hygiene profession has been a major player in these efforts (see Chapters 1 and 2). Progress has been made over the past decade in increasing the use of dental services, especially among poor and near-poor children, and in reducing the rich-poor gap in the utilization of services and access to care for children. In 2016, the percentage of Medicaid and CHIP children aged 2 to 17 years who had a dental visit was 50.4% compared with 35.3% in 2006.[37]

Transforming to an Oral Health Interprofessional Workforce Model

The inability of oral healthcare workforce capacity to meet the needs of a changing society is a matter of maldistribution and, in some instances, a shortage of oral healthcare providers (see Chapter 5), directly impacting access to and utilization of services. This provides an opportunity to explore new delivery models such as expanded care dental hygienists and mid-level providers or dental therapists[12] (see Chapter 2). It also presents a chance to transform healthcare delivery to an *interprofessional collaborative practice* (ICP) model (see Chapters 2 and 11). In ICP, multiple healthcare practitioners, including oral, collaborate to provide patient-centered care, prevention, education, and risk reduction to strengthen health outcomes in a comprehensive *primary care model*.[38] This allows for the introduction of oral care into currently underserved geographic areas.

Accountable care organizations (ACOs) are models created by the ACA to reduce the cost of health care while improving quality. ACOs are "groups of doctors, hospitals, and other healthcare providers who come together voluntarily to give coordinated high-quality care to their Medicare patients" with the goal of ensuring "that patients get the right care at the right time, while avoiding unnecessary duplication of services and preventing medical errors."[39]

When an ACO delivers high-quality care at an overall lower cost to the Medicare program, it shares in the savings.[39] A review of studies published in 2016 through 2018 revealed that ACOs have improved health equity by increasing access to care for specific population groups, improved health outcomes, and produced significant savings which grew over time. This is especially true of physician-group-led ACOs compared with hospital-integrated ACOs, with no or limited down-side risk. For example, from 2012 to 2014, savings of $156 to $474 per ACO beneficiary were realized by physician-group-led ACOs, depending on the length of time beneficiaries were enrolled.[40] In this emerging practice model, dental therapists, dental hygienists, and dentists are integrated with nondental providers, physicians, nurses, and others to deliver coordinated, high-quality preventive and primary oral health care.[41]

The convergence of health professionals can substantially increase workforce capacity by developing integrated health homes using telehealth systems to enable people to communicate across distances, emphasizing prevention and early intervention, and providing cost-effective care for otherwise underserved rural populations.[42] (See Chapter 5 for an expanded discussion of teledentistry.) Although few ACOs currently integrate oral health care, this is expected to increase.[41] However, limitations still exist in dental hygiene scope of practice and supervisory statutes in numerous states that will impede their complete incorporation into this cost-effective interprofessional healthcare delivery model nationally.[12,21,22]

Even so, the dental hygiene profession is rapidly transforming within this interprofessional health workforce model, which is beginning to result in expanded professional opportunities (see Chapter 2). Some recent changes include the following:[12,43,44]

- Mid-level providers are increasing access to care, especially for underserved populations.
- Medical offices, hospitals, and community health centers are using dental hygienists.
- Corporate entities are hiring dental hygienists for myriad positions, including research, sales, and health promotion.

A notable initiative in relation to these trends is the integration of interprofessional education into the Commission on Dental Accreditation standards for dental hygiene programs.[45]

LEADERSHIP

Continued leadership is needed in dentistry and dental hygiene to eliminate oral health disparities and ensure access to oral health services for all. A dental hygiene professional *leader* works within the community to develop consensus on what *oral health care for all* might look like,[2,46] enabling others to see the problem firsthand and participating in implementing solutions. A leader challenges *the way things have always been done* and seeks new ways to maximize resources and productivity while remaining mindful of ethical decision-making processes and commitment to quality care.[9,46]

Leadership is the foundation for fulfilling social and professional responsibilities to society[46] (Figure 9.6). Dental hygiene leaders function at various levels and in different capacities to improve the public's oral health. Regardless of the level or

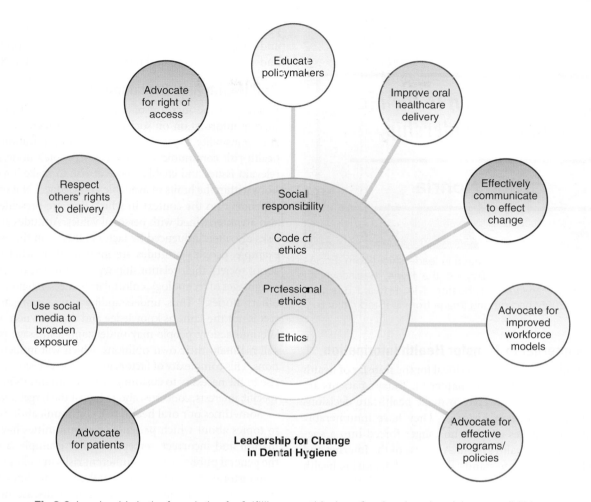

Fig 9.6 Leadership is the foundation for fulfilling our ethical, professional, and social responsibilities.

capacity, leaders demonstrate certain actions in relation to the specific issues discussed in this and other chapters (see Box 9.4).

Dental hygienists have an ethical and professional responsibility to lead and advocate for change to improve the oral health of the public as it relates to whatever professional role they are involved in[9] (see Chapter 2). Furthermore, meeting these leadership responsibilities requires involvement with one's professional organization.[9] The ADHA and its state constituents and local societies provide all dental hygienists opportunities for leadership in promoting the oral health of the public at various levels. They serve as resources of current professional information and enable an informed response to professional issues. In addition, dental hygienists in public health positions have opportunities to lead change through various dental public health organizations highlighted throughout this textbook.

The Role of Communication in Leadership

Dental hygiene leadership embraces the concepts of social responsibility, professionalism, ethics, and communication. The first three concepts have already been addressed. The ability to communicate effectively with patients, community members, other community leaders, public health advocates, colleagues, other health professionals, and government officials, as well as friends and neighbors, is also an essential attribute of leadership (Figure 9.7).

Successful communication in a culturally competent and sensitive manner helps to reduce disparities and promotes oral health and wellness (see Chapter 10). The ability to communicate with community leaders and stakeholders improves the delivery of appropriate care and increases the likelihood that programs, services, and policies will be supported by the community and be relevant to diverse populations, resulting in improved outcomes and reduced disparities.[47] Effective oral and written communication not only improve others' understanding of the issues; they also influence how others view the profession. Thus, communication can impact the success of advocating for initiatives designed to improve the oral health of the public.

BOX 9.4 Actions Demonstrated by Dental Hygiene Leaders

- Advocating for changes in oral healthcare practice that can bring about improved oral health and increased access to oral health care.
- Modeling public health practice by ensuring equal access to care and not tolerating prejudice against any person seeking care.
- Encouraging other professionals in the community to participate in health promotion and disease prevention activities and to celebrate successes.
- Staying abreast of current research and critically evaluating scientific literature in relation to quality oral health care, effective preventive and therapeutic measures, and changes in infrastructure, workforce, and policies to improve the delivery of oral health care.
- Respecting all healthcare providers in the community and forging collaborative relationships to facilitate providing overall health care for the public.
- Working within the profession to ensure continued competency, lifelong learning, and maintenance of quality standards of practice.

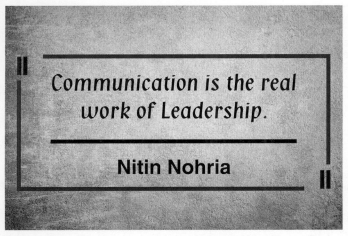

Fig 9.7 The role of communication in leadership. (From: Eccles RG, Nohria N, Berkley JD. Beyond the Hype: Rediscovering the Essence of Management. Boston, MA: Harvard Business School Press; 2005; background image from © iStock/littleclie.)

Use of the Internet to Transfer Health Information

Effective communication is also critical for the transfer of health information to the public (see Chapter 8). Today's patients are more informed and empowered to make healthcare decisions than at any other time in history.[48] They have innumerably more healthcare choices and are no longer forced into a specific local practice or health system. Also, use of the Internet and **social media** have become standard means of acquiring health and healthcare information[48] (see Guiding Principles).

GUIDING PRINCIPLES

The Use of Social Media for Healthcare Communication

- There were 3.48 billion social media users worldwide in 2020, representing a 9% growth since 2019.[49]
- Google receives 63,000 searches per second on any given day,[50] and 7% are health related.[51]
- Approximately 80% of health consumers use the Internet to access health-related consumer reviews such as reviews of treatments or providers.[48]
- Almost 65% of patients say that a strong online presence will influence their choosing one provider over another.[48]
- The majority of patients are likely to trust information posted online by healthcare providers.[52]
- More than half of patients who searched for online information before consulting a healthcare provider discussed the obtained information with the provider and found the provider willing to discuss this information.[53]
- As many as 60% of physicians feel that social media improves the quality of care they provide to their patients.[54]

The *Healthy People* initiative has stressed the importance of health communication and the use of health information technology since 2020.[33] In addition, greater use of social media by oral health professionals has been suggested.[48,52,54] By using information technology effectively, efficiently, and securely, oral health professionals can reinforce the oral healthcare provider/

patient partnership in both face-to-face and virtual associations and be at the forefront of technological innovation for patient-and-family-centered oral health care (see Chapters 8 and 10).

Oral Health Risk Communication

Inherent in the increase of interprofessional collaboration and sharing information on social media is an increased professional responsibility for oral health risk communication. Successful health risk communication increases people's understanding of relevant issues and enables those at risk to make informed decisions within the limits of available knowledge.[55] Not only are risks dependent on the context in which they are presented, but they also are intertwined with personal values. Attitudes about certain risks are often influenced by factors other than the evidence. For example, people's attitudes are influenced by what they believe about society, their relationship with nature, the benefits and disadvantages of technology, cultural influences, religious beliefs, and others' stories.[56] Thus, understanding a message regarding health risk is not the same as knowledge and does not necessarily translate into action; people may understand a message perfectly but still maintain their own opinions, which will influence their actions. This complexity of factors involved in decision-making gives rise to the necessity to customize risk communication to meet the specific interests, concerns, and habits of the target audiences.[57]

Sometimes our oral health risk communication is in relation to topics about which patients or communities have misinformation and incorrect perceptions. For example, a segment of the general public perceives inherent risks in radiographs, amalgam restorations, biofilms in dental unit water lines, instrument sterilization techniques, transmission of disease in the dental environment, and still, community water fluoridation. It is the oral health professional's responsibility to be knowledgeable about current evidence-based research regarding such issues, as well as the publicized misinformation, and to communicate risk in relation to individuals' oral health behaviors and treatment decisions associated with the issues (Figure 9.8).[9,54]

Effectively communicating for shared decision-making depends on respecting beliefs, gathering information consistent with the public's point of view, and then providing a professional account of the evidence underlying sound health decisions

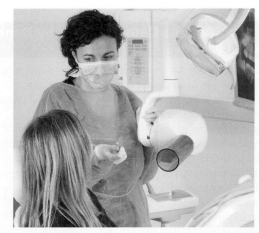

Fig 9.8 An oral health professional talks to a patient about the risks associated with dental radiographs. (© iStock.com.)

and treatment modalities. In this way, oral health professionals can (1) ensure compliance with recommended protocols, regardless of the practice or community setting, (2) minimize risks, (3) communicate pertinent and accurate health information to the public, (4) reduce misinformation, and (5) enable others to make good decisions that will promote oral health for themselves and others. Thus, effective oral health risk communication can impact oral health outcomes.[55]

The means by which health professionals must communicate oral health risks has changed.[56] Because of multiple sources of information through social media and other forms of technology, people are now exposed to more diverse forms of information, some of which are inaccurate. Thus, individuals now need to be able to filter, interpret, and make sense of the information they are given, in increasingly sophisticated ways. This places the burden on oral health professionals to be familiar with evidence-based oral health information and the inaccurate information that is available to the public[58] (see Chapter 7). In addition, oral health professionals are ethically bound to communicate with patients, community leaders, policymakers, and stakeholders in a way that enables them to make sound, informed decisions via a process of shared decision-making.[9,58] The use of social media provides a means for oral health professionals to carry out this responsibility in a form that is acceptable and easily accessible to the public.

SUMMARY

The dental hygienist is a professional. Inherent in the professional role is the responsibility to make ethical decisions to practice dental hygiene in ways that will improve the oral health for the public and increase access to oral health services for all populations. Dental hygienists have a social and professional responsibility to (1) apply interprofessional collaborative leadership to uphold the ethical standards of the dental hygiene profession, (2) advocate for changes to the oral healthcare system that will improve oral healthcare delivery, (3) recognize how determinants of health, overall health, and risk factors for oral diseases and conditions influence oral health, (4) continually use effective health promotion communication skills to advance optimal oral health for all, (5) apply evidence-based practices to improve oral health, (6) advocate for policies to address access-to-care initiatives, and (7) provide leadership for these and other critical public health and professional issues.

APPLYING YOUR KNOWLEDGE

1. Watch and discuss *What If Our Healthcare System Kept Us Healthy?* with Rebecca Onie on TED Talk at http://www.ted.com/talks/rebecca_onie_what_if_our_healthcare_system_kept_us_healthy. Answer the following questions:
   a. What are the strengths and weakness of the U.S. healthcare system?
   b. As a future oral health professional, what did you personally gain from this TED Talk?
   c. Did your perspective change on the social and civic responsibility of the access-to-care issue?
   d. Are there viable interprofessional solutions to the challenges of reaching those who are excluded from our healthcare system?

2. Read the book *Nickel and Dimed* by Barbara Ehrenreich and published by Metropolitan Books (ISBN 0-8050-6388-9). This is a timeless ethnographic portrayal of the working poor and a societal consciousness-raising call to action toward social and civic responsibility. Answer the discussion questions at http://barbaraehrenreich.com/website/nickel_and_dimed_reading_group_guide.htm.

3. Research the legislative agenda of your state dental hygiene association. Develop a plan to advocate for an issue that is part of the agenda and present it in class.

4. Research leadership to identify ways to develop yourself as a leader in your profession of dental hygiene. Develop five professional development goals that you can carry out over the next 5 years in relation to leadership.

LEARNING OBJECTIVES AND COMPETENCIES

This chapter addresses the following community dental health learning objectives and competencies for dental hygienists that are presented in the *ADEA Compendium of Curriculum Guidelines for Allied Dental Education Programs*:

Learning Objectives
- Define the range of personal, social, economic and environmental factors that influence health status, that is, determinants of health.
- Describe the state of oral health in the U.S.
- Describe the dental care delivery system in the U.S.
- Evaluate the role of the government in financing dental care.
- Summarize the legislative process.
- Describe the responsibilities of dental hygienists in the U.S.
- Describe dental labor force use of and access to dental care.
- Analyze need, supply, demand and use of dental care as it pertains to utilization.

Competencies
- Promoting the values of good oral and general health and wellness to the public and organizations within and outside the professions.
- Recognizing the responsibility and demonstrating the ability to communicate professional knowledge verbally and in writing.
- Accepting responsibility for solving problems and making decisions based on accepted scientific principles.
- Advocating for consumer groups, businesses and government agencies to support healthcare issues.

COMMUNITY CASE

Umbrella Health (UH) is a for-profit organization whose mission it is to reduce dental caries in school-aged children, especially children whose families are of low SES. With the goal of increasing oral healthcare access and utilization via a school-based program, UH is interested in piloting a project to provide comprehensive preventive and primary oral health care to low SES children within the elementary school environment. They anticipate the program will prove to be sustainable and continue long term. A team of dental hygienists will provide oral healthcare services utilizing mobile equipment. The efficiency of the program will be increased by using teledentistry communication between the dental hygienists and the collaborating dentist hired specifically for the program, for remote consultation, diagnosis, and referral for follow-up dental treatment. The company has approached the school district administrators for approval of a pilot project in your area. Additionally, UH has asked the local and state dental hygiene professional associations for their support of this innovative initiative. As president of your local dental hygiene society, you have been asked by UH to advocate for the program.

1. What is the first action you should take relative to your social and professional responsibility as a licensed dental hygienist to ensure that this organization is credible?
   a. Research the UH organization's mission, vision, credentials, and financials.
   b. Meet with the UH stakeholders to discuss the program.
   c. Contact UH patients about their satisfaction with oral health services provided by the organization.
   d. Speak with dental hygienists who you know through the dental hygiene society and who have previously worked for UH.

2. If the decision of the local dental hygiene professional association is to support the UH pilot project, what would be your first action as president in promoting the proposed oral health initiative?
   a. Seek federal grant support for the pilot project.
   b. Meet with school administrators and teachers to explain the program and offer assistance in educating parents about this oral health initiative.

   c. Investigate the state statute concerning a licensed dental hygienist providing oral healthcare services in a school-based program.
   d. Meet with your executive board members for feedback and support.

3. What professional responsibility is met by your involvement and participation as a representative of your local dental hygiene society in this initiative?
   a. Confidentiality of patient and client information.
   b. Advocacy in relation to policy development.
   c. Professional leadership in advocating for improved oral health.
   d. Exploration of an interprofessional collaborative practice model.

4. You sense public reluctance to support this project because it takes valuable student-teacher contact time away from the students. How do you respond to the parents' query, "So why provide dental treatment during school time?"
   a. Share evidence-based research results that 50 million hours of school time are lost annually because of dental disease and that school performance is positively correlated to oral health.
   b. Inform parents they can choose not to allow their children to participate if they are concerned about the issue of student-teacher contact time.
   c. Take a vote of parents to determine the level of parental support for the program.
   d. Ignore the parents' concern for now because the decision to move forward with the program should be made by the school administration, not the parents.

5. The school-based program described is an example of which of the following?
   a. Application of the iron triangle of health care.
   b. An oral health policy.
   c. Addressing the right to access to oral health care.
   d. A dental safety net provider.

REFERENCES

1. U.S. Constitution Preamble. Cornell University Law School, Legal Information Institute. Available at: <https://www.law.cornell.edu/constitution/preamble>; [Accessed July 2019].
2. U.S. Department of Health and Human Services. Oral Health in America: A Report of the Surgeon General. Rockville, MD: U.S. Department of Health and Human Services, National Institute of Dental and Craniofacial Research, National Institutes of Health; 2000. Available at: <https://www.cdc.gov/oralhealth/publications/sgr2000_05.htm>; [Accessed July 2019].
3. Social Determinants of Health. Geneva, Switzerland: World Health Organization; 2020. Available at: <https://www.who.int/health-topics/social-determinants-of-health#tab=tab_3>; [Accessed July 2019].
4. Fontenot K, Semega J, Kollar M. Income and Poverty in the United States: 2017. U.S. Census Bureau; 2018 Sept 12. Available at: <https://www.census.gov/library/publications/2018/demo/p60-263.html>; [Accessed July 2019].
5. Key Facts about the Uninsured Population. The Kaiser Commission on Medicaid and the Uninsured; 2018 Dec 7. Available at: <https://www.kff.org/uninsured/fact-sheet/key-facts-about-the-uninsured-population/>; [Accessed July 2019].
6. Blumenthal D, Collins SR. Healthcare coverage under the Affordable Care Act—A progress report. N Engl J Med 2014;371:275. Available at: <http://www.nejm.org/doi/full/10.1056/NEJMhpr1405667>; [Accessed July 2019].
7. Eiber C, Nowak S. The Effect of Eliminating the Individual Mandate Penalty and the Role of Behavioral Factors. The Commonwealth Fund; July 11, 2018. Available at: <https://www.commonwealthfund.org/publications/fund-reports/2018/jul/eliminating-individual-mandate-penalty-behavioral-factors>; [Accessed July 2019].

8. Jost T. The Tax bill and The Individual Mandate: What Happened, and What Does it Mean? Health Affairs Blog; 2017 Dec 20. Available at: <https://www.healthaffairs.org/do/10.1377/hblog20171220.323429/full/>; [Accessed December 2019].

9. Code of Ethics for Dental Hygienists. Chicago, IL: American Dental Hygienists' Association; 2018. Available at: <https://www.adha.org/resources-docs/7611_Bylaws_and_Code_of_Ethics.pdf>; [Accessed July 2019].

10. Healthy Communities Mean a Better Economy. Blue Cross Blue Shield; 2017 Jan 12. Available at: <https://www.bcbs.com/the-health-of-america/articles/healthy-communities-mean-better-economy>; [Accessed April 2020].

11. Who has dental benefits today? Dental Benefits Basics. Dallas, TX: National Association of Dental Plans; 2017.Available at: <https://www.nadp.org/Dental_Benefits_Basics/Dental_BB_1.aspx>; [Accessed February 2020].

12. Bersell C. Access to Oral Health Care: A National Crisis and Call for Reform. J Dent Hyg 2017;91(1):6–14.

13. Senate Bill 1423: Medicare and Medicaid Dental, Vision, Hearing Benefit Act of 2019. Available at: <https://www.govtrack.us/congress/bills/116/s1423>; [Accessed July 2019].

14. Compulsory Education Laws: Background. FindLaw; 2019. Available at: <https://education.findlaw.com/education-options/compulsory-education-laws-background.html>; [Accessed October 2019].

15. ADEA Position Paper:. Statement on the Roles and Responsibilities of Academic Dental Institutions in Improving the Oral Health Status of All Americans 2004. J Dent Educ 2011;75:988–95.

16. Preamble to the Constitution of the World Health Organization. Adopted by the International 16 Health Conference, New York, June 1946; entered into force April 1948. Geneva, Switzerland: World Health Organization. Available at: <https://www.who.int/governance/eb/who_constitution_en.pdf>; [Accessed July 2019].

17. The Universal Declaration of Human Rights, Article 25. United Nations; 1948. Available at: <http://www.un.org/en/documents/udhr/>; [Accessed July 2019].

18. Health Systems Strengthening Glossary. Geneva, Switzerland: World Health Organization. Available at: <https://www.who.int/healthsystems/Glossary_January2011.pdf?ua=1>; [Accessed November 2020].

19. Comprehensive Health Planning and Public Health Services Amendments of 1966, Public Law 89-749. Washington, DC: U.S. Congress. Available at: <http://www.gpo.gov/fdsys/pkg/STATUTE-80/pdf/STATUTE-80-Pg1180.pdf>; [Accessed July 2019].

20. Lewis W. What is the Iron Triangle of Health Care? MOREHealth; 2017 May 18. Available at: <https://medium.com/more-health/what-is-the-iron-triangle-of-health-care-9ce6f5276077>; [Accessed October 2019].

21. Reforming America's Healthcare System Through Choice and Competition. Washington, D.C.: Department of Health and Human Services, Department of the Treasury, Department of Labor; December 2018. Available at: <https://www.hhs.gov/sites/default/files/Reforming-Americas-Healthcare-System-Through-Choice-and-Competition.pdf>; [Accessed September 2019].

22. Delaronde S. The Iron Triangle of Health Care: Access, Cost and Quality 2019. Available at: <https://www.3mhisinsideangle.com/blog-post/the-iron-triangle-of-health-care-access-cost-and-quality/>; [Accessed September 2019].

23. American Dental Education Association Data Brief Examining American Dental Safety Net 2018. Available at: <https://www.adea.org/policy/white-papers/Dental-Safety-Net.aspx>; [Accessed July 2019].

24. Health System Governance. Geneva, Switzerland: World Health Organization; 2020. Available at: <https://www.who.int/health-topics/health-systems-governance#tab=tab_1>; [Accessed March 2020].

25. CDC Policy Process. Atlanta, GA: Centers for Disease Control and Prevention; 2015 May 29. Available at: < https://www.cdc.gov/policy/analysis/process/index.html>. [Accessed February 2020].

26. Kamal R, Cox C. U.S. health system is performing better, though still lagging behind other countries. Peterson-Kaiser Health System Tracker; 2019 Mar 29. Available at: <https://www.healthsystemtracker.org/brief/u-s-health-system-is-performing-better-though-still-lagging-behind-other-countries/>; [Accessed October 2019].

27. Heron M. Deaths: Leading Causes of Death for 2017. Atlanta GA: Centers for Disease Control and Prevention, National Center for Health Statistics, National Vital Statistics Reports. NVSR 2019 Jun 24;68(6)e76. Available at: <https://www.cdc.gov/nchs/data/nvsr/nvsr68/nvsr68_06-508.pdf>; [Accessed July 2019].

28. Artiga S. Hinton E. Beyond Health Care: The Role of Social Determinants in Promoting Health and Health Equity (Issue Brief). Henry J. Kaiser Family Foundation; 2018 May 10. Available at: <https://www.kff.org/disparities-policy/issue-brief/beyond-health-care-the-role-of-social-determinants-in-promoting-health-and-health-equity/>; [Accessed October 2019].

29. Institute of Clinical System Improvement. Going Beyond Clinical Walls: Solving Complex Problems. Robert Wood Foundation; 2014. Available at: <www.nrhi.org/uploads/going-beyond-clinical-walls-solving-complex-problems.pdf>; [Accessed December 2019].

30. Health Equity. Atlanta, GA: Centers for Disease Control and Prevention, National Center for Chronic Disease Prevention and Health Promotion; 2019 Aug 28. Available from: <http://www.cdc.gov/chronicdisease/healthequity/>; [Accessed July 2019].

31. Health Information Privacy. Department of Health and Human Services, Office for Civil Rights Headquarters. Available at: <https://www.hhs.gov/hipaa/index.html>; [Accessed October 2019].

32. Healthy People 2020. Rockville, MD: Office of Disease Prevention and Health Promotion; 2020 Mar 31. Available at: <http://www.healthypeople.gov/>; [Accessed March 2020].

33. Report #7: Assessment and Recommendations for Proposed Objectives for Healthy People 2030. Healthy People 2020. Rockville, MD: Secretary's Advisory Committee for Healthy People 2030; 2019. Available at: <https://www.healthypeople.gov/sites/default/files/Report%207_Reviewing%20Assessing%20Set%20of%20HP2030%20Objectives_Formatted%20EO_508_05.21.pdf>; [Accessed March 2020].

34. Orgera K, Atiga S. Disparities in Health and Health Care: Five Key Questions and Answers. Henry K. Kaiser Foundation Disparities Policy; 2018 Aug. Available at: <https://www.kff.org/disparities-policy/issue-brief/disparities-in-health-and-health-care-five-key-questions-and-answers>; [Accessed December 2019].

35. Children's Dental Health Project. How the Affordable Care Act Moved Oral Health Forward (Blog Post). Teeth Matter; 2018 Mar 23. Available at: <https://www.cdhp.org/blog/502-how-the-affordable-care-act-moved-oral-health-forward>; [Accessed December 2019].

36. DentaQuest Foundation Annual Report; 2014 Apr. Available at: <http://www.dentaquestfoundation.org/sites/default/files/annual_reports/Paths%20to%20Prevention.pdf>; [Accessed April 2020].

37. Dental Visits - Oral and Dental Health: FastStats Table 78. Atlanta, GA: Centers for Disease Control and Prevention, National Center for Health Statistics; 2017. Available at: <https://www.cdc.gov/nchs/fastats/dental.htm>; [Accessed July 2019].

38. Cole JR, Dodge WW, Findley JS, et al. Interprofessional collaborative practice: How could dentistry participate? J Dent Educ 2018;82(5):441–5. Available at: <http://www.jdentaled.org/content/82/5/441>; [Accessed October 2019].

39. Accountable Care Organizations (ACOs). Baltimore, MD: Centers for Medicare and Medicaid Services; 2020 Feb 11. Available at: <https://www.cms.gov/Medicare/Medicare-Fee-for-Service-Payment/ACO>; [Accessed April 2020].

40. Overview of Research on ACO Performance. Washington, D.C.: National Association of ACOs; 2018. Available at: <https://www.naacos.com/assets/docs/pdf/NAACOS-ACO-PerformanceResearchReport7.19.18edited.pdf>; [Accessed April 2020].

41. Wilson K. Connecting Mouth to Body: Integrating Oral Health into ACOs. Boston, MA: Community Catalyst; 2017 Sep 11. Available at: <https://www.communitycatalyst.org/blog/connecting-mouth-to-the-body-integrating-oral-health-into-acos#.XoS1lnJOlhF>; [Accessed April 2020].

42. White Paper Teledentistry: How Technology Can Facilitate Access to Care. Reno, NV: Association of State and Territorial Dental Directors; 2019 Mar. Available at: <https://www.astdd.org/docs/teledentistry-how-technology-can-facilitate-access-to-care-3-4-19.pdf>; [Accessed December 2019].

43. Fried JL, Maxey HL, Battani K, Gurenlian JR, Byrd TO, Brunick A. Preparing the Future Dental Hygiene Workforce: Knowledge, Skills, and Reform. J Dent Educ 2017;81(9):e45–52. Available at: <http://www.jdentaled.org/content/81/9/eS45>; [Accessed October 2019].

44. American Dental Hygienists' Association. What Can a Career in Dental Hygiene Offer You? Available at: <https://www.ada.org/~/media/ADA/Education%20and%20Careers/Files/hygienist_fact.pdf?la=en>; [Accessed July 2019].

45. Changes to Accreditation Standards for Dental Hygiene Education Programs. Available at: <https://www.adha.org/changes-to-accreditation-standards-for-dental-hygiene-education-programs>; [Accessed December 2019].

46. Tanner KG. Identifying Leadership Development Needs of Dental Hygienists Using an Online Delphi Technique (Dissertation). Ann Arbor, MI: ProQuest LLC; 2019. Available at: <https://search.proquest.com/openview/9cb59c1bc7f4a8f5d9c62e1f394ad45a/1?pq-origsite=gscholar&cbl=18750&diss=y>; [Accessed October 2019].

47. Berlinger N, Berlinger A. Cultural and Moral Distress: What's the Connection and Why Does it Matter? AMA J Ethics 2017;19(6):608–16. Available at: <https://journalofethics.ama-assn.org/sites/journalofethics.ama-assn.org/files/2019-07/msoc1-1706.pdf>; [Accessed July 2019].

48. Hainla, L. The Top 5 Patient Healthcare Trends in 2018. Dreamgrow; 2018 Jul 9. Available at: <https://www.dreamgrow.com/21-social-media-marketing-statistics/>; [Accessed July 2019].

49. Thompson, J. The Top 5 Patient Trends in 2019. Patient Value Journey (Blog Post). ReferralMD; 2019. Available at: <https://getreferralmd.com/2019/01/the-top-5-patient-healthcare-trends-for-2019/>; [Accessed July 2019].

50. 63 Fascinating Google Search Statistics. SES Tribunal; 2018 Sep 26. Available at: <https://seotribunal.com/blog/google-stats-and-facts/>; [Accessed February 2020].

51. Drees J. Google receives more than 1 billion health questions every day. Health IT; 2019 Mar 11. Available at: <https://www.beckershospitalreview.com/healthcare-information-technology/google-receives-more-than-1-billion-health-questions-every-day.html>; [Accessed February 2020].

52. Mulin R. PwC Report on the Impact of Social Media in Healthcare (Blog Post). HealthIT Answers; 2012. Available at: <http://www.hitechanswers.net/social-media-likes-healthcare/>; [Accessed July 2019].

53. Tan SS, Goonawardene N. Internet health information seeking and the patient-physician relationship: A systematic review. J Med Internet Res 2017;19(1):e9. Available at: <https://www.ncbi.nlm.nih.gov/pmc/articles/PMC5290294/>; [Accessed February 2020].

54. Warden C. 30 Outstanding Statistics & Figures on How Social Media Has Impacted the Health Care Industry (Blog Post). Referral MD; n.d. Available at: < https://getreferralmd.com/2017/01/30-facts-statistics-on-social-media-and-healthcare/>; [Accessed July 2019].

55. Risk Communication. Atlanta, GA: Centers for Disease Control and Prevention, Gateway to Health Communication & Social Marketing Practice; 2019 Mar 19. Available at: <http://www.cdc.gov/healthcommunication/risks/index.html>; [Accessed July 2019].

56. Resnick L. Making health decisions. Mindsets, numbers, and stories (Blog Post). Harvard Health Publications, Harvard Medical School, Harvard Health Blog; 2011. Available at: <http://www.health.harvard.edu/blog/making-health-decisions-mindsets-numbers-and-stories-201112123946>; [Accessed July 2019].

57. Ellis LD. The Need for Effective Risk Communication Strategies in Today's Complex Information Environment. Harvard T. H. Chan School of Public Health; 2018 Jan 5. Available at: <https://www.hsph.harvard.edu/ecpe/effective-risk-communication-strategies/>; [Accessed February 2020].

58. Strategy 61: Shared Decisionmaking. Agency for Healthcare Research and Quality; 2017 Oct. Available at: <https://www.ahrq.gov/cahps/quality-improvement/improvement-guide/6-strategies-for-improving/communication/strategy6i-shared-decision-making.html>; [Accessed February 2020].

ADDITIONAL RESOURCES

All Eyes Engaged: National Interprofessional Initiative on Oral Health (NIIOH), 2012 Symposium, Denta Quest, 2014—YouTube video
http://www.niioh.org/symposium-oral-health-and-primary-care
Oral Health Atlas
https://www.fdiworlddental.org/resources/oral-health-atlas/oral-health-atlas-2015
Schoolhouse Rock—How a Bill Becomes a Law—YouTube video
https://www.youtube.com/watch?v=Otbml6WIQPo
Summary of HIPPA Privacy Rule
https://www.hhs.gov/hipaa/for-professionals/privacy/laws-regulations/index.html

10

Cultural Competence

Faizan Kabani and Christine French Beatty

OBJECTIVES

1. Describe key demographic, social, and cultural shifts and trends influencing oral health among culturally diverse groups in the United States (U.S.).
2. Describe oral health disparities in the nation and relate them to the diversity of the population.
3. Describe the components of culture and how culture is formed, and explain how culture affects health.
4. Explain the importance of culture and cultural competence in relation to oral health care.
5. Describe the role of federal and state guidelines and requirements in relation to cultural competence in health care.
6. Describe, compare, and contrast models that are used in the development of cultural competence.

7. Describe, compare, and contrast models that can be used to apply strategies and approaches that enhance cross-cultural encounters and cross-cultural communication in oral healthcare settings.
8. Describe, compare, and contrast patient- and-family-centered care and cultural competence; discuss the role and responsibility of the dental hygienist with respect to cultural competence and the provision of culturally competent oral health care.
9. Describe health literacy and its relationship to culture, cultural competence, and oral health; explain the role of the dental hygienist in improving health literacy and describe culturally competent ways to increase health literacy of the population.

OPENING STATEMENTS: The Role of Culture in the Status and Future of Oral Health

- Closing the gap on oral health disparities among diverse cultural groups will lead to better oral health for our nation and is a responsibility of all healthcare providers.[1]
- Race, ethnicity, socioeconomic status (SES) levels, disability, national origin, religion, sex, gender identity, sexual orientation, language, age, and other cultural factors are powerful social determinants of oral health status, access to oral healthcare services, and quality of oral health care.[2]
- Providing culturally and linguistically appropriate services (CLAS) contributes to reducing health disparities and inequities.[3]
- We must commit ourselves to contributing to the establishment of a society in which respect for human dignity and equality are valued.[1]
- There are important variations among and within people from the same country or culture,[3] and there are cultural variations among generations.[4]
- Profound oral health disparities exist in the U.S., with children from low-income families and other vulnerable populations facing up to two times the rate of dental caries experience and untreated tooth decay compared with their more affluent peers.[1]
- Two of the five overarching goals of *Healthy People 2030* relate to culture; they are (1) to eliminate health disparities, achieve health equity, and attain health literacy to improve the health and well-being for all and (2) to create social, physical, and economic environments that promote attaining full potential for health and well-being for all.[5]
- A common goal for all oral health professionals is to provide the best oral care to all patients, which involves identifying ways to prevent and control oral diseases and conditions for members of all cultural groups.[1]

TODAY'S EVOLVING DIVERSE POPULATION

The U.S. is highly diverse as evidenced in neighborhoods, schools, and communities. Diversity extends to integral parts of our existence such as race, culture, SES, language, religion, veteran status, and national origin, to name a few. Diversity also extends to lifestyles, traditions, personal and family histories, ages, abilities, and other dimensions that constitute who we are. In most communities, multiple languages are spoken in schools, workplaces, and homes. All these components are fundamental in interpersonal interactions and community relationships.

In the past, societies primarily had a monocultural and monolingual, assimilation-based perspective. People were expected to give up the values, norms, and beliefs of their societies of origin in favor of new opportunities.[6] Over the years, our nation has transitioned from a "melting pot" to a "salad bowl" paradigm that focuses on valuing and celebrating unique identities.[6] **Cultural diversity** in the U.S. is more realistically an intricate and interdependent mosaic, consisting of diverse unique identities that all contribute to the larger contemporary "American" identity.[6]

The concept of pluralism encompasses acceptance and respect. It means understanding that each individual is unique and recognizing our individual differences. These dissimilarities can be along the various cultural dimensions of race, ethnicity, gender, sexual orientation, SES, age, physical abilities, religious

TABLE 10.1 Distribution and Percentage Change of Race and Ethnicity in the U.S. Population, by Sex, 2010 to 2018

Race/Ethnicity (Percent in 2018)	PERCENT CHANGE	
	Male	Female
White, NHL[a] (60,4%)	0.4	−0.2
Black or African American, NHL[a] (12.5%)	8.2	7.5
American Indian and Alaskan Native, NHL[a] (0.7%)	6.6	7.0
Asian, NHL[a] (5.7%)	28.0	27.5
Native Hawaiian or Other Pacific Islander, NHL[a] (0.2%)	17.7	18.2
Multiracial, NHL[a] (2.2%)	28.2	25.7
Hispanic or Latino (18.3%)	18.0	19.2

[a]Not Hispanic or Latino.
(From Jordan J, Iriondo J. Population Estimates Show Aging Across Race Groups Differs (Tables 2b, 2c). Washington, DC: U.S. Census Bureau; June 2019. Available at: <https://www.census.gov/newsroom/press-releases/2019/estimates-characteristics.html>; [Accessed July 2019].)

beliefs, political beliefs, or other ideologies. Respect for diversity involves the exploration of these differences in a safe, positive, and nurturing environment. It is about moving beyond simple tolerance to embracing and celebrating the rich dimensions of diversity contained within each individual.[7]

The U.S. has continued to become more multiracial, multicultural, multigenerational, and multilingual. According to U.S. Census Bureau estimates, all minority populations outgrew the non-Hispanic white population from 2010 to 2018.[8] Table 10.1 presents the racial/ethnic population distribution in 2018 and the percentage change from 2010 to 2018.[8]

More important is the increase in members of the population who speak a language other than English at home. Self-reported data from the American Community Survey conducted in 2017 by the Census Bureau revealed that an estimated one in five (21.8%) U.S. residents speak a foreign language at home, which has reportedly doubled over the last three decades[9] (Table 10.2). In the five largest American cities, nearly half (48.2%) of residents speak a foreign language at home[9], and, of those who do, 39% self-reported that they speak English "less than very well."[9] These data vary by state with a range of 2% to 44%.[9] However, more than 20% of the population in more than one fourth of the states speaks a foreign language at home, and these data represent an increase in all except six states.[9]

Race, ethnicity, and cultural differences have great significance for all who live in the U.S. There continue to be efforts by individuals, communities, and organizations in both civil society and government entities to promote concepts of cultural competence, cultural diversity, cultural sensitivity, cultural pluralism, and multiculturalism. These inclusive ideas are being incorporated into health care, business, education, and governmental policies. In health care these concepts have implications for how health care is delivered to clients and communities whose cultures and languages vary from those of their healthcare providers.[7] The clients may have different beliefs, values, attitudes, behaviors, and other cultural characteristics.

Three reasons for a healthcare provider to be in the constant pursuit of cultural competence are (1) the societal realities of a changing world, (2) the influence of culture and ethnicity on human growth and development, and (3) the challenge of providing effective and quality health care to all people.[1] These reasons indicate the need and importance of cultural competence, including the significance of developing the necessary skills to communicate and collaborate with persons of other cultures.

Oral Health Disparities of a Diverse Population

In 2000, *Oral Health in America: A Report of the Surgeon General* was published; it is focused on oral health issues. The report served as a reminder that in spite of significant improvements in oral health during the 20th century, serious challenges remained, significant oral health issues still existed, and profound disparities in oral health endured.[1] Two more recent national reports, *Advancing Oral Health in America*[10] and *Improving Access to Oral Health Care for Vulnerable and Underserved Populations*,[11] both published in 2011, reinforced the facts of continuing significant oral health issues and oral health disparities in our nation. In fact, two of the organizing principles of *Advancing Oral Health in America* were to improve oral health literacy and cultural competence and to reduce oral health disparities.[10] In 2020, the U.S. Surgeon General's office announced that an update to the report on oral health published in 2000 was underway.[12] This report will (1) document progress over the past two decades, (2) describe current key oral health issues, (3) articulate a strategic vision for the future, and (4) call upon all Americans to take action.[12]

Health disparities have been defined by the Centers for Disease Control and Prevention (CDC) as "preventable differences in the burden of disease, injury, violence, or opportunities to achieve optimal health that are experienced by socially disadvantaged populations. Populations can be defined by

TABLE 10.2 Linguistic Diversity in the United States: Percentage of Population That Speak a Language Other Than English at Home, 1980–2017

1980	1990	2000	2010	2017	Percent Growth 1980 to 2017
11.0%	13.8%	17.9%	20.6%	21.8%	98.2%

Note: Data for 1980, 1990, and 2000 are from decennial census; data for 2010 and 2017 are from American Community Survey data.
(From Zeigler K, Camarota SA. Almost Half Speak a Foreign Language in America's Largest Cities: Nationally, One in Five Spoke a Language Other than English in 2017. Washington, DC: Center for Immigration Studies; 2018 Sept. Available at: <https://cis.org/Report/Almost-Half-Speak-Foreign-Language-Americas-Largest-Cities>; [Accessed July 2019].)

factors such as race or ethnicity, gender, education or income, disability, geographic location (e.g., rural or urban), or sexual orientation."[13]

Special population groups, such as infants and young children, the poor, those living in rural areas, the homeless, persons with disabilities, racial and ethnic minorities, the institutionalized, and frail older adults, experience a greater burden of oral and craniofacial diseases.[1,14] Marked disparities also exist in access to oral health care and use of preventive services, each vital to the establishment and maintenance of optimal oral health.[1,14] It is understood in the health, medical, and dental communities that there is a critical need to eliminate disparities in oral health care among the diverse populations in the U.S.[1,14] In response to these issues, greater emphasis has been placed on efforts to increase access to oral health care to reduce disparities.[14]

Disparities in health status, including oral health, are compounded by reduced access to care. However, although increased use of healthcare services can reduce disease and contribute to improved health status, this is not the complete picture.[15] Powerful, complex relationships exist among health and biology, genetics, individual behavior, SES, the physical environment, discrimination, racism, literacy levels, and legislative policies in relation to health status.[2,15] These factors that influence an individual's or population's health are known as **determinants of health**.[13–15] (See Chapter 3 for a discussion of the determinants of health.)

In an attempt to reduce disparities, *Healthy People 2030* has emphasized these determinants of health, especially the social determinants, many of which are socially and culturally bound.[5,16] Culture has been shown to impact many of these determinants as they relate to oral health, including the workforce.[1,10,14,17]

The National Partnership for Action to End Health Disparities in collaboration with the U.S. Department of Health and Human Services (DHHS) Office on Minority Health (OMH) has suggested five actions for individuals and groups to address disparities in their communities[18] (Box 10.1). These actions reflect an advocacy role for oral health professionals, which is critical to be able to make a difference at the community level (Figure 10.1). The collaborating partners also developed a Toolkit for Community Action, which has practical ideas about how to carry out the suggested actions (see Additional Resources at the end of this chapter).

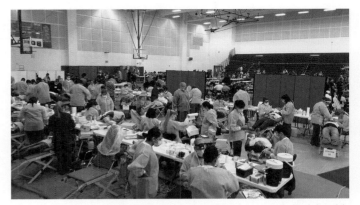

Fig. 10.1 A nonprofit collaborates with the state oral health program to bring healthcare services, including oral health care, to South Texas border towns along the United States-Mexico border. Various healthcare organizations and individuals in the state volunteer to provide free oral healthcare services to this underserved population. (Courtesy Christina Horton.)

CONSIDERING CULTURE

Healthcare access problems include several components. Two important factors are (1) an individual's perception of a given illness and (2) the decision to seek health care, both of which are influenced by culture.[19] A primary requirement in providing culturally sensitive health care is a basic knowledge of the health status and needs of the population groups being served.[19] Historically, many of the healthcare providers serving ethnic populations have been members of the same ethnic/racial groups.[20] However, there is a need for all healthcare providers to have multicultural skills to be able to deliver care to an increasingly diverse population.[20]

Healthcare providers traditionally have their own expectations about how health care should be delivered and how patients should respond to care. Yet, to be able to work effectively with a multicultural population, the healthcare workforce must alter their traditional ways of interacting with patients and communities.[14] To be able to impact determinants of health and thus reduce health disparities, they must be knowledgeable of and attentive to cultural differences and have the communication skills to be able to interact with members of different cultural groups.[7,20]

What Is Culture?

Culture is an integrated pattern of human behavior that includes thoughts, communications, languages, practices, beliefs, values, customs, courtesies, rituals, manners of interacting, roles, relationships, and expected behaviors of a racial, ethnic, religious, or social group, as well as the ability to transmit these to succeeding generations.[21] As such, culture involves a specific set of social, educational, religious, and professional behaviors, practices, and values that individuals learn and adopt while participating in groups with whom they usually interact daily.[7]

In common terms, culture is what we live every day, our daily cross-cultural interactions at work, school, or in our community. It is the lens through which we view the world and form our opinions, thoughts, aspirations, and goals. Culture is both inherent and learned; it is a shared way of interpreting the world.[7,22] Culture is simple yet complex, common yet unique,

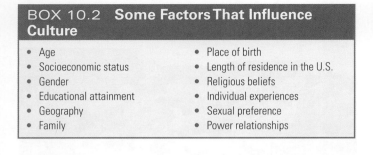

and constantly evolving based on life experiences.[7] Several factors that influence culture are listed in Box 10.2.

Why Consider Culture?

As the U.S. becomes a more racially and ethnically diverse nation, healthcare systems and oral healthcare providers need to respond to the wide diversity present in modern societies.[7,22] Cultural competence is necessary to be able to provide appropriate services to all individuals and communities. Given our modern technologies, it is also a skill we need for global survival. Historically, the challenges of insufficient cultural competence for cross-cultural collaboration go back to the earliest beginnings of humanity.

Every human culture teaches its members to value their beliefs, morals, and views as the best or ideal; unfortunately, in some cases, cultures teach that only their beliefs are acceptable. The resulting lack of cultural interchange and adaptation can lead to **ethnocentrism**—judging other cultures by one's own standards, not accepting other groups, and considering other cultures inferior.[23] Ethnocentrism can lead to making false assumptions about cultural differences, forming premature judgments, and producing divisions among members of different ethnicities, races, and religious groups in society.[23] Ethnocentric individuals believe that they are better than other individuals for reasons based solely on their heritage. Ultimately, ethnocentrism is related to problems of racism and prejudice.[23]

It is possible to incorporate culture into daily activities, such as reading, movies, television, social interactions, community events, and social outings. Exposure to multiple cultures has value to accomplish the following:

- Understand and appreciate the values, attitudes, and behaviors of others
- Avoid stereotypes and biases that can undermine efforts
- Focus on commonalities rather than differences
- Be able to develop and deliver services that are responsive to the individual needs of patients and clients

Effect of Culture on Health and Health-Related Factors

Health is culture-bound. This means that culture influences the conceptions, perceptions, expressions, and approaches to health, healthy living, sickness, and disabilities at both the individual and community levels[15,19] (see Guiding Principles). Also influenced are attitudes toward healthcare providers and facilities and how health information is communicated.[22] Culture can even influence healthcare-seeking behaviors, preferences for traditional versus nontraditional approaches to health care, and perceptions regarding the role of family in health care.[19,24]

Some of these issues relate to oral health, as well as overall health. Although there are standards of care that are followed during patient treatment, individualizing patient care necessitates understanding these cultural differences in relation to health issues.[24] This approach is considered a hallmark of quality of care.

A cross-cultural approach to health care and healing does not eliminate the foundation of Western medical methods. Instead it expands and enhances the ways that we assess and deliver healthcare services by acknowledging, appreciating, and incorporating the beliefs, values, rituals, symbols, and standards of conduct that belong to the community with whom we work and that may also affect their health status. The cross-cultural approach combines medical science and social science for the most effective outcomes.[24]

CULTURAL COMPETENCE

Cultural competence is critical to reducing oral health disparities and improving access to high-quality oral health care.[22] **Cultural competence** in health care is the ability of healthcare providers to deliver services that are appropriately sensitive to the health beliefs, practices, and cultural and linguistic needs of diverse patients.[7] It is a developmental process that occurs over an extended period. Thus, one can be at various levels of awareness, knowledge, and skills along a continuum in relation to applying cultural competence in different settings and situations.[22]

Included in cultural competence is the adaptation of oral health promotion, disease prevention, and clinical oral health services to meet the patient's social, cultural, and linguistic needs.[1,10,11,20] All people must be treated in a culturally competent manner, but this may provide a greater challenge for specific groups, such as children, older adults, people with disabilities, unfamiliar ethnic and racial groups, and low-SES groups (Figures 10.2 and 10.3).[1,10,11,20] Because culture impacts oral health and oral health care, cultural awareness and competence among oral health professionals is paramount.[20]

Community and Organizational Cultural Competence

Cultural competence is required at the individual, organization, and community levels.[20,22] When applied as a framework,

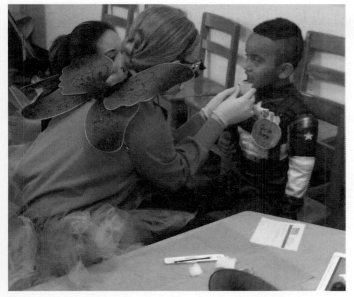

Fig. 10.2 Cultural competence is critical to dental hygiene students as they provide preventive services and oral health education to children and their families in a nonprofit preschool that serves a multiracial, low-income population whose primary language and English proficiency vary. (Courtesy Schelli Stedke.)

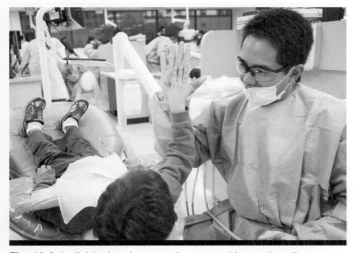

Fig. 10.3 Individuals who must be treated in a culturally competent manner include children, older adults, and individuals with disabilities. (Courtesy Hannah Olowokere.)

cultural competence enables the healthcare system and associated agencies and organizations to understand the needs of groups accessing health information and health care.[25] Although it is important to focus on the culture of a group or community, it is also imperative to keep in mind that cultural competence involves learning useful general information about a culture while at the same time being aware and open to variations and individual differences.[4] One should not fall into the trap of stereotyping all members of a specific ethnic or cultural group; people are individuals even when they share commonalities.[4]

The National Institute on Minority Health and Health Disparities (NIMHD) is the nation's leading governmental research agency specifically charged with the responsibility to improve minority health and eliminate health disparities. The NIMHD has identified the following broad strategies to improve cultural competence and promote health equity in our nation:[26]

1. Ensure a strategic focus on communities at greatest risk.
2. Reduce disparities in access to quality health care.
3. Increase the capacity of the prevention workforce to identify and address disparities.
4. Support research to identify effective strategies to eliminate health disparities.
5. Standardize and collect data to better identify and address disparities.

The NIMHD has identified ways that state and local health departments; businesses and employers; healthcare systems, organizations, insurers, and clinicians; academic institutions; community organizations; and individuals and families can assist in carrying out these recommendations.[26] To meet these goals, organizations must have the capacity to value diversity, conduct self-assessment, manage the dynamics of differences, acquire and institutionalize cultural knowledge, and adapt to diversity in the cultural contexts of the communities they serve.[25,26] In addition, organizations must incorporate principles of cultural competence in all aspects of policymaking, administration, practice, and service delivery and systematically involve clients, stakeholders, and the communities being served.[22,25,26]

As a result of the public health community calling for increased efforts to develop cultural competence in the national and local infrastructure over the last several decades,[1,10,11,20,26] oral healthcare professional societies and organizations have developed standards, initiatives, or statements encouraging, and in some cases requiring, the workforce they serve to be culturally sensitive and culturally competent in relation to oral health care.[27–33] In addition, because of efforts over the last few decades, many materials for this type of training are now available from the National Center for Cultural Competence (NCCC), the OMH of the DHHS, and other recognized national organizations and universities. The NCCC has a training site, the Curricula Enhancement Module Series, as well as multiple other resources and links to other sites and resources on their website. The OMH has resources on health disparities, health conditions and issues affecting racial and ethnic minorities, and organizational capacity-building to improve healthcare services for minority groups. See References and Additional Resources at the end of this chapter for supplemental materials.

Current and future leaders require specific training to increase their cultural competence to improve the health of our nation. National initiatives have called for greater emphasis on cultural competence in overall and oral health professional education programs. Several accrediting agencies for healthcare training programs, including the Association of Medical Colleges, the Association of Schools of Public Health, the American Association of Colleges of Nursing, and the National Association of Social Workers, have all developed competency documents that highlight strategies and resources for training students in cultural competence.[34–36] This significant initiative is also integrated into oral healthcare education programs. The Commission on Dental Accreditation includes cultural competence as an integral part of accreditation standards to dental, dental hygiene, dental therapy, and dental assisting education program.[29]

BOX 10.3   National Standards for Culturally and Linguistically Appropriate Services in Health and Health Care (National CLAS Standards), 2013

Principal Standard

1. Provide effective, equitable, understandable and respectful quality care and services that are responsive to diverse cultural health beliefs and practices, preferred languages, health literacy, and other communication needs.

Governance, Leadership, and Workforce

2. Advance and sustain organizational governance and leadership that promotes CLAS and health equity through policy, practices, and allocated resources.
3. Recruit, promote, and support a culturally and linguistically diverse governance, leadership, and workforce that are responsive to the population in the service area.
4. Educate and train governance, leadership, and workforce in culturally and linguistically appropriate policies and practices on an ongoing basis.

Communication and Language Assistance

5. Offer language assistance to individuals who have limited English proficiency and/or other communication needs, at no cost to them, to facilitate timely access to all health care and services.
6. Inform all individuals of the availability of language assistance services clearly and in their preferred language, verbally and in writing.
7. Ensure the competence of individuals providing language assistance, recognizing that the use of untrained individuals and minors as interpreters should be avoided.

8. Provide easy-to-understand print and multimedia materials and signage in the languages commonly used by the populations in the service area.

Engagement, Continuous Improvement, and Accountability

9. Establish culturally and linguistically appropriate goals, policies, and management accountability and infuse them throughout the organization's planning and operations.
10. Conduct ongoing assessments of the organization's CLAS-related activities and integrate CLAS-related measures into assessment measures and continuous quality improvement activities.
11. Collect and maintain accurate and reliable demographic data to monitor and evaluate the effect of CLAS on health equity and outcomes and to inform service delivery.
12. Conduct regular assessments of community health assets and needs and use the results to plan and implement services that respond to the cultural and linguistic diversity of populations in the service area.
13. Partner with the community to design, implement, and evaluate policies, practices, and services to ensure cultural and linguistic appropriateness.
14. Create conflict and grievance resolution processes that are culturally and linguistically appropriate to identify, prevent, and resolve conflicts or complaints.
15. Communicate the organization's progress in implementing and sustaining CLAS to all stakeholders, constituents, and the general public.

(From The National CLAS Standards. Rockville, MD: U.S. Department of Health and Human Services, Office of Minority Health; 2013. Available at: <https://thinkculturalhealth.hhs.gov/assets/pdfs/EnhancedNationalCLASStandards.pdf>; [Accessed July 2019].)

Culturally and Linguistically Appropriate Services

The OMH of the DHHS published the latest version of the National Standards for Culturally and Linguistically Appropriate Services in Health and Health Care (**National CLAS Standards**) in 2013 (Box 10.3), the purpose of which was to "to advance health equity, improve quality, and help eliminate healthcare disparities by establishing a blueprint for individuals as well as health and healthcare organizations to implement culturally and linguistically appropriate services."[3,37] These standards include a broad definition of culture, including groups identified by geographic, religious, spiritual, biological, and sociological characteristics; a broad audience, including health and healthcare organizations; an explicit definition of health, including physical, mental, social, and spiritual well-being; and a broad scope of recipients, including all individuals and groups involved with health and healthcare organizations, not just patients and consumers.[3,37]

An implementation guide for the National CLAS Standards can be accessed from the OMH website to help federal and state health agencies, community healthcare systems and organizations, policymakers, national organizations, and others advance and sustain culturally and linguistically appropriate services within health and healthcare organizations[3,37] (see Additional Resources at the end of this chapter). The CLAS standards are not legislated but are mandated in some cases for recipients of federal funds. State agencies have embraced the importance of cultural and linguistic competence since the initial standards were released. A number of states have proposed or passed legislation pertaining to training in cultural competence for one or more segments of the state's health professionals, and at least

six states have mandated some form of cultural and linguistic competence for either all or a component of their healthcare workforce.[3,37]

Developing Cultural Competence

Models and curricula abound that describe how cultural competence is acquired for implementation in patient encounters, in organizations and systems, and in community outreach. Some of these models can be used also to evaluate the effectiveness of cultural competencies in these settings. The following are a few examples of models that can be implemented in various settings for cross-cultural encounters to ensure that culturally competent attitudes, knowledge, and behaviors are implemented when providing oral health care in a multicultural clinical or community setting.

Cultural Competence Education Model

The Cultural Competence Education Model is a conceptual model that focuses on the process of developing knowledge and skills relative to cultural competence in healthcare practices to be able to deliver quality care[38] (Figure 10.4). This model is designed as a tool to foster understanding, acceptance, and constructive relations between persons of various cultures. The model is framed on the following three areas of intervention:[38]

- Self-assessment/self-exploration: To become aware of one's own cultural heritage and increase acceptance of different values, attitudes, and beliefs.
- Knowledge: To understand that one culture is not intrinsically superior to another and to recognize individual and group differences and similarities.

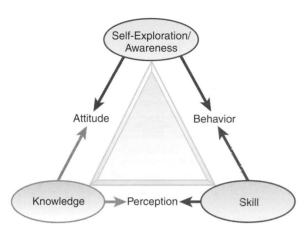

Fig. 10.4 Cultural Competence Education Model.

- Skill: To master appropriate and sensitive strategies and skills in communicating and interacting with persons from different cultures and to seek information about various cultures within a society.

As depicted in Figure 10.4, these three areas in various combinations impact attitude, perception, and behavior. Behaviors are adapted and implemented through self-exploration/awareness and skill development. The development of skills and knowledge affects perception about people of diverse cultures. Attitude is explored, enhanced, and broadened by self-exploration/awareness of and increased knowledge about diversity and the importance of culture to our daily lives. The value of self-assessment and self-exploration have been demonstrated in the development of cultural competence, and they are part of many current training programs and curricula.[39]

Purnell Model for Cultural Competence

The Purnell Model for Cultural Competence is a classic, holistic, complex organizing framework presented to understand culture as a means of guiding the development of cultural competence among healthcare teams of all disciplines who are providing care for multicultural populations in a variety of primary, secondary, and tertiary settings.[40,41] It can be used to learn about one's own culture and the cultures of patients, families, communities, and society. The model can be used in individual one-on-one settings, communities, or organizations.[40,41]

As depicted in Figure 10.5, the Purnell model has an outer rim that represents the global society, a second rim that represents the community, a third rim that represents the family, and an inner rim that represents the individual. The interior of the figure contains 12 cultural domains that are not intended to stand alone because they affect one another.[40,41] These cultural domains that make up the heart of the cultural experience and identity are described in Box 10.4. Oral healthcare providers can use this model to explore their own cultural beliefs, attitudes, values, practices, and behaviors, and to understand those of others. Within this model the development of cultural competence is conceptualized as an upward curve of learning and practice, moving through four levels of achievement of cultural competence[40,41] (see Figure 10.6).

Cultural Competence Continuum

Less complex than the Purnell model, the **Cultural Competence Continuum** is extensively referenced in cultural competence literature and widely used in training programs.[42] Originally presented by Cross et al.[43] in a 1989 monograph entitled *Towards a Culturally Competent System of Care, Volume 1*, the model was revised in 2004 by the NCCC.[42] It still serves as a guide today for systems and organizations to conduct self-assessment and to use the results to set goals and plan for meaningful growth.[42] The model can be used also by individuals to self-assess and plan for their own personal development in relation to cultural competence. Oral healthcare practitioners can use the descriptors of the steps on the continuum to challenge their growth toward becoming more culturally competent.

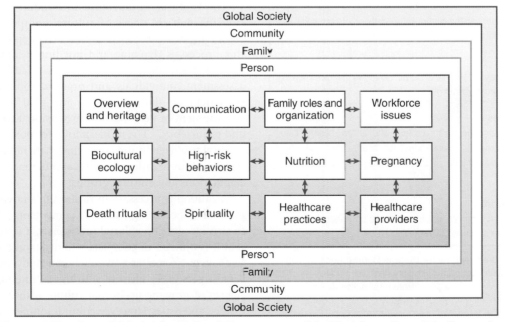

Fig. 10.5 The Purnell Model for Cultural Competence. (Modified from Purnell L. Transcultural healthcare: A culturally competent approach. Philadelphia: F.A. Davis; 2013.)

BOX 10.4 Twelve Cultural Domains in the Purnell Model for Cultural Competence

Overview/Heritage

Concepts related to country of origin and current residence, economics, politics, reasons for emigration, educational status, and occupations.

Communication

Concepts related to verbal and nonverbal variations in communication, use of language, and expression.

Family Roles and Organization

Concepts related to gender and sexual orientation roles, family structure and roles, social status, lifestyle and priorities, and developmental tasks of children and adolescents.

Workforce Issues

Concepts related to autonomy, acculturation, assimilation, gender roles, ethnic communication styles, individualism, and healthcare practices from the country of origin.

Biocultural Ecology

Includes variations in ethnic and racial origins, genetic predisposition, heredity, endemic and topographical diseases, and differences in how the body metabolizes drugs.

High-Risk Behaviors

Includes the use of tobacco, alcohol, and recreational drugs; lack of physical activity; nonuse of safety measures such as seatbelts and helmets; and high-risk sexual practices.

Nutrition

Includes having adequate food; the meaning of food; food choices, rituals, and taboos; and how food and food substances are used during illness and for health promotion and wellness.

Pregnancy and Childbearing

Includes fertility practices; methods for birth control; views toward pregnancy; and prescriptive, restrictive, and taboo practices related to pregnancy, birthing, and postpartum treatment.

Death Rituals

Includes how the individual and the culture view death, rituals and behaviors to prepare for death, burial practices, and bereavement behaviors.

Spirituality

Includes religious practices and the use of prayer, behaviors that give meaning to life, and individual sources of strength.

Healthcare Practices

Includes the focus of traditional versus alternative health care; biomedical beliefs; individual responsibility for health; self-medication practices; and views toward mental illness, chronicity, organ donation, and transplantation.

Healthcare Practitioner

Includes the status, use, and perceptions of healthcare providers; the gender of the healthcare provider may also have significance.

(From Purnell Model: Purnell Model for Cultural Competence by Larry Purnell. Silver Spring, MD: National Association of School Nurses; 2013. Available at: <https://www.nasn.org/nasn/nasn-resources/practice-topics/cultural-competency/cultural-competency-purnell-model>; [Accessed October 2020]; used with permission from Larry Purnell.)

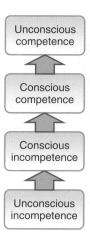

Fig. 10.6 Levels of achievement of cultural competence. (From Purnell Model: Purnell Model for Cultural Competence by Larry Purnell. Silver Spring, MD: National Association of School Nurses; 2013. Available at: <https://www.nasn.org/nasn/nasn-resources/practice-topics/cultural-competency/cultural-competency-purnell-model>: [Accessed October 2020].)

The Cultural Competence Continuum is based on a foundational definition of cultural competence, also originally developed by Cross et al. and modified by the NCCC, that describes the following necessary characteristics of culturally competent individuals and organizations:[42]

- Have a defined set of values and principles, and demonstrate behaviors, attitudes, policies, and structures that enable them to work effectively cross-culturally.
- Have the capacity to (1) value diversity, (2) conduct self-assessment, (3) manage the dynamics of difference, (4) acquire and institutionalize cultural knowledge, and (5) adapt to diversity and the cultural contexts of communities they serve.
- Incorporate the above in all aspects of policymaking, administration, and practice and service delivery, systematically involving consumers, families, and communities.

The Cultural Competence Continuum involves a progression through six stages of cultural competence development, which are described in Box 10.5.[42] As depicted in Figure 10.7, this process is dynamic and not linear, although it has been described and depicted by some as a ladder.[42] Through self-assessment, individuals and organizations can evaluate their placement on the continuum and plan for progress toward development of personal and professional cultural competence and proficiency.[42] The model allows for positive progress even if cultural proficiency and competence are not achieved. Also, it is possible to be at different stages at different times with different populations and cultural groups.

A caution is necessary in relation to studying cultures for the purpose of becoming culturally competent. Although the goal is to strive to develop cultural proficiency, it is important to realize that it is difficult to completely understand a culture that is not one's own. No matter how much you study another culture, you cannot personally identify with the culture nor share the experiences of growing up in that culture with its shared traditions, history, and issues. However, cultural competence can be achieved over time.

BOX 10.5 Description of the Six Stages of the Cultural Competence Continuum

Cultural Destructiveness

Characterized by attitudes, policies, structures, and practices within a system or organization that are destructive to a cultural group.

Cultural Incapacity

The inability of systems and organizations to respond effectively to the needs, interests, and preferences of culturally and linguistically diverse groups; characteristics include but are not limited to institutional or systemic bias, discriminatory practices, disproportionate allocation of resources, and lower expectations for some cultural, ethnic, or racial groups.

Cultural Blindness

An expressed philosophy of viewing and treating all people as the same; characteristics may include encouragement of assimilation by policies or personnel, ignorance of cultural strengths, attitudes that blame consumers for their circumstances, minimal to no value toward cultural and linguistic competence, lack of workforce diversity, and few structures and resources dedicated to acquiring cultural knowledge.

Cultural Precompetence

A level of organizational awareness of their strengths and areas for growth to respond effectively to culturally and linguistically diverse populations; characteristics include but are not limited to expressly valuing the delivery of high-quality services and supports to culturally and linguistically diverse populations, commitment to human and civil rights, hiring practices that support a diverse workforce, tendency for token representation on governing boards, and no clear plan for achieving organizational cultural competence.

Cultural Competence

Demonstration by systems and organizations that exemplify cultural competence demonstrate an acceptance and respect for cultural differences and they practice the following:

- Create a mission statement for the organization that articulates principles, rationale, and values for cultural and linguistic competence in all aspects of the organization.
- Implement specific evidence-based practices, policies, and procedures that integrate cultural and linguistic competence into each core function of the organization.
- Implement policies and procedures to recruit, hire, regularly train, and maintain a diverse and culturally and linguistically competent workforce.
- Dedicate resources for both individual and organizational self-assessment and development of cultural and linguistic competence.
- Develop the capacity to collect and analyze data using variables that have a meaningful impact on culturally and linguistically diverse groups.
- Exercise principles of community engagement that result in the reciprocal transfer of knowledge and skills between all collaborators, partners, and key stakeholders.

Cultural Proficiency

Systems and organizations hold culture in high esteem, use this as a foundation to guide all of their endeavors, and practice the following:

- Continue to add to the knowledge base within the field of cultural and linguistic competence by conducting research and developing new treatments, interventions, and approaches for health and health care in policy, education, and the delivery of care.
- Employ faculty and/or staff, consultants, and consumers with expertise in cultural and linguistic competence in health and healthcare practice, education, and research.
- Publish and disseminate promising and evidence-based health and healthcare practices, interventions, training, education models, and health promotion materials that are adapted to the cultural and linguistic contexts of populations served.
- Support and mentor other organizations as they progress along the cultural competence continuum.
- Actively pursue resource development to continually enhance and expand the organization's capacities in cultural and linguistic competence.
- Advocate with, and on behalf of, populations who are traditionally unserved and underserved.
- Establish and maintain partnerships with diverse constituency groups, which span the boundaries of the traditional health and mental healthcare arenas, to eliminate racial and ethnic disparities in health and mental health.

(From Tawara D. Goode, National Center for Cultural Competence Georgetown University Center for Child and Human Development, University Center for Excellence in Developmental Disabilities, 2004 as adapted from: Cross T, Bazron B, Dennis K, Isaacs, M. Towards a Culturally Competent System of Care, Volume 1. Washington, DC: CASSP Technical Assistance Center, Center for Child Health and Mental Health Policy, Georgetown University Child Development Center; 1989. Included with permission of the Georgetown University National Center for Cultural Competence, Georgetown University Center for Child & Human Development, Georgetown University Medical Center.)

Various federal government and other agencies have focused resources on the development of a culturally competent workforce. Multiple resources are available for individual development of cultural competence and for training in cultural competencies in healthcare organizations. The NCCC has developed a number of educational self-assessment tools based on these and other models to help healthcare providers develop cultural competence and linguistic skills. See the References and Additional Resources at the end of this chapter.

CULTURALLY COMPETENT PATIENT CARE

Cross-cultural encounters often are challenging because they reflect situations that are unfamiliar to daily living and beliefs. They also can provide opportunities for personal growth and development in cultural competence (Figure 10.8).

Effective Cross-Cultural Communication

Cross-cultural communication is a key to successful cross-cultural encounters. **Cross-cultural communication** refers to the effective communication with someone of a different culture. The importance of patient communication and linguistic skills in relation to cultural competence and health outcomes has been emphasized in the literature.[7,10,25] It has also been reflected in the *Healthy People* initiative for decades and is embedded in the objectives in the Health Communication topic area of *Healthy People 2030*.[16,44,45] According to the report *Advancing Oral Health in America*, "As the U.S. population grows more diverse, more will need to be understood about the importance of cultural competence in communication. For example, the cultural and linguistic misunderstandings in health care can be a contributing factor to adverse events such as unnecessary emergency room visits and longer hospital stays."[10]

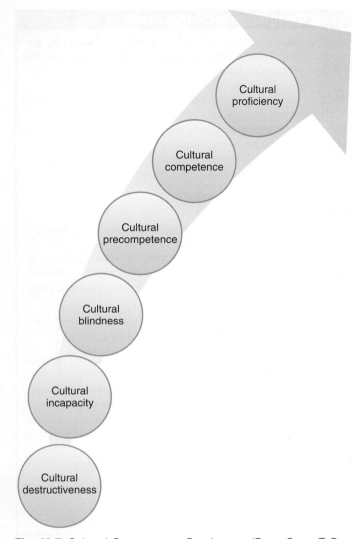

Fig. 10.7 Cultural Competence Continuum. (From Cross T, Bazron B, Dennis K, Isaacs M. Towards a Culturally Competent System of Care, Volume 1. Washington, DC: CASSP Technical Assistance Center, Center for Child Health and Mental Health Policy, Georgetown University Child Development Center; 1989.)

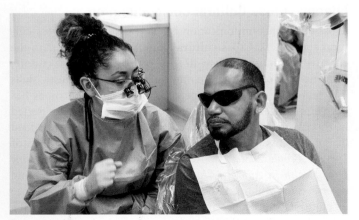

Fig. 10.8 Experiences with cross-cultural encounters in alternative practice settings can help dental hygienists develop cultural competence. (Courtesy Texas A&M College of Dentistry.)

Oral health professionals experience daily cross-cultural interactions with patients that can help them practice and refine their cross-cultural communication skills. In the process, one can learn about the way of life of individuals, families, and communities to better understand the cultural influences on their oral health.[2,10] Some actions to assist with effective cross-cultural communication are listed in the Guiding Principles.

GUIDING PRINCIPLES

Actions That Foster Effective Cross-Cultural Communication

- Communicate in a language that is clear and at the client's level of understanding; send clear messages and provide complete instructions.
- Learn another language if clients are non-English speaking or if they are unable to speak and are proficient in sign language; even learning some basic terminology will assist with communication and denotes respect, interest, and caring.
- Use translators when necessary.
- Use technology, such as assistive technology devices, as needed.
- Define any dental terminology; avoid jargon.
- Listen well to the client's questions and stories.
- Carefully observe the client's body language.
- Look beyond the superficial.
- Be patient, persistent, and, most important, flexible.
- Recognize your own cultural biases.
- Emphasize common ground; do not focus on differences but on similarities.
- Withhold judgment; accept others' differences.
- Empathize; treat each person as an individual.
- Use active listening.
- Do not assume understanding; ask for clarification.
- Always communicate in a respectful manner.

Linguistic competence can also be considered in relation to an organization. According to the NCCC, linguistic competence is defined as "the capacity of an organization and its personnel to communicate effectively, and convey information in a manner that is easily understood by diverse groups, including persons of limited English proficiency, those who have low literacy skills or are not literate, individuals with disabilities, and those who are deaf or hard of hearing."[25] Linguistic competence involves responding to the health literacy needs of the populations served. To be considered linguistically competent, organizations must have policies, structures, practices, procedures, and dedicated resources to support linguistic competence.[25]

Models of Communication for Cross-Cultural Encounters

Several effective models are described in the literature that can be helpful in improving cross-cultural communication to improve the management of cross-cultural encounters in healthcare settings. Such models can be used for training by organizations, for inclusion in health professions educational program curricula, and for self-development of cultural competence. Two of these are the LEARN Model (see Box 10.6)[46] and the RESPECT Model (see Box 10.7).[47] Both of these classic models apply specific behaviors and attitudes to the communication process during cross-cultural encounters and are still in use today.[48]

An explanatory model is a way of exploring the sociocultural context of health conditions with patients.[49] Kleinman

BOX 10.6 LEARN Model of Cross-Cultural Communication

Listen — with sympathy and understanding to the patient's perception of the problem.

Explain — your perceptions of the problem and your strategy for treatment.

Acknowledge — and discuss the differences and similarities between these perceptions.

Recommend — treatment while remembering the patient's cultural parameters.

Negotiate — agreement; strive to understand the patient's explanatory model so the treatment fits into their cultural framework.

(From Berlin E, Fowkes WA. A teaching framework for cross-cultural health care. West J Med 1983;39:934-938. Available at: <https://www.ncbi.nlm.nih.gov/pubmed/6666112>; [Accessed July 2019].)

BOX 10.8 Questions Suggested for Kleinman's Explanatory Model of Illness

1. What do you think caused your problem?
2. Why do you think it started when it did?
3. What do you think your sickness does to you?
4. How severe is your sickness? Do you think it will last a long time, or will it be better soon in your opinion?
5. What kind of treatment do you think you should receive?
6. What are the most important results you hope to receive from this treatment?
7. What are the chief problems your sickness has caused for you?
8. What do you fear most about your sickness?

(From Kandula N. The Patient Explanatory Model. Northwestern Now. Evanston, IL: Northwestern University; 2013 June 13. Available at <http://www.northwestern.edu/newscenter/stories/2013/06/opinion-health-blog-kandula-.html>; [Accessed October 2019].)

introduced the Kleinman Explanatory Model of Illness in the 1970s as a way to better understand how people view their illness in terms of how it happens, what causes it, how it affects them, and what will make them feel better.[50] Still in use today, this model consists of an individualized approach of asking the patient or client and family a series of what, why, how, and who questions to seek information relevant to the health condition (Box 10.8).[49] Especially recommended for application to multicultural healthcare encounters, it can also be applied to understanding the health concerns of all patients.[49] The wording and number of questions can be adapted according to the patient, the health condition, and the setting.[49] The model can be applied easily to oral conditions.

Another model similar to Kleinman's model is called the ETHNIC Model (Box 10.9).[51] Also still in use today, this model is especially helpful to use with a population that believes in alternative medicine, and it too can be adapted to oral health conditions.[52] Use of these or similar models by dental hygienists can increase communication and elicit responses, including culture-specific answers, to help in diagnosis, treatment planning, patient management, and motivation toward behavior change.[53]

All these models are designed for use in clinical encounters in private, community, and organizational systems to communicate with patients (Figure 10.9). They foster creativity when interacting with patients and families in diverse communities. Of particular importance to this chapter is their value when adapted for application to oral health care for multicultural

BOX 10.7 RESPECT Model of Cross-Cultural Communication

Rapport
- Connect on a social level.
- Seek the patient's point of view.
- Consciously attempt to suspend judgment.
- Recognize and avoid making assumptions.

Empathy
- Be empathic.
- Remember that the patient has come to you for help.
- Seek out and understand the patient's rationale for their behaviors or illness.
- Verbally acknowledge and legitimize the patient's feelings.

Support
- Ask about and try to understand barriers to care and compliance.
- Help the patient overcome barriers.
- Involve family members if appropriate.
- Reassure the patient you are and will be available to help.

Partnership
- Be flexible with regard to issues of control.
- Negotiate roles when necessary.
- Stress that you will be working together to address medical problems.
- Reinforce the partnership.

Explanations
- Use simple language, pictures, maps, and other means of explanation.
- Check often for understanding.
- Use verbal clarification techniques.
- Use the patient's language.

Cultural Competence
- Respect the patient and their culture and beliefs.
- Understand that the patient's view of you may be identified by ethnic or cultural stereotypes.
- Be aware of your own biases and preconceptions.
- Know your limitations in addressing medical issues across cultures.
- Understand your personal style and recognize when it may not be working with a given patient.

Trust
- Remember that self-disclosure may be an issue for some patients who are not accustomed to Western medical approaches.
- Take the necessary time and consciously work to establish trust.
- Fulfill promises.
- Follow through with commitments.

(From Welch M. Enhancing Awareness and Improving Cultural Competence in Health Care. A Partnership Guide for Teaching Diversity and Cross-Cultural Concepts in Health Professional Training. San Francisco, CA: University of California at San Francisco; 1998.)

BOX 10.9   ETHNIC Model of Cross-Cultural Communication

Explanation
- Patient's perception of the illness/problem.

Treatment
- Treatments, home remedies, and other medicines previously tried by the patient.

Healers
- Previous advice sought from alternative/folk healers, friends, or other people (nondoctors).

Negotiate
- Finding mutually acceptable options that do not contradict, but rather incorporate patient's beliefs.

Intervention
- Agreeing on an intervention that may include incorporation of alternative treatments, spirituality, healers, and other cultural practices.

Collaboration
- Collaborating with patient, family, other healthcare professionals, healers, and community resources.

(From Warren NS. Cultural and Spiritual Mnemonic Tools for use in Genetic Counseling. Chicago, IL: National Society of Genetic Counselors, Engelberg Foundation; 2010. Available at: <https://www.geneticcounselingtoolkit.com/pdf_files/Cultural%20and%20 Spiritual%20Mnemonic%20Tools%2011.06.09.pdf>; [Accessed July 2019].)

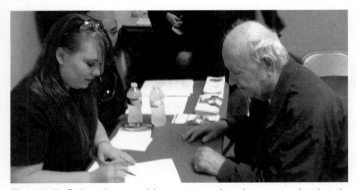

Fig. 10.9 Culturally sensitive cross-cultural communication is important during cross-cultural encounters such as this one with an indigent older adult client at a community soup kitchen. Homeless and low-income individuals without access to dental care receive an oral health intake, screening, oral health counseling, and a referral to connect them with oral health services in the community. (Courtesy Our Daily Bread, Denton, Texas.)

populations to increase cultural competence of oral healthcare practitioners and organizations.[51] Adaptation can be accomplished by rephrasing questions to make them specific to oral health conditions and oral healthcare situations.

Written Communications

Effective communication also involves the ability to use written communications well, which requires consideration of several factors. First is the literacy level. Written materials should be written at the literacy level of the intended audience, using vocabulary and sentence structure that is understandable, and including images as needed to help with understanding.[25,54] If individuals cannot read or have difficulty reading, they may require adaptation of written materials for delivery in the preferred mode of the audience being served.[25,54] This may involve the use of alternative communication methods such as audio, Braille, or enlarged print.[25,54] The second factor to consider is language. To maximize understanding, written materials should be in the preferred language of the population being served.[25,54]

Sometimes it is necessary to translate health communications, health forms, and other materials from English to another language. In this case, professional translators should be used who have the necessary writing skills, fluency in English and the other language, and cultural knowledge to produce a culturally and linguistically appropriate translation that is easy for the intended readers to understand and use.[55] The translator should also have some knowledge of the subject matter of the materials being translated.[55] Three methods of translation are suggested in the Centers for Medicare & Medicaid Services translation guidelines (Box 10.10). The best method to use should be based on available resources and may depend on the material being translated and its purpose.[55] For example, a full, formal back-translation may be required for legal documents, but simple one-way translations may be adequate for patient forms, informational leaflets, and oral health education materials.

BOX 10.10   Three Methods of Translating Written Materials

1. Create it separately in each language
   - Write an original version of the written material from scratch in each language
   - Not an actual translation
   - Good method to use if the material has not been created in English yet
   - Faster and possibly less costly if an English version is not available
2. One-way translation
   - English version is translated by a professional translator
   - Single version of the translation
     - Simplest and least expensive method
   - Should involve additional bilingual people who are familiar with the cultural and language patterns of the intended readers, to review, edit, and proofread the translated material
   - Multiple versions of the translation
   - Translated by different translators and reconciled to produce the final version
   - More expensive and time consuming
     - May be unnecessary if a single translation is done professionally with adequate review
3. Two-way or "back" translation
   - One person translates English version to another language, a second person translates it back to English, and a third person compares the two English versions and edits and rewrites the translated version as needed
   - More time consuming and more costly than one-way translation

(From McGee J. Toolkit for Making Written Material Clear and Effective, Section 5: Detailed Guidelines for Translation, Part 11: Understanding and Using the Toolkit Guidelines for Culturally Appropriate Translation. Washington, DC: Centers for Medicare & Medicaid Services; 2010. Available at: <http://www.cms.gov/Outreach-and-Education/Outreach/ WrittenMaterialsToolkit/Downloads/ToolkitPart11.pdf>; [Accessed July 2019].)

Patient- and Family-Centered Care

Effective communication is at the heart of **patient- and family-centered care** (PAFCC), a concept that has become the standard in the healthcare industry. In this approach, patients and their families are recognized as essential allies in achieving safe, high-quality health care. Patients are listened to, their perspectives and choices are honored, and their personal contexts are incorporated into the planning and delivery of healthcare services.[56] PAFCC is described in relation to individual patients, healthcare providers, and healthcare organizations or systems.[55] Patients are more active in consultations and treatment decisions. Healthcare providers are more mindful, informative, empathetic, and collaborative. Respect, compassion, concern, shared decision-making, and communication are seen as basic elements for PAFCC care.[56]

In addition, healthcare systems that focus on PAFCC do not burden providers with issues of productivity and overloaded schedules at the expense of quality care. Rather, organizational policies strengthen the patient-clinician relationship, promote communication about things that matter, help patients know more about their health, and facilitate patients' involvement in their own care.[57] PAFCC is evidence-based in its consideration of the patient's and family's preferences, goals, and situational needs[58] (Figure 10.10).

PAFCC and cultural competence have been compared; both aim to improve the quality of health care, although each emphasizes different aspects of quality.[59] The main goal of PAFCC care has been to provide individualized care with an emphasis on personal relationships. However, the primary aim of striving for cultural competence has been to increase health equity and reduce disparities. Nevertheless, at the core of both PAFCC and cultural competence is the emphasis on seeing the patient as a unique person. Both depend on the PAFCC approach and address individual patients' preferences and goals, thus complementing

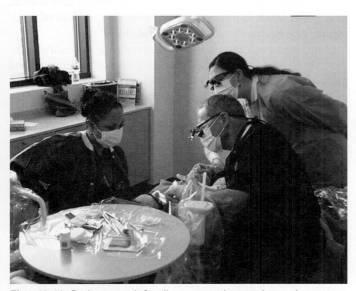

Fig. 10.10 Patient- and family-centered care is as important in community settings as it is in private settings. (Courtesy Christina Horton.)

each other in striving for quality of care. Box 10.11 presents the overlap between PAFCC and cultural competence at both the interpersonal and healthcare systems levels.[59]

The American Academy of Pediatric Dentistry (AAPD) developed a research brief and policy document in 2013 on PAFCC.[60] In this brief, the AAPD discussed principles of PAFCC and oral care in the context of cultural competence (see Box 10.12). These AAPD principles demonstrate that cultural competence is integral to the concept of PAFCC and that in some cases the family is an essential component of this concept.

The AAPD also expressed concern that the individualized, PAFCC approach required for cultural competence and PAFCC may be compromised by the changes in oral health care that are coming about as a result of the Affordable Care Act (ACA).[60] As the system becomes overburdened with additional numbers of patients on Medicaid, it will be important to have policies in place to protect patient- and family-centered practices. The role of oral health professional advocates working in private, corporate, and community-based settings includes encouragement of culturally competent and PAFCC at all levels.[29-33,61]

HEALTH LITERACY

Culturally competent oral health care involves taking into consideration the oral health literacy of the population being served.[62] Oral health literacy is important to the discussion of culturally competent oral health care because low oral health literacy is arguably associated with critical issues and problems[62-54] (see Guiding Principles).

BOX 10.12   Principles of Patient- and Family-Centered Oral Care

Respect and Cultural Competence
- Cultural sensitivity toward the family
- Respectfully considering the family's needs and preferences
- Advocating services with the purpose of building on the family's strengths

Integration and Coordination of Care
- Multidisciplinary teams working together to deliver care
- Successfully facilitating care among these multidisciplinary teams to improve collaborative efforts and access to care

Communication and Information Sharing
- Maintaining open communication among the healthcare team and between the team and family
- Enhancing health literacy

Quality of Care
- Providing high quality, evidence-based health care to patients and their families
- Gaining feedback from families and the healthcare team

Whole-Person and Comprehensive Care
- Ensuring the patient's physical and mental healthcare needs are met
- Placing an emphasis on health promotion

(From Patient Centered Care. Chicago, IL: American Academy of Pediatric Dentistry, Pediatric Oral Health Research & Policy Center; 2013. Available at: <http://www.aapd.org/assets/1/7/PatientCenteredCarePolicyBrief.pdf>; [Accessed July 2019].)

GUIDING PRINCIPLES

Critical Health Issues and Problems That Relate to Health Literacy

- Lower oral health status
- Greater oral health disparities
- Reduced oral health knowledge
- Higher risk of oral diseases and conditions
- Lower rates of adopting healthy behaviors
- Less frequent utilization of preventive oral health services
- Poorer outcomes and higher hospitalization rates
- Lower rates of dental insurance
- Higher overall oral healthcare costs
- Lower rates of participation in dental public health programs

According to the CDC, the ACA has defined **health literacy** as "the degree to which an individual has the capacity to obtain, communicate, process, and understand basic health information and services to make appropriate health decisions."[65] It is dependent on culture, context, knowledge, certain skills, SES, and other factors.[66] Health literacy is not just about knowledge. It involves having complex skills that are necessary to accomplish the following:[62]

1. Find health information and health services.
2. Process the meaning and usefulness of the information found.
3. Navigate the healthcare system, including filling out complex forms, locating providers and services, and making appointments.
4. Share personal information with providers, such as health history and current medications.
5. Engage in self-care and management of chronic disease.
6. Understand mathematical concepts such as probability and risk.
7. Apply numeracy skills such as reading nutrition labels and computing deductibles and copays.

Low health literacy is most commonly seen in individuals who are older adults; racial and ethnic minorities; the less educated, specifically those with less than a high school or general education development (GED) diploma; those with lower general literacy and numeracy skills; those of low SES; nonnative English speakers; and the medically compromised.[62] However, health literacy does not necessarily equate with literacy skills; a person may have outstanding literacy skills and not possess health literacy.[67,68] According to the Center for Health Care Strategies, an estimated 90 million Americans are considered to have low health literacy.[69] This means that a significant proportion of Americans struggle to understand fundamental health information such as health history forms, consent forms, home care and medication instructions, postoperative instructions, and drug labels.

In 2012, an initial collaborative effort took place between the dental and medical communities representing the public, private, and educational sectors to explore the issue of oral health literacy. A second health literacy workshop convened in December 2018, focusing on integrating oral and overall health through shared health literacy practices. Some of the discussion topics pertinent to health literacy were strategies to integrate health literacy at all levels of patient care, the role of health literacy in shaping public policy, organizing public health literacy campaigns, and training and educating health professionals on health literacy.[70] The continuing collaboration between these two communities at the practice, organizational, educational, and policy levels is important to solving the problem of inadequate oral health literacy in the population.[71]

Improvement of oral health literacy is a necessary component of interventions designed to improve oral health and reduce oral health disparities.[66] Knowing that many populations in the U.S. have low oral health literacy, the oral health literacy of the priority population must be considered to increase the potential for successful outcomes.[66] A population's understanding of and willingness to participate in oral health programs must be addressed.[66] Also, developing oral health messages at the appropriate literacy level and targeted to the language and cultural norms of specific populations will help to promote oral health literacy.[62,66]

A number of initiatives at the federal level demonstrate the current emphasis on health literacy. One is the inclusion of specific objectives related to improving health literacy in the topic area Health Communication of the *Healthy People* initiative, starting in the 2010 edition.[44,45] Another is a report published

BOX 10.13 Attributes of a Health Literate Organization

1. Has leadership that makes health literacy integral to its mission, structure, and operations.
2. Integrates health literacy into strategic and operational planning, quality improvement, goals, and measures.
3. Prepares the workforce to address health literacy issues and monitors progress.
4. Provides easy access to health information and services and help in finding the way in facilities.
5. Addresses health literacy in high-risk situations, such as emergency preparedness, crisis and emergency response, and clinical emergencies or transitions.
6. Communicates clearly available health services and costs.
7. Includes members of groups served in the design, implementation, and evaluation of health information and services.
8. Meets the needs of audiences with a range of health literacy skills while avoiding stigmatization.
9. Uses health literacy strategies in oral communication.
10. Designs and distributes print, audiovisual, and social media content that is easy to understand and act upon.

(From Attributes of a Health Literate Organization. Atlanta, GA: Centers for Disease Control and Prevention; 2019 October 17. Available at: <https://www.cdc.gov/healthliteracy/planact/steps/ndex.html>; [Accessed October 2019].)

in 2012 by the Institute of Medicine in which a workgroup identified 10 attributes of a health literate organization.[72] A **health literate organization** was defined as one that "makes it easier for people to navigate, understand, and use information and services to take care of their health."[72] The attributes were developed as guidelines for healthcare organizations to be able to make sure that the population gets the greatest benefit possible from the healthcare information and services provided (Box 10.13). The Office of the Associate Director for Communication at the CDC offers an interpretation of these 10 attributes to apply them to organizations engaged in public health efforts.[73]

The Plain Writing Act passed by the federal government in 2010 mandated that federal government agencies use plain language in written materials, with the goal of making health information clear for low literacy readers.[74] Important to the improvement of health literacy, **plain language** is clear, concise, well-organized, and follows other best practices appropriate to the subject or field and intended audience.[74] Plain language is not unprofessional writing or a method of "dumbing down" or "talking down" to the reader.[75,76] The use of plain language results in clear writing that tells the reader exactly what they need to know without using unnecessary words or expressions,[75,76] making it easier to understand and use health information.[75,76] Federal guidelines for plain language can be used by all healthcare organizations and workforce to assist in writing materials that consumers can understand.[75,76]

Another federal government initiative was the passage in 2000 of an executive order that required federal agencies to examine the services they provided, identify the need for services to those with limited English proficiency, and develop and implement a system to provide those services so persons with limited English proficiency could have meaningful access to them.[77] This has resulted in the development of various programs and resources, many of which are highlighted in this chapter.

The Office of Disease Prevention and Health Promotion endorses a Health Literate Care Model that weaves principles of health literacy throughout all aspects of the healthcare experience.[78] The model identifies essential competencies of health literacy among patients/families, healthcare teams, healthcare organizations/systems, and community partners. According to the model, the integration of health literacy across all dimensions (access, knowledge, and behavior) can lead to improved health outcomes.[78] Figure 10.11 presents an application of the Health Literate Care Model to oral health care that illustrates the multidirectional relationship among these essential stakeholders in achieving improved oral health outcomes. In this model, health literate healthcare systems and organizations use self-management support and link to supportive systems in addition to demonstrating the attributes of health literate organizations presented in Box 10.13.

In 2012, Sorensen et al.[79] reported on the development of a comprehensive conceptual and logical model of health literacy. The model identified 12 dimensions of health literacy, based on the four competencies of health literacy (accessing, understanding, appraising, and applying health information) in three domains (health care, disease prevention, and health promotion). According to the creators of the model, it can support the practice of health care, disease prevention, and health promotion by serving as a basis for developing interventions that will enhance health literacy.[79] The model can contribute also to the development of health literacy measurement tools for use in health literacy program evaluation and research.[79] It can be applied to oral health literacy (Table 10.3) to provide a framework for oral health practitioners to use in the process of assessing the oral health literacy needs of patients and clients and in designing programs and messages to improve their oral health literacy.

The expectation is that oral health literacy will continue to be a major strategy focused on the improvement of oral health and reduction of oral health disparities.[71] Both oral healthcare professionals and patients are key stakeholders in improving oral health literacy and need to work together to ensure effective communication.[62] Necessary skills must be developed to clearly communicate oral health information and teach patients and clients the health literacy skills they need to be wise oral health consumers and make sound oral health decisions. Some ways to accomplish this are listed in Box 10.14. Resources to help with this important task are included in the References and Additional Resources at the end of this chapter.

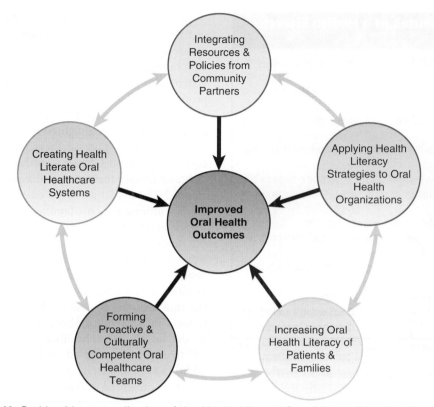

Fig. 10.11 Oral healthcare application of the Health Literate Care Model. (Modified from Koh H, Brach C, Harris LM, Parchman ML. A Proposed Health Literate Care Model Would Constitute A Systems Approach to Improving Patients' Engagement in Care. Health Affairs 2018;2:357-367; Health Literate Care Model. Washington, DC: Office of Disease Prevention and Health Promotion; 2019. Available at: <https://health.gov/communication/interactiveHLCM/>; [Accessed July 2019].)

	ACTION/COMPETENCE RELEVANT TO ORAL HEALTH INFORMATION			
Healthcare Domains	**Access/Obtain**	**Understand/Derive Meaning**	**Process/Appraise**	**Apply/Use**
Oral health care	Ability to access information on oral health issues	Ability to understand oral health information and derive meaning	Ability to interpret and evaluate oral health information	Ability to make informed decisions on oral health issues
Oral disease prevention	Ability to access information on risk factors for oral health	Ability to understand information on risk factors for oral health and derive meaning	Ability to interpret and evaluate information on oral health risk factors	Ability to make informed decisions on oral health risk factors
Oral health promotion	Ability to update oneself on determinants of oral health in the social and physical environment	Ability to understand information on determinants of oral health in the social and physical environment and derive meaning	Ability to interpret and evaluate information on oral health determinants in the social and physical environment	Ability to make informed decisions on social and environmental oral health determinants

TABLE 10.3   Model of Twelve Dimensions of Health Literacy Applied to Oral Health

(Modified from Sorensen K, Van den Broucke S, Fullam J, et al. Health literacy and public health: a systematic review and integration of definitions and models. BMC Public Health (online) 2012;12:80e. doi:10.1186/1471-2458-12-80. Available at: <http://www.biomedcentral.com/1471-2458/12/80>; [Accessed July 2019].)

BOX 10.14 Ways to Improve Oral Health Literacy of the Population

- Consider which information and services work best for different situations and people so they can act in an informed manner.
- Consider the best means of providing information and services for different situations and people.
- Develop health information materials at the appropriate literacy level and targeted to the language and cultural norms of specific populations.
- Use plain language to communicate health information.
- Use lay language rather than technical language to communicate health information.
- Convey information in the client's primary language, using a translator when needed.

- Verify understanding of what people are explicitly and implicitly asking for.
- Take time to check a patient's or client's recall and comprehension of new concepts.
- Provide assistance in learning basic numeric skills such as calculating doses or understanding concepts like risk.
- Aid people in finding providers and services and in filling out complex forms.
- Provide families with access to educational materials and support programs to help them understand and achieve treatment objectives and outcomes.
- Develop a workforce whose members represent the culture of the population being served or have been trained to be culturally competent.

SUMMARY

To become a culturally competent oral healthcare provider, it is important to apply cultural competence to all levels of oral health promotion and disease prevention, for example, individual, family, community, education, organizations, administration, programs, and policies. It is up to the oral healthcare delivery system and individual oral healthcare providers to value, implement, support, and foster cultural competence in every encounter made with a client and in all organizational decisions. This is true for dental hygienists in all roles and career paths, including clinician, health educator, educator, consultant, advocate, researcher, administrator, and entrepreneur, and practicing in all settings. As oral healthcare providers, it is vital to appreciate the key role that culture plays in the general and oral health of the public we serve. It is also important to develop cultural competence to enhance our ability to positively influence the overall and oral health of our patients and clients in both individual and group encounters in private, corporate, and community settings. We must not allow cultural barriers to limit our ability to meet the oral health needs of the public or reduce their opportunities to benefit from the services we can provide. This chapter reviews the concepts of culture and cultural competence and provides helpful guidelines and tools to understand culture and assess and develop cultural competence. Health literacy is discussed in relation to cultural competence as are ways to improve health literacy of the population.

APPLYING YOUR KNOWLEDGE

1. Choose an ethnicity or race other than your own. Apply the Purnell Model for Cultural Competence to understand the culture of the group you selected and to compare and contrast it to your own culture. Give a 10-minute presentation in class to describe what you learned.
2. Search online or find print journals that focus on cultural competence. Compare the journal articles and identify which you think will be the most useful in your interaction with patients of diverse cultures. Write a list of 10 points that you can share with your classmates.
3. Conduct a discussion in your class on the importance of cultural competence and discuss ways that you can apply culturally competent skills in your clinical setting and your community activities.
4. Think about folklore or ethnic traditions. Write down a family tradition or ethnic tradition practiced in your family. It is encouraged that you select health or healthcare-related traditions. Share with your class and learn from your peers the differences and similarities in traditions among diverse cultures.
5. Review the website of the NCCC at https://nccc.georgetown.edu/assessments/. Complete one of the self-assessments. Share with your class what you learned from completing the self-assessment.
6. Review the Toolkit for Community Action developed by the National Partnership for Action to End Health Disparities at https://minorityhealth.hhs.gov/npa/files/Plans/Toolkit/NPA_Toolkit.pdf. Study the ideas proposed to carry out the suggested actions to address health disparities in the community. Pick one and describe how you could implement it in your own community in relation to oral health.
7. Complete the online Cultural Competency Program for Oral Health Professionals developed by the Office of Minority Health to gain essential knowledge and skills on improving basic cultural and linguistic competencies (https://oral-health.thinkculturalhealth.hhs.gov/).

LEARNING OBJECTIVES AND COMPETENCIES

This chapter addresses the following community dental health learning objectives and competencies for dental hygienists that are presented in the ADEA Compendium of Curriculum Guidelines for Allied Dental Education Programs:

Learning Objectives
- Describe cultural diversity.
- Describe the effect culture has on oral health and dental hygiene care.

Competencies
- Providing health education and preventive counseling to a variety of population groups.

COMMUNITY CASE

You are the dental hygienist in a community/migrant health center. You have been asked by Dr. Nisa Rumi, the health center director, to participate in applying for a grant to fund an interdisciplinary project for Vietnamese older adult clients of the health center that includes a component of developing cultural competence of the workforce caring for this population. The grant will focus on health promotion and disease prevention. One of the key criteria of the grant is to take into consideration the use of alternative or folk medicine by the population served.

1. All of the following EXCEPT one are important factors to learn about the community to enhance the cultural competence of the proposed grant. Which is the EXCEPTION?
   a. Social network and social support
   b. Tooth loss
   c. Dietary patterns
   d. Ability and use of English language

2. The grant requires that a model be applied to the development of cultural competence of the oral healthcare workforce that will be caring for the population. In addition, progress of cultural competence development must be tracked and reported to the agency that is offering the grant. Which of the following models would be most suitable for these purposes?
   a. Cultural Competence Continuum
   b. Cultural Competence Education Model
   c. LEARN Model
   d. Purnell Model for Cultural Competence

3. You are planning interdisciplinary service training for the health professionals who will be gathering and recording the data collected for the grant. All of the following EXCEPT one are factors that need to be included in the training to enhance cross-cultural communication with the clients during data collection. Which is the EXCEPTION?

   a. Be patient and flexible to make clients comfortable
   b. Observe clients' body language to improve communication
   c. Use technical discipline-specific terminology during communication to avoid misunderstanding and confusion
   d. Listen well to clients' questions and stories to establish rapport

4. Oral healthcare personnel will be trained in culturally competent communication skills in an attempt to improve the use of preventive oral healthcare services by the population. The grant requires that a model be used to design and implement training strategies. Which of the following models would be most appropriate for this purpose and with this priority population?
   a. LEARN Model
   b. RESPECT Model
   c. Kleinman Explanatory Model of Illness
   d. ETHNIC Model

5. Oral health educational materials will need to be created for the priority population. Existing materials written in English are available for translation. The grant criteria limit the resources used for this purpose. Which of the following translation methods should be incorporated into the grant application?
   a. Development of materials in both English and Vietnamese
   b. Use of one-way translation
   c. Use of two-way translation
   d. Translation by an English-speaking staff member who is taking Vietnamese classes
   e. Use of verbal communication instead of translated written materials in this case

REFERENCES

1. U.S. Department of Health and Human Services. Oral Health in America: A Report of the Surgeon General. Rockville, MD: U.S. Department of Health and Human Services, National Institutes of Health, National Institute of Dental and Craniofacial Research; 2000. Available at: <https://www.nidcr.nih.gov/sites/default/files/2017-10/hck1ocv.%40www.surgeon.fullrpt.pdf>; [Accessed July 2019].

2. Social Determinants of Health: Know What Affects Health. Centers for Disease Control and Prevention. Atlanta, GA: U.S. Department of Health & Human Services; 2018. Available at: <https://www.cdc.gov/socialdeterminants/index.htm>; [Accessed September 2019].

3. National Standards for Culturally and Linguistically Appropriate Services (CLAS) in Health and Health Care. Rockville, MD: U.S. Department of Health and Human Services, Office of Minority Health; 2013. Available at: <https://thinkculturalhealth.hhs.gov/

assets/pdfs/EnhancedNationalCLASStandards.pdf>; [Accessed July 2019].

4. In: Coreil J, Mull JD, editors. Anthropology and Primary Health Care. New York, NY: Westview Press; 2018.

5. Healthy People 2030 Framework. What is the Healthy People 2030 Framework? Rockville, MD: Office of Disease Prevention and Health Promotion; 2020 Mar 29. Available at: <https://www.healthypeople.gov/2020/About-Healthy-People/Development-Healthy-People-2030/Framework>; [Accessed March 2020].

6. Setiloane KT. Beyond the melting pot and salad bowl views of cultural diversity: advancing cultural diversity education of nutrition educators. J Nutr Educ Behav 2016;48:664–8. Available at: <https://www.ncbi.nlm.nih.gov/pubmed/27324670>; [Accessed July 2019].

7. Cultural Respect. Bethesda, MD: National Institutes of Health, Office of Communications & Public Liaison; 2017. Available at: <https://www.nih.gov/institutes-nih/nih-office-director/office-communications-public-liaison/clear-communication/cultural-respect>; [Accessed July 2019].

8. Jordan J, Iriondo J. Population Estimates Show Aging Across Race Groups Differs. Washington, DC: U.S. Census Bureau; June 2019. Available at: <https://www.census.gov/newsroom/press-releases/2019/estimates-characteristics.html.>; [Accessed July 2019].

9. Zeigler K, Camarota SA. Almost Half Speak a Foreign Language in America's Largest Cities: Nationally, One in Five Spoke a Language Other than English in 2017. Washington, DC: Center for Immigration Studies; 2018 September. Available at: <https://cis.org/Report/Almost-Half-Speak-Foreign-Language-Americas-Largest-Cities.>; [Accessed July 2019].

10. Institute of Medicine of the National Academies, Committee on an Oral Health Initiative. Advancing Oral Health in America. Washington, DC: National Academies Press; 2011. Available at: <http://www.hrsa.gov/publichealth/clinical/oralhealth/advancingoralhealth.pdf>; [Accessed July 2019].

11. Institute of Medicine, National Research Council. Improving Access to Oral Health Care for Vulnerable and Underserved Populations. Washington, DC: National Academies Press; 2011. Available at: <https://www.hrsa.gov/sites/default/files/publichealth/clinical/oralhealth/improvingaccess.pdf>; [Accessed July 2019].

12. New Surgeon General's Report on Oral Health. Bethesda, MD: National Institute of Dental and Craniofacial Research; August 2020. Available at <https://www.nidcr.nih.gov/news-events/2020-surgeon-generals-report-oral-health>; [Accessed October 2020].

13. Health Disparities Among Youth. Atlanta, GA: Centers for Disease Control and Prevention; 2020. Available at: <https://www.cdc.gov/healthyyouth/disparities/index.htm>; [Accessed October 2020].

14. Fischer DJ, O'Hayre M, Kusiak JW, et al. Oral health disparities: a perspective from the National Institute of Dental and Craniofacial Research. Am J Public Health 2017;107(S1):S36–8. Available at: <https://www.ncbi.nlm.nih.gov/pmc/articles/PMC5497869/>; [Accessed September 2019].

15. The Determinants of Health. Health Impact Assessment. Geneva, Switzerland: World Health Organization; 2019. Available at: <https://www.who.int/hia/evidence/doh/en/>; [Accessed July 2019].

16. Report #7: Assessment and Recommendations for Proposed Objectives for Healthy People 2030. Healthy People 2020. Rockville, MD: Secretary's Advisory Committee for Healthy People 2030; 2019. Available at: <https://www.healthypeople.gov/sites/default/files/Report%207_Reviewing%20Assessing%20Set%20of%20HP2030%20Objectives_Formatted%20EO_508_05.21.pdf>; [Accessed July 2019].

17. American Dental Education Association. Statement of ADEA policy on diversity and inclusion. J Dent Educ 2017;81(7):893–894. Available at: <https://www.ncbi.nlm.nih.gov/pubmed/28668799>; [Accessed July 2019].

18. National Partnership for Action to End Health Disparities: Toolkit for Community Action. Department of Health & Human Services and National Partnership for Action to End Health Disparities; 2017. Available at: <https://www.minorityhealth.hhs.gov/npa/files/Plans/Toolkit/NPA_Toolkit_092617.pdf>; [Accessed July 2019].

19. Ejike CN. The Influence of Culture on the Use of Healthcare Services by Refugees in Southcentral Kentucky: A Mixed Study. Dissertations; 2017:Paper 116. Available at: <http://digitalcommons.wku.edu/diss/116>; [Accessed March 2020].

20. Cultural Competency Program for Oral Health Providers. Rockville, MD: U.S. Department of Health and Human Services, Office of Minority Health; 2019. Available at: <https://thinkcultural-health.hhs.gov/education/oral-health-providers>; [Accessed July 2019].

21. Culture. Merriam-Webster; 2019. Available at: <https://www.merriam-webster.com/dictionary/culture>; [Accessed July 2019].

22. Cultural Competence. Atlanta, GA: Centers for Disease Control and Prevention, National Prevention Information Network; 2015. Available at: <https://npin.cdc.gov/pages/cultural-competence#general>; [Accessed July 2019].

23. Logan S, Steel Z, Hunt C. Intercultural willingness to communicate within health services: investigating anxiety, uncertainty, ethnocentrism and help seeking behaviour. Int J Intercult Relat 2016;54:77–86. Available at: <https://www.sciencedirect.com/science/article/abs/pii/S0147176716302486>; [Accessed July 2019].

24. Hawley ST, Morris AM. Cultural challenges to engaging patients in shared decision making. Patient Educ Couns 2017;100(1):18–24. Available at: <https://www.ncbi.nlm.nih.gov/pubmed/27461943>; [Accessed July 2019].

25. Conceptual Frameworks/Models, Guiding Values and Principles. Washington, DC: National Center for Cultural Competence, n.d. Available at: <https://nccc.georgetown.edu/foundations/framework.php>; [Accessed July 2019].

26. Scientific Advancement Plan. Bethesda, MD: National Institutes of Health, National Institute on Minority Health and Health Disparities; 2019. Available at: <https://www.nimhd.nih.gov/about/overview/scientific-advancement.html>; [Accessed July 2019].

27. Introduction to the ASTDD Best Practices Project. Reno, NV: Association of State & Territorial Dental Directors; n.d. Available at: <http://www.astdd.org/introduction-to-the-project/>; [Accessed July 2019].

28. National Dental Hygiene Research Agenda. Chicago, IL: American Dental Hygienists' Association; 2016. Available at: <https://www.adha.org/resources-docs/7111_National_Dental_Hygiene_Research_Agenda.pdf>; [Accessed July 2019].

29. Current Accreditation Standards. Chicago, IL: Commission on Dental Accreditation; 2019. Available at: <https://www.ada.org/en/coda/current-accreditation-standards>; [Accessed July 2019].

30. ADEA Core Competencies for Graduate Dental Hygiene Education. Washington, DC: American Dental Education Association and American Dental Hygienists' Association; 2011. Available at: <https://www.adea.org/uploadedFiles/ADEA/Content_Conversion_Final/about_adea/governance/ADEA_Core_Competencies_for_Graduate_Dental_Hygiene_Education.pdf>; [Accessed July 2019].

31. ADEA Compendium of Curriculum Guidelines: Allied Dental Education Program [Revised Ed.]. Washington, DC: American Dental Education Association; 2016. Available at: <https://www.

adea.org/CADPD/Compendium-Revised-2016.pdf>; [Accessed July 2019].

32. American Dental Education Association. ADEA foundation knowledge and skills for the new general dentist. J Dent Educ 2017;81(7):848–52. Available at: <https://www.ncbi.nlm.nih.gov/pubmed/28668790>; [Accessed July 2019].

33. CDHC Education and Training. Chicago, IL: American Dental Association; 2019. Available at: <http://www.ada.org/en/public-programs/action-for-dental-health/community-dental-health-co-ordinators/cdhc-education-and-training>; [Accessed July 2019].

34. Cultural Competence Education for Students in Medicine and Public Health: Report of an Expert Panel. Washington, DC: Association of American Medical Colleges and Association of Schools of Public Health; 2012. Available at: <https://www.pcpcc.org/sites/default/files/resources/Cultural%20Competence%20Education%20for%20Students%20in%20Medicine%20%26%20Public%20Health.pdf>; [Accessed July 2019].

35. Cultural Competency in Baccalaureate Nursing Education. Washington, DC: American Association of Colleges of Nursing; 2008. Available at: <https://www.aacnnursing.org/Portals/42/AcademicNursing/CurriculumGuidelines/Cultural-Competency-Bacc-Edu.pdf>; [Accessed July 2019].

36. National Association of Social Workers: Standards and Indicators for Cultural Competence in Social Work Practice. Washington, DC: National Association of Social Workers (2003). Available at: <https://www.socialworkers.org/Practice/Practice-Standards-Guidelines>; [Accessed July 2019].

37. National CLAS Standards: Fact Sheet. Rockville, MD: U.S. Department of Health and Human Services, Office of Minority Health; n.d. Available at: <https://thinkculturalhealth.hhs.gov/pdfs/NationalCLASStandardsFactSheet.pdf>; [Accessed July 2019].

38. Wells SA, Black RM. Cultural Competency for Health Professionals. Bethesda, MD: American Occupational Therapy Association; 2000. Available at: <https://books.google.com/books/about/Cultural_Competency_for_Health_Professio.html?id=hN6nQAAACAAJ>; [Accessed February 2020].

39. Self-Assessments. Washington, DC: National Center for Cultural Competence; n.d. Available at: <https://nccc.georgetown.edu/assessments/>; [Accessed July 2019].

40. Purnell L. The Purnell model for cultural competence. J Transcult Nurs 2002;13(3):193–6. Available at: <https://www.ncbi.nlm.nih.gov/pubmed/12113149>; [Accessed July 2019].

41. Purnell L. The Purnell model for cultural competence. J Multicult Nurs Health 2005;11(2):7–15. Available at: <https://www.researchgate.net/profile/Larry_Purnell/publication/11265758_The_Purnell_Model_for_Cultural_Competence/links/00b495330173a7096d000000/The-Purnell-Model-for-Cultural-Competence.pdf>; [Accessed July 2019].

42. Goode TD. Cultural Competence Continuum (revised). Washington, DC: National Center for Cultural Competence, Georgetown University Center for Child and Human Development; 2004. Available at: <https://nccc.georgetown.edu/curricula/documents/TheContinuumRevised.doc>; [Accessed July 2019].

43. Cross T, Bazron B, Dennis K, et al. Towards a Culturally Competent System of Care, vol. 1. Washington, DC: CASSP Technical Assistance Center, Center for Child Health and Mental Health Policy, Georgetown University Child Development Center; 1989. Available at: <https://files.eric.ed.gov/fulltext/ED330171.pdf>; [Accessed July 2019].

44. Healthy People 2020. Rockville, MD: Office of Disease Prevention and Health Promotion; 2020. Available at: <https://www.healthy-people.gov/2020/>; [Accessed October 2020].

45. Healthy People 2010 Final Review. Hyattsville, MD: National Center for Health Statistics. Available at: <https://www.cdc.gov/nchs/data/hpdata2010/hp2010_final_review.pdf>; [Accessed March 2020].

46. Berlin E, Fowkes WA. A teaching framework for cross-cultural health care-application in family practice. West J Med 1983;39:934–8. Available at: <https://www.ncbi.nlm.nih.gov/pmc/articles/PMC1011028/>; [Accessed July 2019].

47. Welch M. Enhancing Awareness and Improving Cultural Competence in Health Care. A Partnership Guide for Teaching Diversity and Cross-Cultural Concepts in Health Professions Training. San Francisco, CA: University of California at San Francisco; 1998.

48. The L.E.A.R.N. and R. E.S.P.E.C.T. Models of Cross-Cultural Communication. Buffalo, NY: State University of New York, University at Buffalo, School of Public Health and Health Professions, Center for International Rehabilitation Research Information and Exchange; 2017. Available at: <http://cirrie-sphhp.webapps.buffalo.edu/culture/curriculum/resources/models.php>; [Accessed July 2019].

49. Davidoff F. Understanding contexts: how explanatory theories can help. Implement Sci 2019;14(23):1–9. Available at: <https://implementationscience.biomedcentral.com/articles/10.1186/s13012-019-0872-8>; [Accessed July 2019].

50. Kleinman A. Concepts and a model for the comparison of medical systems as cultural systems. Soc Sci Med Part B: Med Anthropol 1978;12:85–93. Available at: <https://www.ncbi.nlm.nih.gov/pubmed/358402>; [Accessed July 2019].

51. Levin SJ, Like RC, Gottlieb JW. ETHNIC: A framework for culturally competent clinical practice. Patient Care 2000;34(9 Special Issue):188–9.

52. Butler M, McCreedy E, Schwer N, et al. Improving Cultural Competence to Reduce Health Disparities (Comparative Effectiveness Reviews, No. 170, Table 21, Cultural competence models)Rockville, MD: Agency for Healthcare Research and Quality; 2016 Mar. Available at: <https://www.ncbi.nlm.nih.gov/books/NBK361115/table/ch5.t1/>; [Accessed July 2019].

53. Daugherty HN, Kearney RC. Measuring the impact of cultural competence training for dental hygiene students. J Dent Hyg 2017;91(5):48–54. Available at: <https://www.ncbi.nlm.nih.gov/pubmed/29118279>; [Accessed July 2019].

54. Brega AG, Barnard J, Mabachi NM, et al. (University of Colorado Anschutz Medical Campus, Colorado Health Outcomes Program). AHRQ Health Literacy Universal Precautions Toolkit, 2nd ed., AHRQ Pub No. 15-0023-EF. Rockville, MD: Agency for Healthcare Research and Quality; 2015 Jan.

55. Toolkit for Making Written Material Clear and Effective, Section 5: Detailed Guidelines for Translation, Part 11: Understanding and Using the Toolkit Guidelines for Culturally Appropriate Translation. Washington, DC: Centers for Medicare & Medicaid Services; 2010. Available at: <https://www.cms.gov/Outreach-and-Education/Outreach/WrittenMaterialsToolkit/downloads/ToolkitPart11.pdf>; [Accessed July 2019].

56. Patient-and-Family-Centered Care. Institute for Patient-and-Family-Centered Care. Bethesda, MD; 2019. Available at: <https://www.ipfcc.org/about/pfcc.html>; [Accessed July 2019].

57. Lee HL, Chalmers NI, Brow A, et al. Person-centered care model in dentistry. BMC Oral Health 2018;18(1):198. Available at: <https://www.ncbi.nlm.nih.gov/pubmed/30497465>; [Accessed July 2019].

58. About EBD. Chicago, IL; American Dental Association Center for Evidence-Based Dentistry; 2019. Available at: <https://ebd.ada.org/en/about>; [Accessed July 2019].

59. Ahmed S, Siad FM, Manalili K, et al. How to measure cultural competence when evaluating patient-centered care: a

scoping review. BMJ Open 2018;8:e021525. doi: 10.1136/bmjopen-2018-021525. Available at: <https://www.ncbi.nlm.nih.gov/pubmed/30018098>; [Accessed July 2019].

60. Patient Centered Care. Chicago, IL: American Academy of Pediatric Dentistry, Pediatric Oral Health Research & Policy Center; 2013. Available at: <http://www.aapd.org/assets/1/7/PatientCenteredCarePolicyBrief.pdf>; [Accessed July 2019].

61. Code of Ethics for Dental Hygienists. In: Bylaws & Code of Ethics, 35-38. Chicago, IL: American Dental Hygienists' Association; 2018. Available at: <https://www.adha.org/resources-docs/7611_Bylaws_and_Code_of_Ethics.pdf>. [Accessed July 2019].

62. Health Literacy. Bethesda, MD: National Institutes of Health, National Library of Medicine; 2019. Available at: <https://nnlm.gov/initiatives/topics/health-literacy>; [Accessed July 2019].

63. Health Literacy. Bethesda, MD: National Institutes of Health, Office of Communications & Public Liaison; 2018. Available at: <https://www.nih.gov/institutes-nih/nih-office-director/office-communications-public-liaison/clear-communication/health-literacy>; [Accessed July 2019].

64. Firmino RT, Martins CC, Faria LS, et al. Association of oral health literacy with oral health behaviors, perception, knowledge, and dental treatment related outcomes: a systematic review and meta-analysis. J Public Health Dent 2018;78:231–45. Available at: <https://www.ncbi.nlm.nih.gov/pubmed/29498754>; [Accessed July 2019].

65. What is Health Literacy? Atlanta, GA: Centers for Disease Control and Prevention; 2019. Available at: <https://www.cdc.gov/health-literacy/learn/index.html#:~:text=The%20Patient%20Protection%20and%20Affordable,to%20make%20appropriate%20health%20decisions>; [Accessed March 2020].

66. Health Literacy. Rockville, MD: Health Resources & Services Administration, Office of Health Equity; 2019. Available at: <https://www.hrsa.gov/about/organization/bureaus/ohe/health-literacy/index.html>; [Accessed July 2019].

67. National Action Plan to Improve Health Literacy. Washington, DC: Office of Disease Prevention and Health Promotion; 2010. Available at: <https://health.gov/communication/HLActionPlan/pdf/Health_Literacy_Action_Plan.pdf>; [Accessed July 2019].

68. Addressing Literacy and Health Literacy. Washington, DC: National Center for Cultural Competence. Available at: <https://nccc.georgetown.edu/bias/module-4/4.php>; [Accessed July 2019].

69. Health Literacy Fact Sheet. Trenton, NJ: Center for Health Care Strategies; 2013. Available at: <https://www.chcs.org/media/CHCS_Health_Literacy_Fact_Sheets_2013_1.pdf>; [Accessed March 2020].

70. National Academies of Sciences, Engineering, and Medicine. Integrating Oral and General Health Through Health Literacy Practices: Proceedings of a Workshop. Washington, DC: The National Academies Press; 2019. Available at: <https://doi.org/10.17226/25468>; [Accessed March 2020].

71. Atchison KA, Rozier RG, Weintraub J. Integration of Oral Health and Primary Care: Communication, Coordination, and Referral. 2018. Available at: <https://nam.edu/wp-content/uploads/2018/10/Integration-of-Oral-Health-and-Primary-Care.pdf>; [Accessed March 2020].

72. Brach C, Keller D, Hernandez LM, et al. Ten attributes of health literate health care organizations: a discussion paper. Washington, DC: Institute of Medicine of the National Academies; 2012. Available at: <https://nam.edu/wp-content/uploads/2015/06/BPH_Ten_HLit_Attributes.pdf>; [Accessed July 2019].

73. Attributes of a health literate organization. Atlanta, GA: Centers for Disease Control & Prevention; 2019. Available at: <https://www.cdc.gov/healthliteracy/planact/steps/index.html>; [Accessed October 2019].

74. Plain Writing Act, 5 U.S.C. § 105 et seq.; 2010. Available at: <https://www.govinfo.gov/content/pkg/USCODE-2011-title5/pdf/USCODE-2011-title5-partI-chap3-sec301.pdf>; [Accessed July 2019].

75. Checklist for Plain Language. Washington, DC: Plain Language Action and Information Network (PLAIN); n.d. Available at: <https://plainlanguage.gov/resources/checklists/checklist/>; [Accessed March 2020].

76. Federal Plain Language Guidelines. Washington, DC: Plain Language Action and Information Network (PLAIN); 2011. Available at: <https://www.plainlanguage.gov/media/FederalPLGuidelines.pdf>; [Accessed July 2019].

77. Enforcement of Title VI of the Civil Rights Act of 1964–National Origin Discrimination Against Persons with Limited English Proficiency; Policy Guidance. Fed Reg 2001, Tues March 20;66(54)15765-15766. Available at: <https://www.govinfo.gov/content/pkg/FR-2001-03-20/pdf/01-6918.pdf>; [Accessed July 2019].

78. Health Literate Care Model. Washington, DC: Office of Disease Prevention and Health Promotion; 2019. Available at: <https://health.gov/communication/interactiveHLCM/>; [Accessed July 2019].

79. Sorensen K, Van den Broucke S, Fullam J, et al. Health literacy and public health: A systematic review and integration of definitions and models. BMC Public Health (online) 2012;12:80e. doi: 10.1186/1471-2458-12-80. Available at: <http://www.biomedcentral.com/1471-2458/12/80>; [Accessed September 2019].

ADDITIONAL RESOURCES

An Implementation Checklist for the National CLAS Standards
https://thinkculturalhealth.hhs.gov/assets/pdfs/AnImplementationChecklistfortheNationalCLASStandards.pdf
Centers for Disease Control and Prevention (CDC)
http://www.cdc.gov/
Community Tool Box
http://ctb.ku.edu/en
Cultural Competence Program for Oral Health Professionals
https://oralhealth.thinkculturalhealth.hhs.gov/
Curricula Enhancement Module Series
https://nccc.georgetown.edu/curricula/modules.html
Diversity RX: Culturally Competent Care
http://www.diversityrx.org/topic-areas/culturally-competent-care
National Center for Cultural Competence
https://nccc.georgetown.edu/
Toolkit for Community Action, National Partnership for Action to End Health Disparities
https://minorityhealth.hhs.gov/npa/files/plans/toolkit/npa_toolkit.pdf

BOOKS

Dore AK, Eisenhardt AB. Cultural Learning in Healthcare: Recognizing & Navigating Differences. Atlanta, GA: North American Business Press; 2015.
Papadopoulos I. Culturally Competent Compassion: A Guide for Healthcare Students and Practitioners. New York, NY: Routledge Publishing; 2018.

11

Service-Learning: Preparing Dental Hygienists for Collaborative Practice

Schelli Stedke and Christine French Beatty

OBJECTIVES

1. Describe the benefits of experiential learning and specifically of service-learning compared to other forms of experiential learning.
2. Discuss and apply the components and distinguishing characteristics of service-learning.
3. Discuss the value of integrating service-learning with interprofessional collaborations.
4. Discuss the purpose and strategies for risk management in service-learning.
5. Apply service-learning to community oral health practice and integrate public health resources in service-learning.

OPENING STATEMENTS: Benefits of Service-Learning to Students:

- Gaining the ability to transfer and apply knowledge learned in a classroom setting to a "real-world" environment.
- Exposure to opportunities that enable further development and practice of communication skills, mutual objective formation, and leadership skills while working in a group setting.
- Beginning to understand the needs of one's community.
- Applying the concept of social responsibility in a learning environment, which can lead to greater interest in long-term service within the community.
- Participation in experiential learning outside the traditional classroom, which encourages collaboration, critical thinking, and decision-making.
- Through reflections of experiences, enhanced understanding of the importance of contemplation of the service-learning activity to draw personal meaning and opportunity for self-development from the experience.
- Realization of the importance of collaboration among the students, community, academic institution, and possibly other healthcare providers in the development of a service-learning project to meet a specific goal.
- In an interprofessional collaborative service setting, gaining awareness and knowledge of the responsibilities, skills, and knowledge of other healthcare professions while sharing one's own knowledge and experiences.
- The opportunity to use existing community resources and strengths to mutually benefit oneself and the community while empowering community members and organizations to act as co-educators of students.[1]

INTRODUCTION

As a student, preparing for the public health workforce in a rapidly changing dental hygiene profession is arguably one of your most important learning opportunities because it will contribute to advancing your career options. The American Dental Hygienists' Association (ADHA) has collaborated with other entities that are committed to improving oral health care based on the needs of the public and according to a plan that addresses dental hygiene professional and educational changes that are needed to meet the challenges of the 21st century.[2] Included in these necessary changes is the preparation of future dental hygienists by dental hygiene programs that will enable them to take advantage of opportunities in evolving integrated healthcare systems. The ADHA also outlines strategies that will contribute to expanded oral healthcare services for those most in need. In addition, the ADHA and governmental agencies stress the need for collaboration among healthcare professions, creating a workforce that is prepared to deliver care to a diverse population as described in Chapter 10.[2,3]

It is clear that the future of dental hygiene is in the public health workforce and that intentionality and well-led initiatives are necessary for the continued development of the profession.[2–5] Current educational standards require that dental hygiene graduates be able to competently collaborate with other healthcare professionals[5] (Figure 11.1). Curriculum requirements are designed to prepare dental hygienists to work in a changing public health environment that involves such collaboration.

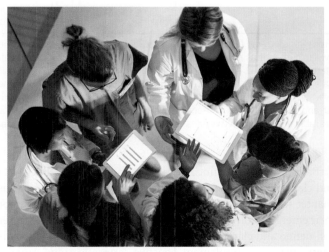

Fig 11.1 Dental hygiene and other healthcare professions students collaborate on patient care treatment plans with the goal of providing better overall care with more positive patient outcomes. (@ iStock.com/Cecilie_Arcurs.)

TABLE 11.1   Key Initiatives for Change Impacting the Dental Hygiene Profession and Response of the American Dental Hygienists' Association (ADHA)

Initiative for Change	Summary	ADHA Response
The Access-To-Care Crisis	More than 46 million people in the U.S. live in dental health professional shortage areas and lack access to basic oral health care.	Apply the increased and nontraditional use of dental hygienists to promote access to oral health care, particularly for underserved populations, as demonstrated in innovative programs.
Changing Demographics and Complexity of Care	Demographic trends indicate the U.S. population is changing, with an increase in underserved individuals and demographic groups that are underrepresented in both patient and practitioner populations. In addition, complex healthcare needs that involve behavioral, financial, cultural, and medical issues must be addressed.	Address shortage areas by improving the primary oral health workforce through alternative workforce models, including expanding the role of dental hygienists and dental therapists.
Future Oral Health Workforce Projections	Demand for oral healthcare services continues to grow. The lack of availability of those who provide services puts a greater demand on dental hygienists, requiring that their scope of practice be fully utilized and their supervision be relaxed to adequately meet oral health needs of the public.	Explore and advocate for the changing role of the dental hygienist as an integrated member of the oral healthcare team, which may somewhat ameliorate dentist shortages by maximizing productivity of the existing oral health workforce. Relax their supervision regulations and increase their scope of practice to reflect their educational preparation and abilities.
Emerging Technology	In recent years advancements in dental technology have helped oral health professionals collaborate, diagnose, manage, and provide services in distant locations. This process of networking, information-sharing, consultation, and analysis is called telehealth and includes teledentistry.	Educate dental hygienists in future technology needs, including the use of technology for information-sharing and communication, to promote their use of digital information, especially remotely, to be able to improve access to care. Also, change regulations to allow for the full utilization of dental hygienists in telehealth situations.
Direct Access	Direct access allows dental hygienists to provide various levels of services based on their assessment without the specific authorization of a dentist; currently, 42 states have varying provisions for direct access.	Continue to develop creative and useful models and change regulations to be able to meet the needs of the public (see examples highlighted in Chapters 2 and 6).
Scope of Practice	Dental hygienists continue to seek the opportunity to practice to the full extent of their educational capabilities. Levels of supervision and regulation vary greatly from state to state with very few states being self-regulated.	Continue to promote self-regulation which allows professions to evolve and effect change within their own profession.
Dental Hygiene Diagnosis	In 2017, a revision was proposed to the Commission on Dental Accreditation dental hygiene accreditation standards to include the dental hygiene diagnosis, with the intent of reflecting the competence and educational preparedness of dental hygienists. This change would have mirrored the purpose of the process of care and clarified the capabilities of dental hygienists in the healthcare setting. The proposal was not accepted, but as the delivery of care model evolves in each state and direct access by dental hygienists becomes more common, it will need to be revisited.	ADHA policy supports dental hygiene curricula that leads to competency in the dental hygiene process of care, including the dental hygiene diagnosis, deeming it a "necessary and intrinsic element of dental hygiene education and scope of practice." With changes in technology, research that supports the oral-systemic link, the complexity and evolution of the healthcare delivery system, and regulations for dental hygienists, educational standards and curricula require modification to provide a broader focus to meet the oral healthcare challenges of the 21st century.

(From Transforming Dental Hygiene Education and the Profession for the 21st Century. Chicago, IL: American Dental Hygienists' Association; 2015. Available at: <https://www.adha.org/resources-docs/Transforming_Dental_Hygiene_Education.pdf>; [Accessed December 2019]; Direct Access States. Chicago, IL: American Dental Hygienists' Association; 2020. Available at: <https://www.adha.org/resources-docs/7513_Direct_Access_to_Care_from_DH.pdf>; [Accessed March 2020]; Proposed Dental Hygiene Standards Revisions. Chicago, IL: Commission on Dental Accreditation; 2017. Available at: <https://www.ada.org/~/media/CODA/Files/2017%20ADA%20Annual%20Meeting%20Material/appendix9_proposed_DH_Standards_2-8d_and_2-13.pdf?la=en>; [Accessed April 2020]; Dental Hygiene Diagnosis (Policy Statement). American Dental Hygienists' Association; 2015. Available at: <https://www.adha.org/resources-docs/7111_Dental_Hygiene_Diagnosis_Position_Paper.pdf>; [Accessed April 2020].)

Based on more defined initiatives for change (Table 11.1) and clearer roadmaps directing the future of the profession, this chapter focuses on helping dental hygiene students prepare for their emerging roles in the public health workforce.[2] The chapter will define and clarify experiential learning models to help students create and implement effective service-learning projects that integrate public health resources and interprofessional considerations. The chapter can be used as a bridge to prepare dental hygienists for advancing models of healthcare delivery, which have been discussed in previous chapters. For example,

Chapters 1 and 2 discussed the importance and current direction of preparing students for **interprofessional collaborative practice** (ICP or IPP). These chapters also addressed the emergence of different workforce models and alternative care providers in the medical and dental profession with the intent of using them in alternative settings to better meet the public's healthcare needs.[6–8]

The emphasis on ICP has necessitated a shift from profession-specific education and training to educating health professions students in an interprofessional collaborative model, referred to as **interprofessional education** (IPE).[4] IPE prepares graduates to work with various other health disciplines to strengthen identified community health issues that cut across the disciplines. Team-based health professional education requires skill sets conducive to this interdisciplinary approach.[4] Collaboration at the student level with health professional students from other disciplines will be critical. Community oral health service-learning programs can provide an opportunity for academic exercises that will help students prepare for this future role in ICP.[2-4]

One of the focuses of this chapter is the planning and implementation of community-based experiences and team-based collaborative projects that will help prepare students for these emerging roles in dental hygiene practice.[3,8] It also focuses on the use of service-learning for community-based instruction and additionally provides instruction to augment the dental hygiene student's public health awareness and ability to use public health resources. Finally, the chapter concludes with an opportunity to connect service-learning instruction with public health practice and resources through simulation exercises.

This chapter has value for faculty and students alike, to learn about service-learning and to identify ways to incorporate it into a community oral health course. Along with the Community Health Program Planning Process presented in Chapter 3 (Figure 3.7) and Chapter 6 (Table 6.3) and the health promotion theories and communication information in Chapter 8, this chapter is useful in designing, planning, implementing, and evaluating assigned community-based service-learning projects. The chapter provides information on the processes, procedures, and strategies of service-learning, as well as ideas and resources to apply to these assignments.

EXPERIENTIAL LEARNING

Also commonly referred to as practical learning or real-world learning, **experiential learning** originated from the grassroots research of educational theorists such as John Dewey, Kurt Lewin, Jean Piaget, and Carl Rogers.[9] According to these educational researchers, hands-on learning was at the center of the best learning experiences. Historically, dental hygiene students have provided a form of experiential learning known as community service to instruct populations about oral health. Educational methods used to prepare dental hygiene students to provide instruction in these instances were limited in magnitude; they were taught to deliver basic oral health educational facts. The benefits of this method proved to be useful in preparing dental hygiene students to deliver oral health messages, but they were oversimplified and deficient in preparing students to anticipate or meet the needs of the public's oral health challenges.

An example of oral health education delivered as community service is dental hygiene students staffing and displaying information at a table at a local health fair. In this situation, students interact with people who stop by their table. This delivery mode has a limited effect in expanding the students' perspectives regarding the community in which they interact. In this setting, how could the dental hygiene students anticipate the needs of their audience? A higher level of experiential learning is needed to prepare dental hygiene students to fulfill the oral health challenges of a rapidly diversifying population while contributing to the current national oral health agenda.[3,6,7]

A Dental Hygiene Example of Experiential Learning

The community service example just mentioned can be contrasted with the following example of experiential learning in a dental hygiene course. In this example, first-year dental hygiene students enrolled in a dental radiology course learn how to interpret radiographic findings, but they are discouraged by their performance on quizzes. After the mid-term examination, the faculty member initiates a collaborative project with an elementary school teacher in which the dental hygiene students will teach some of the concepts they are learning to the elementary school students (Figure 11.2). The faculty member explains to the dental hygiene students that they will be able to connect their didactic learning with the elementary school students' real needs that have been identified by their teacher.

For the dental hygiene faculty member, the purpose of the experiential assignment is to enhance the dental hygiene students' comprehension of the radiology course material. Because active learning is an important principle in educational theory and because dental hygiene students will have to construct much of the elementary school learning experience themselves (*active learning*), chances are that they will benefit from this assignment by increasing their comprehension of the radiology course content. Not only do they have to assess the needs of the elementary school students as specified by the elementary school teacher, but they have to decide how to teach the content and how to evaluate the effectiveness of their teaching. This initiative is a collaborative project in contrast to traditional teaching and learning methods such as lectures, reading assignments, and even radiographic interpretation exercises. Engagement in an active learning experience enhances these traditional methods.

In this way, experiential learning can be used to change the focus of learning, shifting it from the confines of the classroom to the community, while maintaining a key focus on adding to the student's knowledge base. Routine learning methods can be supplemented with purposeful, active, and work-based learning opportunities within the community. At the same time, to ensure that the course objectives are met, the dental hygiene students apply their program planning skills with guidance from

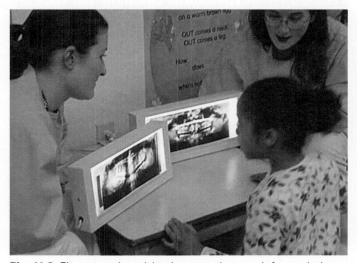

Fig 11.2 First-year dental hygiene students reinforce their acquired radiographic interpretation skills by teaching others. (Courtesy Sheranita Hemphill.)

their faculty and from the community partner (the elementary school teacher in the example given).

Authenticity of Experiential Learning

Experiential learning takes place in authentic situations.[9] A Women, Infants, and Children (WIC) facility is a good example of a service-learning setting in which a broader understanding of oral health is necessary to effect change for a lifetime. For example, to learn about the social determinants of oral health in a community oral health course, a typical strategy is to show an image of a woman standing in line at a local WIC facility, followed by dental hygiene students documenting their thoughts about this woman and small group discussions to explore the social determinants of oral health. However, without actually interacting with the woman, how can they really know what her visits to the WIC facility signify? Perhaps she is seeking nutritional provisions for her child, but is that all?

However, if the dental hygiene students are assigned to actually assist women at a WIC facility, the students will have to use their learned skills to see beyond the obvious. They will have to apply cognitive skills, such as the recall of facts regarding the mission of the public health facility. They will also need to construe oral health needs that the mother and her family may have and that may not be obvious and clear-cut; the reality is bigger than the image. In this case, the dental hygiene students will likely learn much more from having to construct strategies to assist these women and their families. They will brainstorm, share ideas, and possibly remind each other to be thoughtful and use evidence-based information in their discussions rather than anecdotal, opinionated fragments of thought. In essence, they will learn through experience—and the learning environment will become part of the learning experience.[9,10]

Experiential learning is an umbrella term that refers to various models of learning in which experience governs the educational process for the student. Another example is to learn about fluoride varnish programs by actually participating in one in a community setting (Figure 11.3). The experiential learning

Fig 11.3 A dental hygiene student applies fluoride varnish during a service-learning varnish project planned and implemented by her classmates. (Courtesy Christine French Beatty.)

literature is extremely optimistic about the results of linking academic learning outcomes to experiential learning in community-based settings (see Guiding Principles).[11,12]

GUIDING PRINCIPLES
Experiential Learning Outcomes

- Connects classroom learning with authentic situations
- Continuously reinforces learned knowledge and skills through practical experience
- Challenges the student to think critically in addressing real needs
- Increases aptitude when applied in various populations
- Enhances the skills of the dental hygiene workforce

Several well-known experiential learning methods are used in the dental hygiene curriculum (Box 11.1), which vary in

BOX 11.1 Experiential Learning Methods

Service-Learning
Students participate in a teaching/learning method that stresses collaborative planning and implementation of projects. It is structured in in a way that combines community service with preparation and reflection, and it focuses on applying course content to enhance learning. Students engaged in **service-learning** provide community service in response to community-identified concerns and learn about the context in which service is provided, the connection between the service and their academic coursework, and their roles as citizens.

Community Service
Through **community service**, students provide a service to the community, primarily focused on the community's needs. It may or may not have a curriculum connection; the student may provide the service for reasons other than an academic requirement (e.g., club or sorority requirement, religious duty).

Clinical Rotation
Clinical rotation is a curriculum-based activity that includes clinical experiences to enhance the student's skills, knowledge, and expertise. This may incorporate service-learning, depending on the objectives and outcomes desired. This could be a clinical rotation site where students provide patient care and interact with other health professions students and faculty to gain the best patient outcome. Two examples of this would be the CATCH 1 for Health and Stroke Center programs described in this chapter.

Practicum/Internship
A **practicum/internship** is typically longer than a clinical rotation and may incorporate service-learning, depending on the objectives and outcomes desired. An example of a practicum/internship that incorporates service-learning would be placing a dental hygiene student at a Head Start Center to help develop programs for staff, children and parents. An example that does not include service-learning would be the assignment of senior-level dental hygiene students to various public health agencies, higher education institutions, and governmental agencies for the practical experience of on-the-job exposure and training.

Volunteerism
Students provide a service to the community, primarily benefiting the community. **Volunteerism** is not necessarily associated with an academic course. Examples include assisting at the concession stand at an athletic event and participating in a secondary education tutoring program.

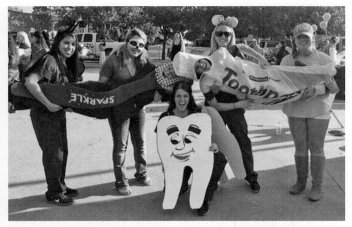

Fig 11.4 Student American Dental Hygienists' Association members provide community service by participating in a Halloween carnival. (Courtesy Charlene Dickinson.)

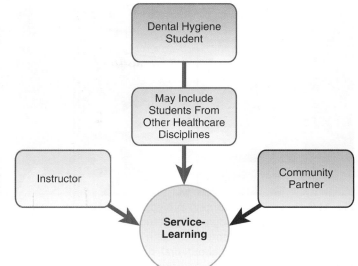

Fig 11.5 Collaborators in service-learning. (Modified from What is Service-Learning? Starting Point: Teaching Entry Level Geoscience. Northfield, MN: Carleton College Science Education Resource Center; 2018 May 7. Available at: <https://serc.carleton.edu/introgeo/service/what.html>; [Accessed April 2020].)

their purpose. The earlier examples related to assisting WIC participants and applying radiology concepts to teach elementary school students are examples of service-learning, having the advantage of fulfilling multiple purposes and enhancing student learning at various levels.[13] Some experiential learning methods do not have a curriculum connection and do not have the same learning value as service-learning,[14] for example, community service projects organized and conducted by student ADHA members (Figure 11.4).

SERVICE-LEARNING

This chapter is focused on the experiential learning model of service-learning. By its nature, service-learning is a teaching and learning method that stresses collaborative planning between the dental hygiene student, the dental hygiene program faculty, and the community partner. More recently, students from other health disciplines may also be included in this learning model to reflect interprofessional education (Figure 11.5). Widely used in educating health professions students, service-learning involves production of an implementation project that is mutually beneficial for everyone involved in the collaborative arrangement.[1] The definition of service-learning is characterized by certain features, all of which are of equal importance:[12]

1. Promotes collaboration between community partners, students, and health professions educational institutions (Figure 11.6).
2. Emphasizes the importance of the community partner self-identifying requests for community service and being actively involved in the service project.
3. Articulates the significance of faculty-assured educational outcomes for the benefit of students.

Service-learning is not a superficial academic exercise in which lessons are taught by dental hygiene students with little observed or learned by them in the process; instead, educational opportunities are purposively built into their service-learning experiences (Figure 11.7). Students are challenged to create unique opportunities for their community partners that will be mutually beneficial[1] (see Guiding Principles).

GUIDING PRINCIPLES
Creative and Unique Ideas That Can Be Integrated Into Service-Learning Projects

- Develop a brochure listing community oral health resources, including safety net facilities.
- Plan and conduct a Basic Screening Survey (BSS) and issue oral health report cards.
- Identify public and private dental facilities that are currently accepting public health insurance (Medicaid and Children's Health Insurance Program [CHIP]) and assist families in finding dental homes.
- Collaborate with local law enforcement officers and students to promote child safety by performing bite impressions for use in identifying children.
- Help the community assess the adequacy of their water fluoridation.
- Develop and implement oral health lesson plans for allied health students or other health professionals (e.g., medical doctors, physician assistants, nurse practitioners, nurses).

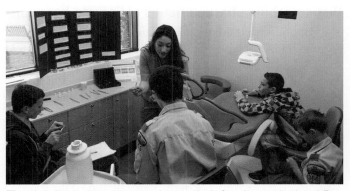

Fig 11.6 Dental hygiene students, their faculty, and a local Boy Scout troop collaborate in a service-learning project in which the scouts learn about oral health and the oral health professions, and students learn about the scouting organization and the scouts' learning needs. (Courtesy Christina Horton.)

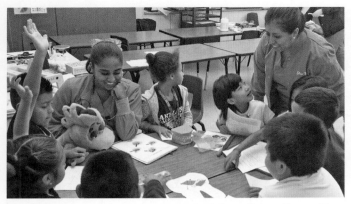

Fig 11.7 In a service-learning project in collaboration with a school-based sealant program operated by the dental clinic of a local faith-based community health center, dental hygiene students teach children about oral health, oral hygiene, and the importance of sealants and fluoride, while learning about the health center, the needs of the children, and how to conduct a sealant program. (Courtesy Terri Patrick.)

Components of Service-Learning

Sometimes service-learning is described as a combination of a community service project and academic coursework. But this definition is incomplete because it does not fully describe that the service-learning process contains specific and ordered components. The very structure of the term service-learning, whereby the two words are separated by a hyphen, implies equality between the service component (what is received by the community partner) and the learning component (what is received by the dental hygiene student, in this case).[15] Also, when the term *service-learning* is used, both words should be presented in matching fashion: the "s" in service and the "l" in learning are always written in identical fashion, either capitalized or in lower-case letters. The hyphen emphasizes the connection between the service and learning components. In essence, service-learning experiences are jointly structured between the community partner and the academic component. The configuration of the term service-learning denotes the importance of ensuring that the needs of both the community partner and the dental hygiene student are addressed.[1,12,16,17]

Distinguishing Characteristics of Service-Learning

The Community Health Program Planning Process detailed and illustrated in Chapter 3 (Figure 3.7) and Chapter 6 (Table 6.3) and the health promotion theories and communication information in Chapter 8 are applied to provide the necessary structure to assure a successful service-learning project. For example, this involves the student identifying the community group's needs, creating goals and objectives, brainstorming activities, identifying roles, developing action and contingency plans, setting timelines, and planning formative and summative, quantitative and qualitative evaluation.[18–20]

Formative evaluation involves examining the service-learning project while it is in-process (think of forming), and summative evaluation involves a formal end-project review of the service-learning project outcomes (think of summary). Using both methods helps to ensure permanence or institutionalization of the service-learning project in the dental hygiene program, thus assuring that valuable service-learning experiences can continue with future cohorts of dental hygiene students.

The full impact of experiential learning will not be realized if the service-learning experience does not follow this structure. Leaving out or re-arranging any one or more program planning steps will reduce the learning value of the service-learning project. In addition, skill sets such as leadership and active listening are essential to preparing and implementing a service-learning project.

In addition, distinct features of service-learning differentiate it from other experiential learning methods: collaboration, orientation, mutual objective formation, reflection, and student evaluation.[12,15,16] These features are universally accepted as ideals that must be present to characterize an experiential learning project as service-learning.

Collaboration

Collaboration means working together to accomplish a goal. Other words that may come to mind when thinking about collaboration include joint effort, teamwork, or partnership. In service-learning projects, the program is jointly planned by the dental hygiene course instructor, the community partner, and the dental hygiene students.[14] Beginning in the initial stages of identifying a service-learning project, this collaboration among all these parties is necessary to ensure that the needs of all are met. The faculty member is interested in assuring that student learning objectives are considered, the community partner is interested in ensuring that the organization's service needs are met, and the dental hygiene students are interested in applying their oral health education knowledge and skills to benefit the community.

With traditional community service projects, dental hygiene faculty members have typically initiated the communications leading to a community service experience for the students. The faculty member contacted an agency representative and asked about placing dental hygiene students in the organization to gain community experience. However, with service-learning, any of the collaborators can initiate the contact and request. The community agency can contact the faculty member to request the services of the dental hygiene students. Likewise, the student can initiate the discussion by contacting an agency to discuss the possibility of developing a mutually beneficial project and then seeking approval from the faculty member.

Collaboration continues throughout all phases of the service-learning process. The expectation of equally balanced interests is a classic feature of service-learning.[12,16] Achieving this balance for all interested parties requires deliberate attention to collaboration during the implementation of all steps of the program planning process as well as carefully carrying out each step correctly.

Orientation

A formal orientation involving all collaborating parties concerning the program being considered for development minimizes disruptions to the service-learning program.[15] Scheduled before the program planning process is initiated, the overall agenda for the orientation should be for all parties to become familiar with each other's programs, clarify expectations, formulate a time line, review risk management policies and procedures, and deal with any other questions or issues pertinent to the service-learning project. It is important for the dental hygiene students, the agency (collaborative partner), and the dental hygiene faculty member to become acquainted with each other's program mission, objectives, population demographics, constraints, guidelines, operations, and facilities. Clear communication and face-to-face meetings are good approaches to gain insight to the different perspectives.

Mutual Objective Formation

The method of developing **objectives** (see Chapter 6) for the service-learning experience is another unique characteristic of service-learning.[21] Using a process of *mutual objective formation*, a service objective (SO) and a learning objective (LO) are combined effectively to create a service-learning objective (S-LO), as depicted in Figure 11.8. What the community partner wants from the dental hygiene students is referred to as the SO, which is a uniquely expressed need that flows directly from the mission and purposes of the collaborating partner[12,18] (Figure 11.9). A course objective from the community course syllabus is selected as the LO for the service-learning experience (Figure 11.10). Then the community partner, the dental hygiene student(s), and the dental hygiene faculty member collaborate to purposefully combine the SO and the LO to form the S-LO (Figure 11.11). This systematic development of the S-LO and further explanations of the SO, LO, and S-LO are presented in Figure 11.12.

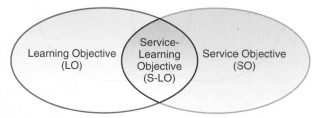

Fig 11.8 Relationship of the service objective (SO), learning objective (LO), and service-learning objective (S-LO).

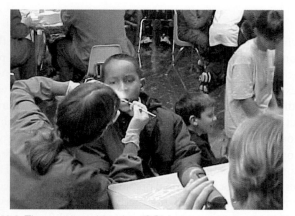

Fig 11.9 The service objective (SO) is to provide oral health services for the underserved population at this school. (Courtesy Sheranita Hemphill.)

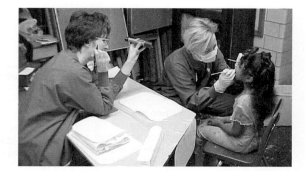

Fig 11.10 The learning objective (LO) is to be able to apply screening techniques and indexes to survey a priority population in the community. (Courtesy Sheranita Hemphill.)

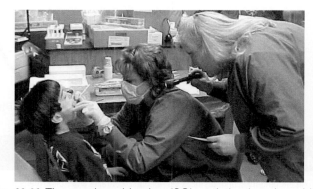

Fig 11.11 The service objective (SO) and the learning objective (LO) are combined as a service-learning objective (S-LO) in the implementation of this service-learning project. (Courtesy Sheranita Hemphill.)

The collaborators working together to combine the SO and LO in creating the S-LO is critical to the service-learning process because it supports the integrity of the service-learning experience and illustrates its mutually beneficial nature.[15,16] The effort involved in honoring the collaborative process of developing the SOs, LOs, and S-LOs will serve to build a close working relationship between the community partner and the dental hygiene students. The example in Box 11.2 illustrates this process of collaboration in mutual objective formation.

Reflection

A service project completed to meet a course requirement without **reflection** is not truly service-learning and does not result in the same learning outcome. The aim of service-learning reflection is to deliberately draw meaning from the experience.[19,20,22–25] Symbolized by the hyphen in service-learning, reflection provides the opportunity for students to process the service-learning experience and consider its implications in the context of learning and growing.[15] As an act of learning in the college environment, critical student reflection should purposefully interconnect with the academic course objectives and the meaningful service to the community, and should include all the related agreeable and disagreeable experiences, thoughts, observations, and perceptions related to the service-learning activity (see Figure 11.13). As a student, you are encouraged to reflect on the impact the service-learning project has on you individually. Besides academic learning,

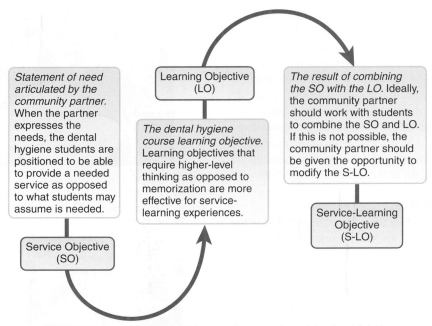

Fig 11.12 Development of the service-learning objective (*S-LO*).

BOX 11.2   Example of the Process of Mutual Objective Formation

- An elementary school district's school nurse contacts a dental hygiene faculty member for assistance in securing dental homes for children needing immediate dental care. The faculty member meets with the school nurse to discuss a possible collaboration.
- The faculty member and school nurse collaborate to present the project of finding dental homes for low socioeconomic status (SES) public elementary school children to the school administration and teachers.
- The school personnel are satisfied because this meets the needs of the school; the summarized service objective (SO) is to keep children healthy for classroom learning.
- The dental hygiene faculty member's goals are met by actively engaging students in a project to advocate for populations with no or inadequate access to oral health care.
- The dental hygiene students are equally satisfied because they have the opportunity to apply their program planning skills. After considering the service-learning activity, they select which one or more course learning objectives (LOs) to apply to the school's SO.
- After informing the school nurse of their LOs, the students and the school nurse meet to collaborate on combining their respective objectives to develop the service-learning objectives (S-LOs), which are then presented to the faculty member for approval.
- The planning for the service-learning program can now proceed.

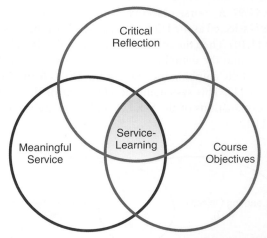

Fig 11.13 The role of reflection in service-learning. (Modified from What is Service-Learning? Starting Point: Teaching Entry Level Geoscience. Northfield, MN: Carleton College Science Education Resource Center; 2018 May 7. Available at: <https://serc.carleton.edu/introgeo/service/what.html>; [Accessed April 2020].)

---

service-learning can significantly impact you in the following areas:[14,15,23]

- Personal growth such as self-identity, spiritual growth, moral development, and sense of self-efficacy
- A sense of caring and commitment to service
- Social responsibility and citizenship skills
- Ability to achieve social change
- Critical thinking, decision-making, and leadership skills
- Application of learning to the "real world"

Personal and civic perspectives are expected and encouraged in this reflection process.[15,23] However, this exercise in reflection should not turn into a political venting session or a campaign to convince others of one's position or opinion. As a student reflecting on your learning experience, you should not assume a position of authority or influence over others. You should state what the experience meant to you in relation to the specific LOs without the need to sway others' thoughts, and you should be curious about others' perspectives. Reflection is not about being right.

You cannot separate your overall experiences from your personal feelings, your prior experiences, and who you are as a person. Yet you cannot expect others to share your views. Herein lies the need for exceptional preparation to engage in effective communication and dialogue. Successful reflection of service-learning cannot occur without them (see Box 11.3).

Dental hygiene faculty members are instrumental in assisting students to connect the course objectives with the actual experience by posing critical questions for reflection. Questions

BOX 11.3 Effective Communication and Dialogue During Reflection

- Engage in introspective thinking; really listen to your inner thoughts, feelings, and prejudices; think deeply.
- Speak carefully; use I messages rather than they or them messages.
- Speak specifically; avoid generalizations.
- Focus on quality interaction; accept personal responsibility and trust others to do the same.
- Avoid adversarial vocabulary.
- Speak to the entire group; avoid singling out any one person.
- Nurture openness and curiosity about others' perspectives; speak and listen with conscious intention for real communication.
- Be quiet; reflect, process, and reduce tension within the conversation.
- Let go of the need to be right; share your perspective without trying to convince others.

BOX 11.4 Examples of Ways Students Can Present Their Service-Learning Projects

- Have community partners facilitate prepared or impromptu discussions.
- Present a poster session and invite the entire college and community.
- Have senior students present experiences to junior students at roundtable discussions.
- Incorporate audiovisuals into any reflection method.
- Guide students in journaling the connections, challenges, context, and continuity of the service-learning experience.
- Create a website to highlight the continuous nature of the program's service-learning efforts.
- Develop an evaluation instrument to be implemented in future service-learning programs.
- Publish an article in a dental hygiene magazine, newsletter website, or blog.

GUIDING PRINCIPLES

Dental Hygiene Students' Reflective Comments Relative to Their Service-Learning Project

"We watched our faculty interact with our community partners and speakers, and we learned that a key ingredient to successful navigation of service-learning projects is making everyone feel equally important and responsible for its success."

"The initial discussions that we had with the teacher were very important. I learned the status of the children's oral health and frequency of their dental visits. The teacher gave us a realistic idea of what was going on with the children's oral hygiene at home. She informed us that some of her students already had dental crowns, and she believed that they weren't learning at home what they needed to know to properly take care of their teeth."

"The observation meeting that we had before our service-learning project was instrumental in preparing our lesson plans. From that meeting, we learned that we need to change our initial ideas of what we might teach because the teacher had explicit expectations of what she wanted her class to learn from us."

"One thing that I would do differently is to make sure that the group had a physical activity to take home with them to show their guardians. I now realize the importance of making oral health a family matter."

"Even though service-learning is a balanced approach to teaching and learning, I still think that the dental hygiene students got the most from the experience. I listened deeply to my peers, and every one of them stated that they learned so much about their selected course objectives."

"Now I know what it means to be 'socially accountable.' It sounds intellectual in the textbook and on the syllabus; this project made me really see the devastation right in front of me."

"From some of the children, we got the impression that their parents are not involved with their oral health, so it was quite an eye opener. This made us really want to talk to the parents, so we initiated a contest to see which classroom could get the most parental involvement."

"I learned, *really* learned, what formative evaluation is. I had to use it. Many of the kids asked more questions than we thought they would. We had to think on our feet and make adjustments during our presentations."

"At first, we didn't understand why we needed to write a summary report to the principal and school nurse, but it turned out to be a fun project because we completed it as a class project. The final document was spectacular. Since we conducted pre- and posttests, we were able to include descriptive data and graphs, and we printed the report letter using color ink cartridges. The final report was impressive."

"As a direct result of this experience, we feel humbled and would love to continue this type of volunteer work throughout our careers as dental hygienists."

must be carefully constructed with the objectives in mind. The purpose of the reflection is to encourage the student's understanding and appreciation of the connection between the course content, the community oral health issues, the sociocultural environment in which they exist, and relevant civic issues (see the Opening Statements). Reflection also has the aim of helping the student identify the personal impact the service-learning project has had on them. Students are encouraged to reflect deeply in relation to all these areas. The goal is to assist the student in identifying and remembering how their perspectives were challenged and enhanced and how the experience affected their lifetime learning journey.[20,23] Reflection should be incorporated into the student's presentation of their service-learning project, which can take various forms[23,25] (see Box 11.4).

As a student, you will find that reflection is critical to your learning process. A review of the benefits of service-learning in the Opening Statements of this chapter may help you focus your reflections. Also, examples of dental hygiene students' reflection comments in the Guiding Principles will enhance your understanding of reflection.

Evaluation of Student Learning

Another unique characteristic of service-learning is the involvement of multiple stakeholders in the assessment of student learning: the faculty member, the community partner, and the student in the form of self-assessment.[16,22] Receiving quality feedback from the faculty and community partners impacts students' self-reported learning and commitment to community engagement.[23]

Use of both formative evaluation and summative evaluation is recommended.[23] Students should use formative feedback to address problems that might arise during the semester to avoid any negative impact on the project. Summative feedback can help improve partnerships, future project designs, and campus-community relations.

BENEFITS OF SERVICE-LEARNING FOR INTERPROFESSIONAL COLLABORATION

Interprofessional Collaborative Practice

The narrow focus on discipline-specific employment settings for health professionals, including oral health professionals, is changing.[2,3] Emergent models of delivering oral health (see Chapter 2) will necessitate that oral health professionals be able to integrate into the growing interprofessional teamwork landscape of healthcare delivery. Endorsements from reputable organizations and expert panels position future oral health professionals as key members of ICP teams.[4]

ICP requires health professionals to enter the workforce ready to integrate into teams of mixed healthcare professionals for the purpose of cooperating to achieve the best health outcomes for patients and communities. National indicators have clearly pointed to the need for a transformation from discipline-specific practice to interprofessional practice to bring about better health outcomes.[2-4] This includes the dental hygiene profession, which is evolving in its delivery systems.[2] Dental hygienists will be in a primary position to address the public's oral health issues within the existing and emerging scope of practice.[2,3]

The movement to position oral health as an integral part of overall health is supported by research, which suggests that higher education health professional programs incorporate IPE into their curricula through collaboration. Many current health professions educational standards, including dental hygiene, require competence of graduates in communication and collaboration with other members of the healthcare team to support comprehensive patient care.[2,5] Several examples in the literature use service-learning as the experiential learning model for IPE.

Interprofessional Strategies in Service-Learning

One of the goals for this chapter is to illustrate how the use of service-learning in the dental hygiene curriculum can be implemented to prepare graduates for the healthcare team-oriented approach in planning, developing, and delivering relevant oral health messages and providing community-based oral health services. Nurses, physical therapists, physician assistants, respiratory therapists, and other healthcare professionals will also graduate capable of working in their discipline's scope of practice, but none will be able to stay abreast of the combined knowledge that each discipline produces, and which all patients will need. Thus, a crucial need exists and will continue to grow for fully functional interprofessional healthcare teams.[3,4]

The International Education Collaborative (IPEC) developed and recently updated four core competencies considered necessary for students, existing healthcare institutions, and health professions educational institutions to prepare for effective interprofessional collaborative teamwork (Table 11.2).[4] Each of these competencies can be incorporated into interprofessional service-learning experiences to enhance learning experiences and provide meaningful outcomes.[4] The updated competencies reflect changes that have occurred in the healthcare system, indicating the vision that ICP is the best way to deliver safe, high-quality, accessible, patient-centered care.[4]

Evolution From Traditional to Collaborative Experiential Learning in Dental Hygiene Curricula

Traditionally, dental hygiene students have been involved in many forms of experiential learning, including community service, clinical rotations, and observations. However, some of these models were typically designed to benefit the dental hygiene students exclusively. Generally, the projects were conceived entirely by the dental hygiene curriculum committee, and they focused on oral health issues, almost at the exclusion of overall health concerns. The projects were implemented at the convenience of the dental hygiene academic calendar and overseen exclusively by the dental hygiene department with little or no input from those receiving the care. The dental hygiene students received academic credit for completing specific tasks, and the outcome was not widely shared.

Recent educational requirements command educational institutions to further develop initiatives through core educational competencies. These competencies require increased communication with other healthcare providers, the public, and organizations within and outside the profession to promote overall health and optimal treatment.[5] Developing programs within educational curricula that involve service-learning and include ICP will help prepare graduates to fulfill the forecasted needs and employment opportunities of an evolving profession. Service-learning is one way to begin addressing the overall and oral access-to-care crisis and makes way for early interactions of dental hygiene students with community partners,

TABLE 11.2 Core Competencies for Interprofessional Collaborative Practice	
Competency Domains	**Competencies**
Values/Ethics for Interprofessional Practice	Work with individuals of other professions to maintain a climate of mutual respect and shared values.
Roles/Responsibilities	Use the knowledge of one's own role and those of other professions to appropriately assess and address the healthcare needs of patients and to promote and advance the health of populations.
Interprofessional Communication	Communicate with patients, families, communities, and professionals in health and other fields in a responsive and responsible manner that supports a team approach to the promotion and maintenance of health and the prevention and treatment of disease.
Teams and Teamwork	Apply relationship-building values and the principles of team dynamics to perform effectively in different team roles to plan, deliver, and evaluate patient/population-centered care and population health programs and policies that are safe, timely, efficient, effective, and equitable.

other healthcare professions students and faculty, and vulnerable population groups in need.[2,3,13,24,26] In this way, service-learning prepares tomorrow's workforce through timely collaborative opportunities.[2-4]

Interprofessional Collaborative Practice and Service-Learning

An ideal framework is afforded by service-learning to provide health professions students with the opportunity to experience ICP while still in school. Such experiences are critical to the process of preparing them with the mind-set and skills needed to move into ICP upon graduation as they enter the healthcare workforce.[4] Exposing students to service-learning combined with IPE and ICP has the potential to assist them in transitioning seamlessly upon graduation into the role of a collaborative practitioner prepared to impact the public's oral health challenges.[2,4] Two interprofessional collaborative service-learning projects are presented to illustrate ICP and IPE. The first is an IPE initiative that demonstrates dental hygiene and speech and language pathology (SLP) students successfully applying their joint knowledge in a collaborative learning environment (Figure 11.14). In this instance, the students provide their discipline-specific professional services to patients that have suffered a cerebrovascular accident (CVA) at a stroke center while working together to improve communication with the patient to render the best possible care. Patients frequently have difficulty with oral communication after their CVA and suffer from partial paralysis which can impede necessary daily oral hygiene.[27]

The SLP students work with the patients regularly to regain lost communication skills through intensive speech and language therapy sessions. For the interprofessional activity, patients receive a thorough oral examination, home care education, and an oral prophylaxis if indicated, while SLP students work collaboratively with the dental hygiene students to provide communication support. At the same time, dental hygiene students rotate through a speech and language therapy session to learn more about the role of a speech and language pathologist. Students have reported that they experienced a greater understanding of the role of the other healthcare provider and felt more confident interacting with healthcare providers from other disciplines after this experience. In addition, dental hygiene students have gained confidence communicating with CVA patients. An unforeseen outcome of this experience has been the anecdotal reporting of SLP students that they increased their knowledge of their own oral health while participating in the collaborative oral hygiene education sessions.

The second IPE example is a school-based program called CATCH 1 for Health (CATCH 1), which provides elementary school-aged children a comprehensive screening and referral, including a physical examination, hearing assessment, vision assessment, and oral health assessment (Figure 11.15). Professional healthcare students from area colleges, including medical, nursing, dental hygiene, speech pathology, audiology, public health, and social work students, participate in this collaborative interprofessional practice experience.

The purpose of CATCH 1 is to provide a broad health screening service to underserved children while fostering

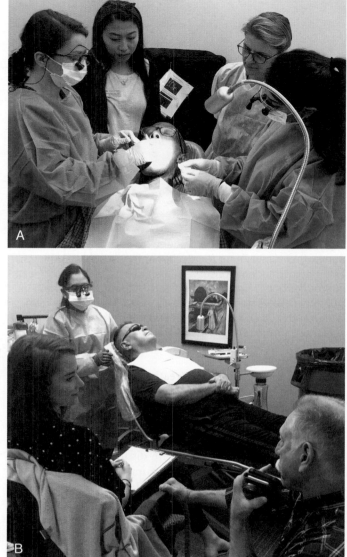

Fig 11.14 Dental hygiene and speech and language pathology (SLP) students work together in an interprofessional education program at a stroke center to treat patients who have suffered a cerebrovascular accident (CVA), while they also learn about the other's health discipline. (A) Two dental hygiene students treat a CVA patient with a SLP student and a dental hygiene faculty member observing from behind; the faculty member supervises and explains the procedure to the SLP student. (B) A dental hygiene student treats a CVA patient who has limited comprehension and speech while the SLP student records data and supports the communication process with the patient; at the same time, they teach the patient's caregiver how to help the patient with his oral health needs. (Courtesy Charlene Dickinson.)

an interprofessional environment among health professions students and supporting the Centers for Disease Control and Prevention (CDC) Whole School, Whole Community, Whole Child model for school-based health programs (see Chapter 6).[28] This program reinforces the notion that as health care continues to evolve, it is critical that students receive education and clinical experiences interacting with other

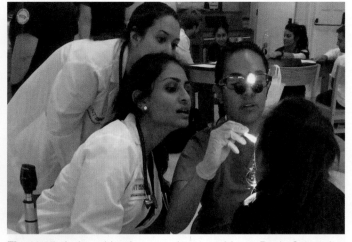

Fig 11.15 A dental hygiene student provides a Basic Screening Survey oral assessment for an elementary school student while two medical students observe as part of the CATCH 1 for Health Interprofessional Education Project. This interprofessional collaboration allows dental hygiene students to learn about medical issues and problems of the head and neck region while medical students learn to recognize oral problems.

healthcare team members in treating and educating a diverse population.

During the 2017 to 2019 period, the CATCH 1 program screened and collected information from approximately 350 elementary school students in a mid-sized urban Title 1 elementary school in a large city with distinct urban and suburban neighborhoods and bordering rural areas. Data have been collected and analyzed from the children screened, including statistics about the percentage of children that are economically disadvantaged and their racial and demographic characteristics, language predominance, food allergy plans, authorized medication for asthma, and oral health needs. In addition, children have been referred for treatment as needed. At the same time, research is being conducted on the various health professions students' attitudes and perceptions related to working in an interprofessional collaborative environment.

RISK MANAGEMENT IN SERVICE-LEARNING

When a person plans to travel, they typically consider obstacles that might be encountered and impede progress. These potential difficulties frequently are not immense, but even small complications can be a hindrance to meeting one's goals. Hence, it is wise to have an alternate plan in case of problems. For instance, if you volunteered to pick up your niece during rush hour to transport her to a sporting event 35 miles outside of the city, you would consider alternate routes in case of traffic congestion. You would ensure that your vehicle had enough gas, that children wore their seatbelts, and that you had the necessary personal identification and cash or a credit card. This thoughtful process of preplanning is an important step in managing possibilities.

Managing possibilities is another way to think of **risk management**. Alternate plans in case of possible problems are referred to by several terms, such as a contingency plan,

emergency plan, or incident plan. These can be thought of as what-if plans. In the same way, situations can occur in the process of a service-learning experience. Although planning for service-learning is not devoid of situational challenges, risk management suggests that such challenges or exposures can be managed through thoughtful preplanning and organization.[29,30] Risk management can have various roles in relation to service-learning (see Box 11.5).[29,31]

Leaders in the field of experiential learning suggest that all stakeholders involved in service-learning should also be involved in planning for risk management.[30] Academic institutions and community partners are likely to have their own risk management departments that serve as institutional clearinghouses with primary responsibility for guiding the risk management procedures when service-learning is implemented. The overall goal of having a formal approval process is to ensure that everyone involved in the service-learning program is aware of each other's expectations and responsibilities.

In educational institutions, this formal process for service-learning typically requires action from the initiating faculty member, the institution, the community partner, and the students. Academic institutions may require community partners to sign affiliation agreements; likewise, community partners may have similar agreements and policy documents that require faculty and student signatures. A faculty member typically initiates the process by learning what is needed to safeguard the educational experience for students. A number of issues should be considered for inclusion in risk management discussions when preparing for service-learning experiences (Box 11.6). Checklists can be used to organize risk management strategies.

The likelihood and severity of the risks of service-learning must be considered in the process of risk management.[29] The issue of risks for students, faculty, academic institutions, community agencies, and community members should be discussed openly, and strategies should be developed and distributed to all parties. Contingency planning, documentation, and continual review are prudent components of risk management related to experiential learning.

Students and professionals alike are legally accountable for their actions. Legal liability is a crucial consideration that

---

BOX 11.5 Purposes of Risk Management in Service-Learning

- Provides a means for an institution to manage risk to maximize its ability to meet learning objectives.
- Offers a way to avoid problems that can lead to failure while maintaining the value of programs that may involve risk.
- Helps institutions and community partners make sound decisions that safeguard the well-being of students, employees, and clients while adhering to government regulations.
- Establishes a system to manage challenges and resources to maintain safety and quality, which is critical to sustaining service-learning experiences and ongoing relationships with community partners.
- Increases accountability and responsibility for allotted resources, including financial.

BOX 11.6   Risk Management Considerations

- University-community agency affiliation agreement
- Student acknowledgment/agreement before participation
- Confidentiality and Health Information Portability and Accountability Act (HIPAA) compliance agreement
- Special insurance policies
- Policies/procedures
- Contact information
- Emergency procedures
- Background checks
- Student misconduct
- Travel, transportation, and parking
- Approval of lesson plan
- Storage of personal items
- Orientation checklist
- Assessment and evaluation procedures and documentation
- Scope of practice
- Supervision procedures and requirements
- Attendance policies

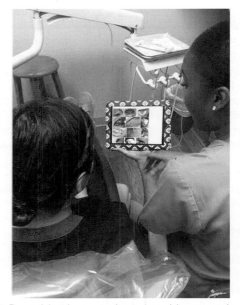

Fig 11.16 Dental hygiene students provide screening, training in self-assessment, and education about oral and pharyngeal cancer (OPC) and the need for regular screening for OPC in a service-learning project completed in collaboration with a local community dental clinic and the Oral Cancer Foundation. (Courtesy Leticia Silva, Deandrea Doddy, and Afua Ampem.)

is acknowledged and thoughtfully considered by responsible institutions before sanctioning experiential learning experiences such as service-learning. Initially, a student's awareness of an institution's risk management processes and procedures may be vague, but students' levels of awareness should increase through the process. This is an important learning experience in relation to working in the community after graduation, where risk management is the standard in educational and healthcare organizations.[30] To minimize legal liability, whether in a service-learning experience in college or later in a community-based project involving practicing dental hygienists, risk management is a key strategy to assure success and sustainability of community oral health initiatives.

SERVICE-LEARNING TO REINFORCE COMMUNITY ORAL HEALTH LEARNING

Learning the processes involved in assessment, program planning, and improvement of oral health can be enhanced with service-learning.[18] Well-constructed service-learning projects can be the learning platform for students to study the leading health indicators, oral health indicators, and determinants of health—especially social determinants—as they impact vulnerable populations. Opportunities are provided to locate and apply local, state, and national oral health surveillance findings and national oral health objectives (Figure 11.16).

In addition, service-learning also provides a form of role-play through which dental hygiene students can safely explore issues of access to care, health equity, and health disparities. Constructing service-learning projects can be instrumental in learning more deeply about the public health issues addressed throughout this textbook. Through service-learning, dental hygiene students can increase their public health knowledge, social awareness, and teamwork potential, as well as improve the oral health of their local communities.[2,4,32]

Public Health Resources

Various public health resources are important to community oral health practice (see Box 11.7). Integrating these resources into service-learning and other community projects will provide additional application of learning about the resources themselves and about the public health process. Use of reputable and national resources adds a dimension of consistency to community oral health projects and a standard measure for assessing the success of course and service-learning project objectives, as well as program objectives, when working in the community after graduation. Additional resources are listed in the References and Additional Resources at the end of this and other chapters and in Appendices A and D. All these resources can help in planning and designing service-learning and other community oral health projects.

Learning Opportunities

The Applying Your Knowledge section of this chapter provides opportunities to apply the service-learning concepts discussed throughout the chapter. By completing the exercises there, you will have the chance to increase your understanding of how to operationalize service-learning to get the most from the service-learning projects you will be assigned. The purpose of these activities is to provide practice in developing S-LOs and creating a lesson plan for a service-learning project, as well as an opportunity to reflect on your learning experiences. These exercises will challenge you to gain a deeper understanding of how to lay the groundwork for a successful service-learning project. Your faculty may modify the assignments to fit the course needs for your maximum value and success.

BOX 11.7   Resources for Service-Learning Projects

Healthy People 2030 (https://www.healthypeople.gov/)
- Science-based national health objectives for the current decade, including oral health objectives, to improve overall and oral health for all ages (see Chapter 4).
- Easily searchable website containing baseline data, targets for improvement, and available progress data related to all health objectives.
- Encourages use of information by individuals, groups, and organizations to improve the community's health; contains ideas about how others have used this resource to improve the health of their communities.
- Provides common, measurable standards by which to evaluate success in meeting the national oral health objectives, which can be implemented easily in service-learning lesson plans and service projects.

State and Local Oral Health Programs
- Website search of one's own state health department to learn about the state's public health and oral health infrastructure and capacity (see Chapters 4 and 5).
- Provides information about the oral health program in the state, including the mission, goals, priorities, and initiatives of the state oral health program as well as the state's preventive programs and potential funding opportunities.
- Provides consumer information through which residents can access information to help them find a dental home, learn about services available, or learn about oral health topics.
- Has water fluoridation status and information for the state (also see fluoridation status by state at https://www.cdc.gov/fluoridation/statistics/2016stats.htm and by water district at https://nccd.cdc.gov/doh_mwf/Default/Default.aspx).
- May provide opportunities for professionals, consumers, and teachers to request educational materials, possibly at low cost or free of charge to professionals for training purposes and for one's own service-learning projects.

Association of State and Territorial Dental Directors (https://www.astdd.org/)
- A national dental public health organization whose membership includes each of the state directors for oral health, representing a strong governmental presence regarding issues, core functions, and best practices for community oral health practice.
- Central location to access a myriad of resources to assist in community-based initiatives, including program development (see Chapters 3 and 6).
- Source of information about the Basic Screening Survey (BSS) for Children and Adults (see Chapter 4), containing everything that a team of dental hygienists would need to conduct a screening survey or to instruct school and agency personnel how to conduct these basic screening surveys.

National Oral Health Surveillance System (https://www.cdc.gov/oralhealthdata/overview/nohss.html)
- Collection of specific oral health data and information from every state, compiled to monitor changes in the oral health indicators over time (see Chapter 4).
- A searchable database to find data relative to oral health status and trends and to compare state oral health information.
- Useful for lesson planning purposes to view descriptive statistics that can be used for needs assessment and for inclusion in presentations to vividly and graphically illustrate oral health points (e.g., a state's ranking relative to the various oral indicators, such as dental visits, teeth cleaning, tooth loss, dental sealants, caries experience, untreated tooth decay, water fluoridation, and oral and pharyngeal cancer).

National Maternal and Child Oral Health Resource Center (https://www.mchoralhealth.org/)
- Supports health professionals, program administrators, educators, policymakers, and others with the goal of improving oral health services for infants, children, adolescents, and their families.
- Gathers, develops, and shares high-quality and valuable information and materials related to current and emerging dental public health issues to provide a comprehensive source of information and other resources for community oral health program planning.
- Interconnected and collaborates with countless organizations, including federal, state, and local agencies; national and state organizations and associations; and foundations.

Centers for Disease Control and Prevention (https://www.cdc.gov/)
- The nation's major health promotion agency responsible for monitoring, protecting, and improving the public's health.
- Conducts critical science related to epidemiology, provides surveillance, delivers health information, operates laboratory systems, and is involved in response-readiness activities.
- Linked to numerous other health- and oral health-related agencies to strengthen its value as a resource.
- Through its Division of Oral Health (DOH; https://www.cdc.gov/oralhealth/index.htm), works with state oral health programs and other organizations to improve access to oral health information, guides infection control, and promotes proven oral health strategies.
- Searchable DOH website with an A-Z index of hundreds of health topics, including health promotion, occupational health, health literacy, oral cancer, and multiple other oral health topics.

SUMMARY

Traditional methods of community-based outreach such as community service, volunteerism, clinical rotations, and field experiences, although limited in scope, are useful in the dental hygiene educational experience. However, these dental hygiene community outreach efforts can be enhanced by using the effective experiential instructional method of service-learning.

Service-learning emphasizes partnership stability via collaboration among students, faculty, and community partners throughout the process, starting with the initial planning. This results in continuity of services, which contributes to the success of future service-learning programs. Thus, service-learning can become institutionalized as a vehicle to accomplish the articulated desires of community partners and to meet dental hygiene students' academic course requirements.

In allowing students to tailor their own learning opportunities to improve in self-identified areas of importance, service-learning can transform learning by challenging and compelling them to become more active or involved in their own learning. Service-learning can also greatly impact oral health literacy and the oral health of the community. It is a powerful method in IPE to prepare dental hygienists for ICP, an important consideration as healthcare delivery systems evolve into this practice model. Learning activities are provided in the chapter for practice in applying service-learning to community oral health.

APPLYING YOUR KNOWLEDGE

Set A. Service-Learning Objectives Exercises

Exercise 1 is to define the following terms. As you progress with this assignment, your definition will take on greater clarity. Use this chapter and the glossary to define these terms. You will also find definitions on the Internet by searching key words such as "define service-learning," and you can use the list of additional resources at the end of this chapter.

1. Service-learning
2. Learning objective
3. Service objective
4. Service-learning objective
5. Reflection

Exercise 2 is a service-learning grid exercise presenting an opportunity to improve your skills of creating mutual objectives; you will practice combining SOs with LOs to build S-LOs in Table 11.3. The first two examples are completed for you.

Exercise 3 is a dental radiology service-learning assignment. This exercise will help you develop a specific S-LO based on the given information, now that you have a better understanding of the terms in exercise 1 and the process in Exercise 2. Follow the three steps below to develop one meaningful S-LO and record on a separate sheet of paper.

1. Pretending you are an elementary school teacher, think of a concept that you would want a dental hygiene student to teach to your class. This is the SO (service to be provided). The following example of a SO is recorded in Table 11.4: *The teacher wants the third-grade class to learn how the dentist finds tooth decay.* Record your example of a SO (what the teacher wants) on your separate sheet of paper.

TABLE 11.3 Exercise 2: Building Service-Learning Objectives

Example Number	Service Objective (SO)	Learning Objective (LO)	Service-Learning Objective (S-LO)
1	Dental hygiene students will support the school nurse with follow-up and dental referral services, including the identification of resources.	Dental hygiene students will demonstrate knowledge of health and nonhealth barriers to dental hygiene services.	Dental hygiene students will learn about the health and nonhealth barriers to dental hygiene services by assisting the school nurse with follow-up and dental referrals.
2	Children and parents will receive age-appropriate and culturally sensitive oral health education.	Dental hygiene students will prepare oral health education lessons for children in inner-city public schools.	Dental hygiene students will prepare and present age-appropriate and culturally sensitive oral health education to families.
3	Adolescents will be able to list the oral health consequences of a diet high in sugar	Dental hygiene students will demonstrate skills in communicating effectively with adolescents.	
4	Adolescent minority youth at the Jefferson House will be encouraged to consider careers in dental hygiene.	First- and second-year dental hygiene students will demonstrate an understanding of basic principles of adolescent learning, including behavior management.	
5	Schoolteachers will learn basic pediatric oral health information that will assist them in recognizing the need for urgent dental treatment.	Dental hygiene students will be able to demonstrate effective skills and knowledge when communicating with schoolteachers.	
6	The older adults will receive a confirmation of oral findings.	Dental hygiene students will demonstrate knowledge and skills in collecting and analyzing the results of an older adult Basic Screening Survey.	
7	The participants will receive an oral health report card that illustrates the results of a screening.	Dental hygiene students will develop a reporting instrument that will convey the results of oral screening.	

TABLE 11.4 Exercise 4: Creating Measurable Service-Learning Objectives

Service Objective (SO): What the Community Partner Wants	Learning Objective (LO): Academic Course Objective	Service-Learning Objective (S-LO): Combination of SO and LO
1. The teacher wants the third-grade class to learn how the dentist finds tooth decay.	The dental hygiene students will be able to identify dental caries on radiographs.	At the end of this presentation, the third-grade students will be able to correctly identify three out of four areas of severe tooth decay on bitewing radiographs. Performance verb: Identify; Condition: At the end of this presentation; Criterion measure: 75% accuracy
2. The teacher wants the fifth-grade class to learn how dental braces work.	The dental hygiene students will be able to...	At the end of this presentation, the... Performance verb: Condition: Criterion measure:
3. The teacher wants the sixth-grade students to learn how to protect their teeth and mouths during sports activities.	The dental hygiene students will be able to...	At the end of this presentation, the... Performance verb: Condition: Criterion measure:

> ## BOX 11.8   Selected Dental Radiology Course Objectives
>
> **Imaging Techniques**
> 1. Compare and contrast intraoral and extraoral imaging criteria and techniques; identify the technique used to produce an image.
> 2. Compare and contrast traditional imaging with digital imaging.
> 3. Define and use terminology.
>
> **Anatomy**
> 1. Describe the normal radiographic appearance of teeth and the supporting structures.
> 2. Identify anatomic structures on a radiographic image.
> 3. Define and use terminology.
>
> **Interpretation**
> 1. Identify radiographic appearance of restorative materials and foreign objects.
> 2. Identify dental caries.
> 3. Identify and describe radiographic bone loss.
> 4. Recognize the appearance of trauma, lesions, and other disturbances.
> 5. Systematically interpret and present radiographic findings.
> 6. Define and use terminology.

2. Next, review the list of selected approved academic dental radiology course objectives (Box 11.8) with the purpose of selecting one that you, as a dental hygiene student, want to teach to a group of elementary schoolchildren. This is not a comprehensive list of radiology course objectives. It includes only objectives that are appropriate for this assignment, and those that are too complex have been excluded. The academic course objective you choose is the LO (what you would be learning related to dental radiology). The following example of a LO is provided in Table 11.4 for guidance: *The dental hygiene students will be able to identify radiographic dental caries.* Record your LO (academic course objective) on your separate sheet of paper.

3. Now combine the teacher's concept (the SO) and the dental hygiene course objective (the LO) to make one complete statement (the S-LO) and record it. This combined statement (the S-LO) is an amalgamation of the community partner's wishes and the dental hygiene academic course objective. This process may take a few attempts before you get it just right. The following example of a combination objective (S-LO) is provided in Table 11.4 for guidance: *At the end of the presentation, the third-grade students will be able to correctly identify three out of four areas of severe tooth decay on bitewing radiographs.* Record your S-LO (combination objective) on your separate sheet of paper.

Exercise 4 consists of practice developing measurable S-LOs in Table 11.4. This exercise will increase your ability to write more meaningful objectives. You will practice writing objectives that are specific and measurable to determine quantifiable outcomes. Refer to Chapter 6 Goals and Objectives section for a discussion of how to write effective, measurable objectives. In this instance, not only will you develop LOs and S-LOs for the

SOs provided in Table 11.4, you will also include a performance verb, condition, and criterion measure for each of the S-LOs as described in Chapter 6. Notice the performance verb, condition, and criterion measure in the S-LO example provided in Table 11.4. Your instructor may have you complete additional activities to increase proficiency and comfort with this skill.

Set B: Service-Learning Lesson Plan Development Exercise

This exercise will provide you the opportunity to develop the initial steps of creating a service-learning lesson plan. (See Figure 11.17 for the template for this exercise.) This activity can be combined with information provided in Chapter 3, including Figure 3.7; Chapter 6 Program Planning Process section, Tables 6.3 and 6.7, and Box 6.17; and Chapter 8 to prepare a complete lesson plan, which is a comprehensive sketch of what is planned for a teaching situation. It is comprehensive in that it is detailed, to the point that someone else could teach your lesson from the outline of the plan. However, it is referred to as a sketch because it does not include an exact account of the dialogue that will be used to teach the lesson. You can think of a lesson plan as a roadmap for how to get from point A to point B that includes time for each of your desired pursuits along the way such as meal detours, entertainment, lodging, weather forecasts, and so on. Your instructor may revise this template to fit the needs of the course, institution, or community.

In the template that lists the initial steps for creating a service-learning lesson plan in Figure 11.17, there is a place for basic information about the presenter and the community partner, and a description of the audience. Beneath this heading, there is a place to document the overall **goal** of the lesson (see Box 6.5 in Chapter 6) and the SOs, LOs, and S-LOs. After this section, there is an area to indicate the concepts, teaching strategies, and time frame needed for each activity and to cite the resources used to develop the lesson plan. The second page of Figure 11.17 is a reflection exercise for you to assess and reflect upon the effectiveness of your service-learning project during and after implementation. This reflection should be based on your formative and summative evaluation of the project and also include your own thoughts, perceptions, observations, and experiences in carrying out the lesson plan. This exercise will help you determine the effectiveness of your SOs, LOs, and S-LOs and of the implementation of the service-learning project. It will also focus on your own personal learning from the service-learning experience.

Your instructor may assign this exercise as an individual project or a small group activity, as a part of the development and reflection of your service-learning project. In either case, the self-explanatory template should be followed to begin the outline of the lesson plan. Also, your instructor may assign or allow you to self-select a population or community partner for your lesson plan. After you have completed this exercise, you can learn from each other by sharing your experiences in class.

Student Hygienists _____ Date _____

Agency _____   Contact Person _____

Address _____ Phone _____ Email _____

Audience _____   Age(s) _____

GOAL: (write one overall goal statement here)

Service Objectives	Learning Objectives	Service-Learning Objectives
What the community partner wants	*Academic course objective from the syllabus*	*The combined SOs and LOs*

Identify the teaching concept, strategy, and time for each of the objectives.

Concepts	Strategies	Time

Identify materials needed for each of the concepts and strategies.

List citations for the resources used.

Fig 11.17 Template for the initial steps of lesson plan development.

LEARNING OBJECTIVES AND COMPETENCIES

This chapter addresses the following community dental health learning objectives and competencies for dental hygienists that are presented in the *ADEA Compendium of Curriculum Guidelines for Allied Dental Education Programs*:

Learning Objectives
- Identify and use community dental health activities related to prevention and control of oral conditions and promotion of health.
- Develop a dental public health program plan.

Competencies
- Providing health education and preventive counseling to a variety of population groups.
- Promoting the values of good oral and general health and wellness to the public and organizations within and outside the professions.
- Advocating for consumer groups, businesses, and government agencies to support healthcare issues.
- Assessing, planning, implementing, and evaluating community-based oral health programs.
- Providing dental hygiene services in a variety of settings, including offices, hospitals, clinics, extended care facilities, community programs, and schools.
- Accepting responsibility for solving problems and making decisions based on accepted scientific principles.

Reflection Exercises

Your instructor may ask you to complete a mixture of the following exercises. They may ask you to use a sheet of paper, blog, or discussion forum to respond to the questions individually or in a small group. Using roundtables or other presentation formats to share responses is also encouraged.

Assessing SO, LO, and Service-Learning

1. What did you learn about the LO that you wouldn't have learned from a straight lecture? You might approach this task by thinking about what you knew about the LO initially.

2. Describe your view of the relationship between the LO and the instructional experience. In other words, how were the LO and SO related? What process did you use to integrate the two?

3. Explain why you think you accomplished or did not accomplish the LO.

4. Now explain why you think you accomplished or did not accomplish the SO.

5. A second way to address this task is to fill in the blanks for the following statement below:

   • As a result of this service-learning experience, I believe that the SO _____ was _____ based on the following _____.

   • As a result of this service-learning experience, I believe that the LO _____ was _____ based on the following _____.

Short Responses

1. What did you know about the situation before you experienced it?

2. What one thing would have helped you prepare for the experience better?

3. What would you do differently and why?

4. What made you feel secure in the experience?

5. How did you feel when the presentation was completed?

6. Who do you think got the most from the assignment and why?

7. How prepared was the community partner for your visit?

8. How well did you understand the task?

9. What worked? Why did it work?

10. What did not work? What could have made it better?

11. What further comments, questions, or observations would you like to share?

Fig 11.17 (*Continued*)

COMMUNITY CASE

The local dental society and the local dental hygiene program collaborated on the Give Kids a Smile (GKS) national event to provide dental treatment for children in the community. The dental hygiene department at Your Community College and volunteers from the dental society conducted a massive oral screening on underserved children in the area. The results revealed that 60% of the 250 children aged 7 to 13 years had an urgent need for dental treatment, and 75% had never visited the dentist. The dental hygiene faculty, local dentists, and dental hygiene students want to provide dental services for this group of children. You are a student in the dental hygiene program, and you have agreed to serve as a member of the GKS planning committee. The committee members consist of community members, agency members, dental hygiene faculty, dental hygiene advisory board members, and dentists from the local dental society.

1. Which resource is the best one to assist the group in developing program objectives for the event?
   a. *Healthy People 2030*
   b. National Oral Health Surveillance System
   c. Association of State and Territorial Dental Directors
   d. Basic Screening Survey

2. Which of the following experiential learning methods for student involvement will provide equal benefit to the students and to the children?
   a. Community service by helping in a future service project
   b. Volunteering to chair the planning committee
   c. A service-learning project with the children and parents
   d. A clinical rotation to a follow-up GKS treatment day

3. In the development of this community dental program, which category of evaluation will your committee use to make modifications during the planning and implementation of the program?
   a. Summative evaluation
   b. Formative evaluation
   c. Normative evaluation
   d. Impact evaluation
4. What type of objective is the following: "Dental hygiene students will be able to identify five major sources of public health financing for oral health services"?
   a. A service objective
   b. A learning objective

c. A service-learning objective
d. Both a learning and a service-learning objective

5. At what point should you approach the chair of the committee about using this experience as your required service-learning experience?
   a. Before the next meeting of the planning committee
   b. After you have met with the planning committee and discussed your interest with your course instructor
   c. After the planning committee has met to make plans for the treatment phase of the GKS program
   d. After the planning committee has been oriented to the purpose and mission of GKS

REFERENCES

1. Engaging Students in Learning: Service-learning. Seattle, WA: University of Washington Center for Teaching and Learning; 2020. Available at: <https://www.washington.edu/teaching/topics/engaging-students-in-learning/>; [Accessed March 2020].
2. Transforming Dental Hygiene Education and the Profession for the 21st Century. Chicago, IL: American Dental Hygienists' Association; 2015. Available at: <https://www.adha.org/resources-docs/Transforming_Dental_Hygiene_Education.pdf>; [Accessed December 2019].
3. Reforming America's Healthcare System Through Choice and Competition. Washington, DC: Department of Health and Human Services, Department of the Treasury, Department of Labor; 2018 Dec. Available at: <https://www.hhs.gov/sites/default/files/Reforming-Americas-Healthcare-System-Through-Choice-and-Competition.pdf>; [Accessed September 2019].
4. Core Competencies for Interprofessional Collaborative Practice: 2016 Update. Washington, DC: Interprofessional Education Collaborative; 2016. Available at: <https://hsc.unm.edu/ipe/resources/ipec-2016-core-competencies.pdf>; Accessed December 2019].
5. Accreditation Standards for Dental Hygiene Education Programs. Chicago, IL: Commission on Dental Accreditation; 2018. Available at: <https://www.ada.org/~/media/CODA/Files/2019_dental_hygiene_standards.pdf?la=en>; [Accessed December 2019].
6. Advocacy. Chicago, IL: American Dental Hygienists' Association; n.d. Available at: <https://www.adha.org/advocacy>; [Accessed December 2019].
7. ADHA Policy Manual. Chicago, IL: American Dental Hygienists' Association; 2018 Jun. Available at: <https://www.adha.org/resources-docs/7614_Policy_Manual.pdf>; [Accessed December 2019].
8. Minjarez, J, Nuzzo, S. Dental Therapists: Sinking Our Teeth into Innovative Workforce Reform. Tallahassee, FL: The James Madison Institute; 2018. Available at: <https://www.jamesmadison.org/dental-therapists-sinking-our-teeth-into-innovative-workforce-reform/>; [Accessed October 2019].
9. Seaman J, Quay J, Brown M. The evolution of experiential learning: Tracing lines of research in the JEE. J Exp Educ 2017;40(Suppl.):1–20. Available at: <https://dx.doi.org/10.1177/1053825916689268>; [Accessed December 2019].
10. Service-Learning and Experiential Education. Starting Point: Teaching Entry Level Geoscience; 2018. Available at: <https://serc.carleton.edu/introgeo/service/experiential.html>; [Accessed December 2019].
11. Nierenberg S, Hughes LP, Warunek M, et al. Nursing and dental students reflections on interprofessional practice after a service-learning experience in Appalachia. J Dent Educ 2018;82(5):454–61. Available at: <https://pubmed.ncbi.nlm.nih.gov/29717068/>; [Accessed December 2019].
12. Bandy J. What is Service Learning or Community Engagement? Nashville, TN: Vanderbilt University Center for Teaching; 2019. Available at: <https://cft.vanderbilt.edu/guides-sub-pages/teaching-through-community-engagement/>; [Accessed December 2019].
13. Allen HB, Gunaldo TP, Schwartz E. Creating awareness for the social determinants of health: dental hygiene and nursing student interprofessional service-learning experiences. J Dent Hyg 2019;93(3):22–8. Available at: <https://jdh.adha.org/content/93/3/22>; [Accessed April 2020].
14. What is Service-Learning? Baltimore: MD: John Hopkins University; n.d. Available at: <https://source.jhu.edu/publications-and-resources/service-learning-toolkit/what-is-service-learning.html>; [Accessed December 2019].
15. What is Service-Learning? Starting Point: Teaching Entry Level Geoscience; 2018. Available at: <https://serc.carleton.edu/introgeo/service/what.html>; [Accessed December 2019].
16. Service-Learning Assessment & Evaluation. Cullowhee, NC: Western Carolina University; n.d. Available at: <https://www.wcu.edu/learn/academic-enrichment/center-for-service-learning/service-learning-forms-resources/service-learning-assessment-evaluation.aspx>; [Accessed December 2019].
17. Mason MR, Dunens E. Service-learning as a practical introduction to undergraduate public health: benefits for student outcomes and accreditation. Front Public Health 2019;7:63. Available at: <https://www.ncbi.nlm.nih.gov/pmc/articles/PMC6454065/>; [Accessed December 2019].
18. Program Planning Resource. The Community Guide. Available at: <https://www.thecommunityguide.org/content/program-planning-resource>; [Accessed December 2019].
19. Reflection. Community Engaged Learning, Teaching, and Scholarship: Service Learning. New Orleans, LA: Loyola University. Available at: <http://www.loyno.edu/engage/reflection>; [Accessed April 2020].
20. Service Learning. Seattle, WA: University of Washington Center for Teaching and Learning; 2019. Available at: <https://www.

washington.edu/teaching/topics/engaging-students-in-learning/service-learning/>; [Accessed December 2019].

21. Learning Objectives (for Service Learning). Community Engaged Learning, Teaching, and Scholarship: Service Learning. New Orleans, LA: Loyola University. Available at: <http://www.loyno.edu/engage/learning-objectives>; [Accessed April 2020].

22. Wolpert-Gawron H. What the Heck Is Service Learning? Edutopia; 2016. Available at: <https://www.edutopia.org/blog/what-heck-service-learning-heather-wolpert-gawron>; [Accessed December 2019].

23. Bandy J. Best Practices in Community Engaged Teaching. Nashville, TN: Vanderbilt University Center for Teaching; 2019. Available at: <https://cft.vanderbilt.edu//cft/guides-sub-pages/best-practices-in-community-engaged-teaching/>; [Accessed December 2019].

24. Temple A, Mast ME. Interprofessional Education through service learning with undergraduate health administration and nursing students. JHAE 2016 Winter; 6:21(e). Available at: <https://www.ingentaconnect.com/contentone/aupha/jhae/2016/00000033/00000001/art00002?crawler=true>; [Accessed April 2020].

25. How to Use Service-Learning. Starting Point: Teaching Entry Level Geoscience. Northfield, MN: Carleton College Science Education Resource Center; 2018. Available at: <https://serc.carleton.edu/introgeo/service/howto.html>; [Accessed December 2019].

26. Lyndon M, Cashell A. Collaboration in health care. JMIRS 2017; 48:207–16. Available at: <https://www.jmirs.org/article/S1939-8654(16)30117-5/pdf>; [Accessed December 2019].

27. Post-stroke Dental Care. Stroke Connection; 2019. Available at: <http://strokeconnection.strokeassociation.org/Winter-2019/Post-stroke-Dental-Care/>; [Accessed December 2019].

28. Whole School, Whole Community, Whole Child. Atlanta, GA: Centers for Disease Control and Prevention; 2020 Feb 10. Available at: <https://www.cdc.gov/healthyschools/wscc/index.htm>; [Accessed April 2020].

29. Yarullin IF, Prichinin AE, Sharipova DY. Risk management of an education project. J Math Educ 2016;11(1):45–56. Available at: <https://www.iejme.com/download/risk-management-of-an-education-project.pdf>; [Accessed December 2019].

30. The Five Keys to Risk Management for Higher Education Boards. Board Effect; 2019. Available at: <https://www.boardeffect.com/blog/five-keys-risk-management-higher-education-boards/>; [Accessed December 2019].

31. School Policy Risk Management. Victoria, Australia: Victoria State Government Education and Training; 2018. Available at: <https://www.education.vic.gov.au/school/principals/spag/governance/Pages/risk.aspx>; [Accessed December 2019].

32. Community Tool Box. Lawrence, KS: University of Kansas; 2019. Available at: <https://ctb.ku.edu/en>; [Accessed December 2019].

ADDITIONAL RESOURCES

American Dental Hygienists' Association
https://www.adha.org/
Community-Campus Partnership for Health
http://ccphealth.org/
Interprofessional Education Collaborative
https://www.ipecollaborative.org/about-ipec.html
Maternal and Child Health Bureau of the Health Resources and
   Services Administration
http://mchb.hrsa.gov/
National Youth Leadership Council
https://www.nylc.org/default.aspx
U.S. Department of Veterans Affairs, Patient Aligned Care Team
   (PACT)
http://www.va.gov/health/services/primarycare/pact/index.asp

BOOK

Gagliardi L. Dental Health Education: Lesson Planning and
   Implementation. 3rd ed. Long Grove, IL: Waveland Press; 2021.

12

Test-Taking Strategies and Community Cases

Christine French Beatty

OBJECTIVES

1. Develop an overview of the National Board Dental Hygiene Examination (NBDHE).
2. Apply tips for examination preparation for the NBDHE.
3. Apply guidelines for answering multiple-choice test items and community testlets.
4. Answer community oral health questions that employ the formats used on the NBDHE.
5. Use critical thinking skills to take a mock NBDHE examination of community testlets for practice.
6. Increase level of personal confidence in preparing for the community section of the NBDHE.

Test taking is a skill. It involves abilities beyond just understanding the material being tested. It is important to be thoroughly familiar with the format of an examination before taking it. For example, in your courses you probably have asked questions about the number and types of questions that will be on a test and the professor's regulations related to the test-taking process.

It is important to develop proficiency in test taking. This chapter is focused on information about the NBDHE to orient you to this important examination. Also included are various test-taking tips designed to help you develop expertise in taking tests (Box 12.1). In addition, Box 12.2 presents the application of some of the logical clues explained in Box 12.1 to help you analyze the correct answers to NBDHE questions.

OVERVIEW OF THE NATIONAL BOARD DENTAL HYGIENE EXAMINATION

The Joint Commission on National Dental Examinations (JCNDE) of the American Dental Association (ADA) is responsible for the development and administration of the NBDHE. The JCNDE contracts with Pearson VUE to administer the NBDHE at test centers across the United States and its territories, and in Canada.[1]

The purpose of this comprehensive, computer-based, pass/fail examination is to help state boards assess the qualifications of individuals who seek licensure to practice dental hygiene.[1,2] The examination assesses the ability to understand important information from basic biomedical, dental, and dental hygiene sciences and the ability to apply it in a problem-solving context.[1,2] NBDHE questions test knowledge and understanding, as well as application, analysis, synthesis, and evaluation of content.

The current NBDHE consists of 350 multiple-choice questions and is administered electronically by a vendor over a 9-hour period with scheduled and optional breaks.[1] The examination includes 200 discipline-based questions and 150 questions based on 12 to 15 dental hygiene patient cases.[1] The major content areas of the examination and associated subjects are presented in Table 12.1.

The NBDHE includes a section of 24 questions related to the community health/research principles content area.[1] Five **community cases** are presented with a series of four or five questions related to each case.[1] The community cases are simulations of the dental hygienist's participation in a particular community oral health program or activity in relation to a specific target population. The questions following each community case require application of information, such as that within this textbook, to select the correct answer.

The community case combined with the associated test items is referred to by the NBDHE as a **testlet**.[1] These five testlets comprehensively represent the content of community health/research principles on the NBDHE (Table 12.1).

National Board Dental Hygiene Examination Question Formats

Multiple-choice items on the NBDHE consist of a stem that poses a problem, followed by a list of three to five possible answers.[1] Only one of these responses is considered the *correct or best answer.*[1] To be able to efficiently answer community questions, it is important to become familiar with the various question formats used consistently on the NBDHE (Box 12.3). Practicing with sample testlets will help you become comfortable with these question formats as well as review content.

BOX 12.1   Test-Taking Tips

1. Relax the night before the examination to allow your mind and body to release tension.
2. Control stress the day of the examination by arriving early. Allow extra time to get to the examination site, and arrange back-up transportation.
3. Be comfortable but alert. Get a good night's sleep, and the morning of the examination, eat a good breakfast with protein for the brain benefits. During the examination wear comfortable clothes, don't slouch – maintain good posture, and sip water throughout the examination.
4. Use your time wisely during the examination. Take the time to determine how many questions are presented and how much time you will need to answer each question or section of questions. Monitor the time you spend on each question, to be certain you will complete the examination.
5. Read directions and questions carefully.
6. Take your time; be careful not to skip questions, misread questions, or mismark answers.
7. Actively reason through each question and read all answers before making your choice.
8. Attempt to answer every question; if you are unsure of an answer, mark or flag that question to enable you to return to it later. On the NBDHE, it is to your advantage to make an educated guess if you do not know the correct or best answer.
9. Attempt to answer the question posed by the stem of a multiple-choice question before you read the alternatives; then read them to find the one that most closely matches your answer.
10. Look for the "best" answer to a multiple-choice question; frequently several will seem correct, but one is the best.
11. Use a process of elimination to answer multiple-choice items. First eliminate the answers that are obviously incorrect, and then focus on the remaining choices to select the best answer.
12. Don't over-think a question; look for the root of the question and answer it accordingly.
13. If you are unsure of the right answer, use logical clues that help you figure it out, but don't allow these clues to misdirect you when you are certain you know the correct answer.
    a. A repeated word or concept: A recurring word or idea in the question and answer to a multiple-choice question can indicate the correct response.
    b. Length of the correct response: Often the longest answer to a multiple-choice question is correct because it provides necessary details.
    c. A similarity in alternatives: You can eliminate similar answers.
    d. Direct opposite of responses: You can eliminate a contradictory answer or one that is a complete opposite to the question.
    e. Use of absolutes or extremes: words such as every, always, all, never, and none may indicate the statement in the stem is false. However, conditional words such as usually, normally, generally, and commonly often mean a statement is true.
14. Take the time to review the test when you have completed it to be certain you have answered all questions, made no errors, and not mismarked any answers.
15. Change answers only if you find you misread the question or come across information in the test that corrects a previous answer.
16. Stay calm; if you find yourself becoming anxious, stop and take a few deep breaths. Don't talk to other students right before the test or during breaks; stress and anxiety can be contagious.

(From Sanders S. 5 tips for passing the National Board Dental Hygiene Examination. Today's RDH, November 10, 2018;e. Available at: <https://www.todaysrdh.com/5-tips-for-passing-the-national-board-dental-hygiene-examination/>; [Accessed December 5, 2019]; Test Taking Tips; 2017. Available at: <https://www.ada.org/~/media/JCNDE/pdfs/nbdhe_examinee_guide.pdf?la=en>; [Accessed December 5, 2019]; Tips for Better Test Taking, n.d. Available at: <http://www.studygs.net/tsttak1.htm>; [Accessed December 5, 2019]].)

BOX 12.2   Application of Logical Clues to Answering Test Questions

The following examples demonstrate how to answer test questions by applying the clues presented in Box 12.1. The answer to each question is provided following the question, along with a rationale based on these clues rather than knowledge of content. Questions relate to health promotion and behavioral change; a knowledge review can be found in Chapter 8. Remember you should apply these clues *only when you are unsure of the correct answer*.

1. Which of the following describes the Stages of Change Theory?
   a. An example of ways to influence changes in public policy
   b. A means of assessing a person's readiness to change and adopt behaviors that lead to a healthy lifestyle
   c. A model that includes key concepts such as reciprocal determination, observational learning, and reinforcement
   d. A way to directly assess how susceptible to periodontitis a patient perceives oneself to be

   The correct answer is b. Answer b repeats the word *change*, which provides a clue. Although answer choice a also includes the word *changes*, the topic is not relevant because the question is supposed to be focused on health promotion and behavioral change. Answer choices c and d have no wording similar to that of the question stem.

2. Which of the following is an example of the tailoring technique that is used in formulating an individual's oral health plan?
   a. Highlighting one or two messages that might apply to your patient
   b. Using photographs of American Indian women for posters in an Indian Health Service clinic
   c. Providing three individualized recommendations based on risk factors identified during a personal risk assessment

   d. Asking a group whether they prefer a video, slides, or a demonstration

   The correct answer is c. This answer uses a similar idea—the concept of individualization—even if one does not connect risk with tailoring. Answer choices b and d can be eliminated; they are opposites of the question stem, referring to a group rather than an individual. Answer choice a uses the vague term *might*, making it a less feasible answer.

3. You have developed a new program to promote oral health to teenage mothers, and you would like to discuss your ideas with other health professionals at an upcoming dental public health conference to determine ways to expand the program. Which of the following formats would be best for this presentation?
   a. Roundtable discussion
   b. Oral presentation
   c. Research poster presentation
   d. Table clinic

   The correct answer is a. This answer repeats the term *discuss* (in *discussion*), reiterating the purpose of the undertaking as stated in the stem.

4. Which of the following strategies would ensure the greatest understanding of how to perform an oral cancer examination in a group of adults?
   a. Distributing a handout with a description and pictures
   b. Using a multimedia presentation
   c. Demonstrating an oral cancer examination, followed by a discussion and a return demonstration of the oral cancer self-examination
   d. Watching a video together, followed by discussion

   The correct answer is c. This answer is considerably longer than answer choices a, b, and d and provides more detail.

TABLE 12.1 Major Areas of the National Board Dental Hygiene Examination and Associated Subjects

Major Areas	Number of Items	Associated Subjects
Scientific Basis for Dental Hygiene Practice	61	• Anatomic Sciences • Physiology • Biochemistry and Nutrition • Microbiology and Immunology • Pathology: General and Oral • Pharmacology
Provision of Clinical Dental Hygiene Services	115	• Assessing Patient Characteristics • Obtaining and Interpreting Radiographs • Planning and Managing Dental Hygiene Care • Performing Periodontal Procedures • Using Preventive Agents • Providing Supportive Treatment Services • Professional Responsibility

Community Health/Research Principles[a]	24	• Promoting Health and Preventing Disease Within Groups
		• Participating in Community Programs
		  • Assessing populations and defining objectives
		  • Designing, implementing, and evaluating programs
		• Analyzing Scientific Literature, Understanding Statistical Concepts, and Applying Research Results

Case-based items	150	Clinical Cases

[a]Some dental hygiene programs have a separate research course; for the purpose of the NBDHE, research content is folded into community oral health content.
(Data from National Board Dental Hygiene Examination (NBDHE) 2020 Candidate Guide. Joint Commission on National Dental Examinations; 2020. Available at: <https://www.ada.org/~/media/JCNDE/pdfs/2019_NBDHE_Guide.pdf?la=en>; [Accessed October 25, 2020]; NBDHE General Information. Joint Commission on National Dental Examinations; 2020. Available at: <https://www.ada.org/en/jcnde/examinations/national-board-dental-hygiene-examination>; [Accessed October 25, 2020]])

BOX 12.3 National Board Dental Hygiene Examination Question Formats

Question

Communicates a problem or set of circumstances, posed as a question.

Example:

What type of graph shows a plot of variables to depict their relationship?

a. Pie chart
b. Histogram
c. Scattergram*
d. Polygon

Completion

Requires the correct completion of a concept or idea.

Example:

A public health dental hygienist who meets with city council members to explain the benefits of fluoridation for the purpose of convincing them to adopt fluoridation for the community is functioning in the role of

a. administrator
b. advocate*

c. clinician
d. researcher

Negative

Used in situations where exceptions to general rules, principles, or appropriate actions exist; standard language applied in the stem, including the use of a word such as EXCEPT or NOT, which is capitalized to bring attention to it.

Example:

Each of the following is important when framing a health education message EXCEPT one. Which is the EXCEPTION?

a. Attempting to connect the message to people's values, beliefs, knowledge, and emotions
b. Using the same message for all members of the population to ensure consistency*
c. Making a message meaningful to the audience by personalizing it
d. Focusing oral health education materials on the specific needs of the audience

* Note: The correct answer to each sample question is italicized.

ANSWERING COMMUNITY CASE QUESTIONS IN TESTLETS

Testing with cases or testlets requires students not only to retrieve knowledge, but also to use **critical thinking** skills to apply knowledge to specific situations. The NBDHE measures your ability to solve problems and make decisions based on both the knowledge you have acquired in your coursework and your critical thinking skills. Your critical thinking skills are just that—thinking about what you know.

In most dental hygiene schools, students have the opportunity to practice critical thinking by applying what they have learned in the community course to projects they conduct in the community. These projects require critical thinking skills to determine the best way to achieve maximum oral health for the selected target population. Studying the "Applying Your

Knowledge" features at the end of each chapter in this textbook is also a good way for students to practice critical thinking skills.

On the NBDHE you will apply information you have learned in your community course to simulated community situations. Thus, when answering the community testlet questions, you must change your train of thought from thinking about clinical practice to thinking about community practice. Recall the definitions and principles from within this textbook and the comparisons of private practice and community oral health practice. Your selection of the correct answer must be what is best for the community as a whole rather than for an individual.

In this community frame of mind, carefully read through the community case described in the testlet. Note the key words and phrases that can guide your thinking through the correct answers. Then begin to read the questions, referring back to the case as you answer the associated questions. Remember the questions are intended to relate only to the case presented, and you must select the best answer in relation to the information in the case. It is also a good idea to reread the case one more time after answering the questions to catch any incorrect answers you may have selected as a result of not recalling important data from the case.

PREPARING FOR THE NATIONAL BOARD DENTAL HYGIENE EXAMINATION

To reduce stress and ensure success, careful preparation is required to take an examination of the magnitude of the NBDHE. In general, as you prepare for it, try to identify your weak areas and concentrate your review on them. Do not cram for it. Rather, have a study strategy and schedule time for review, possibly using a calendar to set aside hours to study weekly. Also plan a location that is conducive to study and where you will have no distractions.

Consider the study methods that work for you. Some people study well in groups, which can be beneficial because you learn other students' ideas and ways to recall, critically think about, and apply information. Other students do better alone, and many students use both methods.

Previous NBDHE questions give you practice in test taking and often cover material that never changes. Alternate your content review periods with practice examinations. Practice test modules and a list of reference texts used to construct NBDHE questions are available on the ADA/JCNDE website.[3] A web search can identify other resources for additional sample examinations.

In addition, become very aware of the regulations of the NBDHE. Study all the information available on the NBDHE and related websites. Read the current NBDHE candidate guide several times. Research where you have to go to take the examination and how long it will take to get there.

As you prepare, take care of yourself by eating well, staying hydrated and getting adequate rest. Also, staying calm is important to your psyche as you study. Remember, you will not know everything. Moreover, a positive attitude always helps!

APPLICATION OF CRITICAL THINKING: SAMPLE COMMUNITY ORAL HEALTH PRACTICE TESTLETS

The following five testlets provide a practice test in community oral health. The number and types of questions are similar to those on the NBDHE in the area of community health/research principles. You need to complete these questions in 35 minutes or less to allow approximately 1 minute each on the other 200 discipline-specific questions on the examination.[1] The correct answers and rationales follow the testlets in this chapter.

Testlet No. 1

You practice dental hygiene in a private dental office that serves a relatively higher socioeconomic status (SES) population of an economically and ethnically diverse, multicultural city of 1.5 million people. The city water supply is not fluoridated; consequently, dental caries experience is prevalent in the overall city population. Most families in the city are of Hispanic descent. You recently assisted the public health dental hygienist in conducting a screening on the children in a local Title 1 elementary school to document their oral health status. Fluoridation was defeated 10 years ago because of a strong antifluoridation campaign. Fluoridation will be on the ballot again in 8 months. The natural level of fluoride (F) in the community water is 0.2 mg/L.

1. As a private practice hygienist, what would be the best thing for you to do to help get the fluoride referendum passed?
   a. Continue educating your patients on the benefits of fluoride
   b. Start calling community leaders
   c. Make a financial contribution to the cause

   d. Contact your local dental hygiene society to help with their unified plan of action
2. All the following political tactics EXCEPT one will be beneficial to ensure that the fluoridation referendum will pass. Which is the EXCEPTION?
   a. Public debate with the antifluoridationists
   b. Analysis of the referendum of 10 years ago
   c. Endorsements by community leaders
   d. Distribution of literature in Spanish and English throughout the community
3. Which of the following methods would be best to communicate to the parents the overall oral needs of their children after the screening?
   a. Sending DMFT index results home with the children
   b. Mailing literature on the importance of children's oral health to the parents
   c. Phoning the parents to report findings of the screening on their children and refer them for treatment
   d. Sending Basic Screening Survey results home with a referral and a list of local community dental clinics
4. How much F should be added to the water to bring the F level to the optimal level recommended by the CDC?
   a. 0.5 mg F
   b. 0.7 mg F
   c. 0.8 mg F
   d. 1 mg F

5. If the fluoridation referendum fails to pass again, which alternative program would be the best one to implement?
   a. Send letters to parents to recommend they take their children to the dentist for fluoride treatments
   b. Give oral hygiene lessons in the classrooms
   c. Initiate a school fluoride varnish program
   d. Implement a sealant program

Testlet No. 2

Upon completion of a community oral health certification program, you are employed as a public health dental hygienist in a local health department to develop the first oral health unit in the department. You are asked to plan, implement, and evaluate a school-based educational and preventive program for selected elementary schools in the school district. The population has a large cohort of recently immigrated Vietnamese families. Your plan includes classroom education and the use of a mobile dental van to provide screenings, cleanings, sealants, fluorides, and referrals to dental homes. Surveillance data will be collected using the DMFT index.

1. All of the following EXCEPT one should be the foundation of planning for this program and guide the emphasis of the program. Which is the EXCEPTION?
   a. *Healthy People 2030* objectives
   b. Guidelines from the Association of State and Territorial Dental Directors
   c. Protocols used in private clinical practice before making the transition to public health practice
   d. The best available evidence related to the interventions selected for the program.
2. The index used to collect data will be helpful to assess which of the following?
   a. The demand for services that are provided by your oral health program
   b. The children's gingival and periodontal status
   c. The need for dental services to be provided by the dental homes
   d. The children's risk of contracting medical conditions
3. In the evaluation phase of the program, you plan to measure the children's performance skills in the area of oral hygiene; this can be accomplished with a(n)
   a. written pretest and posttest.
   b. demonstration of the procedures by the children.
   c. survey of the children's attitudes about oral health, administered orally.
   d. unscheduled measurement of the index at school after lunch.
4. The DMFT scores are correlated with oral hygiene, resulting in a correlation coefficient of 0.30. What is the correct interpretation of these results?
   a. Moderate positive relationship
   b. Weak positive relationship
   c. Moderate negative relationship
   d. Weak negative relationship
5. All of the following programs EXCEPT one would be potential resources for payment for dental services that might be needed by this target population. Which is the EXCEPTION?
   a. Medicare
   b. Medicaid

   c. State Children's Health Insurance Program (CHIP)
   d. Private insurance
6. What is the best method to assure that written educational materials used in the program are effective and culturally appropriate?
   a. Develop materials in both English and Vietnamese
   b. Use one-way translation to translate English materials
   c. Use two-way translation to translate English materials
   d. Have materials translated by a teacher at one of the schools who is studying the Vietnamese language
   e. Use English materials, expecting that the children will be able to translate them for their parents

Testlet No. 3

One of your private practice patients is a nursing home administrator. He requests your assistance in providing an oral health-care program for the patients with Alzheimer's disease who reside at the Manor Care, to improve their oral health. The program is to include education, routine screening, and referrals. Screening data are collected with the BSS, PHP, and oral cancer examinations. The residents are from a lower SES group and have complex health histories. The social worker has consents for dental treatment, if needed, and the center has a vehicle to use for transportation. You collaborate with the local community college that has a dental hygiene program and a nursing program to involve their students in this community program.

1. The first step in planning the program would be to
   a. arrange a time for an in-service for the nursing home staff.
   b. survey attitudes of the staff about oral health to determine what is needed.
   c. arrange a meeting of key nursing home staff to assess needs and determine program goals.
   d. plan an education session for the residents.
2. The screening indicates that there is a need for better oral hygiene and dental restorative treatment. All of the following EXCEPT one are possibilities for dental care for the patients who are mobile. Which is the EXCEPTION?
   a. Ask the dentist and hygienist in your community who use portable equipment to include Manor Care on their list of nursing homes to visit
   b. Check with the nearby dental school to arrange to transport residents to their clinic for dental treatment on a reduced-fee or no-cost basis
   c. Take the residents to a community clinic that bases its fees on a sliding scale
   d. Take the residents to a private practice dentist who accepts Medicare patients
3. Which index is appropriate to use to evaluate improvement in the residents' oral hygiene as a result of the program?
   a. BSS
   b. PHP or BSS
   c. PHP or OHI-S
   d. PHP
4. Six months after initiation of the program, family members are surveyed to determine their satisfaction to be able to adjust program activities if necessary. What type of evaluation is this?
   a. Formative and quantitative
   b. Summative and quantitative

    c. Formative and qualitative

    d. Summative and qualitative

5. Which ethical principle is reflected by the use of consents in this program?

    a. Nonmaleficence

    b. Beneficence

    c. Autonomy

    d. Fidelity

6. Involving the students in the education of the staff about the oral-systemic link for this population incorporates all the following components into the program EXCEPT one. Which is the EXCEPTION?

    a. Interprofessional collaborative practice

    b. Interprofessional education

    c. Service learning

    d. Multicultural focus

Testlet No. 4

You reside in a medium-sized town and work in a community health center dental clinic that serves the region. The regional public health dental hygienist asks for your assistance in assessing, planning, and implementing oral health programs in your town. She is especially concerned about the older adult population and about developing a tobacco awareness program in the middle school. You examine secondary data to be able to provide a clear description or "snapshot" of the community before proceeding with further steps in program planning.

1. All of the following characterize the description or "snapshot" of the community in this case EXCEPT one. Which is the EXCEPTION?

    a. Differs from the community profile

    b. Provides all the data required to proceed with program planning

    c. Briefly describes the features of the community

    d. Is developed by the advisory committee at the beginning of the assessment phase of community health program planning

2. You decide to collect baseline data on the older adults who visit your clinic to document their needs and possibly to use in securing funds for program development for the older adult population in the community. You want to measure gingival health, bleeding, calculus, periodontal pockets, and loss of attachment. Which is the best index for this purpose?

    a. CPITN

    b. OHI-S

    c. GI

    d. PDI

    e. CPI

3. You intend to survey the middle school students in your town to assess their perception of how susceptible they are to addiction and cancer caused by tobacco products. In your prevention program you will present the benefits of not smoking or chewing tobacco and discuss the results of their decisions. Which model of health promotion are you using?

    a. Stages of Change Theory

    b. Social Learning Theory

    c. Community Organization Theory

    d. Health Belief Model

4. Upon completion of your tobacco awareness program, you intend to present the results to other healthcare professionals at a health promotion conference. Which strategy would you choose if you desire to reach a large number of people, have the opportunity to meet other professionals in person that share your professional interests, and have time for interaction, and you do not intend to use audiovisual equipment?

    a. Poster presentation

    b. Roundtable discussion

    c. Oral paper

    d. Web-based presentation

5. You meet with the state dental hygienist about possibly implementing your tobacco awareness program statewide. In attempting to follow the essential services of the public health core functions, she wants to support and implement programs at all levels of prevention. Which level of prevention is represented by your tobacco awareness program?

    a. Primary

    b. Secondary

    c. Tertiary

Testlet No. 5

You are contacted by the administrator of a group home for mentally challenged adults to develop an oral health program for the staff. The administrator has received multiple complaints from the attending caregivers regarding the residents' oral health. Limited manual dexterity abilities of the residents require that they receive assistance with oral hygiene routines; yet complaints of severe resident halitosis and bleeding during normal oral hygiene routines have made the caregivers reluctant to provide assistance. After gathering basic demographic information, you visit the facility to determine the actual oral health status of the residents.

1. You conduct an oral health survey on the residents who have natural teeth, using the GI. The following scores are recorded: 2.50, 2.70, 2.80, 3.0, 2.50, 2.40, and 2.90. The mean GI score of these residents is

    a. 2.50

    b. 2.69

    c. 2.70

    d. 7.0

2. What is the BEST way to assess that daily oral hygiene protocols are being adhered to for the residents?

    a. Assess the values of caregivers by conducting focus groups

    b. Measure the plaque biofilm and gingivitis scores of residents over time

    c. Observe the residents' ability to brush correctly

    d. Observe the caregivers' ability to brush correctly

3. Which of the following is the best use of the dental hygienist in this situation?

    a. Conduct an educational program for the residents regarding daily oral hygiene care

    b. Use portable equipment to provide dental hygiene services to the residents

    c. Present an in-service training program for the staff of the group home

    d. Provide daily oral hygiene care for the residents

4. Which teaching strategy will raise the caregivers' compliance in this situation?
   a. Demonstrate proper oral hygiene procedures
   b. Lecture on the importance of oral hygiene
   c. Show pictures of good oral health versus oral disease
   d. Train them how to maintain their own personal oral hygiene skills

5. What is the best action to take before conducting the screening to assure that the results will be reliable?
   a. Acquire informed consent
   b. Calibrate the examiners
   c. Inform the residents about the screening procedures
   d. Plan how many residents will be screened

ANSWERS AND RATIONALES

The answers and rationales for each answer are presented. Also, chapter cross-references are provided to help you review related information in the text.

Testlet No. 1

1. **d.** A unified plan of action is the best defense against a strong antifluoridation group. Answers a, b, and c are also possibilities of things you can do, but d is best and foremost because it can have the greatest impact (see Chapter 6).

2. **a.** A public debate with antifluoridationists only provides them with an opportunity to reach more people with their scare tactics. In addition, most of their arguments appeal to emotions, making it difficult to have an effective debate. Analysis of any prior fluoridation campaign efforts and getting support of community leaders are key steps in preparing for a campaign. Use of educational materials in the primary languages of the community is crucial (see Chapters 6 and 10).

3. **d.** The Basic Screening Survey (BSS) is an easy tool used for screening that includes an assessment of the immediacy of treatment needs (emergency care, treatment is necessary, or routine care is recommended). The DMFT is more complex, provides more detail than is required for screening, and would not yield results that would be easily understood by the parents. Local community clinics provide the best fee for service for low-income patients, and a Title I school has a high percentage of children from low-income families. It is difficult to reach people by phone, and a follow-up list for referral is important to the screening process for ethical reasons (see Chapters 2, 4, 5, and 6).

4. **a.** The addition of 0.5 mg F to the naturally occurring 0.2 mg F per L of water will result in 0.7 mg F, which is the CDC recommendation for the optimal level (see Chapter 6).

5. **c.** A school fluoride varnish program would be the next choice because it is cost effective and would benefit all the children in reducing dental decay. Sealants are more expensive and do not replace fluoride. Education does not guarantee a reduction in decay. Both sealants and education should be used in conjunction with a community-based fluoride program (see Chapter 6).

Testlet No. 2

1. **c.** Local and state programs should reflect the national priorities that are manifested in the *Healthy People 2030* health objectives. The Association of State and Territorial Dental Directors provides evidence-based guidelines for community oral health program planning that should be referenced when planning local and state programs. Program interventions involve the provision of various preventive oral health services; selection of these interventions should also be based on the best available evidence. Protocols used in private clinical practice do not necessarily transfer to dental public health practice. Populations served by community oral health programs have unique needs, and public health principles must be applied to community-based programs (see Chapters 4, 5, and 6).

2. **c.** An assessment such as that conducted using the Decayed, Missing, Filled Teeth (DMFT) Index determines the need for treatment of dental caries, not the demand, and not the need for treatment unrelated to dental caries. Answers b and d would not be appropriate because the DMFT is an assessment tool for determining dental caries experience, not gingivitis, periodontitis, or risk of medical conditions (see Chapter 4 and Appendix F).

3. **b.** Evaluation of performance is best conducted with an activity or demonstration by the person being evaluated. Knowledge and attitudes do not indicate that the children have developed the necessary oral hygiene skills. Unscheduled measurement of the index would be appropriate to determine compliance with oral hygiene rather than performance, but it would likely be invalidated by timing it immediately after lunch unless the children brush after eating (see Chapters 6 and 8 and Appendix F).

4. **b.** Correlation coefficient results demonstrate the strength and direction of the relationship between two variables. The sign of the coefficient (negative or positive; below or above 0) indicates the direction of the relationship. The value of the coefficient indicates the strength of the relationship: 0.9 to 1.0 is very strong, 0.70 to 0.89 is strong, 0.50 to 0.69 is moderate, 0.26 to 0.49 is weak, and 0.25 and below shows little if any relationship (see Chapter 7).

5. a.   Medicaid, CHIP, and private insurance include dental treatment benefits for children. The Affordable Care Act requires dental insurance coverage for children. Because the scenario did not specify that the population was low income, private dental insurance would likely be available for treatment of children from middle and higher SES families. Medicare is a program for older adults (aged ≥65 years), and it does not cover routine dental services (see Chapter 5).

6. b.   One-way translation is adequate for translating educational materials as long as appropriate translation procedures are used, such as use of a professional translator that is proficient in Vietnamese and English and familiar with the oral health concepts in the materials being translated. Developing materials in both English and Vietnamese is an unnecessary extra expense and effort since English materials are readily available for translation. Two-way translation of educational materials is more expensive than one-way translation; it is not necessary as long as appropriate one-way translation methods are used. The teacher who is studying the Vietnamese language will enhance cross-cultural communication, but they are not a professional translator and likely not familiar with the oral health concepts. Newly immigrated Vietnamese children are unlikely to be able to read English materials well enough to assure understanding of the oral health concepts and to be able to translate them for their parents. In addition, translation by children for parents does not follow the principles of patient- and family-centered oral care (see Chapter 10).

Testlet No. 3

1. c.   Assessment of needs is always the first step in program planning. A meeting with agency staff must take place before implementing any needs assessment activities with the priority population. An educational program with the residents is not feasible for this population of Alzheimer's patients (see Chapters 3 and 8).

2. d.   All of these approaches would be feasible except choice d because Medicare does not offer benefits for routine dental treatment (see Chapter 5).

3. d.   To compare the assessment and evaluation measures to evaluate the program, the same index should be used to measure a condition during the evaluation phase that was used to measure it during the assessment phase. The Patient Hygiene Performance (PHP) index is the only index used to assess oral hygiene in this case, so it should also be used to evaluate the oral hygiene improvement resulting from the program. The Basic Screening Survey (BSS) is a survey method, not an index, and it does not include a measure of oral hygiene. The OHI-S is an oral hygiene index, but it was not used for screening as part of the assessment in this case (see Chapter 4).

4. c.   Measurement of ideas and opinions (satisfaction) is qualitative. Measurement during a program for the purpose of making adjustments is formative (see Chapters 3, 6, and 7).

5. c.   Use of autonomy is agreeing to respect the rights of the residents to self-determine participation in the program. Nonmaleficence, beneficence, and fidelity do not relate to informed consent (see Chapter 9).

6. d.   A multicultural focus is not incorporated by involving the dental hygiene and nursing students in the education of the staff about the oral-systemic link. The program has a multicultural focus (institutionalized older adults, individuals with Alzheimer's disease), regardless of whether the dental hygiene and nursing students are involved. Interprofessional collaborative practice (ICP) encompasses communication among health professions in healthcare delivery, enabling the integration of oral health into overall health, thus emphasizing the oral-systemic link. Interprofessional education occurs when the ICP model is applied to the education of health professional students, whereby they work as a team to provide care for the individual or group. Service learning is the merging of the professional student's provision of community service in response to community-identified concerns with learning about the context in which service is provided (see Chapters 2, 10, and 11).

Testlet No. 4

1. b.   The snapshot is a brief description of the community developed by the advisory committee as one of the first actions taken in the comprehensive assessment step of the community health program planning process. It is generated before collecting assessment data. A community profile, not a snapshot of the community, provides all the data required to proceed with program planning, based on the results of the formal organized community assessment process (see Chapter 3).

2. e.   The Community Periodontal Index (CPI) is a modification of the Community Periodontal Index of Treatment Needs (CPITN) and is used to assess periodontal status by gathering data in all the areas described in the case. The CPITN measures periodontal treatment needs rather than periodontal status. The Periodontal Disease Index (PDI) is not widely used anymore. Also, the PDI and the other indices are specific, not including all the periodontal parameters described in the case. The Gingival Index (GI) measures only gingivitis, and the Oral Hygiene Index-Simplified (OHI-S) measures only plaque biofilm and calculus (see Chapter 4 and Appendix F).

3. **d.** The Health Belief Model (HBM) is the only one listed that includes information on the people's perceptions or beliefs about oral health. Also, one of the key concepts of the HBM is a focus on the benefits of healthy behavior (see Chapter 8).

4. **a.** Poster presentations allow for the most interaction with the largest number of people. This is a popular presentation method at health promotion conferences. Audiovisual equipment is not used, and personal interaction is foremost. A roundtable discussion focuses on in-depth discussion but with a small group of people. An oral paper is presented to a large group, but this format provides limited opportunity for interaction. A web-based presentation can reach a large number of people and provide for interaction electronically, but it will not provide the opportunity to meet other professionals in person (see Chapter 8).

5. **a.** A tobacco awareness program is an example of primary prevention, which is directed at preventing a disease before it occurs. Secondary prevention involves treatment to reduce or eliminate disease in the early stages. Tertiary prevention limits disability from disease in more advanced stages (see Chapters 2 and 6).

Testlet No. 5

1. **b.** To compute the mean, add the scores and divide by the total number of scores (n). The result is 2.685, which rounds to 2.69. Of the other answer choices, 2.50 is the mode, 2.70 is the median, and 7.0 is n (see Chapter 7).

2. **b.** The only real measure of actual oral hygiene routines and their subsequent effectiveness is the residents' oral hygiene over time. Answers a and d assess short-term objectives designed to lead to the final desired outcome, which in this case is improved oral hygiene of the residents. Answer c is inappropriate because the residents' compromised cognitive function limits their ability to perform oral hygiene effectively. As a result, the staff members are expected to assist them with daily oral hygiene (see Chapter 3).

3. **c.** A principle of the role of the dental hygienist in public health is to maximize the effect by educating and training others who can provide education or services directly to the target population (see Chapters 2 and 6).

4. **d.** Training caregivers in personal oral hygiene will provide them an opportunity to experience the benefits of good oral hygiene. After this is valued, the caregivers will be more likely to assist residents with their daily oral hygiene. In addition, this training will increase the caregivers' confidence in their abilities to improve the residents' oral health (self-efficacy), which is also an important factor in compliance. Other answers are worthwhile strategies but are less likely to increase compliance (see Chapters 6 and 8).

5. **b.** Training and calibration of examiners is the best way to assure that the data being collected are reproducible or reliable. Other answers do not relate to reliability of data. Acquiring informed consent is an ethical responsibility. Informing the residents about the screening procedures is good practice to avoid misunderstandings, assure compliance, and provide full disclosure for informed consent. Planning how many residents will be screened is an important part of preparation. Also, if a sample is to be used during screening, planning for an adequate number in the sample is important to assure validity of the data (see Chapters 7 and 9).

REFERENCES

1. National Board Dental Hygiene Examination (NBDHE) 2020 Candidate Guide. Joint Commission on National Dental Examinations; 2020. Available at: <https://www.ada.org/~/media/JCNDE/pdfs/nbdhe_examinee_guide.pdf?la=en>; [Accessed December 5, 2019].
2. National, Regional and State Dental Hygiene Certification Exams. DentalCareersEDU.org; 2020. Available at: <https://www.dentalcareersedu.org/dental-hygienist-examination>; [Accessed October 25, 2020].
3. NBDHE General Information. Joint Commission on National Dental Examinations; 2020. Available at: <https://www.ada.org/en/jcnde/examinations/national-board-dental-hygiene-examination>; [Accessed October 25, 2020].

ADDITIONAL RESOURCE

Blue CM. Comprehensive Review of Dental Hygiene, 9th ed. Maryland Heights, MO: Elsevier; 2021.

Additional Websites for Community Resources and Information for Community Program Planning

In addition to the references at the end of each chapter, resources have been provided in the Additional Resources at the end of most chapters. Other resources for health and oral health information are available from many organizations and governmental agencies. Listed here are various selected professional, nonprofit, community, health, and voluntary organizations; clearinghouses and resource centers; foundations; policy and research centers; programs and initiatives; and healthcare organizations. The National Maternal and Child Oral Health Resource Center and other organizations listed here also link to other organizations and agencies that provide oral health information. Appendix D provides information on federal, state, and local government agencies that can also be helpful as resources for assessment and community programming

Academy of General Dentistry (AGD)
www.agd.org
American Academy of Dental Therapy (AADT)
http://aaofdt.org/
American Academy of Oral and Maxillofacial Pathology (AAOMP)
http://www.aaomp.org/about/position-papers-policies/
American Academy of Pediatric Dentistry (AAPD)
www.aapd.org
American Academy of Pediatrics (AAP)
https://www.aap.org/en-us/Pages/Default.aspx
American Academy of Periodontology (AAP)
www.perio.org
American Association for Dental Research (AADR)
www.aadronline.org
American Association for Health Education (AAHE)
http://www.cnheo.org/aahe.htm
American Association of Endodontists (AAE)
www.aae.org
American Association of Orthodontists (AAO)
www.aaoinfo.org
American Association of Public Health Dentistry (AAPHD)
www.aaphd.org
American Cancer Society
www.cancer.org
American College Health Association (ACHA)
https://www.acha.org/
American College of Prosthodontists (ACP)
www.prosthodontics.org
American Dental Assistants Association (ADAA)
https://www.adaausa.org/
American Dental Association (ADA)
www.ada.org
American Dental Education Association (ADEA)
www.adea.org
American Dental Hygienists' Association (ADHA)
www.adha.org

American Diabetes Association
www.diabetes.org
American Heart Association
www.heart.org
American Medical Association (AMA)
www.ama-assn.org
American Public Health Association (APHA)
www.apha.org
American School Health Association (ASHA)
http://www.ashaweb.org/
Association of State and Territorial Dental Directors (ASTDD)
www.astdd.org
California Dental Association Foundation
https://www.cdafoundation.org/
Children's Dental Health Project
https://www.cdhp.org/
Community Dental Health
https://communitydentalhealth.org/about
Delta Dental Plans Association
https://www.deltadental.com/
FDI World Dental Federation (FDI)
www.fdiworlddental.org
Georgetown University Health Policy Institute
https://hpi.georgetown.edu/#
Health Policy Institute (HPI), American Dental Association
https://www.ada.org/en/science-research/health-policy-institute
Institute for Oral Health (IOH), American Dental Hygienists' Association
https://www.adha.org/ioh-about-us
International Association for Dental Research (IADR)
www.iadr.com
Interprofessional Education Collaborative (IPEC)
https://www.ipecollaborative.org/about-ipec.html
Kaiser Permanente
https://healthy.kaiserpermanente.org/

March of Dimes
https://www.marchofdimes.org/

Mental Health America
https://www.mhanational.org/

My Community Dental Centers
https://www.mydental.org/

National Association of Dental Plans (NADP)
https://www.nadp.org/

National Center for Dental Hygiene Research & Practice (DHNet)
https://dent-web10.usc.edu/dhnet/

National Center for Interprofessional Practice and Education
https://nexusipe.org/

National Dental Practice-Based Research Network
www.nationaldentalpbrn.org

National Maternal and Child Oral Health Resource Center
https://www.mchoralhealth.org/

Pew Charitable Trusts
https://www.pewtrusts.org/en/

Pew Research Center
https://www.pewresearch.org/

Robert Wood Johnson Foundation
https://www.rwjf.org/

Society for Public Health Education (SOPHE)
www.sophe.org

Texas Health Institute, Oral Health
https://www.texashealthinstitute.org/oral-health.html

The Arc of the U.S. (for individuals with intellectual and developmental disabilities)
https://thearc.org/

W. K. Kellogg Foundation
https://www.wkkf.org/who-we-are/overview

Zero to Three (for child development information)
https://www.zerotothree.org/

Community Oral Health Competencies and Learning Objectives

The *ADEA Compendium of Curriculum Guidelines, Allied Dental Education Programs (Revised Edition), 2015-2016 (ADEA Curriculum Guidelines)* published by the American Dental Education Association provides comprehensive guidelines to serve as a curriculum-development aid for the Community Oral Health course in a dental hygiene program in the United States (U.S.). The guidelines include a course overview, educational goals, learning objectives, competencies, definitions, prerequisites, a content outline, educational strategies, learning assessment activities, and other guidelines. The intent is to result in a course that (1) provides a broad understanding of the oral healthcare delivery system and an objective view of the significant social, political, psychological, cultural, and economic forces directing the system, (2) delivers the knowledge and skills necessary to meet specific oral health needs of community groups as distinct from the traditional clinical approach designed to meet the needs of individual patients, and (3) exposes students to the community-based role of the dental hygienist by allowing them to manage access-to-care issues within underserved populations.

The community oral health competencies and learning objectives contained in the *ADEA Curriculum Guidelines* are listed here. These guidelines can be adapted for use by programs in other countries.

COMPETENCIES

1. Providing health education and preventive counseling to a variety of population groups.
2. Promoting the values of good oral and general health and wellness to the public and to organizations within and outside the oral healthcare professions.
3. Identifying services that promote oral health and prevent oral disease and related conditions.
4. Advocating for consumer groups, businesses, and government agencies to support oral healthcare issues.
5. Assessing, planning, implementing, and evaluating community-based oral health programs.
6. Using screening, referral, and education to bring consumers into the oral healthcare delivery system.
7. Providing dental hygiene services in a variety of settings, including offices, hospitals, clinics, extended care facilities, community programs, and schools.
8. Employing current infection prevention and control resources in community-focused healthcare settings.
9. Evaluating reimbursement mechanisms and their impact on access to dental care.

10. Recognizing and using written and electronic sources of information.
11. Evaluating the credibility and potential hazards of dental products and techniques.
12. Evaluating published clinical and basic science research and integrating this information to improve the oral health of the patient.
13. Recognizing the responsibility and demonstrating the ability to communicate professional knowledge verbally and in writing.
14. Accepting responsibility for solving problems and making decisions based on accepted scientific principles.
15. Expanding and contributing to the knowledge base of dental hygiene.

LEARNING OBJECTIVES

1. Explain the history of dental hygiene in relation to dental public health.
2. Define community dental health/dental public health.
3. Define the range of personal, social, economic and environmental factors that influence health status (i.e., determinants of health).
4. Identify and use the currently practiced public health preventive modalities.
5. Defend the need for preventive modalities in dental public health practice.
6. Identify appropriate levels of supplemental fluoride for a community.
7. Describe the history, process, and status of community water fluoridation.
8. Identify and use community dental health activities related to prevention and control of oral conditions and promotion of health.
9. Explain the role of dental providers, with emphasis on the dental hygienist, in activities related to the practice of public health.
10. Describe the state of oral health in the U.S.
11. Describe the dental care delivery system in the U.S.
12. List the government departments and agencies related to oral health and dental hygiene.
13. Compare the federal, state/provincial and local presence of government in dental care delivery.
14. Evaluate the dental hygienist employment opportunity ratio.
15. Describe issues surrounding the use of the dental workforce in relation to access to dental care.

16. Analyze need, supply, demand, and use of dental care as it pertains to utilization.
17. Critique current methods of payment for dental care.
18. Define and apply terminology associated with financing dental care.
19. List the different insurance coverage options available for dental care.
20. Evaluate the role of the government in financing dental care.
21. Describe the demographics, educational preparation, and regulation of dental hygienists in other countries.
22. Compare dental public health programs in other countries.
23. List and define the international professional organizations involved in dental public health.
24. Discuss the regulation of dental hygienists in other countries.
25. Summarize the legislative process.
26. Identify the major bodies of law.
27. Describe the rules and regulations of the dental hygiene scope of practice.
28. Advocate for the use of a dental hygienist without restrictive barriers in scope of practice.
29. Describe the responsibilities of dental hygienists in the U.S.
30. Define oral health in relation to health education and health promotion.
31. Describe health education and health promotion principles.
32. Outline the different learning and motivation theories.
33. Describe how a dental hygienist could best educate a target population.
34. Describe the process of lesson plan development.
35. List and describe teaching strategies.
36. List the characteristics of an effective teacher.
37. Develop and present a lesson plan for oral health education.
38. Identify target (priority) populations to whom dental hygienists may provide services.
39. Describe cultural diversity.
40. Describe the effect culture has on oral health and dental hygiene care.
41. List barriers to obtaining and delivering dental hygiene care.
42. Describe the various program planning paradigms.
43. Describe various dental public health programs.
44. Develop a dental public health program plan.
45. Perform a needs assessment of the target population.
46. Plan a community program based on a needs assessment.
47. Identify possible constraints, alternatives, and evaluation tools for a community program.

48. Plan an evaluation of a community program.
49. Describe the mechanisms of program evaluation.
50. Compare qualitative and quantitative evaluation.
51. Describe and define the goals of various dental indices.
52. Define oral epidemiology and related terms.
53. Describe current epidemiological trends of oral conditions and diseases.
54. Identify the role of host, agent, and environment in the disease process.
55. List and describe the publications reporting oral epidemiology and use appropriate information resources in community dental health.
56. Describe oral epidemiology and its relationship to dental hygiene.
57. Describe the current epidemiological issues of disease.
58. Describe the reasons for conducting research in dental hygiene.
59. Define the purpose of dental hygiene research.
60. List, explain, and describe the various research approaches appropriate in community dental health.
61. Define and describe data analysis and interpretation techniques used in community dental health literature.
62. Identify data by their type and scale of measurement.
63. Define and describe descriptive and inferential statistics.
64. Select and compute appropriate measures of central tendency and measures of dispersion.
65. Describe and construct frequency distributions and graphs.
66. Describe the evolution of dental care product production.
67. Defend the dental hygienist's role in advocating the use of effective dental care products and treatment modalities.
68. Educate the public in dental care product evaluation.
69. Effectively critique oral health research reported in dental publications.
70. Describe dental public health careers.
71. Describe various government-related opportunities for dental public health programs.
72. Define dental hygiene positions in the areas of public health and government.

(From ADEA Compendium of Curriculum Guidelines, Allied Dental Education Programs (Revised Edition), 2015-2016. Washington, DC: American Dental Education Association; 2015. Available at: https://www.adea.org/cadpd/allied-dental-education-resources.aspx; [Accessed April 2020].)

Community Partnerships for Oral Health

APPENDIX C.1 POTENTIAL COMMUNITY PARTNERS

Patients, Clients, and Consumers of Services
- Patients and clients
- Parents and family representatives
- Advocacy groups for patients, clients, and consumers of services
- Advocacy groups for parents and family representatives
- Consumers of services
- Public representatives
- Support groups for patients, clients, and consumers of services
- Support groups for parents and family representatives

Government Agencies and Programs
- State, territorial[1], tribal[2], and local departments of health administrators and staff (e.g., oral health; maternal and child health; Women, Infants, and Children program [WIC]; primary health care; family planning; rural health; health disparities; minority health; human immunodeficiency virus [HIV]; chronic diseases; tobacco control)
- State, territorial[1], tribal[2] and local human service agency staff and administrators (e.g., government hospitals, clinics, and institutions; programs for individuals with mental illness and mental disabilities; programs for individuals with developmental and acquired disabilities; programs for individuals with special healthcare needs [e.g., blind, deaf]; units on senior affairs and aging; departments of corrections)
- Regional councils of governments
- Area Agencies on Aging
- County extension agencies
- Other county and city officials (e.g., working with childcare, youth services, literacy, libraries, older adult and disability services, public transportation, public housing, workforce development)
- Environmental health (e.g., community water supervisors or managers related to community water fluoridation)

Policymakers and Organizations
- U.S. Congress: Senators and representatives
- Legislators: State senators and representatives
- Local government elected officials: County judges, mayors, city councilors, county commissioners
- Policy institutes (e.g., Georgetown University Health Policy Institute, Robert Wood Johnson Foundation, Kaiser Permanente, Pew Research Center)
- Policy advocates (e.g., local legal aid organizations, League of Women Voters [LWU], American Association of Retired Persons [AARP], League of United Latin American Citizens [LULAC], National Association for the Advancement of Colored People [NAACP])

Community Organizations

- Advocacy organizations for clients and consumers of services, including children, individuals with disabilities, HIV, cancer, and other medically compromising conditions, and who are older adults, poor, or homeless (e.g., American Cancer Society, American Heart Association, American Diabetes Association, March of Dimes, Easterseals, Mental Health America, Zero to Three, United Cerebral Palsy Association, The Arc of the U.S., American Red Cross, United Way, National Urban League, Court Appointed Special Advocates [CASA], LWV, and AARP)
- Community action agencies
- Older adult nutrition services and sites
- Early childhood intervention organizations and programs
- National, state, and local information and resource networks (e.g., organizations coordinating nonemergency call centers for government services, United Way helplines, toll-free hotlines, and health information and referral support centers)
- Representatives of consumer and regional advisory groups
- Religious organizations (e.g., churches and other ministries)
- Faith-based organizations (e.g., Catholic Charities, Salvation Army)
- Community centers and neighborhood associations
- State and local coalitions; collaborations; initiatives; outreach staff; and community-based organizations and advocacy organizations for oral health, public health issues, and access to health care (e.g., insuring children and adults; the uninsured; vulnerable groups)
- Foundations and corporate giving programs: international, national, state, and local community grant makers and philanthropy sector administrators and staff
- Local representatives active in collaborative service programs with health and human service agencies that specifically address key issues (e.g., community planning)
- Service organizations for vulnerable population groups (e.g., literacy, older adult and disability services, youth services, veterans, women, public transportation, public housing, workforce development, childcare, food banks, homeless shelters, migrant and seasonal farm workers)
- Administrators and staff for programs and supportive services, including Alzheimer's facilities and care, assisted living, programs for assistive technology and disability aids, senior-care agencies, geriatric and professional care managers, home care services, home maintenance and chore services, hospice care, medical equipment and medical alert programs, nursing homes, assisted living centers, retirement communities that provide health care, older adult health care and house call doctors, and veterans' benefits consultants
- Corporation for National and Community Service, AmeriCorps, Senior Corps, Learn and Serve America, Volunteers in Service to America (VISTA), Youth Service Corps, and City Year
- Business leaders (see later section)
- Unions and organized labor
- Civic organizations: Junior League, Rotary International, Kiwanis, Lions Club, Elks
- Youth groups: Boys and Girls Clubs, YMCA, YWCA, Big Brothers/Big Sisters, Special Olympics
- Media: international, national, state, and local media, via newspapers, television, radio, magazines/journals, Internet, websites, blogs, social media, and social networking (e.g., Facebook, Twitter, Flickr, YouTube, Messenger)

Education-Related Organizations and Groups

- Regional education service centers
- Local school districts and boards: Superintendents, principals, teachers, school nurses, school social workers, parent liaisons
- Local child development and childcare grantees and Head Start grantees and delegate agencies (e.g., Head Start executive directors, Head Start health coordinators)
- Parent-Teacher Associations/Organizations
- Parenting education programs
- Adult education and literacy programs
- Home school programs
- Employment and vocational education programs
- Education-related unions
- Fraternities and sororities

Health and Human Service Providers, Groups, Organizations, and Associations

- Health systems, hospitals and clinics (e.g., rural and community, public, nonprofit, private, children's hospitals, Department of Veterans Affairs hospitals and clinics, county hospital districts)
- Community health centers
- School-based health programs
- Safety-net health and oral health programs (e.g., community dental clinics, nonprofit dental clinics)
- Maternal and Child Health Programs
- State and local health professional associations
- Dentists, dental hyginists, dental therapists, and dental assistants
- Physicians, pediatricians, family physicians, and physician assistants
- Nurses, nurse practitioners, and nurse midwives
- Speech pathologists
- Dieticians
- Nursing home administrators
- Early childhood, early intervention providers
- Social workers, care coordinators, and case managers
- Health educators, community health workers, community health advisors, lay health advocates, outreach educators, community health representatives, peer health promoters, peer health educators, and patient navigators

Third-Party Payers

- Health plans
- Dental insurers
- Managed care organizations
- Health maintenance organizations (HMOs)
- Employers providing dental insurance coverage
- Employers not providing dental insurance coverage
- Medicaid; Children's Health Insurance Program (CHIP)
- Marketplace plans established by the 2010 Patient Protection and Affordable Care Act
- Health insurance coverage high-risk pools, preexisting condition insurance plans, and health insurance exchanges
- Medicare supplement, advantage, and drug plans
- Long-term care insurers
- Health insurance programs and special initiatives reaching out to people with disabilities; veterans and military personnel; families; children; young adults; older adults; early retirees; individuals living in rural areas; Hispanics/Latinos; African Americans; Asian Americans and Pacific Islanders; American Indian and Alaska Natives; small businesses; employers; women; and lesbian, bisexual, gay, transgender, and queer (or questioning; LBGTQ) communities
- Dental benefits plan organizations and associations (e.g., National Association of Dental Plans)

Higher and Professional Education

- Administrators, faculty, staff, and organizations that represent the following:
  - Universities and colleges
  - Dental, dental hygiene, dental therapist, and dental assisting schools
  - Nursing schools
  - Medical schools
- Allied health schools (e.g., occupational therapy, physical therapy, speech and language pathology, and dietetics)
- Schools of public health, community health, and health education
- Schools of public policy and health administration
- Schools of social work
- Law schools

Business Organizations and Retail Outlets

- Airlines
- Banks
- Beauty and barber shops
- Chambers of Commerce (e.g., Women Chamber of Commerce, Hispanic Chamber of Commerce)
- Computer companies and stores
- Grocery stores
- Delicatessens and specialty and ethnic food stores
- Health clubs
- Insurance companies
- Shopping malls
- Maternity stores
- Movie theaters
- Other professionals (e.g., attorneys)

[1]Territorial agencies and organizations include the following territories and jurisdictions: District of Columbia; Pacific-Basin territories and jurisdictions: Territory of American Samoa, Territory of Guam, Republic of the Marshall Islands, Federated States of Micronesia, Commonwealth of the Northern Mariana Islands, and Republic of Palau; and Eastern territories and jurisdictions: Commonwealth of Puerto Rico and U.S. Virgin Islands.
[2]Tribal agencies and organizations include the following: American Indian/Alaska Native tribally designated organizations; Alaska Native Health Corporations; Urban Indian Health Organizations.

APPENDIX C.2 ORAL HEALTH COLLABORATIVE PARTNERSHIPS AND COALITIONS

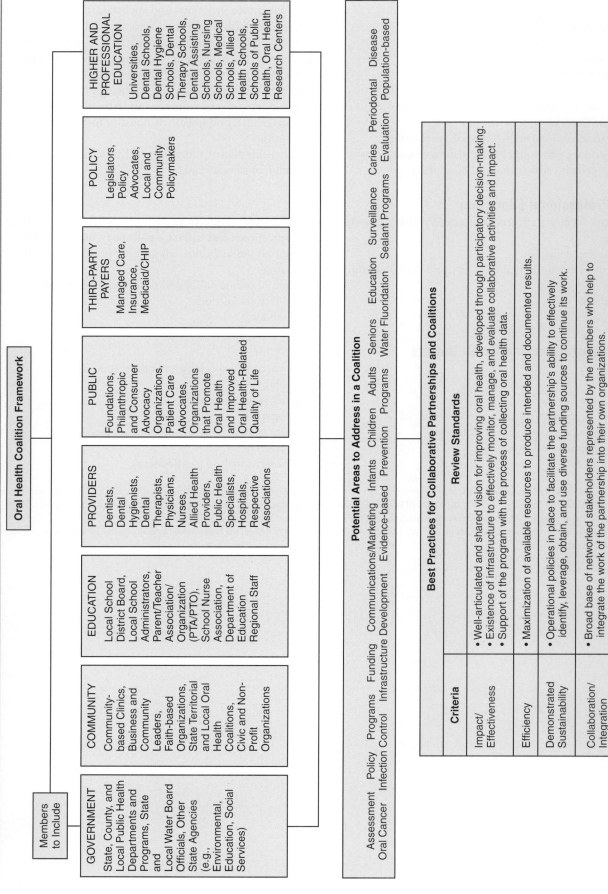

Oral Health Coalition Framework

Members to Include

GOVERNMENT
State, County, and Local Public Health Departments, State and Local Water Board Officials, Other State Agencies (e.g., Environmental, Education, Social Services)

COMMUNITY
Community-based Clinics, Business and Community Leaders, Faith-based Organizations, State Territorial and Local Oral Health Coalitions, Civic and Non-Profit Organizations

EDUCATION
Local School District Board, Local School Administrators, Parent/Teacher Association/Organization (PTA/PTO), School Nurse Association, Department of Education Regional Staff

PROVIDERS
Dentists, Dental Hygienists, Dental Therapists, Physicians, Nurses, Allied Health Providers, Public Health Specialists, Hospitals, Respective Associations

PUBLIC
Foundations, Philanthropic and Consumer Advocacy Organizations, Patient Care Advocates, Organizations that Promote Oral Health and Improved Oral Health-Related Quality of Life

THIRD-PARTY PAYERS
Managed Care, Insurance, Medicaid/CHIP

POLICY
Legislators, Policy Advocates, Local and Community Policymakers

HIGHER AND PROFESSIONAL EDUCATION
Universities, Dental Schools, Dental Hygiene Schools, Dental Therapy Schools, Dental Assisting Schools, Nursing Schools, Medical Schools, Allied Health Schools, Schools of Public Health, Oral Health Research Centers

Potential Areas to Address in a Coalition

Assessment Policy Programs Funding Communications/Marketing Infants Children Adults Seniors Education Surveillance Caries Periodontal Disease
Oral Cancer Infection Control Infrastructure Development Evidence-based Prevention Programs Water Fluoridation Sealant Programs Evaluation Population-based

Best Practices for Collaborative Partnerships and Coalitions

Criteria	Review Standards
Impact/Effectiveness	• Well-articulated and shared vision for improving oral health, developed through participatory decision-making. • Existence of infrastructure to effectively monitor, manage, and evaluate collaborative activities and impact. • Support of the program with the process of collecting oral health data.
Efficiency	• Maximization of available resources to produce intended and documented results.
Demonstrated Sustainability	• Operational policies in place to facilitate the partnership's ability to effectively identify, leverage, obtain, and use diverse funding sources to continue its work.
Collaboration/Integration	• Broad base of networked stakeholders represented by the members who help to integrate the work of the partnership into their own organizations.
Objectives/Rationale	• Goals and objectives that correspond to and support the state, territory, or local area oral health goals, objectives, and initiatives.

(Modified from Best Practice Approach: State and Territorial Oral Health Programs and Collaborative Partnerships. Reno, NV: Association of State and Territorial Dental Directors; March 2020. Available at: <https://www.astdd.org/bestpractices/stohp-partnerships.pdf>; [Accessed April 2020].)

Resources for Community Health Assessment

APPENDIX D.1 EXAMPLES OF GOVERNMENT RESOURCES FOR HEALTH DATA

Listed here are websites for some of the government resources for health and oral health data. These can be supplemented with the resources in Appendix A and the references and resources provided at the end of most chapters.).

Administration for Children and Families (ACF)
www.acf.hhs.gov

Administration for Community Living (ACL; includes aging and disability networks)
https://acl.gov/

Agency for Healthcare Research and Quality (AHRQ)
www.ahrq.gov

Agency for Toxic Substances and Disease Registry (ATSDR)
https://www.atsdr.cdc.gov/

Centers for Disease Control and Prevention (CDC)/Division of Oral Health (DOH)
www.cdc.gov/oralhealth/index.htm

Centers for Medicare & Medicaid Services (CMS)
www.cms.gov

Department of Health & Human Services (DHHS)
www.hhs.gov

Food and Drug Administration (FDA)
https://www.fda.gov/home

Government Grants
www.grants.gov

Health Resources and Services Administration (HRSA)
www.hrsa.gov

Healthy People 2030
https://health.gov/healthypeople

Indian Health Service (IHS) Dental Portal
www.ihs.gov/DOH

My Water's Fluoride (MWF), CDC
https://nccd.cdc.gov/DOH_MWF/Default/Default.aspx

National Center for Health Statistics (NCHS), CDC
www.cdc.gov/nchs/index.htm

National Institute of Dental and Craniofacial Research (NIDCR)
www.nidcr.nih.gov

National Institutes of Health (NIH)
www.nih.gov

National Oral Health Information Clearinghouse (NOHIC), NIDCR
https://health.gov/node/109

National Oral Health Surveillance System (NOHSS), CDC
https://www.cdc.gov/oralhealthdata/overview/nohss.html

Occupational Safety and Health Administration (OSHA)
www.osha.gov

Pan American Health Organization (PAHO)
https://www.paho.org/en/topics/oral-health

Public Health Service (PHS)
https://www.hhs.gov/surgeongeneral/corps/index.html

Substance Abuse and Mental Health Services Administration (SAMHSA)
https://www.samhsa.gov/find-help/national-helpline

Synopses of State Oral Health Programs, CDC
www.cdc.gov/oralhealthdata/overview/synopses/index.html

Water Fluoridation Reporting System (WFRS)
https://www.cdc.gov/fluoridation/data-tools/reporting-system.html

World Health Organization (WHO), Oral Health
https://www.who.int/health-topics/oral-health/#tab=tab_1

APPENDIX D.2 SUMMARY OF DATA COLLECTION METHODS

Method	Instrument	Cost and Time	Advantage
Document Study			
Review and evaluate existing documents or records describing past events or occurrences	Information abstracted from archival sources (raw data, datasets of summary data, printed reports); qualitative or quantitative data from public legislative bodies, governmental officials and agencies, private businesses, professional and community organizations, and nonprofit foundations	$–$$ ◷–◷◷	Data often readily available
Observational Field Study			
Assessment of actual events, objects, or people in "natural" setting	Assessors use checklists, evaluation forms, cameras, tape recorders, rating scales, and observation field notes; qualitative approach with content or situational analysis	$$ ◷◷	Provides first-hand information
Windshield or Walking Tour			
Within community-designated boundaries, observers and recorders drive or walk in community areas at varying times of day and days of the week to assess community activities, interactions, and events through observation, informal conversations, and interactions with community members	Observers and recorders document community characteristics and record information using observational guides, checklists, survey tools, notes, photos, audiotapes, and videotapes; qualitative approach with content or situational analysis; results summarized and displayed through written narratives, tables, diagrams, slide and video shows, maps, and collages	$–$$ ◷–◷◷	Provides first-hand information
Mailed Survey			
Assessment (e.g., surveys, polls, evaluations) conducted by direct mail; adaptations include questionnaire sent home with children from school, telefax surveys, magazine or newsletter surveys, or electronic surveys (using networked computers, email, Internet, websites, blogs, social media, social networking pages, Facebook, Twitter, Flickr)	Self-administered standardized, structured questionnaire with closed- and open-ended questions completed by respondent; quantitative approach with statistical analysis of responses	$–$$ ◷–◷◷	Data can be collected from a large sample
Telephone Interview			
Survey interview conducted by telephone	Interviewer reads structured interview schedule (standardized, questionnaire) with closed- and open-ended questions to respondent; quantitative approach with statistical analysis of responses	$$ ◷	Data can be collected from a large sample
Person-to-Person Interview			
Survey interview conducted face-to-face between a respondent and an interviewer	Structured interview schedule (standardized, questionnaire) with closed- and open-ended questions read to respondent by an interviewer; quantitative approach with statistical analysis of responses	$$–$$$ ◷◷–◷◷◷	Face-to-face communication allows for more in-depth information and overcomes lack of literacy
In-Depth Personal Interview			
Survey conducted face-to-face to learn about life history, events, and experiences	Interviewer uses open-ended, flexible, unstructured nondirective questions; transcriptions of tape recordings used for thematic analysis of content	$$–$$$ ◷◷–◷◷◷	Can be used with a smaller sample with expanded perspectives
Screening Survey			
Rapid assessment using screening procedures	Standardized written criteria and measurements, measuring instruments, and protocols; cursory inspection provides crude estimates; quantitative approach with statistical analysis of results	$$ ◷◷	Can provide practical and uniform information in a short time period

APPENDIX D.2 SUMMARY OF DATA COLLECTION METHODS (*CONT.*)

Method	Instrument	Cost and Time	Advantage
Epidemiological Survey			
Extensive assessment using examination procedures, clinical samples, and clinical tests	Standardized written criteria and measurements, measuring instruments, and protocols; detailed planning of examination conditions, indices, criteria, sampling approaches, personnel training, data collection, data management, and analysis; quantitative approach with statistical analysis of results	$$–$$$ ⊕⊕–⊕⊕⊕	Provides more detailed information
Asset Maps			
Geographic study and mapping that can identify patterns of community characteristics, physical assets, or settings of human activity and interactions	Input and display of data from existing sources or new data onto geographic map using simple materials (map and adhesives or pushpins) or detailed community planning and evaluation computer software (e.g., Geographic Information System [GIS] computer software) and other powerful tools for organizing location, distribution, and mapping of spatial data	$–$$ ⊕–⊕⊕	Provides good overview and visualization of information
Inventories or Directories			
Documenting and cataloging of assets and capacities of individual community members or community resources such as institutions, organizations, and associations	Identify, evaluate, and organize assets and capacities in a community and develop adequate mechanisms for linkages that can produce opportunities for action; such capacities may include assets owned or skills processed by individual community members; may also include sources of mutual aid, connections, and resources among institutions, organizations, and associations in a community	$–$$ ⊕–⊕⊕	Data often have been collected previously
Focus Group			
Guided group discussion provides information on a specific topic from a certain population group	Moderator leads guided group discussions among 6 to 12 individuals over 45 to 90 minutes by using a series of open-ended questions on a preestablished discussion guide; transcriptions from tape recordings and written field notes of discussions used for thematic analysis of content	$$–$$$ ⊕⊕–⊕⊕⊕	Provides varied and ample information
Public Forum or Community Dialogue Event			
Individuals or groups provide verbal input or feedback on specific issues	Moderator solicits, collects, and summarizes written comments or oral testimony; oral testimony recorded by tape recorder or court reporter to generate official record for analysis	$$ ⊕⊕	Provides first-hand and ample information
Community Visioning Process			
Groups of community stakeholders collectively develop shared vision of their community in the future	Through an interactive approach (retreat or workshop format), a skilled facilitator brings individuals together over one or more days and guides participants through the vision process by posing questions and assisting participants to visualize the future community and possibilities for forward advancement; small groups discuss visions and images; creation of document to reflect visions; follow-up meeting held to refine visions and to develop plan for incorporation of visions into community planning process	$$–$$$ ⊕⊕–⊕⊕⊕	Provides varied input for broad-based, ample information
Creative Assessment			
Community members document perceptions of community through creative means	Creative techniques and forums for expression (e.g., photography, film, theater, music, dance, murals, puppet shows, storytelling, drawings) used to convey wide range of perceptions of a community	$$–$$$ ⊕⊕–⊕⊕⊕	Provides interesting and innovative information

$, Inexpensive; $$, moderate cost; $$$, expensive; ⊕, less time consuming; ⊕⊕, moderately time consuming; ⊕⊕⊕, very time consuming.

APPENDIX D.3 EXAMPLES OF INFORMATION FOR A COMMUNITY HEALTH ASSESSMENT

Community Health Measures	Examples
Health status (measurements of natality [births], morbidity [illness], and mortality [deaths])	**Birth statistics:** Age, parity of mother, duration of pregnancy, types of births (single, twin), complications of pregnancy, complications of birth, birth defects, birth weight (e.g., low), premature births, and births to adolescent, older, or unmarried females
	Morbidity statistics: Incidence and prevalence of diseases, conditions, disabilities, injuries (distribution, intensity, and duration) such as unintentional and intentional injuries, homicide, suicide, cancer, heart disease, diabetes, stroke, infectious diseases (communicable), HIV/AIDS, tuberculosis, STD, mental illness, alcohol and drug abuse problems, occupational diseases, disability and decreased independence, developmental disabilities (e.g., cleft lip and/or palate, craniofacial anomalies), and oral diseases or conditions (e.g., dental caries, periodontal diseases, or oral injuries)
	Mortality statistics: Distribution of death rates by age, race/ethnicity, sex, cause, and geographic location; and leading causes of death such as cancer (breast, colon, lung, or oral), heart disease, stroke, homicide, motor vehicle injuries, suicide, unintentional injury, and infant, neonatal, and postneonatal mortality
Health risks and protective factors (identification of patterns of behavioral and nonbehavioral factors)	**Self-rated (self-reported) general and oral health status:** Recent poor health, days of work lost, days of school lost (e.g., caused by dental problems or care), average number of unhealthy days in past month, and satisfaction with quality of life and public health, healthcare, and social service system
	Occupational risks and work disability: Exposure to chemicals and physical, musculoskeletal, psychological, and other forms of stress; loss of mobility; and physical and emotional challenges
	Stress indicators and resources: Drunk driving, robberies, and assaults; access to drugs, recent drug use, and alcoholic beverage outlets; gang problems; family violence (e.g., child abuse and neglect, spouse and elder abuse); emotional issues (e.g., major depression, self-esteem issues, alienation, discrimination, feelings of hope and despair, feelings of anger); social and family support and resources (adaptation and cohesion); life events and stress (e.g., personal, family, job stress)
	Levels of health knowledge, beliefs, attitudes, behaviors, practices, and skills about self-care: Personal care (e.g., toothbrushing with fluoride toothpaste, flossing, health interventions); lifestyle such as physical activity, diet (e.g., amount of sugar), health-related substance use (e.g., tobacco, alcohol, mood-altering drugs), and safety practices (e.g., seat belts, mouthguards); knowledge about location, availability, and appropriate use of local health resources, services, and programs; and family healthcare expenditures
	Use of child and adult preventive health services: Routine dental and medical examinations, dental sealants, fluoride treatments, prenatal care in first trimester, immunizations for children and adults, Pap smears, mammograms, and colon cancer screening
Access to public health, healthcare, and social service system (scope, adequacy, accessibility, and availability of services in a coordinated, integrated system)	**Access to community preventive services (community water fluoridation) and public health services:** Scope and adequacy of local health department covering essential public health services by health providers, (numbers, types, locations, and adequacy), including infrastructure and capacity measures, local voluntary health programs, and operational health promotion and education programs in work sites, schools, and the community (e.g., community water fluoridation; school-based dental sealant programs, fluoride varnish programs, and oral health education; community-based screening and referral; work-site tobacco cessation programs)
	Access to facilities for personal health care: Assessment of numbers, types, location, and adequacy of hospitals; emergency and urgent care, outpatient primary care, oral health care, hearing care, vision care, mental health care, and speech, physical, and occupational therapy facilities; alcohol and drug treatment programs; nursing homes; and community health centers
	Access to health professionals: Adequacy and numbers of educated public health professionals and personal healthcare professionals with expertise and competence; and levels of knowledge, attitudes, behaviors, practices, and skills of public health and personal healthcare professionals
	Access to health insurance and usual sources of health care: Comprehensive benefits with dental insurance and per capita spending (e.g., Medicare, Medicaid, Children's Health Insurance Program [CHIP], private insurance, Supplementary Security Income [SSI])
	Scope and adequacy of local social service programs: Level at which basic human, family, and community needs are addressed

HIV/AIDS, Human immunodeficiency virus/acquired immunodeficiency disease; *STD,* sexually transmitted disease.

APPENDIX D.4 EXAMPLES OF PRIMARY DATA COLLECTION TASKS

Planning

- Determine scope and objectives
- Prepare protocols describing assessment plan
- Select data collection methods
- Establish criteria
- Determine sampling methods and processes
- Obtain approval of authorities
- Plan for personnel and physical arrangements
- Plan for data analysis phase (recording, managing, and analyzing data)
- Plan for data reporting phase
- Prepare budget
- Develop timetable of main activities and responsible staff
- Plan for referral process (for clinical findings detected in health survey)
- Plan and develop consent form
- Translate consent form
- Gain approval of consent form from Institutional Review Board
- Plan and develop data collection instruments
- Develop data collection protocols
- Plan data entry processes
- Plan quality assurance processes for data collection
- Plan and develop training materials for field team

- Plan and develop data collection and entry process (manual collection or direct data entry into personal computer or a mobile device, also known as handheld device, handheld computer, palmtop computer, or personal digital assistant [PDA])
- Translate data collection instruments
- Gain approval of data collection instruments from Institutional Review Board
- Pilot-test consent form and data collection instruments
- Revise consent form and data collection instruments
- Obtain approval of revised consent form and data collection instruments from Institutional Review Board
- Draw sample
- Plan fieldwork and scheduling
- Purchase and organize supplies
- Initiate contact with data collection sites (work through established community networks or organizational structures)
- Organize logistics for data collection, including travel and site requirements
- Train field team
- Calibrate field team
- Implement pilot test of assessment

Implementing

- Contact and recruit participants
- Gain consent of participants
- Record data
- Manage data

- Analyze data
- Maintain quality assurance processes
- Summarize findings
- Report findings

Selected Oral Conditions and Factors Influencing Oral Health That Can Be Assessed in Oral Health Surveys

ORAL CONDITIONS/FACTORS	VARIABLES THAT CAN BE ASSESSED
Craniofacial anomalies, including developmental anomalies	• Cleft lip or cleft palate • Craniofacial anomalies • Oral malformations
Dental caries	• Coronal caries • Early childhood caries • Gross loss of tooth structure • Missing teeth because of caries • Pulpal involvement • Retained roots • Root caries • Untreated tooth (dental) decay
Dental sealants	• Access to community- or school-based sealant program • Dental sealants on specific teeth (permanent first molars, second molars, and lateral incisors; primary molars) • Number of teeth sealed
Dietary intake	• Ability to recognize cariogenicity of specific foods • Bottle- and breast-feeding practices • Food choices and dietary patterns (dietary recall/dietary intake questionnaire) • Frequency of eating (food frequency questionnaire)
Expenses and payment source for oral health services	• Dental care expenses • Dental insurance • Medicaid/Children's Health Insurance Program (CHIP) • Other funding sources for oral healthcare programs and clinics (e.g., local government budget; federal, state, local government grants; foundations; non-profits; health, community, service, religious, business, and healthcare professional organizations)
Fluoride use	• Access to community- or school-based fluoride varnish program • Community water fluoridation • Fluoride supplements • Fluoride toothpaste • Fluoride treatments
Fluorosis	• Associated factors • Prevalence/trends
Malocclusion	• Occlusion and occlusal traits • Orthodontic treatment needs
Medications	• Medications prescribed for dental treatment
Oral and pharyngeal cancer	• Oral cancer diagnosis • Receipt of examination to detect oral cancer • Stage of cancer at time of diagnosis
Oral health knowledge, beliefs, opinions, attitudes, practices, behaviors, and skills	• Community stakeholders and policymakers • General population (children, adolescents, parents, younger and older adults) • Oral healthcare providers • Other healthcare providers

Oral health-related quality of life (OHRQoL)

- Ability to smile and convey a range of emotions through facial expressions with confidence and without pain or discomfort
- Comfort engaging in social interactions
- Difficulty speaking
- Difficulty swallowing
- Effect of oral health on self-esteem
- Inadequate salivary function (e.g., dry mouth, Sjögren's syndrome, xerostomia)
- Lost work, lost school days, activity change due to a dental problem
- Masticatory function (ability to chew)
- Oral comfort when chewing, eating
- Oral comfort when sleeping
- Pain level (e.g., dental, oral, temporomandibular disorder [TMD]; acute and chronic)

Oral healthcare providers

- Oral healthcare provider information (demographics, diversity)
- Oral healthcare provider numbers, distribution, and ratios
- Oral healthcare provider training
- Staffing of oral healthcare providers
- Types of healthcare providers seen

Oral healthcare utilization

- Access to dental care (e.g., cost, travel time, satisfaction)
- Community centers and clinics with oral health services
- Dental care satisfaction
- Dental services by type (e.g., prevention, restorations, extractions, crowns)
- Emergency dental care (e.g., traumatic injuries)
- First dental visit
- Frequency of dental visits
- Last dental visit (indicating when)
- Number of children and other ages with dental home
- Number of dental visits
- Oral health care during pregnancy
- Reason for dental visit
- Reason for last dental visit
- School-based dental programs
- State and local dental programs
- Types of dental providers seen
- Use of hospital emergency room for dental care
- Usual source of dental care

Orofacial injury

- Type of injury (e.g., tooth trauma, fractured bone)
- Type of trauma (e.g., fall, automobile accident, sports injury)

Perceived oral health status and treatment needs

- Satisfaction with teeth and in respect to oral health
- Self-assessment of general oral health status
- Self-perceived need for dental care

Periodontal diseases

- Alveolar bone loss
- Calculus (subgingival, supragingival)
- Furcations
- Gingival bleeding
- Gingival inflammation
- Gingivitis
- Loss of attachment
- Plaque biofilm
- Pocket depths
- Recession
- Tooth mobility
- Treatment need

Preventive care	• Preventive care by clinician • Preventive self-care (e.g., oral hygiene)
Primary/permanent dentition	• Cleaning • Oral debris
Soft tissue lesions	• Mouth sores • Oral herpes • Oral lesions • Oral ulcers • Tongue lesions
TMD	• Clicking/popping • Crepitation • Limited opening and function • Pain
Tobacco	• Smoking cigarettes • Smoking cigars • Smoking pipes • Tobacco cessation counseling by dental professionals • Use of smokeless tobacco (snuff, e-cigarettes, vaping)
Tooth loss/edentulism	• Complete loss of teeth • Denture ownership and use • Missing teeth • Tooth count
Treatment needs	• Dental service needed by type of care (e.g., primary preventive, restorative extraction, dentures, soft tissue lesion, TMD) • Treatment urgency

Common Dental Indexes

Dental Index	Criteria/Interpretation
Dental Caries Indexes Dental caries indexes are cumulative and irreversible:	

Decayed, Missing, Filled (DMF) Index:
• An index used to measure clinically observable coronal caries experience (active caries and treatment resulting from caries) in permanent dentition only; can be scored on teeth (DMFT) or surfaces (DMFS).
• DMFT is recommended for population surveys, and DMFS is recommended for clinical trials because it provides more sensitivity even though it has greater variability.
	• Components of DMF:
	  • D denotes dental caries, including recurrent decay.
	  • M denotes missing (extracted) because of dental caries.
	  • F denotes filled because of caries, and with no current (new or recurrent) decay.
	• Is typically based on 28 teeth (third molars are excluded).
	• Tooth or surface is scored only as one component (e.g., recurrent decay is scored only as D).
	• Teeth missing or filled for reasons other than caries are not scored (e.g., missing because of periodontitis, orthodontic treatment, trauma, surgical removal of impaction, or unerupted; filled because of cosmetic purposes, bridge abutment).
	• Interpretation requires analysis of components as well as total DMF (e.g., a high D and low F reflects high caries experience and low dental utilization, whereas a high F and low D reflects high caries experience but high dental utilization; a high M likely reflects emergent care only).
	• Results can be reported in several ways:
	  • Total DMF = caries experience
	  • D/DMF = rate of decayed teeth or treatment needs (active caries or morbidity)
	  • M/DMF = rate of missing teeth (mortality)
	  • F/DMF = rate of filled teeth

dmf, def, df Indexes:
• Lower case letters represent the DMF as used to measure observable caries experience in the primary dentition: *dmft, deft,* or *dft* for teeth; *dmfs, defs,* or *dfs* for surfaces.
• *dmf* is applied only to primary molars.
• *def* and *df* are scored on all primary teeth; they are modifications of the *dmf* by not counting missing teeth to avoid potential errors because of exfoliation, increasing the reliability compared with the *dmf* but also possibly underestimating caries experience.
• For a mixed dentition, the *DMF* and *dmf, def,* or *df* indexes are scored separately and never combined or added together.
	• Components of *dmf*:
	  • d = decayed with no recurrent caries
	  • m = missing because of caries (not exfoliated)
	  • f = filled because of caries
	• Components of *def*:
	  • d = decayed with no recurrent caries
	  • e = severe caries and *indicated for extraction* (not extracted)
	  • f = filled because of caries
	  • Missing teeth are not scored, regardless of reason
	  • *def* has greater sensitivity than *df* because it allows for two grades of severity of carious lesions.
	• Components of *df*:
	  • d and f are same as for *def* with no differentiation of severity of caries
	  • Missing teeth are not scored, regardless of reason
	  • *df* has greater reliability than *def* because it does not have the subjectivity of scoring the severity of carious lesions
	• Other scoring criteria and interpretation of the *dmf, def,* and *df* indexes are the same as for the DMF.

Root Caries Index (RCI): • Used to measure total root caries experience. • Scored on exposed root surfaces.	• Expressed as a percentage of D and F root surfaces out of the population of at-risk root surfaces. • All exposed root surfaces are scored (four surfaces per tooth: mesial, distal, lingual/palatal, and facial). • Only cavitated lesions are scored as D. • Supra- and subgingival lesions can be reported separately.

Dental Index	Criteria/Interpretation
Classification of Early Childhood Caries (ECC) and Severe Early Childhood Caries (S-ECC): Evaluation of a child's primary dentition (from birth to age 72 months or 6 years) to determine whether one or more surfaces are D (noncavitated or cavitated), M (because of caries), or F (because of caries).	ECC Criterion: • One or more *dmfs* (cavitated or noncavitated) in children younger than 6 years S-ECC Criteria (vary with age): • Younger than 3 years: Any sign of smooth-surface caries • Age 3 years: One or more cavitated *dmfs* in maxillary anterior teeth OR four or more *dmfs* • Age 4 years: One or more cavitated *dmfs* in maxillary anterior teeth OR five or more *dmfs* • Age 5 years: One or more cavitated *dmfs* in maxillary anterior teeth OR six or more *dmfs*
Gingival Indexes Gingival indexes are reversible.	
Gingival Index (GI): • A core index for measuring the severity of marginal gingivitis. • Used to determine prevalence and severity of gingivitis in epidemiological surveys and individual dentition. • Often used in controlled clinical trials of preventive or therapeutic agents. • Measured by clinical observation, by pressing the probe on the gingiva to determine degree of firmness, and by "walking" the probe inside the gingival sulcus to determine bleeding. • Reported as a mean score for the individual, population, or research group.	• *Scoring Criteria:* 0—Normal, healthy gingival tissues 1—Mild inflammation: slight change in color and/or slight edema; no bleeding on probing 2—Moderate inflammation: bleeding on probing and other signs of inflammation 3—Severe inflammation: tendency to spontaneous bleeding and other marked signs of inflammation such as striking redness, edema, and ulceration • *Interpretation of GI:* 0.1–1.0: Mild inflammation 1.1–2.0: Moderate inflammation 2.1–3.0: Severe inflammation • Results can be unreliable and difficult to replicate because of subjectivity of criteria (calibration is critical).
Modified Gingival Index (MGI): • Modification of the GI by eliminating the probing inside the sulcus. • Developed to reduce the probability of disturbing plaque during probing, decrease gingival trauma caused by probing, and minimize the calibration required to control examiner error.	• *Scoring Criteria:* 0—Normal, healthy gingival tissues 1—Mild inflammation involving any portion of but not the entire marginal or papillary gingival unit 2—Mild inflammation involving the entire marginal or papillary gingival unit 3—Moderate inflammation 4—Severe inflammation • The MGI provides a less sensitive measure of gingivitis than the GI because of the elimination of the bleeding-on-probing component.
Sulcus Bleeding Index (SBI): • A complex bleeding index to detect early signs of gingivitis and measure extent of inflammation. • Useful for short-term clinical trials. • Measured by "walking" the probe at the base of the sulcus. • Four gingival units scored for each tooth: labial and lingual marginal gingiva (M units) and mesial and distal papillary gingiva (P units).	• *Scoring Criteria:* 0—Healthy appearance of P and M units; no bleeding on probing 1—Apparently healthy P and M units with no change in color and no swelling, but bleeding from sulcus on probing 2—Bleeding on probing and change of color caused by inflammation; no swelling or macroscopic edema 3—Bleeding on probing and change in color; slight edematous swelling 4—Bleeding on probing and obvious swelling; may have change in color 5—Bleeding on probing, spontaneous bleeding, change in color, and marked swelling with or without ulceration • Results can be unreliable because of subjectivity of criteria (calibration is critical).
Gingival Bleeding Index (GBI): • A simple, easy-to-implement, dichotomous measure of the presence or absence of interproximal bleeding. • Measured by passing unwaxed floss on each side of the papilla, using a C shape and one up and down stroke.	• *Scoring Criteria:* Results are reported by frequency of score based on presence (1) or absence (0) of bleeding. • Each area of gingiva is observed for bleeding for 30 seconds after flossing if bleeding is not immediate or not on the floss. • Because the severity of bleeding is not measured, the GBI is less sensitive than the SBI but more reliable and easier to calibrate.
Eastman Interdental Bleeding Index (EIBI): • A simple, easy-to-implement, dichotomous measure of the presence or absence of interproximal bleeding. • Measured by horizontally inserting a wooden interdental cleaner/stimulator four times, depressing the papilla 1 to 2 mm.	• *Scoring Criteria:* Results are reported by frequency of score based on presence (1) or absence (0) of bleeding. • Each area is observed for bleeding for 15 seconds after insertion of interdental cleaner. • Because the severity of bleeding is not measured, the EIBI is less sensitive than the SBI but is more reliable and easier to calibrate.

Dental Index	Criteria/Interpretation

Periodontal Disease Indexes

These periodontal indexes are cumulative and composite (measure both reversible and irreversible changes within the same index).

Community Periodontal Index (CPI):

- An index used to measure periodontal status of a community.
- Developed by the World Health Organization (WHO); adaptation of the WHO Community Periodontal Index of Treatment Needs (CPITN) by eliminating the treatment need codes from the CPITN; in contrast to the CPITN, the CPI measures only periodontal status, and the CPITN reported periodontal treatment needs as well.
- Sulci/pockets are measured with the WHO specially designed, lightweight probe that has 0.5-, 3.5-, 5.5-, 8.5-, and 11.5-mm markings, a colored area to denote the range of 3.5- to 5.5-mm depth, and a ball tip.
- The Periodontal Screening and Recording® (PSR) system developed by the American Dental Association (ADA) was based on the CPITN and is similar to the CPI.

- To reflect current theory of periodontal conditions, the index consists of two components scored and reported separately:
  - CPI Codes (periodontal status)
  - LOA Codes (loss of attachment; same as clinical attachment loss [CAL])
- Includes measurements of gingival inflammation, bleeding, calculus, clinical attachment loss, and periodontal pockets.
- The CPI divides the teeth into sextants for measurement, with specific teeth scored for each sextant; index teeth differ for children and adults.
  - Adults: Sextant is measured only if two or more teeth are present that are not indicated for extraction; teeth measured are first and second molars in posterior sextants and maxillary right central incisor and mandibular left central incisor in anterior sextants; if a molar is missing, no replacement tooth is selected for the sextant; if no index tooth/teeth is/are present in a sextant, all other teeth in the sextant are scored.
  - Children: Teeth measured are all first molars and maxillary right and mandibular left incisors; pocket depth is not recorded in children younger than age 15 years.
- *Scoring Criteria for CPI Codes:*
  Code 0—Entire colored band visible; healthy periodontal tissues: no bleeding
  Code 1—Entire colored band visible; bleeding upon gentle probing
  Code 2—Entire colored band visible; calculus present; bleeding may or may not be present
  Code 3—Colored band on probe partially hidden by gingival margin denoting 4–5 mm pocket depth
  Code 4—Colored band entirely hidden denoting $\geq$ 6 mm pockets
  If the cementoenamel junction (CEJ) is visible or the CPI is 4, LOA codes 1 to 4 are used.
- *Scoring Criteria for LOA (CAL) Codes:*
  Code 0—0–3 mm LOA: CEJ is covered by gingival margin and CPI score is 0 to 3
  Code 1—3.5–5.5 mm LOA: CEJ is within the colored band on the probe
  Code 2—6–8 mm LOA: CEJ is between the top of the colored band and the 8.5 mm mark on the probe
  Code 3—9–11 mm LOA: CEJ is between the 8.5 and 11.5 mm marks on the probe
  Code 4—LOA $\geq$ 12 mm: CEJ is beyond the highest mark (11.5 mm) on the probe

Periodontal Disease Index (PDI):

- Because the PDI combined measures of reversible and irreversible disease within the same index, it is no longer recommended based on the current understanding that gingivitis and periodontitis are two different disease entities.

- Even so, the PDI has the following current significance:
  - It first introduced the current method of combining recession and pocket depth to determine CAL.
  - The six teeth scored by the PDI (tooth numbers 3, 9, 12, 19, 25, and 28), referred to as the Ramfjord teeth (after Dr. Ramfjord, who developed the index), are considered sensitive for partial mouth scoring of periodontal conditions and are frequently used today with other periodontal measures for partial mouth scoring.
- A disaggregated approach is currently used to measure the various components of the PDI that represent the clinical signs and accumulated destructive results of past disease (bleeding, recession, pocket formation, and CAL).

Dental Index	Criteria/Interpretation
Fluorosis Indexes	
Dean's Fluorosis Index (DFI)/Community Fluorosis Index (CFI): • One of the most universally accepted fluorosis indexes, simple and easy to use, and used to establish prevalence in the population. • Developed by Dean as a classification with six categories, referred to as Dean's Fluorosis Index; later numbers ranging from 0–4 were added to denote the categories for surveillance purposes, and the index was referred to as the Community Fluorosis Index (CFI); today this index is referred to by both names. ***Comparison With Other Fluorosis Indexes:*** The Thylstrup-Fejerskov Index (TFI) and the Tooth Surface Index of Fluorosis (TSIF) are two commonly used modifications of the DFI/CFI; developed for research purposes, both have a wider range of scores and expanded categories for greater sensitivity.	• *Scoring Criteria:* Normal (0)—Enamel presents the usual translucent semivitriform type of structure; surface is smooth, glossy, and usually pale creamy white Questionable (0.5)—Enamel has slight aberrations from the normal translucency, ranging from a few white flecks to occasional white spots; this classification is used when neither the Very Mild nor Normal classification is definitively justified Very mild (1)—Small, opaque, paper-white areas are scattered irregularly and involve less than 25% of the tooth surface; frequently included in this classification are teeth showing no more than about 1-2 mm of white opacity at the cusp tips of premolars or second molars Mild (2)—More extensive white opaque areas in the enamel involving less than 50% of the tooth Moderate (3)—All enamel surfaces of the teeth are affected, and surfaces subject to attrition show wear; brown stain is frequently a disfiguring feature Severe (4)—All enamel surfaces are affected; hypoplasia is so marked that the general form of the tooth may be affected; discrete or confluent pitting is a major diagnostic sign of this classification; brown stains are widespread, and teeth often appear as if corroded • An individual is categorized by classification based on the lesser of the two worst-affected teeth, with anterior and posterior teeth equally weighted. • Prevalence of each category is reported in a population; can be reported as the mean of all scores in the population, or as a percentage of the population scored in each category. • Interpretation: A classification of mild or less is not considered a cosmetic problem, and a mean score of less than 0.6 is not considered a problem for a community.

BIBLIOGRAPHY

Chattopadhyay A. Oral Health Epidemiology: Principles and Practice. Sudbury, MA: Jones and Bartlett; 2011.

Funmilayo ASM, Mojirade AD. Dental fluorosis and its indexes, what's new? IOSR-JDMS 2014;13(7) Ver.III:55-60. Available at: <www.iosrjournals.org/iosr-jdms/papers/Vol13-issue7/Version-3/M013735560.pdf>; [Accessed March 2020].

National Health and Nutrition Examination Survey (NHANES) Oral Health Dental Examiners Manual. Atlanta, GA: Centers for Disease Control and Prevention; January 2020. Available at: <https://wwwn.cdc.gov/nchs/data/nhanes/2019-2020/manuals/2020-Oral-Health-Examiners-Manual-508.pdf>; [Accessed March 2020].

Policy on Early Childhood Caries (ECC). Classifications, Consequences, and Preventive Strategies, 2016. Reference Manual of Pediatric Dentistry, pp. 79–81.

Chicago, IL: American Academy of Pediatric Dentistry; 2020–2021. Available at: <https://www.aapd.org/research/oral-health-policies--recommendations/early-childhood-caries-classifications-consequences-and-preventive-strategies/>; [Accessed November 2020].

Wyche CJ. Indices and scoring methods. In: Boyd LD, Mallonee LF, Wyche CJ, editors. Wilkins' Clinical Practice of the Dental Hygienist. 13th ed., pp. 357–379. Burlington, MA: Jones & Bartlett Learning; 2021.

Abstract A summary or brief description of a report, manuscript, or presentation, placed at the beginning, approximately 100 to 300 words in length, and designed to provide an overview; used to concisely define a research study's purpose, methods, materials, results, and conclusions; also used for community reports such as a community assessment or program outcomes.

Access to oral health care/access to care Assurance that conditions are in place for people to obtain the (oral) health care they need and want, including epidemiological, social, personal, demographic, and psychological conditions, as well as characteristics of the (oral) healthcare system such as availability, accessibility, accommodation, affordability, and acceptability; reported by *Healthy People* as the timely use of personal health services and dental treatment to achieve the best (oral) health outcomes. Also referred to as access to dental care.

Accountable care organization (ACO) A provider-run organization in which participating providers are collectively responsible for the care of an enrolled population and may share in any savings associated with improvements in the quality and efficiency of care.

Acute Referring to a health effect; brief exposure of high intensity, in contrast to chronic.

Administration for Children and Families (ACF) An agency of the DHHS that promotes the economic and social well-being of families, children, individuals, and communities; administers the Head Start program.

Administrator A career path or role of the dental hygienist that involves a supervisory role in which they direct and oversee oral health programs.

Advocate/advocacy A career path or role in which the dental hygienist works to promote change and advance people's health through legislation, public policy, research, and science, in response to seeing problems related to achieving optimal oral health and attempting to develop a solution; may involve helping to create and implement new or revised oral healthcare laws.

Agent factors Biological or mechanical means of causing disease, illness, injury, or disability, including microbial, parasitic, viral, and bacterial pathogens or vectors; physical or mechanical irritants; chemicals; drugs; trauma; and radiation; they interact with host and environmental factors over time in the multifactorial perspective of epidemiology.

Alternate hypothesis A positive statement of the hypothesis that is based on the expectation that sample observations are influenced by some nonrandom cause; accepted if the null hypothesis is rejected.

Alternative practice A setting outside the private office in which the dental hygienist provides oral health services to members of the public who are underserved by the traditional private practice setting.

Analysis of variance (ANOVA) A parametric statistical test used to compare two or more sample mean scores; the only appropriate statistical test for the comparison of three or more mean scores.

Analytic study An epidemiological study that provides information about the association of risk attributes in relation to a disease or condition to establish risk and estimate causality.

Antifluoridationists Opponents of community water fluoridation.

Assessment/Assess A core public health function that includes the regular and systematic collection, assemblage, and analysis of data and communication regarding the oral health of the community; the first step of the program planning or community health improvement process.

Association of State and Territorial Dental Directors (ASTDD) A national dental public health organization whose membership includes each of the state directors for oral health; provides a strong governmental presence regarding issues, core functions, and best practices for community oral health practice and is a central location to access resources for community oral health initiatives.

Assurance A core public health function in which agencies ensure that services necessary to achieve agreed-upon health goals are provided, either by encouraging actions by other entities (private or public sector), by requiring such action through regulation, or by providing services directly.

Bar graph A simple graph in which bars or columns are used to display frequencies of nominal or ordinal data or the value of different but comparable items (categorical data); the bars or columns are separated (do not touch as they do in a histogram) because of the categorical nature of the data.

Baseline Initial observation or value that serves as the basis for comparison with subsequently acquired data in a research study or program evaluation.

Basic Oral Health Survey A simple screening survey model developed by the World Health Organization (WHO) for use in global surveillance; provides a standardized oral health survey method that results in comparable data internationally.

Basic screening/Basic Screening Survey (BSS) A rapid assessment accomplished in a short time by visual detection and providing information about gross dental and oral lesions. The BSS is a simple screening survey model developed by the ASTDD and used in the U.S. for basic screening and referral for dental care; two versions exist, one for older adults and another for preschool- and school-age children. Similar to the WHO Basic Oral Health Survey.

Behavioral Risk Factor Surveillance Survey (BRFSS) A state-specific telephone survey that is developed nationally to assess the practice of behaviors that influence health status; includes questions to assess the use of oral health services.

Best practice approach A public health strategy that is supported by evidence, including research, expert opinion, field lessons, and theoretical rationale, for its effectiveness in reliably leading to a desired result.

Blind study (masking) A research study design in which the examiners and study participants are unaware of group assignment (double blind) or only the examiners are unaware of group assignment (single blind).

Block grant A consolidated grant of federal funds, formerly allocated for specific programs, that a state or local government may use at its discretion for various programs, including health; Maternal and Child Health Services and Preventive Health and Health Services are common block grants for health and oral health services.

Calibration A process used to determine, check, rectify, or adjust a measurement device to increase the accuracy and precision of the measurements. Calibration is applied also to examiners or raters who are involved in data collection to achieve agreement with set criteria and a standard of performance.

Capacity/oral health capacity The ability of the oral healthcare system to implement public health strategies, deliver oral health services, and develop oral health literacy of the public. It consists of fiscal and economic resources, workforce and human resources, physical infrastructure, interorganizational relationships, informational resources, system boundaries and size, governance and decision-making structure, and culture. It is a determinant of performance of an organization and thus oral health outcomes.

Case-control study An epidemiological observational retrospective research study in which two groups from the same population, one with the disease (referred to as cases) and one without the disease (referred to as controls), are compared to identify factors in their history that can be associated with the disease, condition, or outcome (called exposures); can identify risk and trends and suggest possible causes.

Categorical data Nonnumeric data that represent categories.

Centers for Disease Control and Prevention (CDC) A major federal agency of the DHHS Public Health Service that monitors health, informs decision makers about health topics, provides people with information so they can take responsibility for their own health, provides healthcare workers with information on health promotion, and prevents disease and promotes health. Oral health is included in all these activities.

Children's Health Insurance Program (CHIP) A joint federal-state funded program administered by states to provide comprehensive health insurance coverage, including dental, to eligible children, through both Medicaid and separate CHIP programs.

Chi-square test One of the most commonly used nonparametric statistical tests; used to analyze differences in counts and proportions of categorical variables and to test the significance of relationships between variables that have been established by correlation.

Chronic Referring to a health-related state that lasts a long time, in contrast to acute.

Clinical rotation A curriculum-based experiential learning activity that is not necessarily associated with a service outcome and is designed primarily to benefit the student's learning. Students are assigned rotations to gain clinical experiences that enhance knowledge, skills, and expertise; can be used to provide exposure to community settings.

Clinical significance The practical importance of a treatment effect in research; also used to refer to criteria of a measurement instrument being clinically meaningful.

Clinical trial An experimental study that tests the safety, efficacy, and/or effectiveness of procedures, therapies, drugs, or other interventions to prevent, screen for, diagnose, or treat disease in humans.

Clinician A career path or role in which the dental hygienist assesses oral health needs and provides treatment for individuals.

Coalition A cooperative, collaborative effort on the part of many diverse individuals and organizations that reflects a public-private partnership to build systems and develop programs that improve community health.

Cohort study An epidemiological observational longitudinal prospective research study in which a subset of a defined population is observed over time to generate reliable incidence or mortality rates; usually a large population, a study lasting a prolonged period (years), or both; can include a comparison group.

Collaboration The process of working together to accomplish a goal.

Collaborative practice Cooperative working relationship of a dental hygienist with a consulting dentist, without supervision.

Common risk factors approach A method used to create cross-disciplinary health promotion programs sharing common risk factors for disease, based on the fact that many of the risk factors negatively impacting oral health also have a detrimental effect on overall health.

Communication plan Outlines objectives, key messages, activities, evaluation methods, and responsibilities for communication projects or programs.

Community The public or group of people with common interests who live in a specific locality; in relation to community oral health, can be used to refer to a large or small group within the population.

Community cases/scenarios Short descriptions of community oral health real-world situations used as examples; combined with test questions to form testlets by the National Board Dental Hygiene Examination (NBDHE) to test the community health/research principles content area.

Community dental health coordinator A community health worker developed by the American Dental Association (ADA) that focuses on oral health education and disease prevention in underserved rural, urban, and Native American communities to expand access to dental care.

Community health Focuses on studying, protecting, and improving health within a community; frequently used synonymously with public health.

Community oral health/community dental health Community health in relation to oral health; frequently used synonymously with dental public health (see dental public health).

Community oral health assessment A multifaceted process of identifying factors that affect the oral health of a selected population to be able to determine resources and interventions needed for oral health improvement.

Community Organization Theory The process of involving and activating members of a community or subgroup to identify a common problem or goal, to mobilize resources, to implement strategies, and to evaluate their efforts.

Community partnership/community partner An arrangement between or among agencies, organizations, businesses, and/or people that collaborate and combine resources to work toward a unified, common goal; considered a key public health activity in the community program planning process.

Community profile A comprehensive description of the community developed through a formal organized community assessment process.

Community service When used in relation to education of students in community oral health, students providing a service to the community with the primary focus on the community's needs; may or may not have a curriculum connection.

Community trial A quasi-experimental study in which a community, rather than a group of individuals, receives the intervention.

Community water fluoridation The addition of a controlled amount of fluoride to the public water supply to bring it to an optimal level for the purpose of preventing dental caries in the population.

Confidence interval An inferential statistic that estimates the accuracy of a sample statistic representing the population parameter.

Continuous data Numeric data that can be expressed by a large or infinite number of measures along a continuum, such as test scores, thus having real value when expressed as a fraction.

Control group The group of study participants that does not receive the experimental

treatment or intervention for the purpose of comparison to the experimental group.

Convenience sampling Using a group of individuals who are most readily available to be participants in a research study.

Core functions of public health The commonly recognized central tasks of public health identified by the Institute of Medicine that provide the basis for all public health activities. The core functions are assessment, policy development, and assurance.

Correlation statistics A group of statistics that are used to determine whether a variation in one variable may be related to a variation in another variable; used to determine the association or relationship of variables.

Critical thinking The intellectually disciplined process of actively, objectively, and skillfully conceptualizing, applying, analyzing, synthesizing, and/or evaluating information for the purpose of forming a judgment and making a decision. Critical thinking is a core competency of dental hygiene educational programs and required for community oral health practice.

Cross-cultural communication The communication or exchange of information among persons from different cultures, which is necessary in a diverse population.

Cross-cultural encounter Contact and interactions among diverse persons or communities, which occurs with regularity in a diverse population.

Crossover study An observational or controlled experimental study in which study participants receive a sequence of different treatments with a washout period between; has the advantage of exact matching since the study participants serve as their own controls.

Cross-sectional study/survey An observational study that examines the relationship between disease (or other health-related state) and other variables of interest as they exist in a defined representative cross section of the population, observed at one particular time; can identify the frequency of variables without examining relationships; requires a large sample size.

Cultural competence The ability of healthcare providers to deliver services that are respectful of and responsive to the health beliefs, practices, and cultural and linguistic needs of diverse patients and communities, thus helping to fulfill the profession's responsibility to reduce the burden of disease for people of various cultures and backgrounds.

Cultural Competence Continuum A model commonly used for training in the development of cultural competence, consisting of six stages: cultural destructiveness, cultural incapacity, cultural blindness, cultural precompetence, cultural competence, and cultural proficiency. Through self-assessment, individuals and organizations can evaluate their placement on the continuum and plan for and track progress toward developing personal and professional cultural competence and proficiency.

Cultural diversity The degree to which a population consists of diverse individuals from different cultures, taking into account differences such as nationality, ethnicity, race, gender, age, language, and religion.

Culture An integrated pattern of human behavior that includes thoughts, communications, languages, practices, beliefs, values, customs, courtesies, rituals, manners of interacting, roles, relationships, and expected behaviors of a racial, ethnic, religious, or social group.

Data Facts or pieces of information used to calculate, analyze, or plan in the course of community program planning or research.

Data collection The process of gathering information during the assessment or evaluation process of program planning or the measurement of variables in the conduct of research.

Defluoridation Water treatment that reduces the level of fluoride in the community water when it is too high, to make it safe for human consumption.

Demand Healthcare services desired by the individual or community.

Dental care voucher A form authorizing a dental provider to bill the distributing agency for dental services or treatment, whereby payment is guaranteed by the agency that provides the voucher; a means of payment that is available for limited oral health services to low income, uninsured individuals who fall outside the eligibility guidelines for entitlement programs such as Medicaid.

Dental health professional shortage area (dental HPSA) Geographic area or healthcare facility in which the dentist/dental health professional to population ratio is low as designated by the HRSA. HPSAs receive various federal benefits as a result of the designation, including qualifying for funding of a federally qualified health center.

Dental home The ongoing relationship between the oral healthcare provider and the patient that allows for the delivery of comprehensive, continuously accessible, coordinated, and patient- and family-centered oral health care.

Dental hygiene-based dental therapist Dental therapist that has advanced dental therapy training after dental hygiene licensure and extensive dental hygiene experience; has both a dental hygiene and a dental therapy scope of practice; model promoted by the American Dental Hygienists' Association (ADHA).

Dental index An abbreviated rating scale or set of numbers derived from a series of observations of a specified oral disease or condition; used to measure the amount or severity of an oral disease or related condition in a population; dental indexes and dental indices can both be used as the plural form.

Dental public health The science and art of preventing and controlling oral diseases and promoting oral health through organized community efforts; serving the community rather than the individual, the focus is on oral health education of the public, applied research, administration of group dental care programs, and prevention and control of dental diseases on a community basis.

Dental therapist A mid-level oral healthcare provider; the advanced dental therapist has a greater scope of practice and requires less supervision.

Denturist An oral healthcare provider who has direct access to the population and is authorized to fabricate and deliver dentures.

Department of Health and Human Services (DHHS) A department of the federal government presiding over agencies that implement programs to fulfill health goals, including oral health; primarily provides an infrastructure, research, surveillance, and funding for programs that are carried out at the state and local levels.

Dependent variable The variable thought to depend on or to be affected by the independent variable in an experimental or quasi-experimental study; the outcome variable of interest.

Descriptive statistics Category of statistics that are used to describe and summarize data; used to determine information about the sample being studied without generalizing to the population.

Descriptive study A study in which the characteristics of a population are defined, providing information about the naturally occurring health status, behavior, attitudes, or other characteristics of a particular group.

Determinants of health Factors that interact to create circumstances that have a comprehensive influence on collective and personal well-being with a profound effect on health; can be classified as social, physical, economic, environmental, biological, personal, and behavioral, many of which cannot be controlled by the individual.

Dichotomous scale/data A measurement scale that arranges items into either of two mutually exclusive categories; categorical data that possess only two categories.

Dietary fluoride supplements Fluoride drops, tablets, or lozenges used as a source of fluoride to supplement the diet when fluoridated drinking water is not available.

Diffusion of Innovations Theory A theory or concept that assesses how new ideas, products, or services spread within a society or to other groups or how innovations are adopted.

Direct access The dental hygienist's right to initiate treatment based on an assessment of a patient's needs without the specific authorization of a dentist, to treat the patient without the presence of a dentist, and to maintain a provider-patient relationship.

Direct reimbursement The dental hygienist's right to file and be reimbursed for services directly from third-party payers such as Medicaid and private dental insurers.

Direct supervision The level of supervision that requires that the dentist be present, examine the patient to authorize the work to be performed, and check it after.

Discrete data Numeric data with a set of fixed or finite values that can be counted only in whole numbers.

Early and Periodic Screening, Diagnostic, and Treatment (EPSDT) Benefits resulting from the federal mandate to provide comprehensive and preventive healthcare services for children under age 21 years who are enrolled in Medicaid; required dental benefits include relief of pain and infections, restorations, and primary preventive procedures beginning at age 6 months.

Early childhood caries (ECC)/ECC classification The presence of one or more decayed (non-cavitated or cavitated), missing (due to caries), or filled tooth surfaces in any primary tooth in a preschool-age child between birth and 71 months of age (infants through 5 years old). The term Severe Early Childhood Caries (S-ECC) refers to atypical, progressive, acute, or rampant patterns of dental caries. Classification system is used to categorize ECC and S-ECC by age.

Early Head Start Head Start program that serves children from birth to age 3 years.

Ecological approach Concerned with the relations of people to one another and the interactions between people and their physical surroundings, including the interdependence of people and institutions; in relation to epidemiology, referred to as ecoepidemiology.

Ecological study An observational study in which existing group-level data, as opposed to data collected from individuals, are used to relate risk attributes to health or other outcomes.

Empowerment/empowering Enabling individuals or a community to gain mastery in and take control of overall decision-making about achievement of health for themselves or their own community.

Endemic The constant, normal presence of a disease or infectious agent within a given geographic area or population group.

Entrepreneur The career path or role in which a dental hygienist applies imagination and creativity to initiate or finance a new enterprise, many of which have a community focus by serving a vulnerable, underserved priority population.

Environmental factors Physical, sociocultural, sociopolitical, and economic components that interact with host and agent factors over time in the multifactorial perspective of epidemiology.

Epidemic Occurrence of cases of an illness, specific health-related behavior, or other health-related events in a community or region, clearly in excess of normal expectancy; from Greek *epi* (upon), *demos* (people).

Epidemiology The study of the distribution and determinants of health-related states and events in specified populations and its application to the prevention and control of health problems.

Epidemiologic examination A visual/tactile examination accomplished with dental instruments and light source; provides more detailed information than basic screening.

Epidemiologic triangle The graphic representation of the multiple factors that result in disease: agent factors, environmental factors, and host factors, that interact over time.

Eradication   In relation to disease, termination of all transmission of infection by extermination of the infectious agent through surveillance and containment.

Essential public health services/essential public health services to promote oral health   A framework that provides guidelines and describes the roles of public health as applied by many national programs. The ASTDD applied these essential services to develop a framework and guidelines for the roles of state oral health programs in their promotion of oral health; used in the development and evaluation of dental public health activities at the state level and in some cases at the local level.

Ethics/professional ethics   The general science of right and wrong conduct; the code by which the profession regulates actions and sets standards for its members, with the recognition that professionals are accountable for their actions; has application to professional conduct in community oral health practice.

Ethnocentrism   Judging others by one's own cultural standards based on a belief that one's personal cultural group is superior.

Etiology   The science of causes, causality; in common use, cause.

Evaluation/evaluate   The final step of the program planning or community health improvement process during which outcomes are measured against objectives that were developed during the earlier planning stage, for the purpose of judging the effectiveness and efficiency of a program; referred to as summative evaluation. Evaluation can consist also of formative evaluation; use of both summative and formative evaluation is considered good practice in community health practice and service-learning. (See formative evaluation and summative evaluation.)

Evidence-based decision-making   Application of a combination of relevant components to oral healthcare practice: scientific evidence, practitioner's professional expertise and judgment, patient or community preferences or values, and circumstances of the situation.

Experiential learning   An umbrella term that encompasses various models of learning in which experience governs the learning process, including reflection, critical analysis, and synthesis in relation to the experience; essential to learning community oral health concepts and practice.

Experimental group   The sample group of participants in an experimental study that receives the experimental treatment or intervention.

Experimental study   A study intended to discover the effect of a treatment, procedure, or program in a controlled setting. Experimental studies have the greatest control and thus provide the highest level of evidence of all study designs.

Extraneous (confounding) variable   Any relevant variable in a study that is not controlled and can be a source of error in relation to any observed effects in the study outcomes.

Factorial study   An experimental study that simultaneously tests the effect of multiple factors (independent variables or treatments) on the dependent variable and includes an assessment of potential interactions among the treatments.

FDI World Dental Federation (FDI)   An international organization that represents the oral health community in developing a common vision to advance the science and practice of dentistry, address the global oral disease burden, and improve oral health through education, community programs and efforts, and advocacy.

Federal poverty level (FPL)   A measure of income level issued annually by the DHHS and used to determine eligibility for certain programs and benefits; current FPL amounts can be found at www.hhs.gov.

Federally qualified health center (FQHC)   A community health center that serves an underserved area or population as defined by the Health Resources and Services Administration; receives federal funding, enhanced reimbursement from Medicare and Medicaid, and other federal benefits.

Fee-for-service   A payment model in which healthcare services are paid for as itemized in the provider's invoice, patients are able to make healthcare decisions independently, and providers bill for each service separately and have no third-party restrictions on care provided and fees charged; used to describe individual out-of-pocket payment for services by uninsured individuals and payment mechanism in an indemnity insurance plan.

Fluoride mouthrinse program   Weekly rinsing with a fluoride mouthrinse by children, usually in a school setting, in communities that do not have access to water fluoridation.

Fluoride varnish program   Public health program that makes fluoride varnish available to children in communities that do not have access to water fluoridation, or that supplements fluoridation in a population that is at elevated risk for dental caries; administered through health department medical clinics, school-based programs, and other community programs.

Focus group   Small number of people (usually between 6 and 12, but typically 8) brought together with a moderator to discuss a specific topic and produce qualitative data; useful for the purpose of idea generation in community assessment or for evaluation of programs, initiatives, or products such as health messages or communication materials.

Formative evaluation   Evaluation mechanisms conducted during the implementation step of the program planning or community health improvement process to ensure effectiveness of program processes, procedures, and activities and to provide an opportunity for adjustment as needed; sometimes referred to as process evaluation.

Framing health messages   A concept that relates to the cues (e.g., sounds, symbols, words, pictures) that signal how and what to think about a health issue. Gain-framing a message focuses on what is to be gained by adopting the recommended health behavior, and loss-framing is the opposite, focusing on the effect of practicing an unhealthy behavior.

Frequency distribution table   A table that shows the frequency or number of times that values or categories occur in a data distribution.

Frequency polygon   A line graph that portrays a distribution of continuous data.

General supervision   Level of supervision of the dental hygienist in which the dentist does not have to be on the premises, but the patient must be one of record (previously seen by the dentist).

Goal   A broad-based statement of desired change to result from a community oral health program, from which specific objectives are developed.

Hawthorne effect   Change in behavior of research study participants in response to their awareness that they are being observed or to the attention they receive as a result of the procedures of the study; can reduce internal validity of a study and produce an error in research results.

Head Start   A school-readiness program administered by the ACF that is designed to break the cycle of poverty by providing a comprehensive early learning program for preschool aged children of low-income families; oral health is addressed by Head Start.

Health   A state of complete physical, mental, and social well-being and not merely the absence of disease.

Health Belief Model   A health education/health promotion model that attempts to explain and predict health behaviors by focusing on the attitudes and beliefs of individuals; centered on perceptions of susceptibility to the disease, severity of the disease and its effects, benefits or efficacy of the advised action, and tangible or psychological costs of the advised action, referred to as barriers.

Health communication   The use of communication strategies to inform and influence individual decisions that enhance health.

Health disparities   Uneven distribution of the burden of disease such as oral disease throughout the population, especially in the poor, older adults, disabled, and other vulnerable and underserved population groups; considered unfair because it is caused by social or economic disadvantage.

Health education/oral health education   A component of health promotion and the process by which individuals are encouraged to become responsible for their personal health; includes efforts to increase awareness of one's health and to impart sound, evidence-based knowledge and skills to develop and maintain behaviors and attitudes that lead to better health and wellness through prevention. Oral health education is health education in relation to oral diseases and conditions.

Health equity/health inequities   Health equity is achieved when all people have the opportunity to attain their full health potential and no one is disadvantaged from achieving it because of social position or other socially determined circumstances. Health inequities are the unfair, unjust, unnecessary, and avoidable differences in health status seen within and between various populations.

Health information technology The application of computers and telecommunications equipment to health care for the comprehensive management and communication of health information for decision-making related to health issues.

Health Insurance Portability and Accountability Act (HIPAA) Federal regulations governing and protecting the rights and privacy of patients in health care.

Health literacy The degree to which individuals have the capacity to obtain, process, and understand basic health information and services that are needed to make appropriate health decisions.

Health literate organization A healthcare organization that makes it easier for people to navigate, understand, and use information and services to take care of their health.

Health marketing A multidisciplinary area of public health practice that draws from fields such as marketing, communication, and public health promotion to provide a framework of theories, strategies, and techniques for application to public health research, interventions, and communication campaigns; involves creating, communicating, and delivering health information and interventions using client-centered and science-based strategies to prevent disease and protect and promote the health of diverse populations.

Health promotion A broad concept referring to the process of enabling people and communities to increase their control over the determinants of health and thus to improve their own health; moves beyond a focus on individual behavior toward a wide range of social and environmental interventions.

Health Resources and Services Administration (HRSA) The primary federal agency that provides programming designed to improve access to healthcare services for people who are uninsured, isolated, or medically vulnerable.

Healthy People A dynamic national compilation of measurable 10-year health goals and objectives for prevention of disease and promotion of health that identify nationwide health improvement priorities for the current decade and are applicable at the national, state, and local levels; the name includes the current decade (e.g., *Healthy People 2030*).

Histogram A type of graph that depicts the frequency distribution of continuous (ratio or interval scale) data; similar in appearance to a bar graph except the bars of a histogram are joined (touching) to show the continuous nature of the data.

Host factors Influences on a person's susceptibility and resistance to disease that interact with agent and environmental factors over time in the multifactorial perspective of epidemiology.

Hypothesis (research hypothesis) A statement that provides a supposition, prediction, or explanation of the expected outcome of the proposed research. (See null hypothesis and alternate hypothesis.)

Implementation/implement The third step in the program planning or community health improvement process during which the plan is put into action and the plan's activities, personnel, equipment, resources, supplies, and preliminary progress toward program goals are monitored (formative evaluation).

Incidence The rate of illness commencing or of persons falling ill (new cases of disease or health condition) during a designated period in a specified population.

Independent variable The experimental treatment or intervention that is imposed on the experimental group as it is manipulated by the researcher in an experimental or quasi-experimental study to observe its relationship with some other quality.

Indirect supervision The level of supervision that requires that the dentist be present, generally authorize the work to be performed, examine the patient, either before or after work is performed, and be available for consultation during treatment.

Inferential statistics Category of statistics used to make inferences or draw generalizations about the population that are based on the sample data.

Infrastructure/oral health infrastructure The systems, people, relationships, and resources that enable federal, state, and local agencies to perform public health functions and address oral health problems.

Interprofessional collaborative practice/ interdisciplinary collaboration Multiple health workers from different professional backgrounds collaborating to work together with patients, families, caregivers, and communities to deliver the highest quality of care; can facilitate a focus on the oral-systemic link, improve oral and overall health outcomes, and result in empowering communities in relation to health improvement.

Interprofessional education Educating health professions students in an interprofessional collaborative model to prepare health professions graduates to practice using this approach in community settings to address identified community health issues that cut across the disciplines.

Interrater reliability Agreement of measurement findings by two or more examiners

Interval scale A scale of measurement in which differences between values can be quantified in absolute but not relative terms; characterized by having order and equal distance between points on the scale but no absolute 0 value.

Interventions Activities of a community health program designed to bring about the desired results of the community health improvement process.

Intrarater reliability Consistency of measurement findings by one examiner with those previously recorded by the same examiner.

Iron triangle of health care A concept of health care that consists of three essential and competing components of the healthcare system: quality, cost, and access.

Judgmental (purposive) sampling Method of sampling in which the researcher uses personal judgment to select study participants who are believed to best represent the population.

Leading health indicators (LHI) A smaller set of *Healthy People* objectives selected to communicate the highest priority health issues and actions or initiatives for the current decade.

Learning styles The means by which individuals collect and retain knowledge based on personal factors, behaviors, and attitudes that facilitate learning in given situations.

Lesson plan Detailed description of an individual lesson prepared ahead to guide instruction.

License portability The ability of a licensed professional in one state to be recognized to practice in another state, allowing practice across jurisdictional boundaries.

Longitudinal study An observational research method in which data are gathered for the same individuals repeatedly over a period of time.

Managed care A type of health insurance that uses techniques to control the cost of providing benefits, including contracts with providers to deliver care at reduced costs, financial incentives for beneficiaries to use these providers, and control of services provided; the approved providers make up what is referred to as the plan's network.

Mann-Whitney U test A nonparametric statistical test used to compare differences between two independent groups when the dependent variable is either ordinal or is continuous but not normally distributed.

Matching A research method applied during randomization to assure equivalency of research groups on a variable.

Mean Arithmetic average of a group of scores; the sum of the numbers divided by the quantity of scores.

Median The exact middle score or value in a distribution of scores.

Medicaid A joint state-federal financed program that is administered by the states to provide comprehensive medical coverage for individuals within certain income limits; includes dental coverage for children of low-income families and limited dental coverage for adults.

Medical Expenditure Panel Survey (MEPS) A set of large-scale national surveys of families and individuals, their medical providers, and employers across the U.S. on the cost and use of health care and health insurance coverage; includes data on the number of annual dental visits for various population groups.

Medicare A federal health insurance program that provides comprehensive health care for adults ages 65 years and older; not a source of financing oral health care unless it is medically necessary.

Meta-analysis A statistical technique for combining the findings from independent studies; used in systematic literature reviews to provide a higher level of evidence for evidence-based decision-making.

Mode The score or value that occurs most frequently in a data set; only measure of central tendency that can be used with nominal data.

Monitoring/monitor Systematic examination of public health program coverage and delivery for the purpose of assuring the program is proceeding as planned and to provide opportunity to respond by adjusting the program as needed; includes systematic assessment of the extent to which a program is consistent with its design and implementation plan, is reaching its intended target population, and can be justified in terms of a cost-benefit analysis.

Morbidity Any departure, subjective or objective, from a state of physiological or psychological well-being; sickness, illness, and morbid condition are synonymous.

Mortality Related to death caused by an illness or condition.

Multifactorial approach Referring to the concept that a given disease or another outcome may have more than one cause.

Multiple intelligences Different types of intellectual abilities, for example, verbal-linguistic, visual-spatial, and musical, that affect how individuals learn.

Narrative review A nonsystematic, traditional descriptive summary that reviews existing literature; typically includes a biased subset of studies, based on availability or author selection.

National CLAS Standards A comprehensive series of federal guidelines that inform, guide, and facilitate practices related to culturally and linguistically appropriate services (CLAS) for health and health care.

National Health and Nutrition Examination Survey (NHANES) A program of survey research studies that uniquely combines interviews and physical examinations to assess the health and nutritional status of adults and children, including oral diseases and conditions.

National Health Interview Survey (NHIS) A survey that is used to collect data through personal household interviews regarding health status, healthcare costs, and progress toward achieving national health objectives, including oral health.

National Oral Health Surveillance System (NOHSS) A system of oral health data sources designed to monitor the burden of oral disease, the use of the oral healthcare delivery system, and the status of community water fluoridation on both a national and state level; also involves timely communication of oral health findings to responsible parties and the public. A collaborative effort between the CDC, Division of Oral Health, and the ASTDD.

National School Lunch Program Federal government program operated by the Food and Nutrition Service of the U.S. Department of Agriculture that provides free or reduced price lunches to children according to the income level of their families, based on FPL; used as a criterion to target schools for dental public health programs.

Need Those services deemed by the health professional to be necessary based on analysis of assessment data.

Networking Meeting people and interacting with them as a means of cultivating productive relationships for professional development and potential employment.

Nominal scale A scale of measurement that merely allocates data to distinct categories.

Nonparametric statistics The branch of statistics consisting of tests used when assumptions about a normal distribution in the population cannot be met or when the level of measurement is nominal or ordinal; contrasts with parametric statistics.

Normal distribution A theoretical symmetric distribution that is characteristic of data representing most occurrences in the world; results in a bell-shaped curve in which approximately 68% of the population falls within 1 standard deviation (SD) of the mean, approximately 95% falls within 2 SDs of the mean, and approximately 99% lies within 3 SDs of the mean.

Null hypothesis A negatively stated hypothesis that there is no significant difference between specified populations, with any sample observations occurring by chance.

Objective A desired end result of community oral health program activities, described in a specific, measurable way; more specific than a goal.

Observational research A classification of research studies that involves systematic observation of study participants' behaviors, actions, or other exposures to disease-related factors without influencing or interfering with the variables; no variable is manipulated.

Occurrence A general term in epidemiology to describe the frequency of a disease or other attribute or event in a population without distinguishing between prevalence and incidence.

Optimal fluoride level The recommended level of fluoride in the community water supply to prevent dental caries; currently set by the DHHS at 0.7 milligrams of fluoride per liter of water (0.7 mg/L).

Oral health educator/oral health education A career path or role in which the dental hygienist works to prevent disease and to promote oral health through the process of teaching about oral health; oral health education is the process of teaching people about oral health to help them prevent oral disease.

Oral health indicators Quantifiable characteristics of a population used by researchers to describe the oral health of a population; they generally line up with *Healthy People* objectives and are tracked by the National Oral Health Surveillance System.

Oral health–related quality of life (OHRQOL) A multidimensional construct that, with respect to their oral health, reflects (among other things) people's comfort when eating, sleeping, and engaging in social interaction; their self-esteem; and their satisfaction, including people's perspectives of the ways in which oral diseases, conditions, and treatments affect their lives.

Oral paper A method of professional presentation of a topic, usually intended to present new or groundbreaking research.

Ordinal scale A scale of measurement that orders data into categories in rank order; the space between these categories is undefined.

Organizational Change Theory Describes how organizations pass through a series of stages as they initiate change, and how organizational structures and processes influence workers' behavior and motivation for change; the theory is based on several models of change.

Pandemic An epidemic occurring over a very wide area such as multiple continents or worldwide, and usually affecting a large proportion of the population.

Parameter A term relating to a numeric characteristic of the population.

Parametric statistics Branch of statistics consisting of tests that are used when data include interval or ratio scales of measurement, the sample is large and randomized, and the population from which the sample is taken is normally distributed; contrasts with nonparametric statistics.

Patient Protection and Affordable Care Act (ACA) A comprehensive healthcare federal statute reform law passed in 2010 that contains provisions of quality health insurance coverage and other related benefits; also referred to as Affordable Care Act and Obamacare.

Patient- and family-centered care Concept regarded as a standard of care in which patients and their families are recognized as essential allies in achieving safe, high-quality health care; in relation to healthcare decisions affecting them, they are listened to, informed, respected, and involved, and their wishes are honored.

Peer review Process used by scientific journals to validate research and evaluate submitted manuscripts; consists of review by a group of experts in the same field.

Per capita In relation to people taken individually; per person; for each person.

Percentile A statistical measure that represents the value below which a specific percentage of observations fall in a distribution of values.

Pie chart A circular graphic that illustrates numerical proportion by dividing the whole circle or pie into sections; represents parts of a whole.

Pilot study/pilot testing Performance of a preliminary research study or trial run of a community program in preparation for a major study or large-scale community program; provides opportunity to adjust research design or program strategies based on formative evaluation; not useful for evidence-based decision making.

Placebo A variation of a no-treatment control, in which research participants receive a fake treatment that is not active, thus providing no therapeutic value; may lead to a placebo effect, during which a participant may notice or experience a difference because of the expectation of a difference based on not knowing that they are receiving a placebo.

Plain language Clear, concise, to-the-point, and well-organized writing that is grammatically correct and includes complete sentence structure and accurate word usage, making it easy to read, understand, and use; important to the development of health literacy.

Planning/plan An organized response to a community's established needs to reduce or eliminate one or more problems; the second step of the program planning or community health improvement process.

Pluralistic In reference to a healthcare system, a combination of public and private forces that coexist simultaneously, which can result in a fragmented, uncoordinated, and complex system with many elements and entry points.

Policy development A core public health function in which laws and other policies are planned and developed to support community oral health issues.

Population In community health, all the inhabitants of a particular area that are served by public health; can be as small as a local neighborhood, school, or residential facility, or as large as an entire country or region. In research, also referred to as the target population, the entire group or whole unit of individuals from which the sample is drawn and to which the results of an investigation can be generalized.

Population health An approach to health that aims to improve the health outcomes of a defined group of people; utilizes non-traditional partnerships among different sectors of the community to achieve the goal; focuses on three processes: (1) identifying and analyzing the distribution of specific health statuses and outcomes, (2) evaluating clinical, social, economic, behavioral, and environmental factors associated with the outcomes, and (3) implementing a broad scope of interventions to modify the factors associated with health outcomes.

Poster A method of professional presentation of a topic during which the presenter discusses a visual display individually with people who stop to look.

Posttest only study An experimental study in which the dependent variable is measured only after the treatment intervention has been introduced; there is no pretest for comparison.

Poverty A general state of lacking a certain amount of material possessions or money, but also a multifaceted concept that includes social, economic, and political elements and is usually closely related to inequality. Poverty is associated with the undermining of a range of key human attributes, including health.

Power analysis A statistical determination of how many study participants are needed to provide statistical significance; calculated using a specific statistical formula.

Practicum/internship One form of experiential learning that is typically a longer assignment than a clinical rotation. The student may be assigned to work in a particular specialty area for an entire academic quarter or semester.

Pretest-posttest study An experimental study in which the dependent variable is measured before and after the treatment intervention is introduced.

Prevalence The proportion of instances of a given disease or other condition in a given population at a designated time; usually a specified point in time (point prevalence) versus a period of time (period prevalence).

Primary literature Original materials of new information, representing original thinking, reporting a discovery from the time period involved, and not filtered through secondary interpretation or evaluation.

Primary prevention Services that are designed to prevent a disease before it occurs; includes health education, avoidance of disease, and health protection.

Priority populations The populations identified by federal mandate as having priority to target public health efforts: inner-city, rural, low income, minority, women, children, older adults, and those with special healthcare needs, including those who have disabilities, need chronic care, or need end-of-life health care; the populations primarily targeted by public health programs.

Program planning process Model commonly used in dental public health practice that serves as the framework and provides a basic flowchart of steps to assess, plan, implement, and evaluate in the process of community health improvement; provides a systematic approach to the process of community oral health improvement and takes into account the interrelated determinants of oral health.

Proportion Any expression of the amount of disease or health condition, presented as a fraction in relation to the size of the population; the numerator is part of the denominator; can be expressed as a percentage.

Prospective A research design in which outcomes or phenomena are observed over a long period forward in time.

Public health The science and art of preventing disease, prolonging life, and promoting physical health and efficiency within a population through organized community efforts; concerned with protecting the health of entire populations, not just individuals.

Public health problem Health problems addressed by public health, identified according to the public health importance of the problem; the ability to prevent, control, or treat the problem; and the capacity of the health system to implement control measures for the problem.

Public health system The combination of all public, private, and voluntary entities in an area that contribute to the delivery of essential public health services and contribute to the public's health and well being throughout the community; includes public health agencies, healthcare providers, public safety agencies, human service and charity organizations, education and youth development organizations, economic and philanthropic organizations, environmental agencies or organizations, and recreation and arts-related organizations.

Public health solution An effective measure designed to solve a public health problem, focused on health promotion and disease prevention with the community at large.

_p_ value The value that determines the statistical significance of a study by providing the smallest level of significance at which the null hypothesis can be rejected.

Qualitative data Information that reflects the quality or nature of things that cannot be measured or analyzed numerically and must be expressed in words, such as interview responses.

Qualitative research Broad category of research that answers questions of why and how; focuses on exploring issues, understanding phenomena, and answering questions by analyzing qualitative data.

Quantitative data Information that is objective and measurable; can be measured and expressed as a quantity or amount (numbers).

Quantitative research Broad category of research that involves the systematic empirical investigation of observable phenomena through mathematical, computational, or statistical techniques.

Quasi-experimental research Similar to experimental research, but specifically lacks the use of randomization.

Random sampling A sampling technique in which each member of the population has an equal chance of being included in the sample, thus preventing the possibility of selection bias.

Randomization In a controlled experimental study, random (by chance) assignment of the participants to the treatment and control groups.

Range A crude measure of dispersion that provides an expression of the difference between the highest and lowest values in a distribution of scores.

Rate The expression of disease in a population using a standardized denominator and including a time dimension; allows for comparisons.

Ratio The expression of the magnitude of the occurrence of disease exposure or other variable in relation to another, which can be written as a fraction (4/3), with a colon (4:3), or with the word "to" (4 to 3).

Ratio scale A scale of measurement that not only has all the properties of nominal, ordinal, and interval data, but also has an absolute or fixed zero value or point, thus permitting relative comparison of different values.

Refereed journal A journal in which the published articles are written by experts and reviewed by several other experts in the field before acceptance for publication; also referred to as a peer-reviewed or scholarly journal.

Referral An essential component of assessment and screening and an ethical obligation when a need for dental care is observed; without further observation and referral for care, screening is ineffective.

Reflection In relation to learning, giving thought to an experience or encounter to draw meaning from it; a necessary step in the process of service-learning and critical thinking.

Relevant variable A variable that should be controlled because it can influence how the independent variable affects the dependent variable; also called a confounding variable.

Reliability The extent to which a measurement such as an instrument, questionnaire, or dental index gives consistent results at different times;

results of measures are reproducible and stable; an essential component of validity.

Repeated measures   A study design in which the dependent variable is measured several times, usually at posttest; also referred to as a time series study design.

Replication   The repetition of a study with different participants and in different situations to determine if the basic findings of the original study can be generalized further.

Researcher   A career path or role in which the dental hygienist uses scientific methods to acquire knowledge on topics relevant to serving the needs of the public's oral health.

Retrospective   A research design whereby past events are examined in relation to an outcome that is established at the beginning of the study.

Risk factor   An aspect of personal behavior or lifestyle, an environmental exposure, or an inborn or inherited characteristic that is associated with an increased occurrence of disease or other health-related event or condition.

Risk management   In relation to working in the community, a formal process by which an organization identifies and analyzes its risks, establishes goals and objectives to manage risk, and selects and implements measures to address its risks in an organized fashion.

Roundtable discussion   Method of professional presentation of a topic in which the participants sit in a circular pattern at a table to discuss issues relevant to the topic.

Safety net   The array of various unrelated entities, settings, and structures (providers, funders, and programs) developed through government, community, non-profit, and educational institutions and organizations that deliver or support health care to vulnerable populations who have no or limited insurance and cannot afford to pay for services out of pocket.

Sample   A portion or subset of the entire population.

Scattergram   A graph that visually depicts the relationship between two variables.

School-based oral health program   An oral health program that offers services at the school, via school clinics with stationary equipment, in a room in the school building using portable equipment, or in a mobile van parked at the school; may provide one or a combination of the following: screening, sealants, fluoride treatment, oral health education, other primary preventive services, clinical and radiographic examination, restorative services, and extractions.

Scientific method   A series of logical steps followed in the conduct of research through which a problem is identified, a hypothesis is formulated, relevant data are gathered, the hypothesis is empirically tested, and conclusions are drawn.

Scope of practice   The procedures that an oral health professional is permitted to practice according to the state statute.

Secondary literature   Sources of information that provide interpretations and evaluations of primary sources and offer a commentary

on, and discussion of, the evidence previously reported; do not contribute new evidence.

Secondary prevention   Services that are designed to slow the progression of a disease or its sequelae at any point after its inception; includes detection and treatment of disease or injury as soon as possible to halt or slow its progress.

Self-efficacy   Reflects personal confidence in one's ability to exert control over their own motivation, behavior, and social environment.

Service-Learning   An experiential learning method that is a jointly structured learning experience in which the community oral health course learning objectives (LO) and the community partner's service objectives (SO) are deliberately combined to form a service-learning objective (S-LO) for the mutual benefit of the student, the health professional education institution, and the community; involves collaboration and reflection.

Silver diamine fluoride (SDF)   A medicament used to arrest cavitated carious lesions and prevent future caries; especially useful in high risk populations in community settings.

SMART + C objectives   A mnemonic acronym for criteria used as a guide for setting program objectives: Specific, Measurable, Achievable, Relevant, Timed, and Challenging.

Snowball sampling   A sample that is formed by having research participants recruit other participants for a test or study; used in situations where potential participants are hard to locate.

Social determinants of health   Underlying social factors that are shaped by the distribution of money, power, and resources; are influenced by public policy; and impact health. These conditions in the places where people live, learn, work, and play affect a wide range of health risks and outcomes.

Social justice   The view that everyone deserves equal economic, political, and social rights and opportunities.

Social Learning Theory   A health education/health promotion model that is based on the idea that people learn through their own cognitive processing of others' actions that they observe, their inferences about the results of these actions, their imitation of others' behaviors, the judgment of behaviors voiced by others, and environmental influences on behavior. Behavioral change is accomplished through the interaction of behaviors, environmental influences, and personal cognitive processes.

Social marketing   The use of marketing principles to influence human behavior and affect social change for the benefit of society; can be applied to health.

Social media   Computer mediated tools that allow people to create and share information, ideas, and pictures or videos in virtual communities and networks.

Social responsibility   A broad term meaning that people and organizations are expected to behave ethically and with sensitivity toward social, cultural, economic, and environmental

issues; encompasses professionalism, personal and professional ethics, and the role of a profession in the context of the greater society.

Socioeconomic status (SES)   The social standing or status of a person or group in a community or society on a social-economic scale, measured by factors such as education, type of occupation, income, wealth, and place of residence.

Split-mouth study   Research study design in which all participants receive two or more treatments to a separate unit of the mouth; has the advantage of exactly matching the control and experimental groups.

Stages of Change Theory   Health education/health promotion model that is based on three major concepts or assumptions: (1) change is a process or cycle through various stages that occur over time rather than as a single event, (2) people cycle through the various stages of readiness to change and can even relapse, based on the behavior to be changed and the supportive nature of the environment, and (3) to motivate change in health behavior, one must design health education efforts that are based on the individual's current stage of readiness to change.

Stakeholders   People or organizations that have an interest in a decision or activity of an organization, i.e., are invested in a program, are interested in the results of an evaluation, and/or have a stake in what will be done with the results of an evaluation.

Standard deviation   A numerical value that demonstrates how widely individual scores in a group vary around the mean; used with interval and ratio data; computed as the positive square root of the variance.

State oral health program (SOHP)   A state-level dental public health program under the organizational structure of the state health department; also referred to as state dental public health program. In practice, the term is also used to refer to territorial oral health programs.

Statistic   A numeric characteristic of a sample.

Statistical conclusion   The conclusion of a research study founded on the statistical results of the data analysis.

Statistical significance   A value that expresses the probability that the results of data analysis from a given research study could be occurring purely because of chance.

Status   State or condition of a disease or related condition in the population.

Stratified random sampling   The use of random selection of study participants from two or more subdivisions (strata) of the population that possess similar characteristics; recommended for a heterogeneous population.

Summative evaluation   Mechanisms of evaluation that are conducted during the evaluation step of the program planning or community health improvement process to determine the results or outcomes of the program (the change that has occurred as a result of the program). Objectives form the basis for summative evaluation.

Surveillance/oral health surveillance/ surveillance system The ongoing, systematic collection, analysis, and interpretation of health-related data essential to planning, implementing, and evaluating public health practice, closely integrated with the timely dissemination of these data to those responsible for planning, implementing, and evaluating public health practices and programs to prevent and control diseases and conditions. Oral health surveillance is surveillance in relation to oral health conditions and related factors. A surveillance system is the process or procedure that is used to conduct surveillance.

Surveillance, Epidemiology and End Results Program (SEER) A program of the National Institute of Health National Cancer Institute that monitors and provides information on cancer statistics in an effort to reduce the burden of cancer in the U.S. population.

Systematic review A critical assessment and evaluation of all previously published research studies that address a particular issue, using a set of specific criteria to apply an organized, explicit, systematic method of locating, assembling, and evaluating the body of literature; can be completed with or without a meta-analysis.

Systematic sampling Selection of study participants by including every *n*th person from a list or file of the total population.

Tailored health message A health message (health communication) that is designed to be meaningful to a specific individual, based on features unique to that person.

Teledentistry The remote provision of dental care, advice, or treatment through the medium of information technology; can be used for a dentist to remotely supervise or provide consultation to a dental hygienist or dental therapist.

Tertiary literature Sources of information that are a distillation and collection of primary and secondary sources such as almanacs and dictionaries.

Tertiary prevention Services designed to soften the impact of an ongoing illness or injury that has lasting effects by helping people manage long-term, often complex health problems and injuries (e.g., chronic diseases, permanent impairments) to improve as much as possible their ability to function, their quality of life, and their life expectancy.

Testlet The NBDHE test format that combines a community case (scenario) with the associated test items.

Theory A set of interrelated concepts, definitions, and propositions that presents a systematic view of events or situations by specifying relationships among variables to explain and predict the events or situations.

Third-party payment Payment for healthcare services by someone other than the patient. The three parties involved are the patient, the provider of the healthcare service, and the third party, which is the organization that participates in financing the services rendered such as an insurance company, union, or government program.

Time In relation to the epidemiologic triangle and epidemiology, the length of time it takes for damage or symptoms to occur, the duration of time before death or recovery occurs, or the period from infection to the threshold of an epidemic for a population.

Time series graph A graph that illustrates data points at successive time intervals.

Trend Inclination or general direction in which a health condition is changing or developing.

***t*-test** A statistical test used to analyze the difference between two sample mean scores.

Type I alpha (α) error Based on statistical results, rejection of the null hypothesis when it is actually true.

Type II beta (β) error Based on statistical results, acceptance of the null hypothesis when it is actually false.

Unsupervised practice According to state statute, dental hygienists' right to make treatment decisions and provide treatment within their scope of practice without a dentist's supervision.

Validity The degree to which an assessment measures what it is supposed to or intended to measure; the accuracy of a measurement instrument such as a dental index. In research, external validity is the extent to which the results of a study can be generalized to the population, and internal validity is the degree to which a causal conclusion is warranted based on the control of confounding variables and other sources of error.

Variable A characteristic or concept that varies within the population under study.

Variance A numerical value that demonstrates how widely individual scores in a group vary around the mean; used with interval and ratio data.

Volunteer dental services programs Community oral health programs operated by professional and nonprofit organizations through which oral health professionals volunteer to provide oral health services to underserved populations.

Volunteerism Activity in which individuals provide a service to the community that is of major benefit; in the educational arena, not necessarily associated with an academic course.

Washout period The period in a crossover study between the treatments under study, during which study participants receive no treatment to eliminate the effects of a previous treatment.

Water Fluoridation Reporting System (WFRS) An online tool managed by the CDC to track the level of fluoride in local water supplies; provides the data for national surveillance reports of the status of community water fluoridation in the nation.

Web-based presentation The use of computer technology to deliver an online professional presentation of a topic on the web; can involve one or more speakers and connection to the audience via phone lines or computer audio.

Wilcoxon signed-rank test A nonparametric statistic to test the difference between two related or paired data sets using the median as the basis for comparison.

Women, Infants, and Children Special Supplemental Nutrition Program (WIC) A federal program in the Department of Agriculture that provides grants to states to fund local programs that provide supplemental foods, healthcare referrals, and nutrition education for low-income pregnant, breastfeeding, and nonbreastfeeding postpartum women, and to infants and children up to age 5 years who are found to be at nutritional risk; includes nutrition education related to oral health.

World Health Organization (WHO) An international health organization with the primary role of directing and coordinating international health within the United Nations system; primarily focused on serving the needs of developing countries.

INDEX

Page numbers followed by "*f*" indicate figures, "*b*" indicate boxes, and "*t*" indicate tables.